GOLJAN

RAPID REVIEW

PATHOLOGY

ANTHONY W. ALFREY, MD

Associate Professor and Chair
Department of Pathology
Oklahoma State University Center for Health Sciences
Tulsa, OK

GOLJAN

RAPID
REVIEW

PATHOLOGY

SIXTH EDITION

ELSEVIER

Elsevier
1600 John F. Kennedy Blvd.
Ste 1800
Philadelphia, PA 19103-2899

RAPID REVIEW PATHOLOGY, SIXTH EDITION   ISBN: 978-0-323-87057-3

Notice

Practitioners and researchers must always rely on their own experience and knowledge in evaluating and using any information, methods, compounds or experiments described herein. Because of rapid advances in the medical sciences, in particular, independent verification of diagnoses and drug dosages should be made. To the fullest extent of the law, no responsibility is assumed by Elsevier, authors, editors or contributors for any injury and/or damage to persons or property as a matter of products liability, negligence or otherwise, or from any use or operation of any methods, products, instructions, or ideas contained in the material herein.

Previous editions copyrighted 2019, 2014, 2011, 2007, and 2004.

Executive Content Strategist: James T. Merritt
Senior Content Development Specialist: Shilpa Kumar
Publishing Services Manager: Shereen Jameel
Project Manager: Gayathri S
Senior Design Direction: Amy L. Buxton

Printed in India

Last digit is the print number: 9 8 7 6 5 4 3 2 1

Working together
to grow libraries in
developing countries

www.elsevier.com • www.bookaid.org

Preface

The goal for this updated sixth edition is to provide a truly rapid review of pathology for those preparing to take steps 1 or 2 of the USMLE. Those studying for levels 1 or 2 of the COMLEX will also benefit. To this end, I have tried to focus on "high-yield" material with an emphasis on the clinical presentation and the pathogenesis of a disease. As compared to previous editions, the margin notes have been removed. This will allow space for the reviewer to take their own notes. Note that this is meant to be a review, not an in-depth text of pathology. For a deeper understanding of a specific topic, I recommend one of the many references available on ClinicalKey. For treatment options, *Ferri's Clinical Advisor* is a good option. Five-hundred board-quality questions and discussions covering all pertinent subjects throughout the book are also available on Elsevier eBooks+. To activate your Elsevier eBooks+ version, see the PIN page on the inside front cover of the book and follow the instructions to activate your PIN.

Acknowledgments

I first want to thank Dr. Goljan for allowing me to pick up where he left off with the last edition of *Rapid Review Pathology*. None of this would have been possible without his foresight to produce the original Rapid Review many years ago. I also want to give thanks to Jim Merritt, Executive Strategist at Elsevier for promoting this, the sixth edition, for publication. The production of a text requires the assistance of innumerable individuals. I specifically would like to thank Shilpa Kumar, Content Development Specialist as well as the Project Manager, Gayathri S. I would like to also thank those authors who have graciously shared the use of images and diagrams. Finally, thanks to all the medical students who, through the years, have provided valuable insight into the various topics commonly seen on licensing examinations.

Contents

CHAPTER 1
Diagnostic Testing

I. **Purposes of Laboratory Tests**
    A. **Screen for disease**
        1. Must have an effective and safe therapy available.
            a. No reason to identify a disorder if there is no treatment.
        2. Disease must be relatively prevalent within the population.
            a. No reason to screen for rare disorders that are unlikely to be present in a population.
        3. Disease should be detectable before symptoms arise.
        4. Test must have high sensitivity (have few false-negative [FN] test results).
        5. Test must have high specificity (have few false-positive [FP] test results).
    B. **Confirm disease, for example:**
        1. Measurement of cardiac biomarkers (e.g., troponin) to confirm the presence of myocardial injury/infarction.
        2. Urine culture to confirm the presence of a bladder infection.
    C. **Monitor disease, for example:**
        1. Hemoglobin (Hb) A1c to monitor glucose control over the last 8–12 weeks.
        2. Prothrombin time/international normalized ratio to monitor the degree of anticoagulation in a patient receiving warfarin.
II. **Operating Characteristics of Laboratory Tests**
    A. **Two-by-two tables (Fig. 1.1)**
        1. True positive (TP)
            a. Person with disease correctly identified as having the disease.
        2. FN
            a. Person with disease incorrectly identified as being free of disease.
        3. True negative (TN)
            a. Person free of disease correctly identified as being free of disease.
        4. FP
            a. Person free of disease incorrectly identified as having the disease.
    B. **Sensitivity of a test**
        1. Probability of diseased subjects being classified as having disease (i.e., the ability of a test to correctly identify those with a disease).
            a. For example, if 7 of 10 patients with disease have a positive test result, then the test sensitivity is 70%.
        2. Sensitivity percentage $= 100 \times [TP/(TP + FN)]$.
        3. Screening tests should be highly sensitive.
    C. **Specificity of a test**
        1. Probability that nondiseased subjects will be classified as free of disease (i.e., the ability of a test to correctly identify those without the disease).
        2. Specificity percentage $= 100 \times [TN/(TN + FP)]$.
        3. Confirmatory tests should be highly specific.
    D. **Ideal test characteristics**
        1. An ideal test, which does not exist, would have specificity and sensitivity of 100%.
    E. **"Gold-standard" test**
        1. Benchmark by which other tests are compared (i.e., best test).

1

Test result	Specific disease	No disease
+ Test	True positive (TP)	False positive (FP)
− Test	False negative (FN)	True negative (TN)

1.1: Two-by-two table. Those with a specific disease either test positive (true positive—TP) or negative (false negative—FN). Likewise, those free of disease will either test negative (true negative—TN) or positive (false positive—FP).

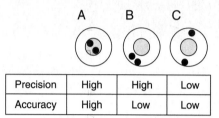

	A	B	C
Precision	High	High	Low
Accuracy	High	Low	Low

1.2: Precision and accuracy of a test. Using a target as an example: Test A has good precision and accuracy; Test B has good precision but is not accurate; Test C is neither precise nor accurate. *(From Goljan E, Sloka K: Rapid review laboratory testing in clinical medicine, St. Louis, 2008, Mosby Elsevier.)*

F. Predictive value of a positive test (positive predictive value - [PPV])
1. Probability of a positive test truly indicating the presence of disease (i.e., the proportion of those with a positive test result who actually have the disease).
2. PPV (%) = 100 × [TP/(TP + FP)].

G. Predictive value of a negative test (negative predictive value - [NPV])
1. Probability that a negative test truly indicates the absence of disease (i.e., the proportion of those with a negative test who are actually free of disease).
2. NPV (%) = 100 × [TN/(TN + FN)].

H. Prevalence
1. Prevalence is the percentage of people with a disease in the population at risk: (TP + FN)/(TP + FN + TN + FP).
2. Prevalence of a disease influences positive and negative predictive values.
3. As the prevalence of a disease increases, the predictive value of a positive test increases (i.e., it is more likely that a positive test indicates the presence of disease).
4. Conversely, as prevalence increases, the predictive value of a negative test decreases (i.e., it is less likely that a negative test indicates the absence of disease).

I. Likelihood ratio (LR)
1. Likelihood that a given test result would be expected in a patient with the target disorder compared with the likelihood that the same result would be expected in a patient without the target disorder.
2. Calculated using a test's sensitivity and specificity.
   a. Because a test may be either positive or negative, an LR for each result is calculated.
3. Positive likelihood ratio (LR+)
   a. Probability of a positive test result when disease is present divided by the probability of a positive test result when disease is absent.
   b. LR+ = sensitivity/(1 − specificity).
4. Negative likelihood ratio (LR−)
   a. Probability of a negative test result when disease is present divided by the probability of a negative test result when disease is absent.
   b. LR− = (1 − sensitivity)/specificity.
5. LR values range from 0 to infinity.
   a. Values > 1 suggest that the disorder is more likely.
   b. Values < 1 suggest that the disorder is less likely.
   c. Value of 1 is of no value (does not change pretest probability).

J. Precision and accuracy (Fig. 1.2)
1. Precision refers to the ability to produce the same test result consistently.
2. When repeat testing reveals similar results, then precision is high and the test is said to be reliable (it reliably gives the same result).
3. Precision is not the same as accuracy, which is the ability of a test to provide a result that is very close to the true value.

GAUSSIAN DISTRIBUTION

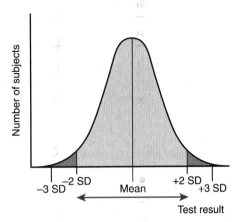

1.3: Normal reference ranges for a specific analyte are commonly ascertained by testing a large pool of healthy volunteers then, assigned as the mean ± 2SD. SD, Standard deviation. *(From Marshall W, Bangert S: Clinical chemistry, ed 6, Philadelphia, 2007, Elsevier. As redrawn in O'Connell TX, Pedigo RA, Blair TE: Crush step I: the ultimate USMLE step I review, Philadelphia, 2014, Saunders Elsevier.)*

III. Reference Ranges
A. Normal (reference) range for a test
1. Laboratory values that are expected to occur in health are usually determined by testing a large pool of healthy volunteers.
2. Once the data are obtained, an average (i.e., mean) and standard deviation (SD) are calculated.
3. Reference ranges are often defined as the mean ± 2SD (Fig. 1.3).
   a. Two SDs above the mean is the upper cutoff.
   b. Two SDs below the mean is the lower cutoff.
   c. For example, a test with a mean of 100 mg/dL and an SD of 5 mg/dL will have a reference range of 90–110 mg/dL (mean ± 2SD).
4. The reference range will exclude 5% of an otherwise healthy population.
   a. In the healthy population, 2.5% of the patients will have an "abnormally" elevated test result while 2.5% will have an "abnormally" low test result.
   b. The take-home point is that laboratory results just slightly out of the normal range do not necessarily indicate the presence of disease. In general, clinical decisions should not be based on a single abnormal laboratory value.
   c. Does the laboratory result fit with the clinical picture? If any doubt, repeat the test.

IV. Preanalytic Variables Affecting Laboratory Results
A. Diet
1. Serum glucose and triglyceride levels rise postprandially as nutrients are absorbed. Accurate measurements require the patient to be fasting for 8–12 hours.
2. Fecal occult blood tests may be falsely positive in those whose recent diet included red meat or certain fruits and vegetables (e.g., horseradish, turnips, and cauliflower).
3. Protein-rich diets increase serum levels of urea, ammonia, and uric acid.
4. Acute alcohol ingestion may elevate plasma urate and triglyceride concentrations.
5. Chronic alcohol ingestion characteristically elevates levels of high-density lipoprotein, gamma-glutamyl transferase, and serum urate.

B. Age
1. Newborns
   a. Hb is largely Hb F, not Hb A, as seen in the adult.
   b. Bilirubin levels rise in the first several days of life with a normal peak at 5 days ("physiologic jaundice") followed by a gradual decline.
2. Males after the age of 50 years
   a. Decreased serum testosterone concentration.
3. Postmenopausal females
   a. Elevated levels of pituitary gonadotropins (e.g., follicle-stimulating hormone).
4. Older adults
   a. Hormone levels (e.g., triiodothyronine and cortisol) decline.
   b. Glomerular filtration rate (GFR) declines with aging.

C. Differences between males and females
1. Males have larger overall muscle mass and therefore higher levels of muscle breakdown products (e.g., creatine kinase and aldolase) compared with females.

2. Premenopausal females have lower Hb, serum iron, and ferritin levels compared with similarly aged males due to monthly menstrual blood loss.

D. Stress (mental and/or physical)
1. Increased adrenocorticotropic hormone, cortisol, and catecholamine levels.

E. Pregnancy
1. "Physiologic anemia of pregnancy" describes a mild normocytic anemia that is a normal finding of pregnancy due to a disproportionate elevation in blood volume in relation to red cell mass (hemodilution effect).
2. Elevated progesterone levels during pregnancy stimulate ventilation, causing a chronic respiratory alkalosis (lower PCO_2) which must be compensated by a metabolic acidosis (decreased serum bicarbonate) to maintain blood pH within the normal range.
3. GFR increases during pregnancy. The associated elevation in creatinine clearance results in slightly lower serum creatinine levels.
4. Increased GFR, in conjunction with reduced tubular reabsorption of glucose, can lead to the urinary excretion of glucose (glucosuria).
5. Alkaline phosphatase may be elevated (isoform released from placenta).
6. Mild elevation in total serum thyroxine (T4) and triiodothyronine (T3) concentrations.
   a. Human chorionic gonadotropin (hCG) and thyroid-stimulating hormone (TSH) have similar structure → cross-stimulation of the TSH receptor by hCG → ↑ thyroid hormone production.
   b. Estrogen-induced increase in thyroxine-binding globulin.
      i. Thus total (bound) thyroid hormone levels are elevated.
      ii. Unbound ("free") levels of T4 and T3 remain normal. The free hormone is the physiologically active form; therefore, patients remain euthyroid.

I. Mechanisms of Cell Injury

A. Hypoxia

1. Hypoxia is defined as inadequate tissue oxygenation. Note that this is not the same as hypoxemia which refers insufficient blood oxygen (<60 mm Hg).
   a. Oxygen is necessary for normal cellular respiration (oxidative phosphorylation, the major source of adenosine triphosphate [ATP]).
2. With hypoxia, the cells are unable to generate adequate energy (ATP). The net result is a failure of several critical cellular processes and, if prolonged, cell injury (Fig. 2.1).
   a. Failure of plasma membrane (e.g., Na^+/K^+ ATPase) pumps
      i. Influx of sodium ions and an influx of water causing cellular swelling (hydropic change).
      ii. Influx of calcium ions activates several enzymes (e.g., proteases, phospholipases, and endonucleases) causing direct toxicity to cellular components.
      iii. Efflux of potassium ions.
   b. Altered energy metabolism
      i. Shift to anaerobic metabolism→buildup of lactic acid (i.e., metabolic acidosis)→acidemia (impaired enzymatic reactions).
   c. Disruption of endoplasmic reticulum
      i. Reduced protein synthesis.
   d. Mitochondrial disruption
      i. Impaired ATP synthesis (further depleting energy stores) and activation of pro-apoptotic pathways.
3. Etiologies
   a. Ischemia (reduced blood flow), usually secondary to cardiac and/or vascular disease.
   b. Decreased oxygen-carrying capacity of blood (e.g., anemia, carbon monoxide poisoning, and methemoglobinemia).
   c. Reduced blood oxygenation (e.g., lung disease).
4. Blood oxygenation (Fig. 2.2)
   a. Oxygenation refers to the passive diffusion of oxygen from the alveolus into the pulmonary capillary. Oxygen then either binds to hemoglobin (Hb) (forming oxyhemoglobin) or is dissolved in the plasma.
      i. Arterial oxygen saturation (SaO_2) is a measure of the percent of Hb that is bound to oxygen.
      ii. Arterial oxygen tension (PaO_2) is a measure of oxygen dissolved in the plasma.
   b. Oxygen content of arterial blood (CaO_2) provides a measure of bound and dissolved oxygen and can be calculated as follows:
      i. $CaO_2 = (1.34 \times Hb) \times (SaO_2/100) + (0.0031 \times PaO_2)$.
         (1) The constant 1.34 is the amount of oxygen (milliliter at 1 atmosphere) bound per gram of Hb (value varies from 1.34 to 1.39, depending on the reference).
         (2) The constant 0.0031 represents the amount of oxygen dissolved in plasma.
         (3) Amount of oxygen dissolved is generally small relative to the amount of oxygen bound to Hb but becomes significant at very high PaO_2, as in a hyperbaric chamber or in severe anemia.
5. Alveolar oxygen tension (PAO_2)
   a. Driving force for the diffusion of oxygen across the alveolar–capillary membrane, calculated using the alveolar gas equation:
      i. $PAO_2 = (FiO_2 \times [P_{atm} - PH_2O]) - (PaCO_2/0.8)$
         $P_{atm} = 760$ mm Hg at sea level; $PH_2O = 47$ mm Hg.
   b. Alveolar–arterial (A–a) oxygen difference
      i. Alveolar to arterial (A–a) oxygen difference (A–a PO_2)

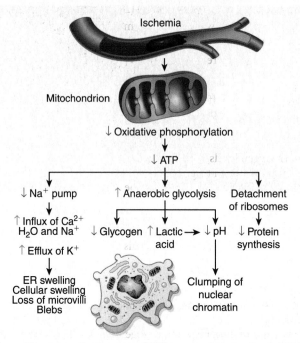

2.1: Hypoxic cell injury. Hypoxia reduces the amount of energy (ATP) generation. Lack of ATP has a variety of detrimental cellular effects. *ATP*, Adenosine triphosphate; *ER*, endoplasmic reticulum. *(From Robbins & Cotran pathologic basis of disease, ed 10, 2021, Fig. 2.24.)*

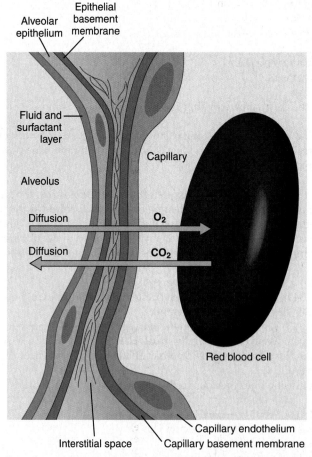

2.2: Oxygenation is the passive diffusion of oxygen across the alveolar–capillary membrane into the pulmonary capillary. Carbon dioxide travels in the opposite direction. *(From Guyton and Hall textbook of medical physiology, ed 14, 2021, Elsevier.)*

(1) Sometimes referred to as the A–a gradient, the A–a PO_2 represents the difference between the average alveolar oxygen tension (PAO_2) and that within the systemic arterial blood (PaO_2).

    (a) A–a PO_2 = PAO_2 − PaO_2

(2) A–a PO_2 increases with age (correction for age is [age/4 + 4]); usually about 10–20 mm Hg.

> On room air, the A–a PO_2 is a measure of the efficiency of oxygen transfer.
> When adjusted for age, an increased A–a PO_2 indicates impaired gas transfer across the alveolus (i.e., impaired oxygenation).

6. Hypoxemia (decreased blood oxygen levels), see Table 2.1
   a. Ventilation–perfusion (V/Q) mismatch (Fig. 2.3)
      i. V/Q mismatch occurs when there is an imbalance between blood flow and ventilation.
      ii. Most common cause of hypoxemia.
      iii. Can be corrected with supplemental oxygen.
      iv. Characterized by an increased A–a difference.
      v. Etiologies include chronic obstructive pulmonary disease, pulmonary vascular disease, and interstitial lung disease.
   b. Shunt
      i. Passage of venous blood that completely bypasses alveoli and is therefore not exposed to alveolar oxygen.
      ii. Etiologies include intrapulmonary shunts (e.g., pulmonary arteriovenous malformation) or intracardiac shunts (e.g., right-to-left shunts).
      iii. Shunts cannot be corrected with supplemental oxygen.
   c. Hypoventilation
      i. Since gases comprise 100% of alveolar content, as the partial pressure of one gas rises, the partial pressure of the others will decrease.
      ii. During hypoventilation, levels of alveolar carbon dioxide ($PACO_2$) rise while levels of alveolar oxygen (PAO_2) decrease (thereby causing a decrease in oxygenation).
      iii. Improves with supplemental oxygen.
   d. High altitude (low inspired partial pressure of oxygen)
      i. Improves with supplemental oxygen.

TABLE 2.1   Hypoxemia

MECHANISM	(A–A) PO_2	RESPONSE TO SUPPLEMENTAL OXYGEN
V/Q mismatch	Increased	Improves
Shunt	Increased	No improvement
Hypoventilation	Normal	Improves
High altitude	Normal	Improves

A–a PO_2, Alveolar to arterial (A–a) oxygen difference; V/Q, ventilation–perfusion.
Reproduced with permission of the © ERS 2022: *European Respiratory Journal* 44(4): 1023–1041; doi:10.1183/09031936.00037014. Published 30 September 2014.

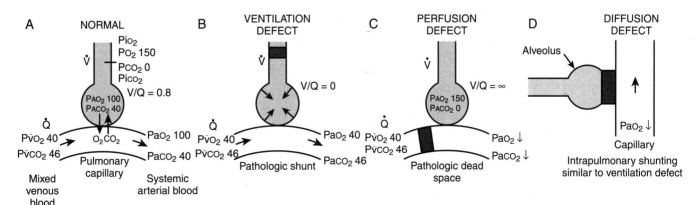

2.3: Diagram demonstrating the effects of ventilation, perfusion, and diffusion defects on blood oxygenation. *PaCO₂*, Partial pressure of arterial carbon dioxide; *PACO₂*, partial pressure of alveolar carbon dioxide; *PaO₂*, partial pressure of arterial oxygen; *PAO₂*, partial pressure of alveolar oxygen; *PCO₂*, partial pressure of carbon dioxide; *PIO₂*, partial pressure of inspired oxygen; *PICO₂*, partial pressure of inspired carbon dioxide; *PO₂*, partial pressure of oxygen; *PVCO₂*, partial pressure of carbon dioxide in mixed venous blood; *PVO₂*, partial pressure of oxygen in mixed venous blood; *V/Q*, ventilation–perfusion. *(Modified from Goljan E, Sloka K: Rapid Review Laboratory Testing in Clinical Medicine, Philadelphia, Mosby Elsevier, 2008, p 76, Fig. 3–5.)*

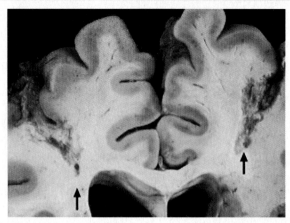

2.4: Watershed infarct. Arrows indicate bilateral infarcts in the watershed zones between the distribution of the anterior cerebral and middle cerebral arteries. *(From Neuropathology, ed 3, 2013, Elsevier.)*

7. Hb-related abnormalities
   a. Anemia (reduction in red cell mass)
      i. Anemia has no effect on oxygenation in the lungs (partial pressure of arterial oxygen [PaO_2] and arterial oxygen saturation [SaO_2] are normal).
         (1) Total oxygen content of blood is reduced (less RBCs available to carry oxygen); thus less O_2 is delivered to the tissues.
   b. Methemoglobin
      i. Methemoglobin refers to oxidized Hb, that is, heme iron in the ferric (Fe^{3+}) state instead of the normal reduced ferrous (Fe^{2+}) state.
      ii. Ferric iron (Fe^{3+}) does not bind to oxygen, regardless of the amount dissolved in plasma; therefore, even though the PaO_2 is normal, the amount of oxygen bound to Hb (SaO_2) is decreased.
      iii. Results in elevated levels of deoxygenated Hb with cyanosis (does not respond to supplemental oxygen).
      iv. Treat with intravenous methylene blue (accelerates the enzymatic reduction of methemoglobin).
      v. Etiologies of methemoglobinemia include drugs (e.g., dapsone, topical anesthetics, nitrates, and nitrites) as well as rare congenital etiologies (e.g., cytochrome b5 reductase deficiency).
   c. Carbon monoxide (CO) poisoning
      i. CO binds to heme very avidly (more than 200 times more avidly than oxygen); forms carboxyhemoglobin.
      ii. Carboxyhemoglobin cannot bind to oxygen; tissue oxygenation is reduced.
      iii. Etiologies of CO poisoning include:
         (1) Exposure to engine exhaust without adequate ventilation.
         (2) Leaky furnaces.
         (3) Smoke inhalation.
      iv. Clinical presentation of CO poisoning
         (1) Headache (first symptom), malaise, dizziness, seizures, syncope, and coma.
         (2) Cherry red discoloration of the skin (insensitive, often late finding).
      v. Diagnosis of CO poisoning
         (1) Compatible history and physical examination.
         (2) Elevated carboxyhemoglobin level.
         (3) Pulse oximetry (SpO_2) cannot be used to screen for CO exposure as it does not differentiate carboxyhemoglobin from oxyhemoglobin.
8. Tissue susceptibility to hypoxia
   a. If hypoxia is severe and/or prolonged, all tissues will be affected.
   b. Tissues that are particularly susceptible include:
      i. Watershed zones (regions in which blood flow between two major arteries do not overlap); for example:
         (1) In the brain, between the distribution of anterior and middle cerebral arteries (Fig. 2.4).
         (2) In the colon, between the distribution of the superior and inferior mesenteric arteries (splenic flexure).
      ii. Tissues at the end of an arterial blood supply
         (1) Renal medulla
         (2) Subendocardial region of heart
         (3) Liver (zone III hepatocytes)
      iii. Neurons
         (1) Of all the cells within the central nervous system, neurons are the most susceptible.
         (2) Particularly susceptible are those within layers III, V, and VI of the cerebral cortex, the Sommer sector of the hippocampus, and Purkinje cells of the cerebellum.

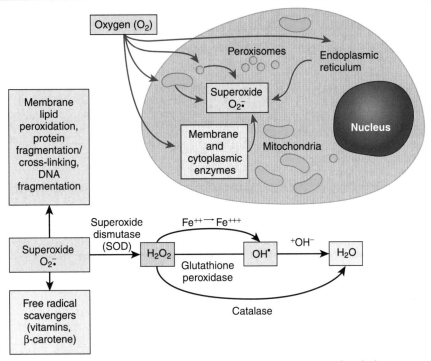

2.5: Production and neutralization of oxygen free radicals. *(From King TS: Elsevier's integrated pathology, 2007, Fig 1.4.)*

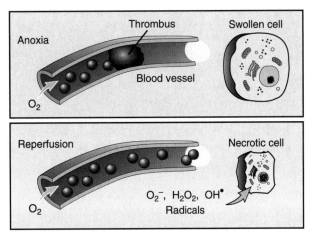

2.6: Reperfusion injury is associated with cell injury secondary to the generation of reactive oxygen species (e.g., O_2^-, H_2O_2, OH·). *(From Pathology for the health professions, ed 4, St. Louis, 2012, Saunders Elsevier.)*

B. Oxidative stress
1. Definition
   a. Cellular injury occurring secondary to an imbalance between pro-oxidants and antioxidants.
   b. Free radicals are chemical species that have an unpaired electron in an outer orbit.
      i. Reactive oxygen species (ROS).
      ii. Reactive nitrogen species.
   c. Unpaired electrons are highly reactive→damage various cellular components (lipids, proteins, and nucleic acid).
2. Formation of free radicals (Fig. 2.5)
   a. Normal metabolic processes (superoxide anion, hydrogen peroxide, and hydroxyl radicals).
   b. Ionizing radiation (hydroxyl radicals).
   c. Carbon tetrachloride (CCl_4)
      i. Once used as a solvent in the dry-cleaning industry, now in limited industrial use.
      ii. Toxicity related to the development of trichloromethyl free radical (CCl_3) by cytochrome P450.
      iii. Causes cellular damage through lipid peroxidation and other pathways.
   d. Reperfusion injury (Fig. 2.6)
      i. Reintroduction of oxygen following an ischemic event leads to the formation of ROS.

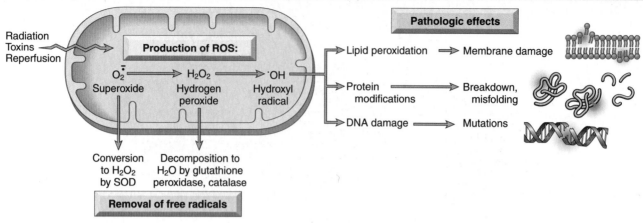

2.7: Creation, removal, and effects of reactive oxygen species. Pathologic effects (i.e., oxidative stress) include damage to cell membranes, proteins (impaired enzymatic activity and protein misfolding), and DNA (thereby predisposing to genetic mutations and potentially, the development of malignancy). *ROS*, Reactive oxygen species; *SOD*, superoxide dismutase. *(From Robbins & Cotran pathologic basis of disease, ed 10, 2021, Elsevier.)*

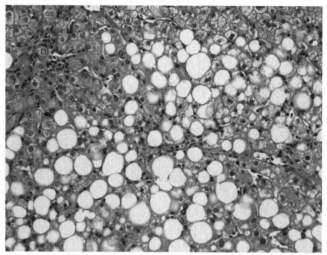

2.8: Steatosis (fat) appears as cytoplasmic vacuoles (clear spaces) because the lipid dissolves during processing. *(From Rosai and Ackerman's surgical pathology, ed 11, 2018, Elsevier.)*

  e. Transition metals (e.g., iron and copper)
    i. Fenton reaction:
       (1) $Fe_2^+ + H_2O_2 \rightarrow Fe_3^+ + OH\cdot + OH^-$.
  3. Prevention of free radical injury
    a. Enzymes
      i. Catalase (hydrogen peroxide → water and oxygen).
      ii. Superoxide dismutase (superoxide anion → oxygen and hydrogen peroxide).
      iii. Glutathione peroxidase (breakdown of hydrogen peroxide).
    b. Binding of metals (e.g., iron–ferritin, copper–ceruloplasmin) prevents the formation of ROS.
    c. Antioxidants (e.g., vitamins A, C, and E) block the formation of free radicals and/or inactivate (scavenge) free radicals.
  4. Effects of free radicals (Fig. 2.7)
    a. Lipid peroxidation (damages cell membranes).
    b. Oxidation of proteins (various effects; inactivation of enzymes and protein misfolding).
    c. Oxidative DNA damage (breaks in DNA and cross-linking of DNA).
II. Intracellular Accumulations
  A. Lipids
    1. Fatty change (steatosis) refers to the accumulation of triglycerides and other fats within tissues (e.g., liver).
    2. Hepatic steatosis (Fig. 2.8) is most commonly associated with alcohol abuse or insulin resistance (e.g., obesity and diabetes mellitus).
    3. Alcoholic steatosis
      a. Alcohol is metabolized primarily in the liver.
         Alcohol $\xrightarrow{\text{alcohol dehydrogenase}}$ Acetaldehyde $\xrightarrow{\text{acetaldehyde dehydrogenase}}$ Acetate

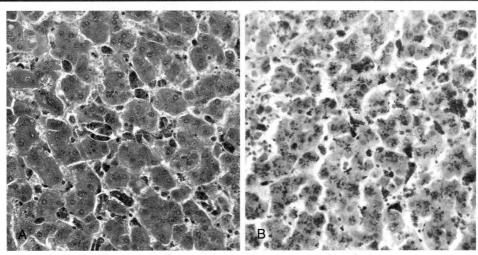

2.9: Hepatic iron overload in a patient with hereditary hemochromatosis. The image on the left shows golden-brown granules of hemosiderin (H&E stain). On the right, hemosiderin appears blue when stained with a special stain (Prussian blue). *(From Pathology for the health professions, ed 4, 2012, Saunders Elsevier.)*

  b. The first step (alcohol dehydrogenase) occurs within the cytoplasm.
  c. The second step (acetaldehyde dehydrogenase) occurs within mitochondria.
  d. Oxidation of alcohol by these pathways causes the reduction of nicotinamide adenine dinucleotide (NAD) to form reduced nicotinamide adenine dinucleotide (NADH).
   i. NAD is needed for the oxidation of fatty acids.
   ii. Altered redox state ($\downarrow$NAD$^+$/NADH ratio) is the major mechanism by which alcohol causes hepatic steatosis.
  e. Hepatic steatosis is reversible within a few weeks of stopping alcohol.
 4. Nonalcoholic steatosis
  a. Insulin resistance (e.g., metabolic syndrome) is thought to be the key mechanism underlying nonalcoholic fatty liver disease in many patients due to changes in lipid metabolism.
   i. Increased release of fatty acids from adipose tissue.
   ii. Decreased uptake of fatty acids by skeletal muscle.
   iii. Increased fatty acid uptake by the liver.
B. Metals (e.g., iron)
 1. Iron is required for heme groups (e.g., Hb and myoglobin) as well as for a variety of iron-containing enzymes.
 2. Free iron is toxic and must be kept in a stored form (ferritin or hemosiderin).
  a. The protein apoferritin binds to free ferrous iron to form ferritin.
  b. Ferritin is water soluble, present within cells and in circulation.
   i. Blood ferritin levels are used as a measure of total body iron stores.
  c. Hemosiderin is a water-insoluble storage form of iron.
   i. Derived as a product of ferritin degradation within lysosomes.
   ii. Unlike ferritin, it does not circulate in serum but can be deposited within tissues and identified on light microscopy.
    (1) On routine hematoxylin and eosin (H&E), hemosiderin appears golden-brown (left side of Fig. 2.9).
    (2) On Prussian blue-stained sections, hemosiderin has a granular blue appearance (right side of Fig. 2.9).
 3. Iron overload
  a. Excess iron deposits within tissues as hemosiderin.
  b. Iron, via the Fenton reaction, leads to the generation of ROS and oxidative injury.
  c. Certain tissues are particularly susceptible, including the liver, heart, and endocrine organs (e.g., pancreas and pituitary gland).
  d. Causes of iron overload include:
   i. Increased intake (e.g., multiple transfusion of red blood cells and excessive ingestion of iron supplements).
   ii. Increased absorption (e.g., hereditary hemochromatosis).
C. Proteins
 1. Examples of intracellular protein deposits include:
  a. Alpha 1-antitrypsin (hepatic damage).
  b. Alpha synuclein (e.g., Parkinson disease and dementia with Lewy bodies).
  c. Beta-amyloid and tau proteins (Alzheimer disease).
D. Calcium
 1. Dystrophic calcification

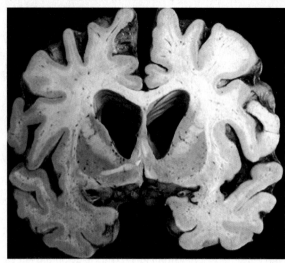

2.10: Atrophy of the brain in a patient with advanced Alzheimer disease. Note ventricular enlargement and widened sulci. *(From Neuropathology, 2014, Fig. 1.)*

      a. Refers to the deposition of calcium within necrotic tissue in the setting of normal serum calcium levels.

      b. Examples include the calcification of atherosclerotic plaques or damaged heart valves.

   2. Metastatic calcification

      a. Calcification of normal tissue (e.g., commonly the deep dermis or subcutaneous tissue) in the setting of hypercalcemia.

         i. Hypercalcemia is usually secondary to hyperparathyroidism (either primary or secondary); commonly a late complication of chronic renal failure.

III. Adaptations to Cell Injury

  A. Atrophy

   1. Definition

      a. Reduction in the size of an organ or tissue secondary to a decrease in cell number and/or size.

   2. Major causes

      a. Cell loss

         i. Advanced Alzheimer disease is an example of atrophy occurring secondary to a loss of cells (Fig. 2.10).

      b. Decreased hormonal stimulation

         i. Vaginal and endometrial atrophy in postmenopausal women as estrogen levels decline.

         ii. Testicular atrophy in those with hypothalamic or pituitary disease (loss of gonadotropin stimulation).

      c. Decreased neural innervation

         i. Skeletal muscle atrophy following the loss of neural innervation (called "denervation atrophy").

      d. Decreased tissue perfusion (ischemia)

         i. Cerebral atrophy in those with reduced cerebral blood flow (e.g., severe atherosclerotic vascular disease).

      e. Inadequate nutrients

         i. Marasmus, chronic inflammatory disease, and cancer.

      f. Increased pressure

         i. Increased pressure (i.e., compression of tissue) impairs blood flow causing ischemia-induced tissue atrophy.

         ii. An example is renal cortical atrophy in those with hydronephrosis.

  B. Hypertrophy

   1. Increase in cell size; leads to an increase in organ size and weight.

   2. Hypertrophy may be physiologic or pathologic.

      a. Physiologic hypertrophy

         i. Skeletal muscle in weightlifters.

      b. Pathologic hypertrophy

         i. Left ventricular hypertrophy in those with systemic hypertension or aortic stenosis (Fig. 2.11).

  C. Hyperplasia

   1. Increased number of normal cells.

   2. Only occurs in tissues whose cells can replicate.

   3. Permanent cells (e.g., neurons and cardiac myocytes) do not undergo hyperplasia because they cannot undergo replication.

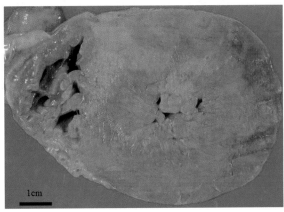

2.11: Left ventricular hypertrophy secondary to pressure overload (systemic hypertension). The left ventricular wall is markedly thickened. *(From Cardiovascular pathology, ed 5, 2022. Fig. 3.3.)*

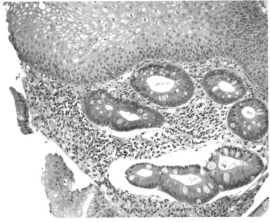

2.12: Intestinal metaplasia of the distal esophagus (Barrett esophagus). *(From Odze and Goldblum surgical pathology of the GI tract, liver, biliary tract and pancreas, ed 3, 2015, Fig. 15.61A.)*

    4. Often secondary to increased hormonal stimulation.
       a. Endometrial gland hyperplasia secondary to elevated serum estrogen.
       b. Prostatic hyperplasia secondary to elevated dihydrotestosterone.
       c. Thyroid enlargement (goiter) secondary to elevated levels of thyroid-stimulating hormone.
    5. May increase one's risk of malignancy.
       a. For example, endometrial hyperplasia is a precursor to endometrial adenocarcinoma.
D. Metaplasia
    1. Definition
       a. Replacement of one fully differentiated cell type by another fully differentiated cell type.
    2. Pathogenesis
       a. Occurs in response to chronic irritation where the new cell type is less sensitive to the stress.
       b. Chronic tissue irritation leads to the release of various cytokines and growth factors that alter gene expression → reprogramming of local tissue stem cells to the new cell type.
       c. Reversible upon removal of the initiating trigger.
    3. Examples:
       a. Intestinal metaplasia of the distal esophagus (Barrett esophagus)
          i.   Squamous epithelium of distal esophagus is replaced by an intestinal-type epithelium with goblet cells and mucus-secreting cells (akin to that of the small intestine).
          ii. Known as Barrett esophagus, intestinal metaplasia of the distal esophagus helps protect against the damaging effects of recurrent gastroesophageal reflux (Fig. 2.12).
          iii. Increased risk of malignant transformation (adenocarcinoma).
       b. Intestinal metaplasia of the stomach
          i.   Secondary to chronic *Helicobacter pylori* gastritis.
          ii. Increased risk of malignant transformation (intestinal-type gastric adenocarcinoma).

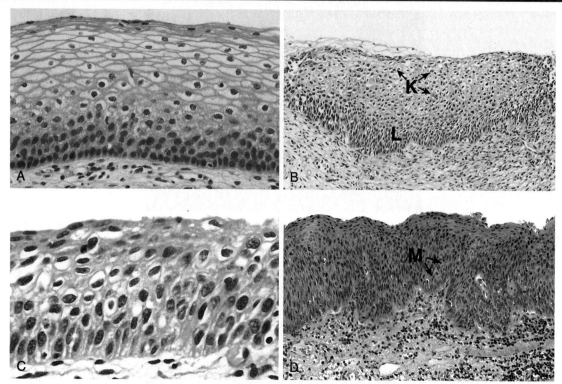

2.13: Dysplasia of the ectocervix: (A) normal ectocervix; (B) low-grade dysplasia of ectocervix/CIN I; *K*, Koilocytes; *L*, lower third of epithelium (C) high-grade dysplasia/CIN II; (D) high-grade dysplasia/CIN III. Note increasing degrees of cytologic atypia with crowded nuclei and increased mitotic figures (*M* in the image) *(From Wheater's pathology: a text, atlas, and review of histopathology, ed 6, 2020, Elsevier.)*

      c. Squamous metaplasia of the bronchial respiratory epithelium
         i.   Ciliated columnar respiratory epithelium is replaced by squamous epithelium due to the chronic irritant effects of smoking.
         ii. Increased risk of bronchogenic squamous cell carcinoma.
      d. Squamous metaplasia of the endocervix
         i.   Normal occurrence at puberty due to lowering of vaginal pH.
      e. Squamous metaplasia of the urinary bladder
         i.   Urothelium replaced by squamous epithelium.
         ii. Seen in those with chronic infection of the bladder (e.g., *Schistosoma haematobium*).
         iii. Increased risk of squamous cell carcinoma of the bladder.

  E. Dysplasia
    1. Defined as "disordered" growth, dysplasia is a potential precursor to cancer (Fig. 2.13).
      a. Recognizable by the cytologic changes (e.g., increased mitotic activity, lack of cellular maturation, and increased nuclear size).
    2. Risk factors for the development of dysplasia include:
      a. Chemical irritants (e.g., cigarette smoke).
      b. Human papilloma virus (HPV) types 16 and 18.
      c. Ultraviolet (UV) light.

IV. Cell Death
  A. Definition
    1. Loss of cells that occurs when unable to adapt to an injury.
    2. Occurs via one of two processes (necrosis or apoptosis).
  B. Necrosis
    1. Irreversible pathologic process secondary to severe injury.
    2. Results in the breakdown of cell membranes and the release of cellular contents into surrounding tissue and/or bloodstream.
      a. "Damage-associated molecular patterns" (DAMPs).
    3. Phagocytosis of cellular debris by tissue-resident macrophages, release of various pro-inflammatory mediators (e.g., tumor necrosis factor and interleukins).
      a. Influx of neutrophils to the site of injury leads to further cell breakdown; due to the release of various enzymes (e.g., proteases).
    4. Causes of necrosis
      a. Ischemia (e.g., acute myocardial infarction and ischemic stroke).

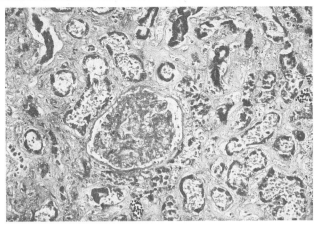

2.14: Coagulative necrosis. Note the loss of cellular and nuclear detail. *(From Underwood's pathology, ed 7, 2019, Elsevier.)*

    b. Physical injury (e.g., burns, frostbite, and radiation).
    c. Infection (microbial toxins and host immune response).
  5. Types of necrosis
    a. Coagulative necrosis (Fig. 2.14)
      i. Type of necrosis in which the cell outlines are preserved, at least for a few days (proteolytic enzymes, as well as structural proteins, are denatured).
      ii. Tissue initially exhibits normal texture. Over the subsequent days, progressive softening occurs as the necrotic cellular debris is removed by macrophages.
      iii. Histologic appearance is variable, depending on the time since the injury. In the first few hours, there are no discernible changes. Over the next few days, there is a progressive loss of nuclear staining and cytoplasmic detail is lost.
    b. Liquefactive necrosis
      i. Type of tissue necrosis characterized by liquefaction.
      ii. Due to the release of digestive enzymes from infiltrating leukocytes.
      iii. Uncommon, most characteristically seen in bacterial abscesses and/or the central nervous system (e.g., following a stroke).
    c. Caseous necrosis
      i. Pattern of "cheese-like" necrosis seen in granulomas; characteristically in association with fungal and/or mycobacterial infection.
    d. Fat necrosis
      i. Enzymatic fat necrosis
        (1) Characteristic of enzyme-mediated necrosis adjacent to an acutely inflamed pancreas (secondary to leakage of lipase from injured pancreatic acinar cells).
        (2) Fatty acids, released by the necrotic adipose tissue, bind to calcium; form chalky yellow-white deposits within and around the pancreas (dystrophic calcification).
        (3) Recognizable on light microscopy as pale pink adipocytes with indistinct cell outlines and loss of nuclei.
      ii. Traumatic fat necrosis
        (1) Characteristically seen following blunt trauma or surgery (e.g., abdomen and female breast).

C. Apoptosis
  1. Defined as "programmed" cell death in which cells that are destined to die undergo a series of enzymatic reactions leading to collapse of the cytoskeleton and fragmentation of the nucleus.
  2. Phagocytosis of cellular debris before the intracellular contents leak out prevents the release of chemotactic factors.
    a. Explains the lack of inflammation with apoptosis.
  3. Normal in some situations, including:
    a. Removal of "webbing" between fingers and toes during embryonic development (Fig. 2.15).
    b. Menses following apoptosis of endometrial tissue following hormonal withdrawal.
  4. Conversely, apoptosis is responsible for the removal of irreversibly damaged cells, for example:
    a. Radiation or chemotherapy → DNA damage → triggers apoptosis of neoplastic cells.
    b. Accumulation of misfolded proteins (e.g., many neurodegenerative diseases) → cell loss via apoptosis.
  5. Activation of apoptosis occurs via one of two mechanisms (Fig. 2.16).
    a. Death receptor (extrinsic) pathway activation
      i. Death receptors, present on the cell surface, are activated upon binding with a specific ligand.
      ii. Tumor necrosis factor receptor 1 (TNFR1) is a major death receptor.

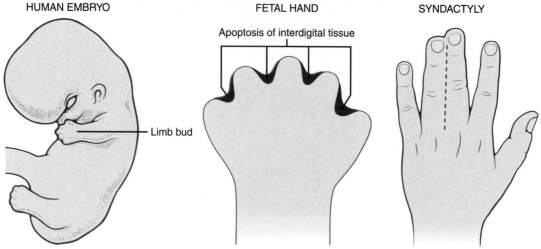

HUMAN EMBRYO   FETAL HAND   SYNDACTYLY

Apoptosis of interdigital tissue

Limb bud

2.15: During embryologic development, apoptosis has a role in the removal of webbing between fingers. In the absence of this effect, the digits remained fused (syndactyly). *(From Pathology for the health professions, ed. 4, St. Louis, 2012, Saunders Elsevier.)*

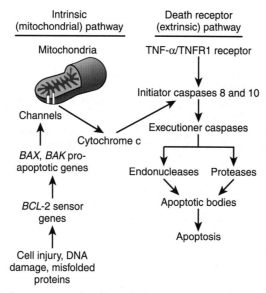

Intrinsic
(mitochondrial) pathway

Death receptor
(extrinsic) pathway

Mitochondria

TNF-α/TNFR1 receptor

Initiator caspases 8 and 10

Channels

Executioner caspases

Cytochrome c

BAX, BAK pro-
apoptotic genes

Endonucleases   Proteases

BCL-2 sensor
genes

Apoptotic bodies

Cell injury, DNA
damage, misfolded
proteins

Apoptosis

2.16: Simplified schematic of apoptosis. Refer to the text for discussion. *TNF*, Tumor necrosis factor; *TNFR*, tumor necrosis factor receptor.

    iii. TNF-α binding to TNFR1 directly activates initiator caspases (caspase-8 and caspase-10).
       (1) Caspases are a family of proteases that have a cysteine residue at their active site and cleave target proteins at specific aspartic acid residues.
    iv. Initiator caspases, in turn, activate effector caspases (proteases and endonucleases) to complete the destruction of the cell.
  b. Intrinsic (mitochondrial) pathway activation
    i. Activated by an increase in the permeability of the mitochondrial outer membrane that, in turn, causes pro-apoptotic molecules (e.g., cytochrome c) to be released into the cytoplasm.
    ii. The integrity of the mitochondrial outer membrane is controlled by the *BCL2* family of proteins.
    iii. This protein family contains both antiapoptotic genes (*BCL2*) and pro-apoptotic (*BAX* and *BAK*) genes.
    iv. Various injurious events (e.g., protein misfolding and free radical injury) activate pro-apoptotic genes (*BAX* and *BAK*).
    v. Once activated, *BAX* and *BAK* form channels in the mitochondrial membrane → releasing cytochrome c into the cytosol → triggering activation of initiator caspase (caspase-9).
    vi. Caspase-9 activates effector caspases (proteases and endonucleases) to cause the execution phase of apoptosis.
  c. Execution phase of apoptosis
    i. Executioner caspases (e.g., caspase-3 and caspase-6), activated by initiator caspases, cause the cell membrane and nucleus to fragment.
    ii. Forms "apoptotic bodies" that are phagocytosed by macrophages. On H&E staining, apoptotic cells have a deeply eosinophilic cytoplasm and a pyknotic, fragmented nucleus.

CHAPTER 3 Inflammation and Repair

I. Acute Inflammation

A. Definition

1. Innate, transient, early response to injury resulting in an influx of neutrophils and macrophages into an area of injury.
2. Acts to rid the body of an offending agent.
3. Denoted by the suffix "itis" (e.g., appendicitis = inflammation of the appendix).
4. Not synonymous with infection.

Cardinal signs of inflammation

- Redness (rubor)
- Heat (calor)
- Swelling (tumor)
- Pain (dolor)
- Loss of function (functio laesa)

B. Stimuli for the development of acute inflammation include:

1. Infections (e.g., bacterial, viral, fungal, and parasitic).
2. Hypersensitivity reactions.
3. Tissue necrosis (e.g., infarction, burns, and trauma).
4. Foreign bodies (e.g., glass, splinters, and suture material).

C. Innate immune response

1. Tissue-resident innate immune cells (e.g., dendritic cells, macrophages, and mast cells) begin the inflammatory process by "sensing" the injurious process.
   a. Molecules (e.g., uric acid, DNA, and RNA) released from damaged cells; collectively referred to as "damage-associated molecular patterns" (DAMPs).
   b. Molecules (e.g., lipopolysaccharide, lipoteichoic acid, and mycolic acid) released from microbial organisms; collectively referred to as "pathogen-associated molecular patterns" (PAMPs).
2. DAMPs and/or PAMPs bind to pattern recognition receptors (PRRs) on innate immune cells.
   a. Examples of PRRs include toll-like receptors, nucleotide-binding oligomerization domain-like receptors, retinoic acid-inducible gene (RIG)-like receptors, and C-type lectin receptors.
3. Binding of PAMPs or DAMPs to the various pathogen recognition receptors triggers the early innate immune response and the release of various pro-inflammatory mediators (e.g., interleukin-1 [IL-1], interleukin-6 [IL-6], and tumor necrosis factor [TNF]).

D. Major components of acute inflammation

1. An early manifestation, due to the release of histamine and other mediators, is arteriolar vasodilation (Fig. 3.1).
   a. Increases blood flow to the region, thereby contributing to the warmth and redness characteristic of acute inflammation.
2. A second manifestation, likewise a result of histamine and other chemical mediators, is endothelial contraction.
   a. Causes small "gaps" to form between cells, thereby allowing for the leakage of plasma fluid into interstitial spaces (edema) (Fig. 3.2).
3. Together, these effects (vasodilation and loss of fluid) cause a slowing of blood flow (called stasis).
   a. White blood cells (WBCs) move toward the periphery of the axial stream (i.e., along the vascular endothelium).
   b. This process, called margination, prepares WBCs for entry into the tissues (called transmigration).
   c. Neutrophils are used in the following discussion as they are the primary leukocyte of acute inflammation.

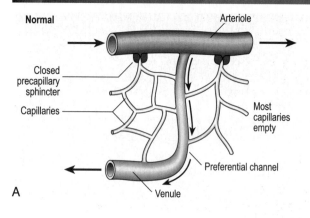

A

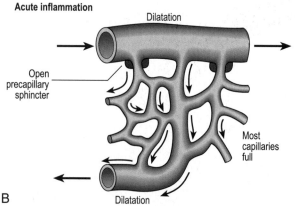

B

3.1: Circulatory changes in acute inflammation. Relaxation of arterioles causes flooding of the capillary network with distention of capillaries and postcapillary venules. *(From Underwood's pathology, ed 7, 2019, Elsevier.)*

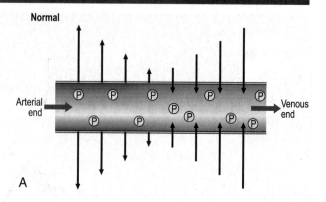

A

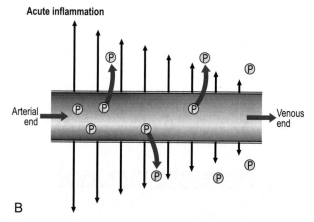

B

3.2: Acute inflammation is associated with the loss of fluid into the extravascular space (edema) Plasma. *(From Underwood's pathology, ed 7, 2019, Elsevier.)*

4. Margination of neutrophils (Fig. 3.3)
   a. Cytokines released in response to the injury (IL-1 and TNF), activate adhesion molecules (selectins) on leukocytes and endothelial cells.
      i. L-selectin on leukocytes; E-selectin, and P-selectin on endothelial cells.
   b. Selectin binding is weak and transient, causes WBCs to "roll" (bind–detach, bind–detach) along the endothelial surface of the vessel.
   c. Subsequent activation of additional adhesion molecules on WBCs (integrins) and endothelial cells (intercellular adhesion molecule and vascular cell adhesion molecule), results in a more robust binding of WBCs to the endothelium.
   d. Now, once firmly bound, neutrophils can transmigrate (cross) into the tissues, primarily through postcapillary venules.
5. Chemotaxis of neutrophils
   a. After exiting the circulation, neutrophils must be directed to the site of injury. This occurs via a chemical gradient (chemotaxis).
      i. Chemotactic mediators include both endogenous (e.g., IL-8, C5a, and leukotriene B4) and exogenous (e.g., bacterial products) factors.
   b. Chemotactic mediators cause neutrophils to extend filopodia, allowing them to move toward the site of injury.
6. Clearance of offending agent
   a. Once at the site of injury, neutrophils begin to clear the offending agent (e.g., bacterium, necrotic cells, etc.) through a process known as phagocytosis.
   b. Phagocytosis is a multistep process that begins by opsonization (Fig. 3.4).
      i. Opsonization is the binding of an opsonin (e.g., immunoglobulin G [IgG] and C3b) to the foreign substance.
      ii. Neutrophils, having membrane receptors for IgG and C3b, are then better able to recognize the foreign substance.
   c. Following recognition, the neutrophil engulfs the microbe (or cellular debris, foreign body, etc.) to form a phagosome.
   d. Subsequent fusion of the phagosome with lysosome forms a "phagolysosome" within which the engulfed material is degraded (Fig. 3.5) by digestive enzymes and reactive oxygen or nitrogen species.

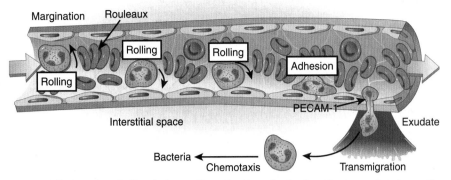

3.3: Neutrophil events in acute inflammation. Rolling is due to the activation of selectin adhesion molecules on the surface of neutrophils, whereas firm adhesion is due to the activation of β2-integrin (CD11a:CD18) adhesion molecules on the surface of neutrophils (not shown). Ligands (attachment sites) for selectin and β2-integrin are located on the surface of endothelial cells (not shown). Neutrophil transmigration through the basement membrane mainly occurs in venules. Neutrophils dissolve the exposed venular basement membrane and transmigrate into the interstitial tissue. This leads to an outpouring of protein-rich fluid (called exudate) along with neutrophils. Once in the interstitial space, chemotactic factors direct the neutrophils to the site of inflammation. *(From Goljan E: Rapid review pathology, ed 4, 2014, Saunders Elsevier, p 37, Fig. 3.3.)*

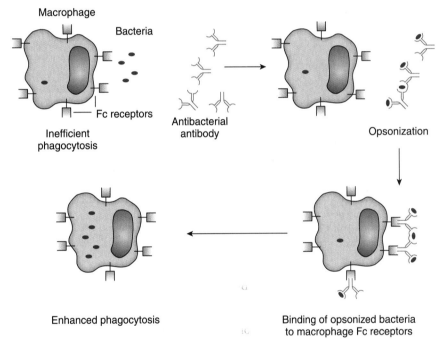

3.4: Opsonization of bacteria by antibody promotes recognition and subsequent phagocytosis. *(From Abbas AK et al., editors: Cellular and molecular immunology, ed 2, Philadelphia, 1994, Saunders, with permission.)*

    i. Nicotinamide adenine dinucleotide phosphate oxidase enzyme complex generates superoxide anion and hydrogen peroxide ("respiratory burst").

    ii. Myeloperoxidase from neutrophilic azurophilic granules converts hydrogen peroxide into hypochlorite (active ingredient in bleach), a potent antimicrobial agent.

E. Patterns of acute inflammation

  1. Purulent (suppurative) inflammation

    a. Characterized by the presence of pus, an exudate comprised neutrophils, necrotic cellular debris, and edema fluid (Fig. 3.6).

    b. Typically, a manifestation of bacterial infections (e.g., *Staphylococcus aureus*).

  2. Abscess

    a. Localized collection of pus with a central area of necrosis surrounded by prominent neutrophilic inflammation.

  3. Fibrinous inflammation

    a. Characterized by a loss of protein-rich fluid through gaps between endothelial cells (leaky blood vessels) to form a fibrin-rich exudate on the tissue surface (Fig. 3.7).

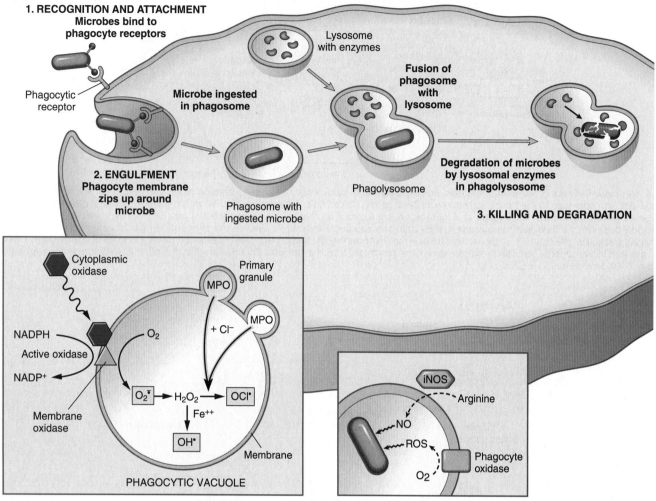

1. RECOGNITION AND ATTACHMENT
Microbes bind to phagocyte receptors

Lysosome with enzymes

Fusion of phagosome with lysosome

Phagocytic receptor

Microbe ingested in phagosome

2. ENGULFMENT
Phagocyte membrane zips up around microbe

Phagosome with ingested microbe

Phagolysosome

Degradation of microbes by lysosomal enzymes in phagolysosome

3. KILLING AND DEGRADATION

Cytoplasmic oxidase

Primary granule

MPO

MPO

NADPH

Active oxidase

NADP$^+$

+ Cl$^-$

O$_2$

Membrane oxidase

$O_2^{\overline{\cdot}}$ → H_2O_2 → OCl$^\bullet$

Fe^{++}

OH$^\bullet$

Membrane

PHAGOCYTIC VACUOLE

iNOS

Arginine

NO

ROS

Phagocyte oxidase

O$_2$

3.5: Phagocytosis and destruction of microbial pathogens involves the formation of phagolysosomes, within which microbes are killed and degraded. $O_2\bullet(-)$, Superoxide anion; •OH, hydroxy radical; iNOS, inducible nitric oxide synthase; MPO, myeloperoxidase; NO, nitric oxide; ROS, reactive oxygen species. (From Robbins & Cotran pathologic basis of disease, ed 10, 2021, Elsevier.)

      i. Typical of inflammatory processes of body cavities (e.g., pericardium and pleura).
   b. If the exudate is not removed, through fibrinolysis and phagocytosis, then fibroblasts may deposit collagen, forming scar tissue.
      i. Constrictive pericarditis (fibrous scarring of pericardium) is an example.
  4. Serous inflammation
   a. Refers to inflammation associated with a thin, watery exudate containing few cells; an example being the collection of serous fluid within skin blisters following a burn injury or viral infection.
F. Systemic effects of inflammation
  1. Fever
   a. Elevation of body temperature; due to the release of fever-inducing substances (called pyrogens).
      i. Pyrogens include both exogenous products (e.g., bacterial lipopolysaccharide) and endogenous products (e.g., IL-1 and TNF).
      ii. IL-1 and TNF enhance prostaglandin production (primarily PGE$_2$) to stimulate the hypothalamus to elevate the body temperature.
  2. Acute phase reactants (APRs)
   a. Proteins whose serum concentrations either increase or decrease by at least 25% during an inflammatory state.
      i. Despite their name, APRs may be seen in association with either acute or chronic inflammatory states.
   b. APRs are synthesized by the liver, primarily in response to IL-6.
      i. IL-1, TNF-α, and interferon-γ (IFN-γ) also stimulate the production of APRs.
   c. Notable APRs that increase during inflammation include:
      i. C-reactive protein
         (1) Highly sensitive; rises quickly with inflammation.
         (2) Often used by clinicians to monitor chronic inflammatory states (e.g., autoimmune disease).

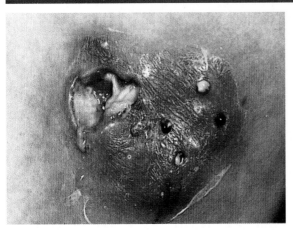

3.6: Purulent inflammation of the skin (pus). *(From Bouloux P: Self-assessment picture tests medicine, Vol 1, London, 1997, Mosby-Wolfe.)*

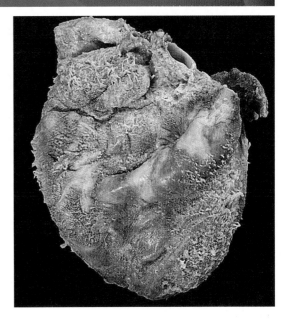

3.7: Fibrinous inflammation (fibrinous pericarditis). *(From Pathology: a color atlas, St. Louis, 2000, Mosby.)*

ii. Hepcidin
(1) By binding to and degrading an iron transporter (ferroportin), hepcidin impairs both the absorption of iron from gut as well as the release of iron from macrophage storage sites in the bone marrow.
(2) Elevated levels, as seen with inflammatory states, explains the pathophysiology underlying anemia of chronic disease/inflammation.
3. Leukocytosis
a. Elevation of the WBC count.
b. Secondary to an increased release of granulocytes from the bone marrow in response to pro-inflammatory cytokines (e.g., IL-1 and TNF) and growth factors released by tissue-resident immune cells.

II. **Chronic Inflammation**
A. **Definition**
1. A response to persistent injurious stimuli or infection lasting weeks to years.
B. **Etiologies include:**
1. Persistent infection (e.g., mycobacteria and fungi).
2. Autoimmune disease (e.g., rheumatoid arthritis and systemic lupus erythematosus).
3. Environmental exposures (e.g., silica and foreign bodies).
C. **Morphologic features**
1. Mononuclear cells (lymphocytes, plasma cells, and macrophages).
2. Tissue injury/destruction (loss of parenchyma → loss of functional tissue).
3. Healing (granulation tissue and fibrosis).
a. Granulation tissue is a type of tissue rich in newly formed blood vessels and activated fibroblasts that acts to fill in the defect (precursor to scar formation).
D. **Granulomatous inflammation**
1. Type of chronic inflammation characterized by collections of activated macrophages and associated lymphocytic inflammation (T cells).
a. Inflammatory focus is known as a granuloma.
2. Characteristically develop in situations in which the offending agent is difficult to eradicate.
a. In some instances, granulomas develop a central area of necrosis—described as "caseous necrosis" due to its cheese-like appearance (characteristic of mycobacterial and fungal infections).
3. Granulomatous inflammation can also arise secondary to noninfectious processes, usually in association with foreign bodies (e.g., suture material and splinters).
a. Other associations include Crohn disease and sarcoidosis (Fig. 3.8).
b. Noninfectious granulomata lack necrosis (i.e., they are noncaseating).
III. **Cell Proliferation**
A. **Cell proliferation and/or regeneration is dependent upon the ability of the cell to replicate.**
1. Examples of cells that can replicate include:
a. Stem cells in epidermis, bone marrow, and gastrointestinal epithelium.

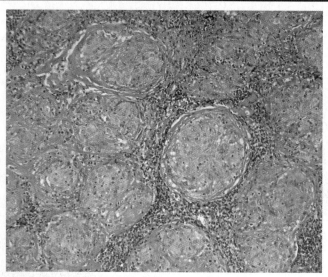

3.8: Granulomatous inflammation. In this image of sarcoidosis, the granulomata are noncaseating (i.e., lack the central area of necrosis). *(From* Hematopathology, *ed 2, 2017, Elsevier.)*

   2. Permanent cells (e.g., neurons and cardiac muscle) cannot regenerate.
      a. Remain in G_0 (quiescent phase, outside of cell cycle).
   B. Entry into the cell cycle requires stimulation by growth factors.
      1. Since these factors stimulate growth, genetic mutations may lead to disease (e.g., cancer).
   C. Examples of growth factors:
      1. Epidermal growth factor (EGF)
         a. EGF acts via binding to a family of EGF receptors (EGFR)Mutations drive growth factor–independent cell replication.
            i. EGFR1 (ERB-B1) mutated in some cancers of the lung, head/neck, brain, and breast.
            ii. EGFR2 (ERB-B2, HER-2) mutated in some breast and other cancers.
      2. Vascular endothelial growth factor (VEGF)
         a. Induced by hypoxia, VEGF stimulates angiogenesis (i.e., new blood vessel growth).
      3. Transforming growth factor-β (TGF-β)
         a. TGF-β stimulates scarring (i.e., fibrosis) following injury as well as certain pathologic conditions.
   D. Process of replication and division into two identical daughter cells, proceeds in a very ordered manner, called the "cell cycle" (Fig. 3.9).
      1. G_1 (gap 1) → S (DNA synthesis) → G_2 (gap 2) → M (mitosis).
   E. Cell cycle regulation
      1. Positive regulators include cyclins and cyclin-dependent kinases (CDKs).
      2. Negative regulators include retinoblastoma (Rb), p53, and CDK inhibitors.
   F. "Checkpoints" are located at the entry into the "S" phase and "M" phases.
      1. Allows cells to "check" for the presence of DNA damage.
      2. If damage is detected at one or the other of these checkpoints, then replication stops.
         a. In the presence of DNA damage, p53 protein accumulates and activates the transcription of several genes including the CDK inhibitor *p21*.
            i. The protein product (p21) is a negative regulator of CDKs; prevents the phosphorylation of Rb (causing cell cycle arrest).
            ii. Allows time for DNA repair to occur.
      3. If the DNA is too severely damaged, then the cell is stimulated to undergo apoptosis (programmed cell death).
      4. Failure of the cell to stop replication in the presence of DNA damage leads to "genetic instability" (a hallmark of malignancy).
IV. Tissue Repair
   A. Repair (healing) of tissue is meant to restore architecture and function.
      1. Requires extracellular matrix (ECM), a protein network with variety of functions, including:
         a. Mechanical support/scaffolding and regulation of cell proliferation.
      2. Disruption of the ECM prevents tissue regeneration/repair.
         a. As an example, full-thickness (third-degree) burns heal by scarring because the loss of skin, basement membrane, and connective tissue infrastructure precludes the regeneration of normal structures.
   B. Steps in scar formation (Fig. 3.10)
      1. WBCs (e.g., neutrophils) enter the site of injury, then degrade, and remove damaged tissue by phagocytosis.
      2. Granulation tissue (fibroblasts, loose connective tissue, blood vessels, and mononuclear cells) proliferation (fills defect).

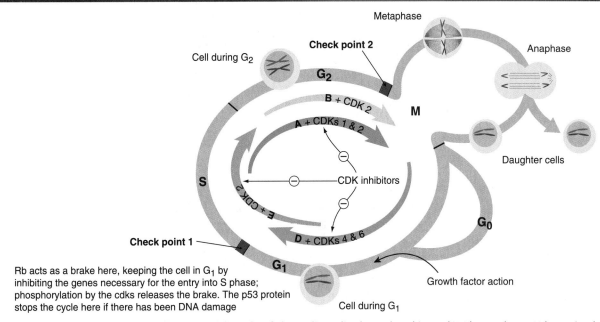

Rb acts as a brake here, keeping the cell in G_1 by inhibiting the genes necessary for the entry into S phase; phosphorylation by the cdks releases the brake. The p53 protein stops the cycle here if there has been DNA damage

3.9: Schematic diagram of the cell cycle showing the role of the cyclin/cyclin-dependent kinase (CDK) complexes. When stimulated by growth factors, a quiescent cell (in G_0 phase) is propelled into G_1 phase in preparation for DNA synthesis. This step is dependent upon the sequential action of cyclin/CDK complexes (which in turn are regulated by CDK inhibitors). In the presence of DNA damage, the tumor suppressor p53 arrests the cycle at check point 1, allowing for repair. If repair fails, the cell normally undergoes programmed cell death (apoptosis). After mitotic division, the daughter cells may enter G_1 or G_0 phase. *Rb*, Retinoblastoma gene. *(From Rang & Dale's pharmacology, ed 9, 2020, Elsevier.)*

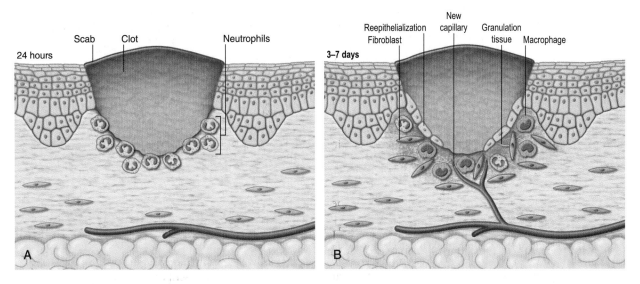

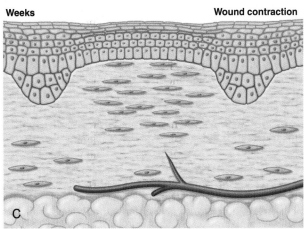

3.10: Steps in wound healing. *(From Plastic surgery: volume 1: principles, ed 4, 2018, Elsevier.)*

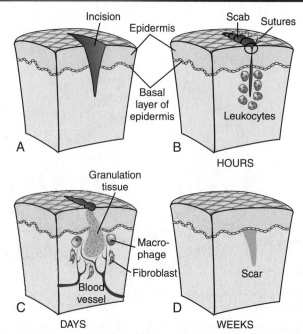

3.11: Wound healing by primary intention. The sequence of events includes an initial fibrin clot (forming a scab), followed by influx of polymorphonuclear leukocytes to remove the injurious agent. Tissue healing begins with the formation of granulation tissue, followed later by collagen deposition (forming a fibrous scar). *(From* Pathology for the health professions, *ed 4, 2012, Saunders Elsevier.)*

   3. Dense fibrous scar tissue formed.
      a. TGF-β stimulates the migration and proliferation of fibroblasts (the cells that deposit collagen to form the scar).
      b. Scar tissue is initially comprised of type III collagen: later remodeled into type I collagen (stronger).

Factors that inhibit normal healing

- Infection (prolongs inflammation which can further damage tissue).
- Diabetes mellitus (decreased tissue perfusion and decreased immune function).
- Nutritional deficiencies (vitamin C for example is required for collagen synthesis).
- Glucocorticoids (inhibit TGF-β, which is required for scar formation).
- Presence of foreign bodies (perpetuate the inflammatory process).

  C. Healing of skin wounds
    1. Healing by primary intention (Fig. 3.11)
      a. Reserved for the healing of clean surgical wounds.
      b. By suturing or skin grafting, the wound edges are brought together to promote the healing process.
    2. Healing by secondary intention (Fig. 3.12)
      a. Reserved for highly contaminated wounds.
      b. Wound is left open to allowing infilling with granulation tissue.
      c. Over time, the wound slowly closes through contraction of myofibroblasts.
    3. Healing by tertiary intention (delayed primary closure)
      a. Contaminated wound is debrided (nonviable tissue removed) and antibiotics provided; followed later by wound closure (suturing, skin grafting).
  D. Abnormal healing of the skin
    1. Keloids are raised scars that grow beyond the borders of the original wound (Fig. 3.13).
    2. Hypertrophic scars are raised scars that remain within the confines of the original wound.
V. Laboratory Findings Associated With Inflammation
  A. Acute inflammation
    1. Neutrophilic leukocytosis
      a. Due to various cytokines (e.g., IL-1) that stimulate the release of postmitotic pool of neutrophils (metamyelocytes, band neutrophils, and segmented neutrophils) from the bone marrow.
      b. Increased band neutrophils (>10% of leukocytes), with or without occasional metamyelocytes is called a "left shift" or a "bandemia" (Fig. 3.14).

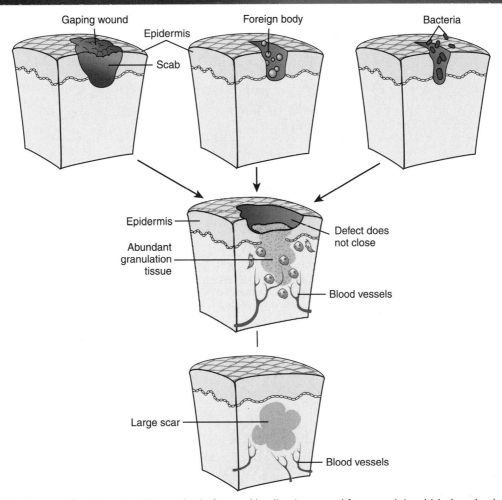

Gaping wound
Epidermis
Scab
Foreign body
Bacteria

Epidermis
Abundant granulation tissue
Defect does not close
Blood vessels

Large scar
Blood vessels

3.12: Wound healing by secondary intention. This method of wound healing is reserved for wounds in which there is a large defect, those that are infected, or those that contain foreign material. The healing is slower because the epithelial cells proliferating from the wound margin take longer to cover the defect. Granulation tissue is more abundant; consequently, scarring is more prominent. *(From* Pathology for the health professions, *ed 4, 2012, Saunders Elsevier.)*

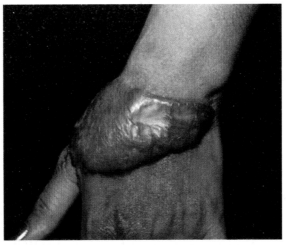

3.13: Keloid formation. Note the raised, thickened scar over the dorsum of the hand. Unlike a hypertrophic scar, keloids grow beyond the borders of the original wound. *(From Lookingbill D, Marks J: Principles of dermatology, ed 3, Philadelphia, 2000, Saunders.)*

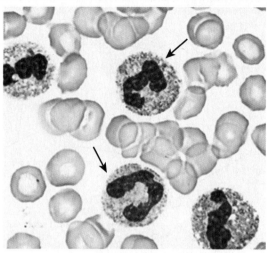

3.14: Absolute leukocytosis with left shift. Arrows point to band neutrophils, which exhibit prominence of the azurophilic granules (toxic granulation). Vacuoles in the cytoplasm represent phagolysosomes. A left shift is due to accelerated release of postmitotic neutrophils from the bone marrow and is defined as >10% band neutrophils or the presence of earlier precursors (e.g., metamyelocytes). *(From Hoffbrand I, Pettit J, Vyas P: Color atlas of clinical hematology, ed 4, Philadelphia, 2010, Mosby Elsevier.)*

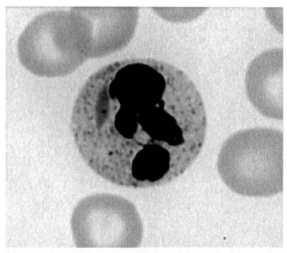

3.15: Neutrophil with a blue gray Döhle inclusion body and toxic granulation in the cytosol. *(From Naeim, F: Atlas of bone marrow and blood pathology, Philadelphia, 2001, Saunders.)*

    2. Toxic granulation
       a. Prominence of dark blue to purple primary granules in metamyelocytes, bands, and segmented neutrophils.
       b. Seen in association with severe inflammatory states, both infectious and noninfectious etiologies.
    3. Döhle bodies
       a. Round to oval, pale, grayish blue inclusions of endoplasmic reticulum (Fig. 3.15).
       b. Found in neutrophils, commonly in association with toxic granulation.
    4. Increased serum IgM
       a. Plasma cells produce antibodies against a specific antigen.
       b. IgM is the first class of antibody produced and thus the predominant immunoglobulin class of acute inflammation; levels usually peak in 7–10 days.
       c. Afterwards, the plasma cell may switch production to a different class of antibody (e.g., IgG) but with the same antigenic specificity (called isotype switching).
  B. Chronic inflammation
    1. Increased monocytes, lymphocytes; IgG predominant immunoglobulin.

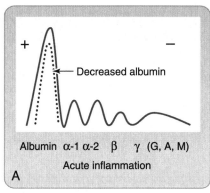

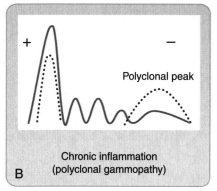

3.16: Serum protein electrophoresis (SPE) in acute inflammation (A) and chronic inflammation (B). Albumin is decreased because of the increased synthesis of acute phase reactants in the liver. The primary difference between acute versus chronic inflammation is the marked increase in IgG antibody production in chronic inflammation producing a diffusely enlarged γ-globulin peak (polyclonal gammopathy). *(From Goljan E, Sloka K: Rapid review laboratory testing in clinical medicine, Philadelphia, 2008, Mosby Elsevier, p 284, Fig. 9-1B and C.)*

C. Erythrocyte sedimentation rate (ESR)
1. ESR measures the rate at which erythrocytes sink (sediment) to the bottom of a tube containing whole blood.
   a. Due to the binding of APRs (e.g., fibrinogen) to erythrocytes, causing them to sediment at a faster rate than would occur in the absence of ongoing inflammation.
   b. Reason why active inflammatory states (e.g., infection, autoimmune disorders, and malignancy) are commonly associated with an elevated ESR.

D. Serum protein electrophoresis in inflammation (Fig. 3.16)
1. In acute inflammation, there is a slight decrease in serum albumin due to the diversion of amino acids for the synthesis of APRs (e.g., fibrinogen).
2. Normal γ-globulin peak because serum IgM is not elevated enough to alter the configuration of the γ-globulin peak.
3. In chronic inflammation, however, not only is there a greater decrease in serum albumin (due to the continued diversion of amino acids for the synthesis of APRs) but γ-globulins are increased as well (due to a marked increase in the synthesis of IgG).
   a. Note that the gamma region is broad because there are many different plasma cell clones producing IgG (called a "polyclonal" gammopathy).

CHAPTER 4

Disorders of the Immune System

I. Normal Immune Response
A. Innate immune response
1. Tissue-resident innate immune cells serve as the first line of defense.
   a. For example, epithelial cells of the skin or mucous membranes serve as a barrier to the entry of infectious agents.
2. As a review (see Chapter 3), recall that macrophages and dendritic cells contain pattern recognition receptors (e.g., toll-like receptors and nucleotide-binding oligomerization domain-like receptors) that recognize certain products of microbes ("pathogen-associated molecular patterns") or necrotic tissue ("damage-associated molecular patterns").
3. Once activated, inflammatory mediators (e.g., interleukin [IL]-1, IL-6, and tumor necrosis factor [TNF]) are released, initiating the host immune response.
   a. Secretion of cytokines (IL-1β, IL-6, and TNF-α) is normally transient; thereby, limiting potential tissue injury.
   b. Overproduction of the various cytokines and other mediators (i.e., dysregulated host immune response) underlies manifestations of sepsis (e.g., septic shock and organ failure).
B. Adaptive immune response (Fig. 4.1)
1. Involves T and B lymphocytes as well as the formation of antibodies against specific molecular structures (antigens).
2. Results in a specific and long-lasting response against specific antigens.
3. In some cases, the immune response may be injurious to self (hypersensitivity reactions [HSRs], discussed later).

II. Major Histocompatibility Complex
A. Encoded by a group of genes on chromosome 6.
1. Also known as human leukocyte antigen (HLA) because they were first identified on leukocytes.
B. Two major classes of major histocompatibility complex (MHC) molecules—class I and class II.
1. Class I MHC molecules are present on all nucleated cells and platelets.
   a. Three genes (*HLA-A*, *HLA-B*, and *HLA-C*).
   b. Antigen presentation in association with MHC class I molecules by CD8+ lymphocytes leads to antigen-specific cytotoxic T-cell responses.
2. Class II MHC molecules are present only on cells of the immune system (e.g., macrophages, B lymphocytes, and dendritic cells).
   a. Encoded in a region called *HLA-D*.
   b. Subregions *HLA-DP*, *HLA-DQ*, and *HLA-DR*.
   c. Class II MHC molecules present antigens to CD4+ T cells.
C. Function of MHC
1. By displaying protein antigens to T cells, MHC molecules direct the appropriate immune response.
   a. Cytotoxic T lymphocyte-mediated response against intracellular microbes or tumor antigens.
   b. Helper T lymphocyte-mediated humoral immune response against extracellular microbes or proteins.
III. Hypersensitivity Reactions
A. Overview of HSR
1. HSRs, which are immune reactions injurious to the host, are often against exogenous antigens (e.g., pollen, food, drugs, pet dander, etc.).
2. Commonly results in skin rashes and itching; some reactions, however, may be lethal due to airway narrowing and/or anaphylactic shock.
   a. Reactions against endogenous antigens (i.e., those present within the host) explain the concept of "autoimmunity."

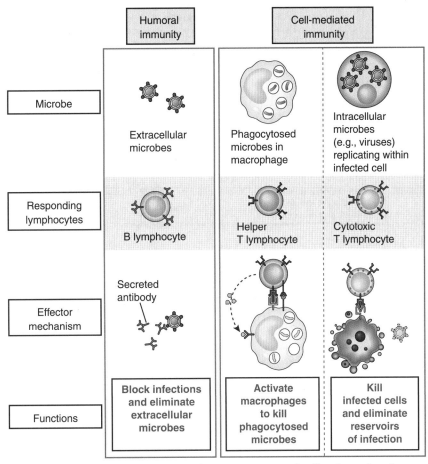

4.1: Types of adaptive immunity. In humoral immunity, B lymphocytes secrete antibodies that primarily target extracellular microbes. In cell-mediated immunity, T lymphocytes activate macrophages to destroy phagocytosed microbes or kill infected cells. *(From Abbas A, Lichtman A: Basic immunology: function and disorders of the immune system, ed 3, Philadelphia, 2011, Saunders Elsevier.)*

B. Type I (immediate) HSR
1. Pathogenesis of immediate hypersensitivity (Fig. 4.2)
   a. Upon initial exposure, antigen-presenting cells present the allergen to naïve CD4+ helper T cells. These cells undergo differentiation into Th2 cells and begin the production of various cytokines.
      i. IL-4 stimulates the production of immunoglobulin E (IgE) antibodies against the specific allergen.
      ii. IL-5 stimulates eosinophil development and activation.
      iii. IL-13 stimulates the secretion of mucus and IgE production.
   b. Lastly, allergen-specific IgE antibodies bind to mast cells.
      i. Derived from the bone marrow, mast cells are located around small blood vessels and nerves, as well as within subepithelial tissues.
   c. Upon reexposure, the allergen binds to preformed IgE molecules bound to mast cells, causing an early phase reaction due to the "degranulation" of mast cells.
      i. Degranulation is characterized by the release of preformed mediators (e.g., histamine, proteases, and heparin) from the mast cell.
      ii. Later, phospholipase A2 is activated (converts membrane phospholipids to arachidonic acid).
      iii. Arachidonic acid is further metabolized by 5-lipoxygenase and cyclooxygenase to leukotrienes and prostaglandins, respectively (worsening the inflammation).
   d. Clinical manifestations
      i. Wheezing (due to bronchospasm).
      ii. Hypotension (due to increased vascular permeability).
      iii. Late phase reaction (sustained inflammatory response occurring hours later, does not require additional antigen exposure).
         (1) Due to the release of IL-5 in response to Th2 activation (IL-5 is a potent eosinophil-activating cytokine).
         (2) Eosinophils release major basic protein and eosinophil cationic protein, both of which contribute to tissue injury.

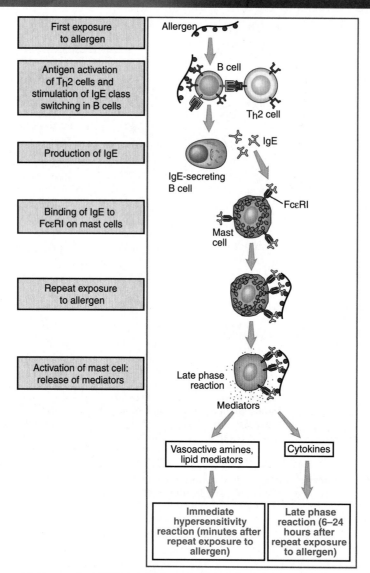

First exposure to allergen

Antigen activation of Th2 cells and stimulation of IgE class switching in B cells

Production of IgE

Binding of IgE to FcεRI on mast cells

Repeat exposure to allergen

Activation of mast cell: release of mediators

Allergen

B cell

Th2 cell

IgE

IgE-secreting B cell

FcεRI

Mast cell

Late phase reaction

Mediators

Vasoactive amines, lipid mediators

Cytokines

Immediate hypersensitivity reaction (minutes after repeat exposure to allergen)

Late phase reaction (6–24 hours after repeat exposure to allergen)

4.2: Type I (immediate) hypersensitivity reactions (HSRs). Initial exposure to allergen stimulates CD4 Th2 reactions and immunoglobulin E (IgE) production. IgE binds to Fc receptors on mast cells. Upon subsequent exposure to the allergen, the IgE molecules are cross-linked, causing the activation of mast cells and the release of preformed mediators (e.g., histamine) that produce an inflammatory reaction. Not shown in the schematic is the late phase reaction, in which the mast cells synthesize and release prostaglandins, leukotrienes, and platelet-activating factor, which prolong the inflammatory response. *(From Abbas A, Lichtman A: Basic immunology: function and disorders of the immune system, ed 3, Philadelphia, 2011, Saunders Elsevier.)*

       (3) Charcot–Leyden crystals, which are sometimes detected in the sputum of asthma patients, represent an eosinophilic protein called galectin-10 (Fig. 4.3).
2. Disorders caused by Type I HSR (Fig. 4.4)
    a. Anaphylaxis
       i. Life-threatening reaction characterized by airway narrowing (due to laryngeal edema, bronchospasm), hypotension (vasodilation-induced loss of systemic vascular resistance), and other manifestations.
    b. Asthma
       i. Reversible airway narrowing characterized by shortness of breath and wheezing; secondary to bronchoconstriction and airway inflammation.
    c. Allergic rhinitis (seasonal allergies and hay fever)
       i. Itchy watery eyes, rhinorrhea, and nasal congestion.
       ii. Associated with increased mucus production, inflammation of nasal passages, and sinuses.
    d. Food allergies
       i. Common precipitants include peanuts, cow's milk, shellfish, tree nuts, and eggs.
3. Laboratory testing in the evaluation of Type I hypersensitivity
    a. Scratch (prick) test

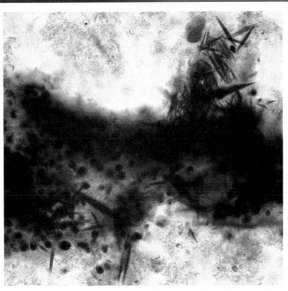

4.3: Charcot–Leyden crystals. *(From Siddique SM, Gilotra NA: Crystal clear: a unique clue to diagnosis in a patient with recurrent nausea and vomiting, Gastroenterology, 147(2):e1–e2, 2014, AGA Institute.)*

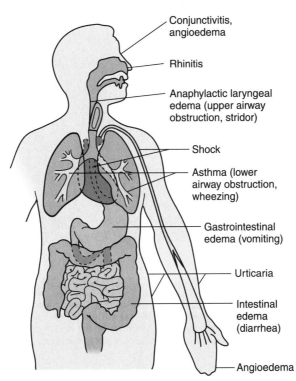

Conjunctivitis, angioedema

Rhinitis

Anaphylactic laryngeal edema (upper airway obstruction, stridor)

Shock

Asthma (lower airway obstruction, wheezing)

Gastrointestinal edema (vomiting)

Urticaria

Intestinal edema (diarrhea)

Angioedema

4.4: Characteristic clinical findings of Type I hypersensitivity reactions. *(From Zitelli B, McIntire S, Nowalk A:* Zitelli and Davis' atlas of pediatric physical diagnosis, *ed 6, 2012, Saunders Elsevier.)*

    i. Best overall sensitivity.
    ii. Positive response is a histamine-mediated wheal and flare reaction after the introduction of an allergen into the skin.
  b. Immunoassays for IgE specific to an allergen
    i. Historically known as the radioallergosorbent test because early immunoassays used radioactivity.
  c. Serum tryptase levels
    i. Tryptase is released from mast cells and basophils.
    ii. Elevated levels expected in Type I HSR.
C. Type II HSR (antibody-mediated cytotoxicity)
  1. Tissue injury occurring as a result of antibody binding to antigens, either on the cell surface or within the extracellular matrix (Fig. 4.5).

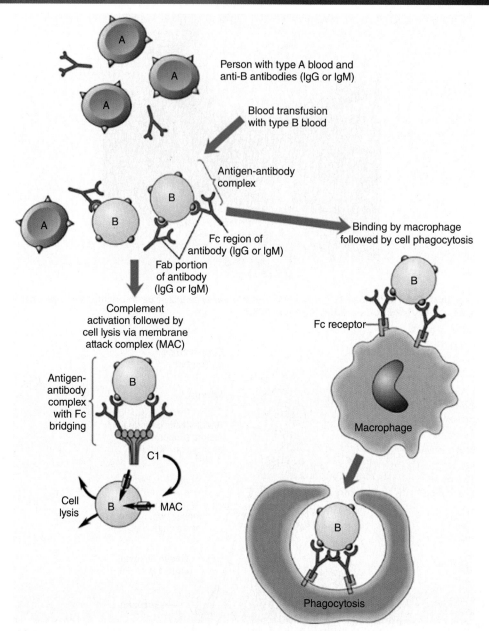

4.5: Type II hypersensitivity reaction. The schematic shows an incompatible blood transfusion where a patient with blood group A inadvertently receives group B blood. Preformed anti-B antibodies attach to the transfused B cells and then bind to Fc receptors on macrophages. The opsonized red cells are then phagocytosed and destroyed. In addition, the activation of complement causes lysis of red blood cells by the membrane attack complex (MAC). *Ig*, Immunoglobulin. *(From Copstead LE, Banasik JL:* Pathophysiology, *ed 5, Philadelphia, 2013, Saunders Elsevier.)*

2. Mechanisms of tissue injury include:
   a. Opsonization and phagocytosis
      i. Opsonized cells (those bound to antibody or complement components) are more easily recognized by phagocytes.
      ii. Once bound to the opsonized cell, the phagocytic cell engulfs, and destroys, the tagged cell.
      iii. Examples:
         (1) Autoimmune hemolytic anemia
            (a) Opsonized erythrocytes are removed by phagocytes in the liver and spleen.
         (2) Immune thrombocytopenia
            (a) Opsonized platelets (removed in a similar manner).
   b. Activation of complement
      i. Binding of antibody to cellular antigen may, in some cases, activate the complement system.
      ii. Complement can cause direct cell destruction via the membrane attack complex (C5–C9).

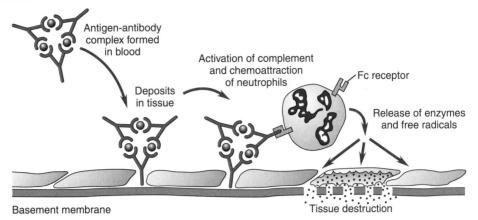

4.6: Type III hypersensitivity reaction. Antigen–antibody immunocomplexes deposit in tissue and activate complement, which attracts neutrophils that release enzymes and free radicals that damage the tissue. *(From Copstead LE, Banasik JL:* Pathophysiology, *ed 5, Philadelphia, 2013, Saunders Elsevier.)*

      iii. Examples:
          (1) In myasthenia gravis, IgG antibodies form against the acetylcholine receptor at the neuromuscular junction. These antibodies block the binding of acetylcholine to the receptor and activate complement. The loss of receptors leads to an inability to fully activate the muscles causing weakness.
          (2) In Goodpasture syndrome, antibodies (usually IgG) form against the noncollagen (NC)-1 domain of the alpha-3 chains of Type IV collagen. Damage to this collagen, which is present within basement membranes of the kidney and lungs, causes renal and pulmonary hemorrhage (i.e., hematuria and hemoptysis).
    c. Antibody-mediated cellular dysfunction
      i. Rather than direct cell injury, antibody binding may interfere with normal cell function (e.g., by either blocking or stimulating receptors).
      ii. For example, Graves disease is characterized by the formation of antibodies that stimulate the thyroid-stimulating hormone (TSH) receptor, thereby causing hyperthyroidism.
  D. Type III HSR (immune complex-mediated)
    1. Antigen–antibody (immune complexes) form, deposit in tissues, and activate complement.
      a. Causes an influx of neutrophils, the release of enzymes/free radicals, and eventually localized tissue injury (Fig. 4.6).
      b. Commonly affects joints, small vessels, and glomeruli (common sites of immune complex deposition).
      c. Because complement proteins are consumed in the process, serum levels of C3 are often used to monitor disease activity (active disease signified by a reduction in complement levels).
    2. An example is systemic lupus erythematosus (SLE).
      a. In SLE, IgG antibodies form against common cellular components (typically DNA and/or DNA-binding proteins). Subsequently, these immune complexes trigger an inflammatory response causing tissue injury at the site of deposition (e.g., glomeruli).
  E. Type IV HSR (delayed-type, T-cell-mediated)
    1. Response delayed until 1–3 days after exposure to the antigen (unique among the HSRs).
    2. Mechanism (Fig. 4.7)
      a. Antigen is taken up, processed, and presented by macrophages or dendritic cells.
      b. Recognition of the antigen by Th1 effector cells is followed by the release of chemokines.
      c. These chemokines recruit macrophages to the site and trigger the release of various injurious cytokines and growth factors (e.g., interferon-γ and TNF) resulting in localized tissue injury.
    3. Example: Tuberculin skin test, poison ivy, and certain metals.
    4. Manifestations include skin erythema and vesiculation.
IV. Transplantation
  A. Types of grafts
    1. Autograft: graft from self to self (e.g., bone, bone marrow, and skin), best survival rate.
    2. Syngeneic (isograft): graft between identical twins.
    3. Allograft: graft between genetically different individuals of the same species.
    4. Xenograft: graft between different species (e.g., pig heart valve into a human).
  B. Transplant rejection (Fig. 4.8)
    1. Hyperacute rejection
      a. Irreversible reaction occurring within minutes to hours of the transplant.
      b. Due to the presence of preformed antibodies against the donor tissue or endothelium that were already present in the recipient's system before transplantation.

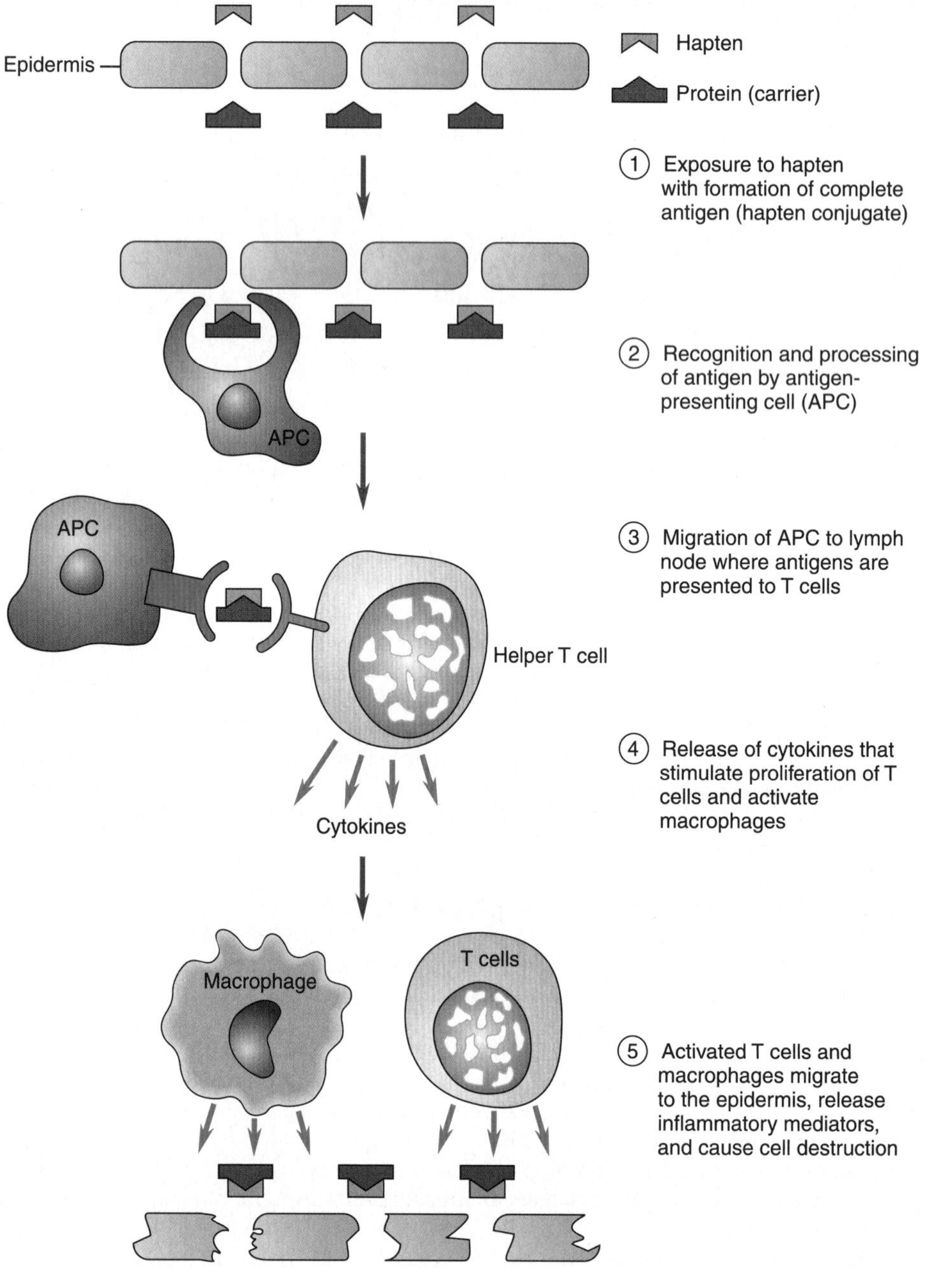

4.7: Type IV hypersensitivity reaction. *(From Copstead LE, Banasik JL:* Pathophysiology, *ed 5, Philadelphia, 2013, Saunders Elsevier.)*

     c. Once the preformed antibodies bind to the transplanted tissue, complement-mediated endothelial injury ensues, causing immediate graft thrombosis and ischemic necrosis.

     d. Uncommon due to pretransplantation screening; requires removal of the transplanted tissue.

  2. Acute rejection

     a. Reaction arising days to weeks after transplantation; involves T cells and antibodies.

     b. Potentially reversible with immunosuppression.

  3. Chronic rejection

     a. Progressive loss of graft function arising in the months to years after transplantation.

     b. Indolent T-cell reaction causing progressive endothelial injury, loss of parenchyma, and fibrosis.

C. Graft-versus-host disease

  1. Due to the engraftment of immunocompetent donor T lymphocytes in an immunologically compromised host.

  2. Donor-derived T cells react against recipient's HLA antigens that are not shared (i.e., those that are foreign to the transplanted T cells).

     a. Injurious to various tissues (e.g., skin, intestinal epithelium, bone marrow, and liver).

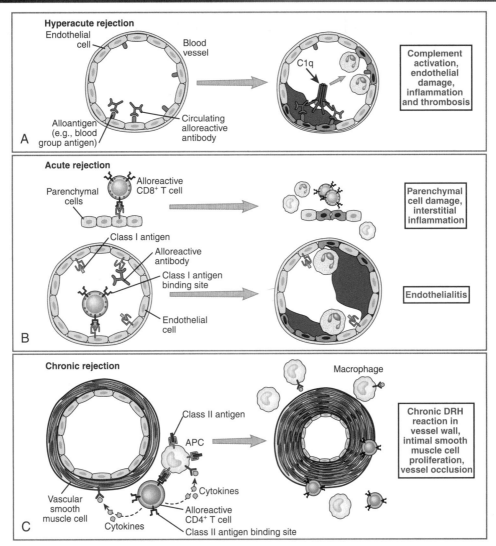

4.8: Mechanisms of graft rejection. (A) In hyperacute rejection, preformed antibodies (e.g., ABO and HLA) react with alloantigens on the vascular endothelium of the graft, activate complement, and trigger rapid intravascular thrombosis and necrosis of the vessel wall. (B) In acute rejection, CD8 T lymphocytes reactive with alloantigens (foreign antigen) on graft endothelial cells and parenchymal cells leading to cellular injury. (C) In chronic rejection, cytokine-induced proliferation of smooth muscle cells and atherosclerosis results in luminal stenosis. Cytokine stimulation of fibroblasts leading to interstitial fibrosis is not shown in the figure. *APC*, antigen-presenting cell. *(From Abbas A, Lichtman A:* Basic immunology: function and disorders of the immune system, *ed 3, Philadelphia, 2011, Saunders Elsevier.)*

3. Key factors
   a. Graft must contain immunologically competent cells.
   b. The host must possess HLA antigens that are not present in the donor graft (i.e., host must appear "foreign" to the graft).
   c. Host must be unable to mount an effective immune response against engrafted T lymphocytes.
4. Clinical findings include:
   a. Rash, possible skin desquamation due to the immunologic reaction against skin epithelia.
   b. Jaundice due to the destruction of small intrahepatic bile ducts.
   c. Diarrhea (may be bloody) due to damage to the gastrointestinal mucosa.

V. **Autoimmune Disease**
   A. **Definition**
      1. Immune reaction against self-antigens that arise when there is a loss of self-tolerance.
      2. Self-antigens include class I and II MHC antigens, nuclear antigens, and cytoplasmic antigens.
   B. **Overview**
      1. In general, autoimmune disorders are more common in women than men.
         a. Believed to occur in genetically predisposed individuals following exposure to some unknown environmental "trigger" (e.g., infection).
         b. Although not everyone will develop the disease, there are certain HLA associations with autoimmune disease (see the below box).

- Ankylosing spondylitis, reactive arthritis (HLA-B27)
- Celiac disease (HLA-DQ2 and HLA-DQ8)
- Hashimoto thyroiditis (HLA-DR3)
- Rheumatoid arthritis (HLA-DRB1)
- Type 1 diabetes mellitus (HLA-DR3 and HLA-DR4)

C. Autoantibodies
1. Serum antinuclear antibody (ANA)
   a. Most sensitive screening test for autoimmune disease.
   b. Antinuclear antibodies are directed against various nuclear antigens (e.g., DNA and histones); detected by indirect immunofluorescence.
   c. Pattern of nuclear fluorescence (e.g., homogeneous, rim, speckled, and nucleolar) is a clue to the type of antibody present.
2. Summary of autoantibodies in various autoimmune disease states (Table 4.1).

D. SLE
1. Definition
   a. Chronic, multisystem, autoimmune disorder characterized by the formation of autoantibodies and tissue injury.
   b. Clinical manifestations often wax and wane.
   c. Analogous to other autoimmune disorders, genetic susceptibility in combination with exposure to an unknown environmental antigen (e.g., viral infection) is thought to underlie the development of the disease.
2. Epidemiology
   a. Most commonly affects females of childbearing age (female/male ratio ~10:1).
      i. Less common in children and older adults.
   b. More prevalent among African Americans and Native Americans.
3. Pathogenesis of tissue injury
   a. Immune complex deposition (Type III HSR)
      i. Antibody against host antigens (e.g., DNA).
      ii. Immune complex formation (e.g., DNA–anti-DNA antibody).
      iii. Activation of complement → tissue injury.
   b. Antibody-mediated cytotoxicity (Type II HSR)
      i. Contributes to the development of various cytopenias (e.g., anemia, leukopenia, and thrombocytopenia).
   c. Antiphospholipid (APL) antibodies
      i. Increased risk of thrombus formation (both arterial and venous) causing strokes, recurrent spontaneous abortions.
4. Clinical manifestations (Fig. 4.9)
   a. Constitutional symptoms
      i. Fatigue, fever, myalgia, and weight loss.
   b. Hematologic abnormalities
      i. Anemia
         (1) Anemia of chronic disease (most common).
         (2) Autoimmune hemolytic anemia (positive Coombs test).
      ii. Leukopenia (lymphopenia).
      iii. Thrombocytopenia.
   c. Arthritis and/or arthralgias
      i. Very common, often one of the earliest manifestations.
      ii. Usually not associated with joint deformity.
   d. Mucocutaneous involvement
      i. Malar "butterfly" rash (Fig. 4.10)
         (1) Erythematous rash over the cheeks and bridge of the nose with sparing of the nasolabial fold.
         (2) Initiated and exacerbated by exposure to ultraviolet light.
         (3) Immunofluorescence shows band-like deposits of immune complexes along the basement membrane.
      ii. Alopecia (partial or complete loss of hair).
   e. Renal injury
      i. Kidney is the most affected visceral organ.
      ii. Due to the deposition of immune complexes within glomeruli.
      iii. Typically, causes diffuse proliferative glomerulonephritis; manifests with hematuria, proteinuria, and hypertension.
      iv. Renal disease is a major cause of death.

TABLE 4.1   Autoantibodies in Autoimmune Disease

AUTOANTIBODIES	DISEASES
Antiacetylcholine receptor	Myasthenia gravis
Antibasement membrane	Goodpasture syndrome
Anticentromere	CREST syndrome
Anti-DNA topoisomerase	Systemic sclerosis (scleroderma)
Anti-dsDNA	Systemic lupus erythematosus (SLE)
Antiendomysial IgA	Celiac disease
Antigliadin IgA	Celiac disease
Antihistone	Drug-induced lupus
Antiinsulin	Type 1 diabetes mellitus
Antiintrinsic factor	Pernicious anemia
Anti-glutamic acid decarboxylase 65	Type 1 diabetes mellitus
Anti-Jo-1 (transfer RNA synthetase)	Polymyositis, dermatomyositis
Antimitochondrial	Primary biliary cholangitis
Antinuclear (ANA)	SLE (sensitive but nonspecific)
	Systemic sclerosis
	CREST syndrome
	Dermatomyositis
	Mixed connective tissue disease
Antiparietal cell	Pernicious anemia
Antiribonucleoprotein (U1-RNP)	Mixed connective tissue disease
Anti-Smith	SLE
Anti-SS-A (Ro)	Sjögren syndrome
Anti-SS-B (La)	Sjögren syndrome
	Hashimoto thyroiditis
Anti-tissue transglutaminase IgA	Celiac disease
Anti-TSH receptor	Graves disease

Anti-dsDNA, Anti-double-stranded DNA; *CREST*, calcinosis, Raynaud phenomenon, esophageal dysfunction, sclerodactyly, telangiectasia; *MCTD*, mixed connective tissue disease; *SLE*, systemic lupus erythematosus; *TSH*, thyroid-stimulating hormone.

    f. Cardiovascular findings
      i. Pericarditis with or without effusion (most common cardiac manifestation).
      ii. Nonbacterial thrombotic endocarditis (Libman-Sacks endocarditis).
        (1) Small sterile vegetations on either side of cardiac valves; may cause deformity of valve and regurgitation.
      iii. Premature atherosclerotic vascular disease (myocardial infarction is another common cause of death).
      iv. Vasculitis
        (1) Most commonly involving small vessels, presents with petechiae, palpable purpura, and superficial ulceration.
    g. Pulmonary manifestations
      i. Pleuritis (with or without effusion).
      ii. Interstitial lung disease.
      iii. Pulmonary hypertension.
    h. Pregnancy complications
      i. Recurrent pregnancy loss (spontaneous abortion) secondary to the APL antibody syndrome.
      ii. Congenital heart block may occur in the offspring of women with SLE in association with anti-Ro/SSA and anti-La/SSB antibodies.
  5. Drug-induced lupus
    a. Highest risk with procainamide and hydralazine.
    b. Manifestations include fever, arthralgias/arthritis, myalgias, rash, and serositis.

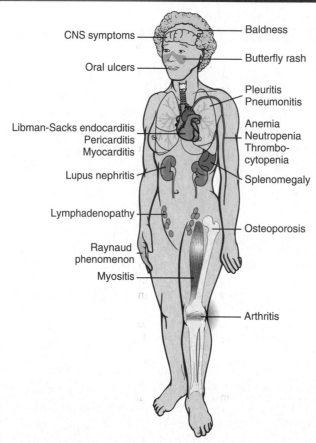

4.9: Clinical and pathologic findings of systemic lupus erythematosus. *CNS*, Central nervous system. *(From* Pathology for the health professions, *ed 4, 2012, Saunders Elsevier.)*

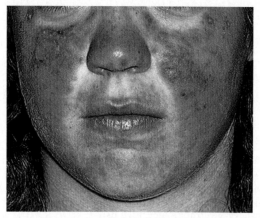

4.10: Malar rash in systemic lupus erythematosus showing the butterfly distribution. *(From Marx J:* Rosen's emergency medicine concepts and clinical practice, *ed 7, Philadelphia, 2010, Mosby Elsevier; taken from Habif TP:* Clinical dermatology, *ed 4, New York, 2004, Mosby.)*

     c. Associated with antihistone antibodies.

     d. Symptoms resolve with discontinuation of drug.

  6. Laboratory testing

    a. Serum ANA

      i. ANA is the best screening test for SLE as it is positive in nearly all patients at some point (i.e., very sensitive).

       (1) A negative ANA test essentially excludes the diagnosis of SLE.

      ii. ANA is not specific for lupus; positive results must be followed by additional testing to evaluate for the presence of autoantibodies that are more specific to lupus.

    b. Anti-dsDNA antibodies

      i. Less sensitive (only present in ~70% of patients) but more specific (~95%) than ANA for the diagnosis of SLE.

      ii. High titer IgG anti-dsDNA is often associated with active glomerulonephritis.

    c. Anti-Smith antibodies

      i. Low sensitivity (not a good screening test) but high specificity (used to confirm the diagnosis of SLE).

    d. Anti-Ro/SSA and anti-La/SSB antibodies

      i. Not specific for SLE, also seen in Sjögren syndrome and other autoimmune disorders.

    e. APL antibodies

      i. Association with strokes and recurrent pregnancy loss.

      ii. Clue is a false-positive serologic test for syphilis (due to antibody binding to cardiolipin used in the test).

    f. Serum complement (e.g., C3 and C4)

      i. Decreased in active disease (due to immune complex-mediated complement activation).

    g. Erythrocyte sedimentation rate (ESR)

      i. Increased in active disease; used to monitor disease activity.

      ii. ESR is better than the CRP for monitoring disease activity in lupus patients.

7. Prognosis

    a. Overall, patients with SLE have higher mortality than the general population.

    b. Major causes of death in the first few years of illness include:

      i. Complications of active disease (e.g., renal disease).

      ii. Infectious complications (due to treatment with immunosuppressive medications).

    c. Longer term complications include:

      i. End-stage renal disease (~10% incidence over 10 years).

      ii. Cardiovascular disease (e.g., myocardial infarction).

      iii. Treatment complications (e.g., infection).

E. Systemic sclerosis (scleroderma)

1. Definition

    a. Multisystemic fibro-inflammatory disorder of the skin and other tissues (e.g., lungs, heart, and gastrointestinal tract) resulting in a variety of clinical manifestations.

2. Epidemiology

    a. More common in females (female-to-male ratio of $\geq$3:1).

    b. Peak onset in the fourth to the fifth decade.

3. Pathogenesis

    a. Underlying etiology is unclear; likely involves genetic and environmental factors (analogous to other autoimmune disorders).

    b. Inflammation and proliferation of vascular smooth muscle cause narrowing of vascular lumens.

    c. Infiltration of activated T cells into tissues associated with the release of various profibrotic cytokines (e.g., transforming growth factor-beta, IL-4, and platelet-derived growth factor).

4. Clinical manifestations

    a. Raynaud phenomenon

      i. Often an early complaint; due to microvascular injury.

      ii. Triggered by exposure to cold and/or emotional stress.

      iii. Vasospasm of digits with episodic digital ischemia.

      iv. Characterized by sequential color change of affected digits (white to blue to red).

    b. Thickening of the skin

      i. Nearly universal, especially involves fingers, hands, neck, and face.

      ii. In later stages of the disease, fingers become tapered and "claw-like" (called sclerodactyly) and the face becomes tightly drawn with radial furrowing around the mouth.

    c. Esophageal fibrosis (causing dysphagia and increased reflux).

    d. Interstitial pulmonary fibrosis and pulmonary hypertension.

5. CREST syndrome (subset of those with limited disease)

    a. C—calcification.

    b. R—Raynaud phenomenon.

    c. E—esophageal dysmotility.

    d. S—sclerodactyly (i.e., tapered and claw-like fingers).

    e. T—telangiectasias (i.e., dilated blood vessels).

6. Laboratory findings in systemic sclerosis and CREST syndrome

    a. ANA test (nearly always positive).

    b. Anti-DNA topoisomerase I (anti-Scl 70); specific, but not sensitive for systemic sclerosis.

    c. Anticentromere antibodies (CREST syndrome).

7. Prognosis

    a. Increased mortality compared to age-matched controls.

    b. Most deaths due to pulmonary complications.

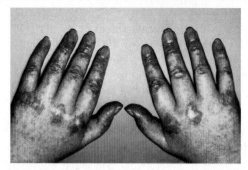

4.11: Dermatomyositis. Note the characteristic purple papules overlying the knuckles and proximal and distal interphalangeal joints (Gottron patches). *(Courtesy of Carol M. Ziminski, MD.)*

  F. **Inflammatory myopathies**
   1. Idiopathic diseases of muscle characterized by proximal muscle weakness and histologic evidence of muscle inflammation.
   2. Most common examples are polymyositis and dermatomyositis.
   3. Polymyositis
       a. Epidemiology
           i. More common in females (2:1); usually adults.
       b. Pathology
           i. Endomysial inflammation by CD8+ cytotoxic T lymphocytes.
       c. Clinical findings
           i. Symmetric, proximal muscle weakness (difficulty climbing stairs or rising from a seated position).
           ii. Dysphagia secondary to weakness of the striated muscle of the upper esophagus and/or oropharyngeal musculature.
           iii. Interstitial lung disease (10% of patients).
       d. Laboratory findings
           i. Elevated levels of muscle enzymes (e.g., creatine kinase and aldolase).
           ii. Antibody findings
               (1) ANA is often elevated (not sensitive or specific).
               (2) Anti-Jo-1 antibody (against histidyl-tRNA synthetase); not sensitive or specific (also seen in dermatomyositis).
   4. Dermatomyositis
       a. Epidemiology
           i. More common in adults, usually arising between 40 and 60 years.
           ii. Occasionally identified in children, usually between the ages of 5 and 10 years.
       b. Pathology
           i. CD4+ lymphocytic infiltrate with injury to capillaries and perifascicular myofibers.
       c. Clinical manifestations
           i. Symmetric proximal muscle weakness (difficulty climbing stairs or rising from a seated position).
           ii. Characteristic cutaneous findings
               (1) Gottren papules (erythematous rash over the knuckles); see Fig. 4.11.
               (2) Heliotrope rash (purple-red discoloration of eyelids).
           iii. Associated with underlying malignancy in some cases.
       d. Laboratory findings
           i. Elevated levels of muscle enzymes (e.g., creatine kinase and aldolase).
           ii. Anti-Jo-1 antibody.
   5. Mixed connective tissue disorder (MCTD)
       a. MCTD is an idiopathic, inflammatory disorder characterized by overlapping features of SLE, systemic sclerosis, and inflammatory myopathies (e.g., polymyositis).
       b. Characteristic autoantibody against U1-ribonuclear protein (U1-RNP).
VI. **Immunodeficiency Disorders**
  A. **Congenital immunodeficiency disorders (Table 4.2).**
  B. **Complement deficiencies**
   1. Rare, associated with increased risk of recurrent bacterial infections and/or SLE.
   2. C3 deficiency (major opsonin of complement system) is associated with severe, recurrent infections with encapsulated bacteria (e.g., *Streptococcus pneumoniae*, *Haemophilus influenzae*, and *Neisseria meningitidis*).

TABLE 4.2   Congenital Immunodeficiency Disorders

DISEASES	DEFECT(S)	CLINICAL FEATURES
B-Cell Disorders		
Bruton agamma-globulinemia	• X-linked • Mutated Bruton tyrosine kinase (*BTK*) gene (important in B-cell receptor signaling; essential for survival and differentiation of immature B cells).	• Small or absent tonsils and lymph nodes. • Maternal antibodies protective from birth to ~6 months. Afterwards, patients develop recurrent upper (otitis media, sinusitis) and lower respiratory tract infections. • *Streptococcus pneumoniae* and *Haemophilus influenzae* are common causes of pneumonia. • GI manifestations include enterovirus infections and giardiasis. • All immunoglobulins markedly decreased.
IgA deficiency	• Failure of B cells to terminally differentiate into plasma cells that secrete IgA.	• Most common primary immunodeficiency disorder. • Often asymptomatic. • Some develop recurrent upper and lower respiratory infections (most common) and/or GI infections (e.g., giardiasis). • Increased risk of atopic disease (e.g., asthma and eczema). • Increased risk of autoimmune disease (e.g., rheumatoid arthritis, SLE, and celiac disease). • Anaphylaxis possible if exposed to blood products containing IgA. • ↓Serum IgA and secretory IgA.
Common variable immunodeficiency	• Etiology unknown. • Presentation often delayed to the third decade.	• Decreased immunoglobulin levels and impaired responses to vaccines. • T-cell deficiency often present as well. • Recurrent upper and lower respiratory tract infections, (e.g., bronchitis, sinusitis, otitis media, and pneumonia); often by encapsulated organisms (e.g., *H. influenzae* and *S. pneumoniae*). • GI infections (e.g., *Giardia*, *Salmonella*, *Shigella*, and *Campylobacter*). • Increased risk for autoimmune disease (ITP and AIHA) and malignancy (malignant lymphoma and gastric cancer). • ↓Serum immunoglobulins.
T-Cell Disorder		
DiGeorge syndrome (thymic hypoplasia)	• Chromosome 22 q11.2 deletion syndrome. • Failure of third and fourth pharyngeal pouches to develop. • Hypoplasia or absence of thymus (site of T-cell maturation) and parathyroid glands.	• Variable immunosuppression dependent upon degree of thymic hypoplasia. • Defective CMI. • Increased viral (e.g., CMV, EBV, and varicella) and fungal (e.g., *Candida* and *Pneumocystis jiroveci*) infections. • Hypocalcemia secondary to hypoparathyroidism. Manifestations include tetany, seizures. • Absent thymic shadow on radiograph. • Danger of GVHD (must irradiate blood prior to transfusion). • Increased incidence congenital heart defects.
Combined B- and T-Cell Disorders		
Hyper-IgM syndrome	• XR (70% of cases). • Mutation in a gene encoding for CD40 ligand. • Interaction of CD40 on B cells with CD40-ligand on activated T cells is required for immunoglobulin class switching. • Net result is decreased production of IgG, IgA, and IgE and increased IgM.	• Recurrent pyogenic infections (decreased IgG for proper opsonization). • *P. jiroveci* pneumonia (lack of CD40-L T-cell interaction with CD40 on monocytes and dendritic cells impairs the production of IL-12 and development of Type 1 T helper cells (thereby impairing cell-mediated immunity).
Severe combined immunodeficiency (SCID)	• X-linked (most common) characterized by mutations in the common γ chain of the IL-2 receptor (shared by the receptors of various interleukins). • **Adenosine deaminase deficiency** (15% of cases): autosomal recessive disorder; lack of the enzyme causes an increase in deoxyadenosine, which is toxic to B and T cells.	• Severe infections of respiratory and GI tract, beginning in early infancy. • Risk of disseminated infections. • Viral pneumonia (e.g., CMV, adenovirus, and RSV) as well as thrush and/or persistent diarrhea develops in infancy. • May develop graft-versus-host disease due to engraftment of maternal T cells in the infant.

(Continued)

TABLE 4.2   Congenital Immunodeficiency Disorders—cont'd

DISEASES	DEFECT(S)	CLINICAL FEATURES
Wiskott–Aldrich syndrome	• X-linked. • Inactivating mutations in *WAS* gene (encodes for a protein involved in cell signaling and cytoskeletal reorganization of hematopoietic cells).	• Eczema, thrombocytopenia, and recurrent infections. • Increased risk for malignancy (leukemia and lymphoma). • Increased risk autoimmune disease. • Immunoglobulins: ↓IgM, normal IgG, ↑IgA, and IgE. • Bone marrow transplantation essential for survival.
Ataxia-telangiectasia	• Autosomal recessive disorder. • Mutation in a gene (*ATM*) that encodes for DNA repair enzymes. • Thymic hypoplasia.	• Cerebellar ataxia, telangiectasia (dilated vessels) in the eyes and skin. • ↑Risk for malignancy. • Defective CMI: ↓total lymphocyte count; defective T-cell function. • Deficient antibody production to viral or bacterial antigens. • Immunoglobulins: ↓IgA 50%–80%; ↓IgE; normal to ↑IgM; ↓IgG2/IgG4; normal to ↓total IgG.

AIHA, Autoimmune hemolytic anemia; *CMI,* cell-mediated immunity; *CMV,* cytomegalovirus; *EBV,* Epstein–Barr virus; *GI,* gastrointestinal; *GVHD,* graft-versus-host disease; *Ig,* immunoglobulin; *ITP,* idiopathic thrombocytopenic purpura; *MCC,* most common cause; *PA,* pernicious anemia; *Rx,* treatment; *SLE,* systemic lupus erythematosus; *SP,* sinopulmonary; *XR,* sex-linked recessive.

3. C5–C9 deficiency is associated with recurrent *Neisseria* infection (especially *N. meningitidis*).
4. C1 inhibitor deficiency is associated with hereditary angioedema.
   a. Angioedema refers to swelling of the deep dermis and subcutaneous tissue, potential for airway obstruction.

C. Secondary immunodeficiency
1. Immunosuppression secondary to another condition
   a. Most common cause is immunosuppressive medications used to prevent organ rejection or in the treatment of autoimmune disease.
2. Human immunodeficiency virus (HIV)
   a. Retrovirus that causes acquired immunodeficiency syndrome (AIDS).
   b. Epidemiology
      i. In developed nations, HIV is more commonly seen in males, often secondary to homosexual contact.
      ii. In developing nations, higher prevalence of females, often secondary to heterosexual contact.
   c. HIV types
      i. HIV-1 (the most common type in the United States).
      ii. HIV-2 (uncommon in the United States; primarily West Africa).
   d. HIV characteristics
      i. Retroviruses (reverse transcriptase converts viral RNA into proviral DNA).
      ii. Three retroviral genes
         (1) The *gag* gene encodes for inner structural proteins.
         (2) The *pol* gene encodes polymerase as well as integrase and protease.
         (3) The *env* gene encodes the viral envelope.
   e. Interaction with host cell (Fig. 4.12)
      i. The HIV surface glycoprotein gp120 binds to CD4 on the host cell and then to a coreceptor (chemokine receptor 5 [CCR5] or chemokine receptor 4 [CXCR4]).
         (1) CD4-positive cells include T helper cells, monocytes, macrophages, and dendritic cells (reason these cells are all susceptible to HIV).
      ii. Binding to the coreceptor induces a conformational change in gp41 → allowing the virus to insert into the cell membrane of the target cell.
      iii. HIV then enters the host cell cytoplasm where the viral reverse transcriptase transcribes the HIV RNA genome into complementary DNA (proviral DNA).
      iv. Virus may remain latent or, in dividing T cells, the proviral DNA enters the nucleus and integrates into the host genome (integrase enzyme) and is transcribed to form new viral particles that then bud from the cell membrane.
   f. HIV transmission
      i. As the viral load increases, so does the risk of transmission (regardless of route).
      ii. Sexual transmission
         (1) In the United States, mostly men who have sex with men; however, heterosexual contact is the major mode worldwide.
         (2) Risk depends on several factors:
            (a) Concomitant sexually transmitted infection increases the risk of transmission (especially when associated with genital ulceration).
            (b) Risk increases in proportion to the number of sexual partners.
            (c) Type of sexual practices: highest risk: anal intercourse (receptive > insertive).

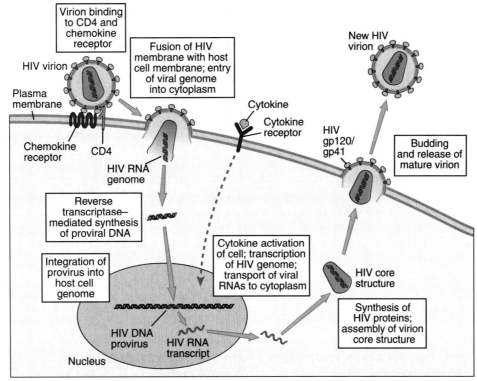

4.12: The life cycle of human immunodeficiency virus type 1 (HIV-1). The sequential steps in HIV reproduction are shown, from initial infection of a host cell to release of a new virus particle (virion). For the sake of clarity, the production and release of only one new virion is shown. An infected cell actually produces many virions, each capable of infecting nearby cells, thereby spreading the infection. *(From Abbas A, Lichtman A: Basic immunology: function and disorders of the immune system, ed 3, Philadelphia, 2011, Saunders Elsevier.)*

    iii. Other modes of transmission
        (1) Sharing of needles (i.e., intravenous drug use).
        (2) Mother-to-child transmission (during birthing or breastfeeding).
           (a) Treatment of HIV-positive women with antiretroviral therapy reduces the risk of transmission to offspring.
        (3) Needlestick injury.
        (4) Transfusion of blood products
           (a) Very rare due to screening of blood products (~1 case per 2 million transfused units).
  g. Pathogenesis
    i. HIV is cytopathic to infected CD4+ lymphocytes; causing incremental loss of cell-mediated immune function (number of CD4+ lymphocytes decline with disease progression).
  h. Diagnosis
    i. Screening: Fourth-generation combination HIV-1/2 immunoassay (detects both HIV-1 and HIV-2 antibodies as well as HIV P24 antigen).
    ii. Confirmatory test: HIV-1/HIV-2 antibody differentiation immunoassay and plasma HIV RNA level.
 i. Natural history of HIV infection (Fig. 4.13)
    i. "Acute retroviral syndrome"
        (1) Some but not all patients develop nonspecific flu-like symptoms (fever, lymphadenopathy, sore throat, rash, diarrhea, weight loss, and headache) 2–4 weeks after infection; spontaneous resolution after a few weeks.
        (2) Early HIV infection is characterized by rapid viral replication (very high viral load) and abrupt decline in CD4+ cells.
        (3) Once viral clearance begins, the viral load drops while CD4 counts rise (though not to baseline).
    ii. Chronic asymptomatic carrier phase
        (1) Lasts several years (usually 8–10) in the absence of antiretroviral therapy.
        (2) CD4 counts are initially >500 cells/mm3 but drop slowly over time.
        (3) Increased incidence of some non-AIDS-defining conditions
           (a) Oral hairy leukoplakia (Epstein–Barr virus [EBV]).
           (b) Oropharyngeal and/or vulvovaginal candidiasis.

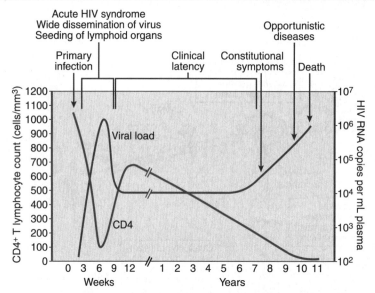

4.13: Viral and immunologic progression of untreated HIV infection. Note the increase in opportunistic infection as the CD4 count declines. *(From Walker BR, Colledge NR, Ralston SH, Penman ID: Davidson's principles and practice of medicine, ed 22, 2014, Churchill Livingstone Elsevier.)*

Acquired immunodeficiency syndrome (AIDS)

Characterized by HIV positivity and a CD4 count ≤200 cells/mm³ and/or the presence of an AIDS-defining condition.
AIDS-defining conditions include:
- *Pneumocystis jiroveci* pneumonia
- Kaposi sarcoma (HHV-8)
- Burkitt lymphoma (EBV)
- Primary CNS lymphoma (EBV)
- Invasive cervical cancer (HPV)

Immunologic abnormalities in AIDS include:
- Lymphopenia (destruction of CD4+ helper T cells)
- Defective cell-mediated immunity
- Anergy (diminished response to TB skin testing)
- Reversal of CD4:CD8 ratio (normally >2 but reverses due to loss of CD4+ T cells)

VII. Amyloidosis
A. Overview
1. Amyloid refers to diseases that share a common feature, the deposition of amyloid within tissue (Fig. 4.14).
2. Amyloid is not a specific protein but rather low molecular weight subunits of a variety of proteins that have become insoluble due to their cross-beta-pleated sheet configuration.
   a. Specific protein varies depending on the clinical situation.
B. Representative types of amyloid protein
1. Amyloid light chain (AL)
   a. Light chains (plasma cell disorders; myeloma).
2. Amyloid-associated (AA)
   a. Derived from proteolysis of serum amyloid A protein; an acute phase reactant elevated in chronic inflammatory conditions (e.g., rheumatoid arthritis and chronic osteomyelitis).
3. Beta-2 microglobulin (dialysis-associated amyloidosis).
4. Transthyretin (systemic senile amyloidosis).
5. β-Amyloid (Aβ) is derived by proteolysis of amyloid precursor protein (APP).
   a. Aβ is found in Alzheimer disease and cerebral amyloid angiopathy (see Chapter 26).
C. Pathogenesis
1. Amyloid fibrils are insoluble; form misfolded proteins that aggregate in and around cells.
D. Clinical manifestations
1. Vary depending upon the type of precursor protein, the tissue distribution, and the amount deposited.
2. Renal effects

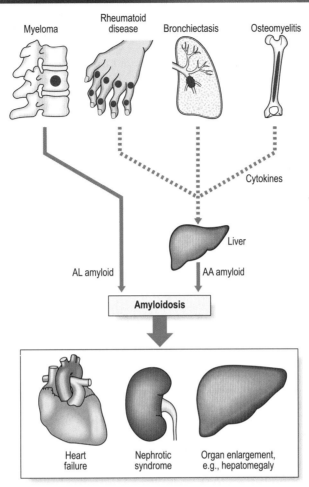

4.14: Common etiologies and clinical manifestations of systemic amyloidosis. In myeloma-associated amyloidosis, the AL amyloid is comprised of immunoglobulin light chains secreted by neoplastic plasma cells. Chronic inflammatory states (e.g., rheumatoid arthritis) can lead to the deposition of AA amyloid, produced by the liver in response to cytokines secreted by chronic inflammatory cells. *(From Underwood's pathology, ed 7, 2019, Fig. 6.13.)*

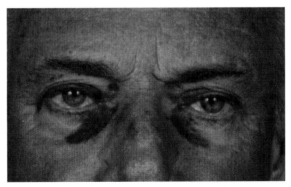

4.15: Periorbital purpura in amyloidosis. *(From Kitchens CS: Purpura and other hematovascular disorders. In Kitchens CS, Konkle BA, Kessler CM, editors: Consultative hemostasis and thrombosis, ed 3, Philadelphia, 2012, Elsevier.)*

    a. Proteinuria
       i. Variable severity, nephrotic range in some cases.
      ii. Severe proteinuria causes generalized pitting edema due to the loss of intravascular oncotic pressure.
  3. Gastrointestinal effects
     a. Macroglossia (enlarged tongue); may interfere with speech and swallowing.
     b. Gastroparesis, constipation, and malabsorption.
  4. Bleeding
     a. Amyloid causes vascular fragility, for example:
       i. Bilateral periorbital ecchymosis, forms after cough or sneeze (Fig. 4.15).
      ii. Lobar hemorrhage in brain (cerebral amyloid angiopathy).

5. Cardiac effects
    a. Restrictive cardiomyopathy (diastolic dysfunction and poor ventricular filling) due to amyloid within myocardium.
    b. Arrhythmias, heart block due to amyloid within the conduction system.
    c. Angina and/or myocardial infarction due to the deposition of amyloid within coronary arteries.
6. Neurologic effects
    a. Symmetrical distal sensory or mixed sensorimotor polyneuropathy.
    b. Autonomic neuropathy (e.g., orthostatic hypotension, diarrhea, and gastroparesis).
E. **Diagnosis**
    1. Abdominal fat pad biopsy often used.
    2. Tissue is stained with Congo red (highlights the amyloid, appear apple-green under polarized light microscopy).

Water, Electrolyte, Acid–Base, and Hemodynamic Disorders

5

I. Body Fluid Homeostasis

A. Body fluid compartments (Fig. 5.1)

1. Total body water (TBW) accounts for ~60% of body weight.
   a. Two-thirds of TBW are within the intracellular fluid (ICF) compartment.
   b. One-third of TBW is within the extracellular fluid (ECF) compartment.
      i. Three-fourths of ECF are around cells (interstitial fluid).
      ii. One-fourth of ECF is intravascular (plasma).

B. Fluid movement in and out of cells (i.e., between ICF and ECF)

1. Dependent upon osmotic gradients (Fig. 5.2).
2. Osmosis is the tendency for water to pass through a semipermeable cell membrane into a solution containing a higher solute concentration.
3. Plasma osmolality (POsm) is a measure of the number of osmotically active particles (osmoles) dissolved in a kilogram of plasma (mOsm/kg).
4. POsm = 2 [serum Na$^+$] + [serum glucose]/18 + serum blood urea nitrogen [BUN]/2.8.
   a. Normal POsm = 275–295 mOsm/kg.
5. Sodium and glucose are restricted to the ECF compartment, whereas urea is free to diffuse between the ECF and the ICF compartments.
   a. Urea therefore has no effect on water movement and is often excluded from the POsm calculation.
6. Effective osmolality (EOsm) = [2 (serum Na$^+$) + (serum glucose/18)].
   a. EOsm is a better reflection of water movement between ECF and ICF compartments.
   b. Sodium and glucose are called "effective osmoles" because they remain in the ECF compartment.
7. Tonicity of a solution
   a. An isotonic solution has the same EOsm as that within cells (ICF compartment). For this reason, there is no net fluid movement between the ECF and ICF compartments.
   b. A hypotonic solution has a lower EOsm than that within cells (ICF compartment). Water moves down its concentration gradient (i.e., into the cell), causing cellular swelling (Fig. 5.2B).
   c. A hypertonic solution has a higher EOsm than that within the cell. Water moves down its concentration gradient (i.e., out of the cell), causing the cell to shrink (Fig. 5.2C).
8. ECF
   a. Sodium is the major osmotically active ion of the ECF compartment; therefore, ECF volume is dependent upon total body sodium (TBNa$^+$).
      i. TBNa$^+$ is the total number of sodium molecules in the body.
      ii. Not the same as serum sodium [Na$^+$], which is the concentration of sodium within the blood.
   b. Decreased TBNa$^+$ causes volume depletion (hypovolemia).
      i. Manifestations of hypovolemia include (Fig. 5.3):
         (1) Dry mucous membranes, thirst.
         (2) Decreased skin turgor (i.e., skin tenting when pinched).
         (3) Postural hypotension (dizziness on standing).
         (4) Weight loss (due to a decrease in sodium-containing fluid).
         (5) Decreased jugular venous pressure.
         (6) Confusion and stupor, decreased urine output, and lack of tears.
         (7) Increased capillary filling time (normal capillary fill time after pinching the fingertip is <2 seconds).

TOTAL BODY WATER

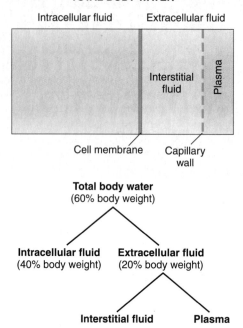

5.1: Body fluid compartments. The intracellular fluid compartment is the largest compartment. The extracellular fluid (ECF) compartment is subdivided into the interstitial fluid compartment and the vascular compartment (plasma). *(From Costanzo LS: Physiology, ed 5, 2014, Saunders Elsevier.)*

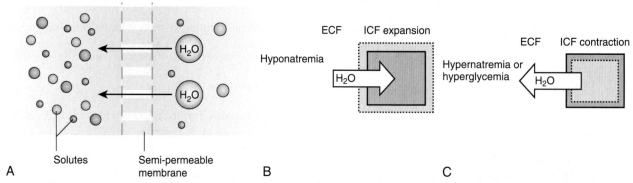

5.2: (A) Osmotic movement of water across a membrane. The membrane is semipermeable, being permeable to water but not all solutes. In this schematic, water moves from low solute concentration (right side of the membrane) to high solute concentration (left side of the membrane). Eventually the solute concentration (osmolality) will be the same on both sides of the membrane. (B) Osmotic shifts in hyponatremia. Note that water moves from the compartment with the lowest solute concentration (extracellular fluid [ECF] compartment) to the compartment with the highest solute concentration (intracellular fluid [ICF] compartment) thereby causing expansion of the ICF compartment. (C) In hypernatremia or hyperglycemia, water moves from the ICF compartment into the ECF compartment by osmosis (ICF compartment contracts). *(A, From Naish J, Court DS: Medical sciences, ed 2, 2015, Saunders Elsevier.)*

    c. Increased $TBNa^+$ causes volume overload (hypervolemia).
       i. Manifestations of hypervolemia include dependent pitting edema.
          (1) Excess of sodium-containing fluid in the interstitial space.
          (2) Fluid moves to dependent portions of the body (e.g., ankles, if standing; sacrum, if supine) due to gravity.
          (3) Pitting edema is characterized by a temporary depression in the skin following gentle pressure.
C. Fluid movement in and out of the vasculature (between ECF compartments)
    1. Fluid movement between vascular and interstitial spaces is driven by Starling forces (not osmosis).
      a. Starling forces (Fig. 5.4)
        i. Hydrostatic pressure refers to the force of fluids against their enclosing barrier.
        ii. Oncotic pressure refers to the osmotic pressure generated by proteins in a solution (albumin is the major protein).
    2. Net direction of fluid movement depends upon the dominant Starling force.
      a. An increase in plasma hydrostatic pressure and/or a decrease in plasma oncotic pressure (e.g., a decrease in serum albumin) is associated with the diffusion of fluid out of the vasculature (capillaries/venules) into the interstitial space.
        i. Causes pitting edema and body cavity effusion (e.g., ascites).

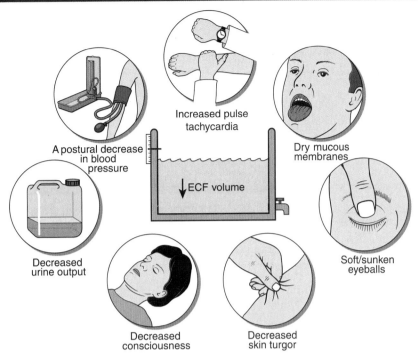

5.3: The clinical features of hypovolemia. *(From Gaw A, Murphy MJ, Srivastava R, Cowan RA, O'Reilly DSJ: Clinical biochemistry: an illustrated colour text, ed 5, 2013, Churchill Livingstone Elsevier.)*

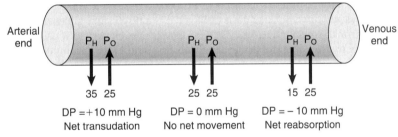

5.4: Starling forces in a capillary/venule. Hydrostatic pressure (P_H) "pushes" fluid out of capillaries/venules, whereas oncotic pressure (P_O) keeps fluid within vessels. On the left of the schematic, P_H is greater than P_O, so fluid leaves the vessel to enter the interstitial space (net transudation). In the middle of the schematic, each pressure is equal and there is no net fluid movement. On the right side of the schematic, P_O is greater than P_H; hence, there is net reabsorption of fluid. *(From Brown T: Rapid review physiology, ed 2, Philadelphia, 2012, Mosby Elsevier.)*

       b. Etiologies of reduced plasma oncotic pressure include:
         i. Cirrhosis (due to the reduction in protein synthesis by the liver).
         ii. Nephrotic syndrome (increased urinary loss of protein).

II. Acid–Base Disorders

A. Overview

1. The pH is the negative logarithm of the hydrogen ion concentration.
2. Normal pH of blood is 7.35–7.45 (must be maintained within this narrow range).
3. Arterial pH below 7.35 is called "acidemia," whereas a pH above 7.45 is called "alkalemia."
    a. The process that drives the pH upward or downward is known as alkalosis or acidosis, respectively.
4. Physiologic control of acid–base status is dependent upon the respiratory system and the kidneys.
    a. Disorders affecting either can lead to an acid–base imbalance.
5. For each primary disorder, the body attempts to compensate to maintain the pH as close to normal as possible.

B. Interpretation of acid–base disorders

1. The pH defines the primary disorder.
    a. If the pH is low, then the primary disorder is acidosis.
    b. If the pH is elevated, then the primary disorder is alkalosis.
    c. The serum bicarbonate and $PaCO_2$ are then evaluated to determine the primary defect (i.e., respiratory, metabolic, or both).
2. Begin by examining the pH.
3. Is it normal (7.35–7.45), low (<7.35), or high (>7.45)?
    a. Then evaluate the partial pressure of carbon dioxide (PCO_2) and the bicarbonate (HCO_3^-).

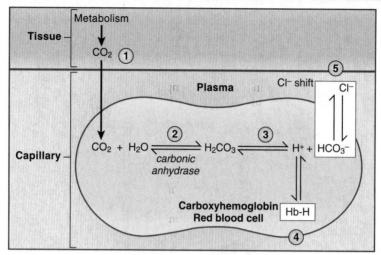

5.5: Transport of carbon dioxide in the blood. *(Modified from Costanzo LS: Physiology, ed 5, 2014, Saunders Elsevier.)*

4. Which one explains the pH?
   a. A low pH (acidemia) can be explained by an elevated PCO_2 (respiratory acidosis) or a low HCO_3^- (metabolic acidosis).
   b. A high pH (alkalemia) can be explained by a low PCO_2 (respiratory alkalosis) or a high HCO_3^- (metabolic alkalosis).
5. Evaluate for compensation.
   a. Compensation for a primary respiratory acidosis (↑ PCO_2) is a metabolic alkalosis (↑ HCO_3^-).
   b. Compensation for a primary respiratory alkalosis (↓ PCO_2) is a metabolic acidosis (↓ HCO_3^-).
   c. Compensation for a primary metabolic acidosis (↓ HCO_3^-) is a respiratory alkalosis (↓ PCO_2).
   d. Compensation for a primary metabolic alkalosis (↑ HCO_3^-) is a respiratory acidosis (↑ PCO_2).
6. When the expected compensation does not occur, the disorder is said to be uncompensated.
   a. If compensation occurs, but does not bring pH into the normal range, a partially compensated disorder is present. Note that full compensation rarely occurs; the exception being chronic respiratory alkalosis (e.g., living at a high altitude).

C. Respiratory acidosis
1. Hypoventilation induced elevation in the partial pressure of carbon dioxide ($PaCO_2$) to >45 mm Hg.
2. Transport of carbon dioxide (CO_2) in the blood (Fig. 5.5).
   a. CO_2 diffuses into red blood cells and combines with H_2O (catalyzed by the enzyme carbonic anhydrase) to form carbonic acid (H_2CO_3) which then dissociates into H^+ and HCO_3^-.
   b. H^+ is buffered by deoxyhemoglobin (Hb-H).
   c. HCO_3^- moves out of the red cell in exchange with Cl^- (called "chloride shift").
3. Etiologies
   a. Airway obstruction
      i. Chronic obstructive pulmonary disease (the most common cause), status asthmaticus.
   b. Lung injury
      i. Acute lung injury, pulmonary edema.
   c. Decreased respiratory drive
      i. Sedative overdose, brainstem lesion.
   d. Disease of neuromuscular function
      i. Guillain–Barre syndrome, myasthenia gravis.
4. Compensation
   a. Renal compensation involves a increase in HCO_3^- (metabolic alkalosis) and takes ~3 days.
   b. In acute respiratory acidosis, the serum bicarbonate is normal to slightly elevated (≤30 mEq/L).
   c. In chronic respiratory acidosis, renal compensation is more complete and thus the serum bicarbonate is higher (>30 mEq/L).
5. Clinical manifestations
   a. Headache, sleepiness, confusion, and anxiety.
   b. Increased cerebral blood flow (potential for cerebral edema).
      i. An elevated level of carbon dioxide in the bloodstream, called hypercapnia (or hypercarbia), causes cerebral vasculature to dilate.
      ii. Note that the opposite effect occurs in the lungs where hypercarbia causes pulmonary vasoconstriction and the development of pulmonary hypertension.

D. Respiratory alkalosis
1. Respiratory alkalosis is characterized by a low PCO_2 (<33 mm Hg).
2. Due to increased alveolar ventilation (rapid, deep breathing) with excessive exhalation of CO_2.
   a. Anxiety (rapid breathing) is the most common cause.
3. Compensation for respiratory alkalosis is a metabolic acidosis (decreased serum HCO_3^-).
   a. Once again, it takes ~3 days for the kidneys to fully compensate.
   b. Before full renal compensation has occurred, the serum bicarbonate will be ≥18 mEq/L (indicating acute respiratory alkalosis).
   c. Conversely, a serum bicarbonate of <18 mEq/L indicates a chronic respiratory alkalosis (i.e., the kidneys had time to respond to the respiratory alkalosis).
4. The reduction in PCO_2 is associated with various physiologic changes.
   a. Increased pH.
   b. Decreased cerebral blood flow (lightheadedness and confusion).
   c. Decreased serum ionized Ca^{2+} concentration.
      i. Alkalosis increases the number of negative charges on albumin (more COO^- groups on acidic amino acids), thereby providing more binding sites for calcium ions.
      ii. As more calcium binds to albumin, free ionized calcium levels drop, the patient develops hypocalcemia, and manifestations of neuromuscular irritability.
         (1) Perioral numbness and tingling, muscle cramps.
            a. Perioral twitching when the facial nerve is tapped (Chvostek sign).
         (2) Carpopedal spasm, laryngospasm, and seizures.
            a. Trousseau's sign (induction of carpopedal spasm after blood pressure cuff is inflated above systolic blood pressure for 3 minutes).

E. Metabolic acidosis
1. Metabolic acidosis is characterized by a reduction of serum bicarbonate to <22 mEq/L.
   a. The compensatory response is to "blow off" CO_2 by increasing ventilation (i.e., respiratory alkalosis [↓ PCO_2]).
2. Pathogenesis
   a. Metabolic acidosis may be due to either of the following:
      i. Addition of an acid (increased anion gap [AG] type of metabolic acidosis—discussed later).
      ii. Loss of, or inability to reclaim, bicarbonate (normal AG type of metabolic acidosis).
   b. To differentiate, one must first calculate the "AG."
3. AG
   a. AG = serum Na^+ − [serum Cl^- + serum HCO_3^-].
   b. Normal is 12 mEq/L ± 2 (represents unmeasured anions that are normally present but not accounted for in the formula; includes phosphate, albumin, and sulfate).
   c. An elevated AG indicates the presence of additional anions that should not be present (e.g., lactate, salicylate, acetoacetate, β-hydroxybutyrate, and others).
   d. Excess H^+ ions of the acid (e.g., lactic acid) are buffered by HCO_3^- (thus serum HCO_3^- is decreased).
      i. $H^+ + HCO_3^- \rightarrow H_2CO_3 \rightarrow H_2O + CO_2$.
   e. If the AG is elevated, determine whether there is an "osmolal gap."

"MUDPILES"

Causes of a high anion gap metabolic acidosis:
- **M**ethanol (metabolized into formic acid)
- **U**remia
- **D**iabetic ketoacidosis (also alcoholic or starvation ketoacidosis)
- **P**ropylene glycol
- **I**soniazid (or iron) overdose
- **L**actic acid
- **E**thylene glycol (metabolized to glycolic acid)
- **S**alicylates (late)

4. Osmolal gap
   a. Difference between the calculated POsm and the measured POsm.
   b. Useful in determining if an increased AG metabolic acidosis is due to the accumulation of nonelectrolyte solutes as seen with toxic ingestion (e.g., ethanol, ethylene glycol, and methanol).
   c. First calculate the POsm.
      i. Calculated POsm = (2 × serum sodium) + (glucose/18) + (BUN/2.8).
   d. Then measure the POsm.
      i. Difference between calculated POsm and measured POsm should be <10 mOsm/kg.

e. If the measured osmolality is more than 10 mOsm/kg greater than the calculated osmolality, then the patient is said to have an elevated osmolal gap.

    i. In general, the most common cause of an elevated osmolar gap is the ingestion of an alcohol, usually ethanol.

    ii. The combination of elevated AG metabolic acidosis and an elevated osmolal gap suggests the ingestion of ethanol, methanol, and/or ethylene glycol.

        (1) Note that isopropyl alcohol causes an elevation of the osmolal gap *but not the AG*.

5. Normal AG metabolic acidosis

    a. In a normal AG metabolic acidosis, the decrease in HCO_3^- anions is matched by an increase in chloride anions.

    b. Etiologies include:

        i. Gastrointestinal losses of bicarbonate (e.g., diarrhea). Recall that bicarbonate is secreted by the pancreas into the duodenum to alkalinize the gastric bolus, thereby preventing the inactivation of digestive enzymes.

        ii. Renal losses of bicarbonate or inability to acidify the urine (e.g., renal tubular acidosis).

6. Clinical manifestations (both increased and normal AG)

    a. Hyperventilation

        i. Kussmaul respirations (deep, slow breathing) to "blow off" CO_2 ($\downarrow PaCO_2$).

    b. Effects of the underlying etiology including:

        i. Renal toxicity of ethylene glycol (calcium oxalate crystals).

        ii. Blindness with methanol ingestion.

F. Metabolic alkalosis

1. Characterized by an elevated serum bicarbonate (>28 mEq/L), due to either a loss of H^+ ions or a gain of HCO_3^- ions.

2. Compensation is a respiratory acidosis ($\uparrow PaCO_2$).

3. Etiologies

    a. Loss of gastric secretions/acid (vomiting, nasogastric suction).

    b. Hypokalemia (e.g., hyperaldosteronism, vomiting, and diuretics).

        i. With hypokalemia, potassium moves out of cells into the ECF. To maintain electroneutrality, hydrogen ions move into cells (causing metabolic alkalosis).

G. Mixed acid–base disorders

1. Presence of two or more primary acid–base disorders occurring concurrently.

2. Clues that suggest a mixed disorder include a normal pH, an extreme acidemia, or an extreme alkalemia.

    a. Example: A patient in cardiorespiratory arrest would have a very low pH because of a combined respiratory acidosis (lack of breathing) and metabolic acidosis (lactate from anaerobic metabolism).

III. Edema

A. Definition

1. Accumulation of excess fluid within the interstitium.

B. Types

1. Transudate: Protein-poor fluid. Due to increased hydrostatic pressure (e.g., heart failure) and/or decreased oncotic pressure (i.e., hypoalbuminemia).

2. Exudate: Protein-rich fluid. Due to increased vascular permeability (e.g., infection, neoplasm) or decreased lymphatic resorption (lymphedema).

C. Pathophysiology

1. Transudates arise from alterations in Starling forces (increased intravascular hydrostatic pressure and/or decreased oncotic pressure).

2. Examples:

    a. Pulmonary edema in those with left-sided heart failure

        i. Increased hydrostatic pressure within the pulmonary vasculature leads to loss of fluid into the pulmonary interstitium and alveoli (i.e., pulmonary edema).

    b. Peripheral edema in those with right-sided heart failure

        i. Increased hydrostatic pressure within the systemic venous system → leakage of fluid into interstitial spaces (most evident in dependent areas of the body; lower legs if ambulatory; sacrum if bedridden).

    c. Portal hypertension

        i. Elevated pressures within the portal vein, most commonly secondary to cirrhosis (altered hepatic architecture impairs the flow of blood through the liver) → leakage of fluid into peritoneum ("ascites").

    d. Hypoalbuminemia

        i. Decreased production (e.g., severe hepatic dysfunction and malnutrition) or increased loss (e.g., nephrotic syndrome).

        ii. Hypoalbuminemia → loss of intravascular oncotic pressure → peripheral edema and ascites.

        iii. Note that both portal hypertension and decreased hepatic protein synthesis contribute to the development of ascites in those with cirrhosis.

    e. Lymphatic obstruction (causes lymphedema)

        i. Radical mastectomy and axillary node dissection with disruption of axillary lymphatics (uncommon today).

        ii. Filariasis (e.g., *Wuchereria bancrofti*).

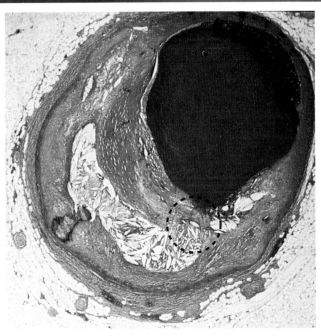

5.6: Coronary artery thrombosis. In this specially stained cross-section of a coronary artery, collagen is blue and the thrombus is red. The red thrombus in the vessel lumen is comprised of platelets held together by fibrin. Directly beneath the thrombus is a fibrous plaque (fibrous cap), which stains blue. Beneath the plaque is necrotic atheromatous debris. The circle shows disruption of the fibrous plaque with cholesterol crystals extending through the wall to the lumen. *(From* Pathology: a color atlas, *St. Louis, 2000, Mosby.)*

    3. Exudates
       a. Increased vascular permeability with leakage of protein-rich fluid from venules into the interstitial spaces (e.g., acute inflammation).
IV. Thrombosis
  A. Definition
    1. Formation or presence of a blood clot (thrombus) within the blood vessel.
    2. Thrombi are comprised of varying proportions of coagulation factors, red blood cells, and platelets.
  B. Risk factors (Virchow triad)
    1. Endothelial injury (e.g., vasculitis and trauma).
    2. Alterations in blood flow (e.g., stasis and turbulent flow).
    3. Hypercoagulable state (inherited or acquired).
  C. Venous thrombi
    1. Comprised primarily of red blood cells with few platelets.
    2. Arise following stasis of blood flow, sometimes in conjunction with a hypercoagulable state.
    3. Most commonly develop within the deep veins of the lower leg, usually the calf (thus the terminology of "deep venous thrombosis" or DVT). Potential for propagation (extension) of the thrombus into the thigh veins (e.g., popliteal vein and femoral vein).
       a. Though uncommon, thrombi may also arise within mesenteric or cerebral veins (e.g., portal vein, hepatic vein, and dural venous sinuses).
    4. DVT causes pain, swelling, and skin discoloration; potential for embolization (see later discussion).
  D. Arterial thrombi
    1. Comprised predominantly of platelets held together by fibrin, usually arise following endothelial injury (often in relation to turbulent blood flow).
    2. Commonly form over disrupted atherosclerotic plaques (Fig. 5.6).
       a. For this reason, arterial thrombi are more likely to develop in locations commonly affected by atherosclerosis (e.g., abdominal aorta and coronary arteries).
    3. Potential for tissue ischemia secondary to obstructed blood flow.
V. Embolism
  A. Definition
    1. Detached mass (e.g., blood clot, fat, and gas) carried through the blood to a distant site.
    2. Most emboli originate from the deep veins of the lower extremities or the left side of the heart.
  B. Clinical manifestations (Fig. 5.7)
    1. Pulmonary embolus

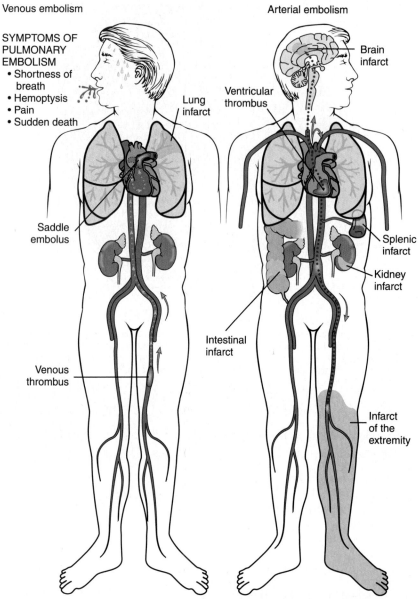

Venous embolism

SYMPTOMS OF
PULMONARY
EMBOLISM
• Shortness of
  breath
• Hemoptysis
• Pain
• Sudden death

Lung
infarct

Saddle
embolus

Venous
thrombus

Arterial embolism

Brain
infarct

Ventricular
thrombus

Splenic
infarct

Kidney
infarct

Intestinal
infarct

Infarct
of the
extremity

5.7: Venous and arterial emboli. On the left, venous emboli commonly lodge within the lung (pulmonary embolus) resulting in a variety of symptoms (e.g., shortness of breath). On the right, note that arterial emboli may occlude arteries throughout the body leading to widespread tissue infarction. (*From* Pathology for the health professions, *ed 4, 2012, Saunders Elsevier.*)

a. Sudden obstruction of a portion of the pulmonary arterial vasculature, usually from a deep venous thrombus that arose within the lower extremity.
  i. Acute onset of dyspnea, tachypnea, chest pain, and cough.
b. Low risk of infarction because the lungs have a dual blood supply (pulmonary and bronchial arteries).
c. Potential for sudden death following occlusion of the pulmonary artery by a large thrombus.
  i. The term "saddle embolus" refers to an embolus overlying the bifurcation of the right and left pulmonary artery branches (analogous to a saddle on a horse); associated with a sudden marked increase in right ventricular afterload.
  ii. Because the right ventricle is not designed to pump against high afterload, obstruction of the pulmonary artery by large thrombus causes a sudden reduction in cardiac output (CO), right ventricular dilatation, and potentially death.
    (1) Dilation of the ventricle is associated with increased wall tension and thus reduced myocardial perfusion (with subendocardial ischemia, right-sided heart failure, and potential for sudden death).
2. Paradoxical embolism
  a. Refers to a venous embolus that crosses from the right to the left side of the heart (e.g., through a patent foramen ovale or atrial septal defect) into the systemic (arterial) circulation.

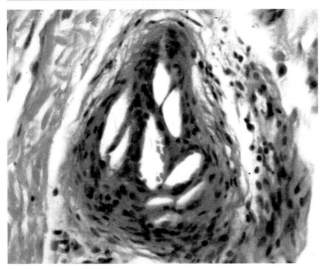

5.8: Cholesterol embolus. The clefts (*white spaces*) represent cholesterol that dissolved during tissue processing.

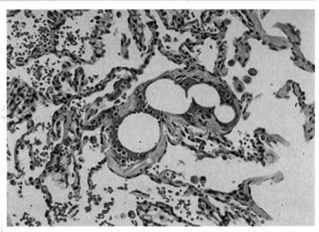

5.9: Fat embolism. Fat globules (*clear spaces*) within a small pulmonary blood vessel in a patient who died following a traumatic fracture of the femur.

3. Systemic embolism
   a. Most originate from the left side of the heart, risk factors include:
      i. Atrial fibrillation
         (1) Predisposes to the formation of intra-atrial clots.
         (2) Risk of systemic embolism resulting in strokes, mesenteric infarct, etc.
      ii. Poor myocardial contractility (e.g., following myocardial infarction)
         (1) Predisposes to the formation of mural fibrin thrombi due to stasis of blood within the ventricular chamber, often in association with endothelial injury.
      iii. Fragments of atherosclerotic plaque ("atheroemboli")
         (1) Commonly from the abdominal aorta or carotid artery.
         (2) Characterized by cholesterol within the embolus on microscopic examination (Fig. 5.8).
   b. Common sites of embolization
      i. Lower extremities.
      ii. Brain (usually through the middle cerebral artery).
      iii. Small intestine (via the superior mesenteric artery).
   c. Complications
      i. Tissue infarction in the area supplied by the affected vessel, resulting in strokes, renal infarct, small intestinal ischemia/infarct, etc.
4. Fat embolism
   a. Secondary to traumatic fracture of a long bone in which marrow fat enters ruptured sinusoids and venules within the marrow.
   b. Embolization of the small fat particles to distant sites leading to the obstruction of blood flow and tissue ischemia.
   c. Symptoms, if they appear, begin 12–72 hours after the traumatic event and may include mental status changes due to involvement of the brain or respiratory distress due to involvement of the lungs (Fig. 5.9).
5. Amniotic fluid embolism
   a. Amniotic fluid may gain access to uterine venous channels, either through a tear in the placental membranes or through a rupture of uterine veins.
   b. Manifestations/complications
      i. Abrupt onset of dyspnea, cyanosis, hypotension, and bleeding.
      ii. Dyspnea due to pulmonary edema and/or acute respiratory distress syndrome.
      iii. Disseminated intravascular coagulation (DIC) secondary to activation of coagulation pathways.
      iv. Cardiac arrest secondary to acute pulmonary vascular obstruction and/or vasoconstriction.
   c. High maternal mortality (>50%)
      i. Autopsy findings include the presence of fetal squamous cells and lanugo hair within the pulmonary vasculature.
6. Decompression sickness
   a. Definition
      i. Type of gas embolism usually in association with deep sea diving.
   b. Pathogenesis
      i. Atmospheric pressure increases with depth, causing nitrogen and other gases to dissolve within the blood and tissues.

      ii. The decrease in ambient pressure, as seen with rapid ascent, allows dissolved gases to reform as gas bubbles within the blood and tissues.

      iii. Stimulates inflammatory cascade, potentially obstructs blood flow.

    c. Clinical manifestations

      i. Severe pain in joints, skeletal muscles, and bones ("the bends").

      ii. Headache, lightheadedness, pulmonary edema, hemorrhage, and atelectasis.

    d. Treatment

      i. Hyperbaric oxygen therapy (causes dissolution of gas bubbles).

VI. Shock

A. Overview

1. Shock refers to a state of inadequate tissue oxygenation secondary to reduced perfusion (which is dependent upon adequate pressures to "push" blood around the body).
2. Mean arterial pressure (MAP) is equal to the diastolic blood pressure (DBP) + 1/3 (systolic BP − diastolic BP).
3. Calculated as the CO multiplied by the peripheral (systemic) vascular resistance (PVR).

Mean arterial pressure (MAP)
$MAP = DBP + 1/3(SBP - DBP)$
$MAP = CO \times PVR$
Cardiac output (CO)
$CO = HR \times SV$

---

4. CO is equal to the heart rate (HR) multiplied by the stroke volume (SV).
5. When one of the variables is decreased, compensatory mechanisms are activated in an attempt to maintain BP.
    a. For example, a reduction in CO (e.g., following an acute myocardial infarction) leads to activation of the sympathetic nervous system via baroreceptors in aortic arch and carotid bodies.
    b. Increased sympathetic outflow → causes compensatory vasoconstriction of peripheral arterioles, thereby increasing PVR and thus MAP.
6. In general, patients develop manifestations of shock with systolic blood pressures of less than 90 mm Hg (or MAP of <60 mm Hg).

B. Major types

1. Hypovolemic shock
    a. Shock occurring as a result of hypovolemic-induced reduction in preload and thus CO.
    b. Usually requires a 20% or more reduction in blood volume (≈1000 mL); most commonly due to massive blood loss (e.g., trauma, gastrointestinal bleed, ruptured abdominal aortic aneurysm).
    c. Pathophysiology
      i. Decreased blood volume → decreased left-ventricular end-diastolic volume (↓ LVEDV) or preload.
      ii. With decreased preload, there is less blood available to be pumped to the body (SV is decreased).
      iii. ↓ SV → ↓ CO → ↓ MAP → ↓ tissue perfusion.
      iv. As a compensatory response, the sympathetic nervous system is activated (i.e., catecholamines, vasopressin, and angiotensin II are released).
        (1) Vasoconstriction of peripheral arterioles leads to an increase in PVR.
      v. Mixed venous oxygen content (MVO_2) is decreased.
        (1) The best indicator of tissue hypoxia.
        (2) Indicates the degree of blood oxygen extraction.
        (3) With hypovolemic shock, blood flow through the microcirculation is slower and more oxygen is extracted by the tissues (MVO_2 is decreased).
      vi. Summary: ↓ CO, ↓ MAP, ↑ PVR, ↓ MVO_2.
    d. Clinical manifestations
      i. Cold and clammy skin (due to vasoconstriction of superficial vessels).
      ii. Hypotension.
      iii. Tachycardia (compensatory response to decreased SV).
      iv. Decreased urine output (decreased renal blood flow and glomerular filtration rate).
    e. Laboratory findings
      i. Increased AG metabolic acidosis (increased lactic acid formed from anaerobic glycolysis).
2. Cardiogenic shock
    a. Marked reduction in CO, due to impaired pumping function of the heart, resulting in decreased tissue perfusion.
      i. Etiologies include myocardial infarction (most common), acute valvular dysfunction, and cardiac arrythmias.
    b. Pathophysiology
      i. Decreased CO (decreased force of contraction) → blood accumulates in the left ventricle → increases left-ventricular end-diastolic pressure (LVEDP) and LVEDV.

TABLE 5.1   Summary of Pathophysiologic Findings Associated With the Various Types of Shock

TYPES OF SHOCK	CO	PVR	LVEDP	MVO$_2$
Hypovolemic	↓	↑	↓	↓
Cardiogenic	↓	↑	↑	↓
Endotoxic (septic)	↑	↓	↓	↑

CO, Cardiac output; *LVEDP*, left-ventricular end-diastolic pressure; *MVO$_2$*, mixed venous oxygen content; *PVR*, peripheral vascular resistance.

     ii. As noted above, with a reduction in CO, there is a compensatory increased sympathetic activity with arteriolar vasoconstriction (increasing PVR).

     iii. MVO2 is decreased (slowed blood flow allows for increased oxygen extraction from the blood).

     iv. Summary: ↓ CO, ↓ MAP, ↑ PVR, ↓ MVO$_2$.

  c. Clinical manifestations

     i. Similar to those in hypovolemic shock (i.e., cold, clammy skin; hypotension; and decreased urine output, lactic acidosis).

3. Distributive shock

  a. Shock occurring secondary to a severe loss of vascular tone (i.e., widespread vascular dilatation).

  b. Etiologies

     i. Sepsis (septic shock)

       (1) Microbial products stimulate the innate immune system to release various vasoactive mediators (e.g., tumor necrosis factor) that cause widespread loss of vascular tone (i.e., decreased PVR).

     ii. Anaphylaxis (anaphylactic shock)

       (1) Systemic release of histamine and other vasoactive substances; usually follows exposure to various allergens (foods, medications, and insect stings) to which the patient has been previously sensitized (Type I hypersensitivity reaction).

  c. Pathophysiology

     i. Since MAP = CO × PVR, a reduction in vascular tone (i.e., PVR) causes a decrease in MAP.

     ii. In an attempt to compensate for the loss of peripheral resistance, increased sympathetic outflow causes an increase in CO (bounding pulses) and blood flow. With increased blood flow, however, there is less time for the tissues to extract oxygen from the blood (MVO$_2$ is increased).

     iii. Summary: ↑ CO, ↓ MAP, ↓ PVR, ↑ MVO$_2$.

  d. Clinical and laboratory findings

     i. Warm skin (due to vasodilation of the superficial blood vessels).

     ii. Hypotension (due to arteriolar vasodilation).

     iii. Bounding pulses (increased CO as a compensatory response to the hypotension).

  e. Complications

     i. Ischemic acute tubular necrosis (acute kidney injury).

     ii. Multiple organ dysfunction syndrome due to widespread tissue hypoxia and associated lack of adequate ATP synthesis.

4. Summary of pathophysiologic findings associated with the various types of shock (Table 5.1).

CHAPTER 6
Genetic and Developmental Disorders

I. Mendelian Disorders

A. Overview

1. Mendelian disorders are diseases caused by mutations in one gene.
2. Different versions of a gene are called alleles.
3. For any given gene, one allele is inherited from the mother and one allele is inherited from the father.
4. Alleles can be "dominant" or "recessive."
   a. The variant, that for a variety of reasons, tends to be expressed over the other is the "dominant" allele, whereas the other is "recessive."
   b. Dominant alleles will show their effect even if the individual only has one copy of the allele.
   c. Recessive alleles only show their effect if the individual has two copies of the allele.
   d. In a few situations (e.g., ABO blood grouping), both alleles are expressed (called codominant).
5. Penetrance
   a. Full penetrance describes the situation in which all individuals with the mutant gene exhibit the disorder.
   b. Incomplete penetrance describes the situation in which some with the mutant gene exhibit the disorder while others are phenotypically normal.
6. Expressivity
   a. Refers to the variations in the clinical presentation of a mutation.
      i. For example, those that inherit the major disease-causing mutation of cystic fibrosis (CF) have variable degrees of pancreatic dysfunction.

B. Autosomal dominant (AD) disorders (Fig. 6.1)

1. In AD disorders, only one mutant gene (A) is required to express the disorder.
   a. Example: Aa × aa → Aa, Aa, aa, aa.
      i. 50% of offspring have the disorder (Aa).
      ii. 50% do not have the disorder (aa).
   b. Males and females are equally affected.
2. Specific AD disorders include:
   a. Familial hypercholesterolemia (FH)
      i. Heterozygous FH is common (~1 in 300), and homozygous FH is rare.
      ii. Characterized by impaired hepatic clearance of low-density lipoprotein (LDL); most commonly due to a mutation in the LDL receptor (*LDLR*) gene.
         (1) Heterozygotes exhibit a two- to threefold elevation of plasma LDL; patients have early onset of atherosclerotic vascular disease (young adulthood).
         (2) Homozygotes exhibit a five- to sixfold elevation of plasma LDL and have onset of atherosclerotic vascular disease (e.g., myocardial infarction) very early in life (teenage years).
   b. Marfan syndrome
      i. Inherited mutation in the *FBN1* gene resulting in decreased levels of the protein fibrillin-1.
         (1) Fibrillin-1 is a major component of microfibrils found in elastic tissue, especially prominent in the aorta, ligaments, and the eye.
      ii. Prevalence of 1 in 5000.
      iii. Clinical manifestations
         (1) Tall stature with long extremities, tapering fingers, and chest wall abnormalities (either pectus excavatum or pigeon-breast deformity).

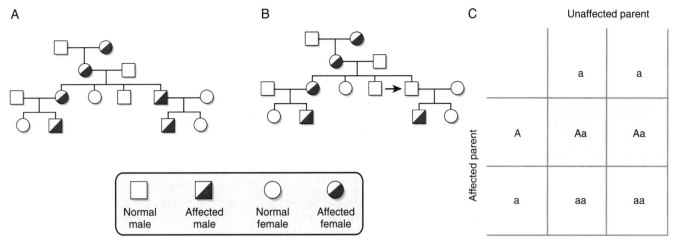

6.1: (A) Pedigree showing complete penetrance in an autosomal dominant disorder. Complete penetrance means that all individuals with the mutant gene express the disease. (B) Incomplete penetrance means that an individual has the mutant gene but does not express the disorder. The unaffected father with the mutant gene (*arrow*) has transmitted the disorder to his son. (C) The Punnett square illustrates the mating of an unaffected parent (aa) with an individual who is heterozygous for an autosomal dominant disease gene (Aa). Note that 50% of the offspring are affected. *(C, From Jorde LB, Carey JC, Bamshad MJ: Medical genetics, ed 4. Philadelphia, 2010, Mosby Elsevier, p 60, Fig. 4.2.)*

      (2) Bilateral subluxation of the lens of the eye (ectopia lentis).

      (3) Cardiovascular abnormalities

          (a) Mitral valve prolapse.

          (b) Dilation of aortic root (risk aortic regurgitation and aortic dissection/rupture).

  c. Neurofibromatosis

    i. Neurofibromatosis type 1 (NF1)

      (1) Due to decreased function or production of neurofibromin (a tumor suppressor protein) secondary to mutations in *NF1 on chromosome 17*.

      (2) Clinical manifestations (in typical order of appearance), include:

          (a) Café-au-lait macules.

          (b) Axillary and/or inguinal freckling.

          (c) Lisch nodules (hamartomas of the iris).

          (d) Neurofibromas (tumors of peripheral nerves).

    ii. Neurofibromatosis type 2 (NF2)

      (1) Due to decreased function or production of merlin (tumor suppressor protein) secondary to mutations in *NF2 on chromsome 22*.

      (2) Clinical manifestations include:

          (a) Tumors of the CNS

            • Bilateral vestibular schwannomas.

            • Meningiomas.

            • Ependymomas.

          (b) Peripheral neuropathies.

          (c) Cataracts and other ocular manifestations (developing in childhood).

  d. Huntington disease

    i. Expansion of cytosine–adenine–guanine (CAG) trinucleotide repeat in the huntingtin (*HTT*) gene on chromosome 4.

    ii. Normal *HTT* alleles contain 6–26 CAG repeats; Huntington disease develops in those with >36 CAG repeats.

    iii. Although the protein (huntingtin) is widely expressed throughout the body, those with Huntington disesase (HD) suffer primarily from neuronal loss in the caudate and putamen.

    iv. Age of onset varies inversely with the number of CAG repeats (though most patients present by 40 years of age).

    v. Manifestations

      (1) Movement abnormality (chorea).

      (2) Psychiatric illness (irritability and depression).

      (3) Dementia.

      (4) Death (usually within 10–20 years of diagnosis).

C. Autosomal recessive (AR) disorders (Fig. 6.2)

  1. In AR disorders, the disease only occurs when there are two mutant alleles of the disease-associated gene (i.e., a disease-associated mutant gene has been inherited from each parent).

    a. Patient must be homozygous for the mutant gene (aa).

    b. Homozygotes (aa) tend to present early in life.

    c. Heterozygotes (Aa) are usually asymptomatic carriers.

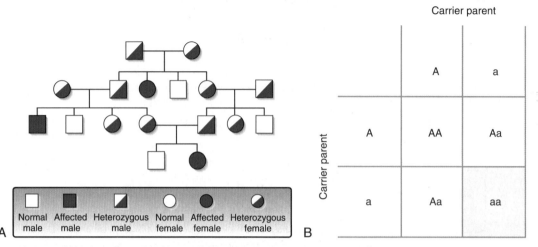

6.2: (A) Pedigree of an autosomal recessive disorder. Both parents must have the mutant gene (a) to transmit the disorder to their children. Approximately 25% of the children of heterozygous parents are normal (AA), 50% are asymptomatic heterozygous carriers (Aa), and 25% express the disorder (aa). (B) The Punnett square illustrates the mating of two heterozygous carriers of an autosomal recessive gene (Aa). Note that 25% of the offspring are affected (aa), 50% are asymptomatic carriers (Aa), and 25% are normal (AA). *(B, From Jorde LB, Carey JC, Bamshad MJ: Medical genetics, ed 4, Philadelphia, 2010, Mosby Elsevier, p 61, Fig. 4.5.)*

2. Risk of transmission
   a. Example: Aa × Aa → AA, Aa, Aa, aa.
      i. 25% of offspring do not have disorder (AA).
      ii. 50% of offspring are asymptomatic carriers (Aa).
      iii. 25% of the offspring have the disorder (aa).
3. Specific AR disorders include:
   a. CF
      i. Multisystem disorder caused by a mutation in the *CFTR* gene on chromosome 7 (the most common mutation is a deletion of phenylalanine at the 508th position).
      ii. Reduced synthesis or activity of the CF transmembrane conductance regulator (CFTR) protein impairs ion channel transport resulting in the production of thickened, viscous secretions involving multiple organ systems.
      iii. Viscous respiratory secretions predispose the patient to recurrent infections (e.g., *Pseudomonas aeruginosa*).
         (1) Major cause of morbidity and mortality.
      iv. Viscous pancreatic secretions predispose to the development of pancreatitis. Eventual loss of pancreatic exocrine function (chronic pancreatitis) leads to steatorrhea and a deficiency of fat-soluble vitamins.
      v. Impaired chloride resorption from sweat (rationale underlying the sweat chloride test).
      vi. Increased risk of meconium ileus due to thickened intestinal mucous.
      vii. Infertility is common due to viscous cervical mucous and impaired sperm transport.
      viii. Confirmatory sweat test (sweat chloride >60 mEq/L is diagnostic of CF).
   b. Sickle cell disease (SCD)
      i. The normal adult hemoglobin (HbA) contains two alpha-globin chains and two beta-globin chains.
      ii. SCD is due to a point mutation in the beta-globin gene (valine substituted for glutamic acid at the sixth position); causing the production of sickle hemoglobin (HbS).
      iii. When deoxygenated, HbS is poorly soluble and forms polymers that distort the shape of red cells ("sickling").
      iv. Sickle red blood cells (RBCs) are susceptible to hemolysis (explaining the chronic anemia) and also become "sticky" with a tendency to adhere to the vascular endothelium, the latter causing vascular occlusion and associated complications, including:
         (1) Bone infarction (avascular necrosis).
         (2) Splenic infarction ("autosplenectomy")
            (a) Loss of splenic function places patients at an increased risk of infection, particularly with encapsulated organisms (e.g., *Streptococcus pneumoniae*, *Haemophilus influenzae*, and *Salmonella* spp.).
         (3) Cerebral infarction (strokes).
         (4) Priapism (obstructed venous drainage from the erect penis).
      v. Those heterozygous for the mutation (i.e., sickle cell trait) are largely asymptomatic because levels of HbS are not high enough to cause spontaneous sickling in most situations.
      vi. Homozygotes (i.e., sickle cell anemia) develop clinical manifestations, usually beginning around 6 months of age as fetal hemoglobin (HbF) is replaced by the abnormal HbS.

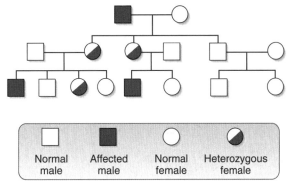

6.3: Pedigree of an X-linked recessive (XR) disorder. The affected male transmits the mutant gene on the X chromosome to both of his daughters and none of his sons. Both daughters are asymptomatic heterozygous carriers of the mutant gene. The daughter with four children has transmitted the mutant gene to 50% of her sons.

      (1) Because it binds to oxygen very avidly, HbF protects against sickling for the first several months of life (HbF prevents the red cells from becoming deoxygenated, thereby preventing sickling).

      (2) Hydroxyurea is sometimes given (increases HbF) in an attempt to reduce sickling.

  c. Tay-Sachs disease

    i. Lysosomal storage disorder caused by deficiency of the enzyme hexosaminidase A (mutation in *HEXA*).

    ii. Loss of motor skills beginning during the first year; progressive neurodegenerative changes resulting in seizures, blindness, and death (usually by 4 years of age).

D. X-linked disorders (Fig. 6.3)

  1. Disorders caused by genetic variants on the X chromosome.

  2. Males, who have only one X chromosome, express the disorder.

    a. Said to be "hemizygous" for the mutant gene as the Y chromosome is not homologous to the X chromosome (hence the term hemizygous).

  3. Affected males transmit the mutant gene to all their daughters.

    a. Daughters are carriers of the mutant gene but are usually asymptomatic because of the paired normal allele from the mother.

    b. Sons that inherit the mutant gene express the disease (they do not have the paired normal homologous allele).

  4. Female carriers transmit the mutant gene to 50% of their offspring.

    a. Each son has a 50% chance of having the disease.

    b. Each daughter has a 50% chance of being a carrier.

      i. In rare cases, the female carrier may be symptomatic due to the inactivation of the maternally derived X chromosome.

  5. Specific X-linked conditions

    a. Hemophilia A

      i. Bleeding disorder due to reduced synthesis of factor VIII (mutation in *F8* gene).

      ii. Prevalence of ~1 in 5000 males.

      iii. Bleeding tendency depends upon factor VIII levels.

        (1) Severe deficiency (<1% factor VIII activity) usually presents during childhood.

      iv. Manifestations include excessive bleeding following circumcision or other medical procedures, bleeding into the joint (hemarthrosis), the brain, or soft tissues.

      v. Female carriers are usually asymptomatic because they are heterozygous for the defect (one normal allele and one abnormal allele) and therefore have adequate factor VIII (~50%) to prevent bleeding in most circumstances.

    b. Hemophilia B

      i. Mutation in *F9* gene resulting in reduced factor IX levels.

      ii. Clinically like hemophilia A but much less common (prevalence of 1 in 30,000 males).

    c. Fragile X syndrome

      i. The most common inherited cause of intellectual disability in males. Females may be affected to a lesser degree.

      ii. Pathogenesis

        (1) Expansion of a CGG trinucleotide repeat with a resultant loss-of-function mutation in the fragile X mental retardation 1 (*FMR1*) gene and thus decreased to absent levels of the fragile X mental retardation protein (FMRP).

      iii. Clinical manifestations

        (1) Decreased intellectual ability and developmental delay (e.g., delayed motor and language skills).

        (2) By adolescence, patients develop long, narrow face with prominent forehead and jaw, large "seashell-shaped" ears, and testicular enlargement.

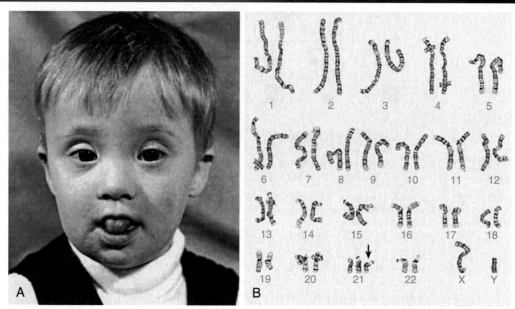

6.4: (A) Face of a child with Down syndrome. (B) Karyotype of a male with trisomy 21. *(From* Nelson Textbook of Pediatrics, *Fig. 98.8. Copyright © 2020 Elsevier Inc.)*

    d. Lesch-Nyhan syndrome
      i.   Motor-behavioral disorder due to mutations in the gene coding for the enzyme hypoxanthine-guanine phosphoribosyl transferase.
      ii. Deficient enzyme activity impairs salvage pathways of purine intermediates (causing hyperuricemia and hyperuricosuria).
      iii. Clinical manifestations
         (1) Gout.
         (2) Urate nephropathy (deposits of urate within renal tubules).
         (3) Intellectual disability.
         (4) Various motor abnormalities.
         (5) Self-mutilating behavior.

II. Chromosomal Disorders
A. Overview
    1. Gametes contain 23 chromosomes.
      a. 22 Autosomes and a single sex chromosome.
    2. Human somatic cells contain 46 chromosomes.
      a. 22 Pairs of homologous autosomes and one pair of sex chromosomes.
    3. Normal chromosome complement
      a. 46, XX for females; 46, XY for males.
B. Autosome chromosomal disorders
    1. Down syndrome (Trisomy 21)
      a. Chromosomal disorder characterized by distinct facial features, multiple malformations, and variable degrees of intellectual disability (Fig. 6.4).
      b. The most common chromosome abnormality among live births (1 in 700).
      c. Most cases are due to meiotic nondisjunction (paired homologous chromosomes fail to separate normally during meiotic division).
      d. Increased maternal age is the major risk factor (extra chromosome 21 is usually of maternal origin).
      e. Clinical manifestations
        i.   Intellectual disability (mild to severe).
        ii. Upslanting palpebral fissures.
        iii. Epicanthic folds.
        iv. Transverse palmar (Simian) crease.
        v. Congenital heart defects (~50% of patients).
          (1) Complete atrioventricular septal defect, ventricular septal defect, and atrial septal defect.
        vi. Intestinal manifestations
          (1) Duodenal atresia and Hirschsprung disease.
        vii. Increased risk of acute leukemia.
        viii. Early-onset Alzheimer disease (usually by the sixth decade)

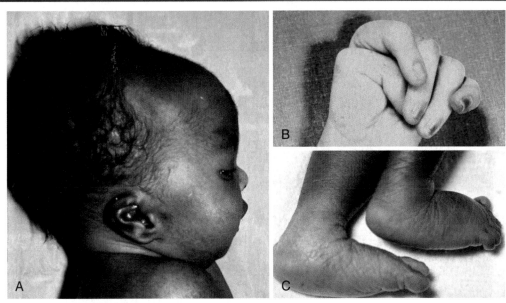

6.5: Physical manifestations of trisomy 18. (A) Prominent occiput and low-set ears. (B) Clenched hand showing the typical pattern of overlapping fingers. (C) Rocker-bottom feet. *(From* Zitelli and Davis' atlas of pediatric physical diagnosis*, ed 7, Fig. 1.24. Copyright © 2018 by Elsevier, Inc.)*

(1) Chromosome 21 contains the *APP* gene, encoding for amyloid precursor protein (cleaved by secretase enzymes to form amyloid beta, a component of senile plaques; see Chapter 26).

  f. Prenatal screening of maternal serum (quadruple test)
    i. Decreased α-fetoprotein (AFP).
    ii. Decreased unconjugated estriol (uE3).
    iii. Increased human chorionic gonadotropin (hCG).
    iv. Increased inhibin A.
  g. Diagnostic confirmatory testing
    i. Cytogenetic and DNA studies.
2. Trisomy 18: Edwards syndrome
  a. Chromosomal disorder caused by the presence of an extra chromosome 18.
  b. Second most common autosomal trisomy (1 in 5500 live births).
  c. Increased risk with advanced maternal age.
  d. Common findings include prominent occiput, low-set and structurally abnormal ears, rocker-bottom feet, clenched fist with overlapping fingers, and congenital heart defects (Fig. 6.5).
  e. Most die in utero or within the first few weeks of life.
3. Trisomy 13 (Patau syndrome)
  a. Incidence of 1 in 15,000 births.
  b. Multiple severe congenital anomalies including holoprosencephaly, polydactyly, congenital heart defects, severe intellectual disability, and early death.
C. **Examples of sex chromosome disorders**
  1. Turner syndrome (45, X)
    a. Chromosomal condition in females characterized by complete or partial absence of a second normal X chromosome.
    b. Most common sex chromosome abnormality in females (~1 in 2500 female births).
    c. Clinical manifestations (Fig. 6.6)
      i. Short stature (cardinal finding; >95% of cases).
      ii. Shield chest (widely spaced nipples).
      iii. Lymphedema in the hands, feet, and neck.
      iv. Webbed neck, cystic hygroma.
      v. Low posterior hairline.
      vi. Increased carrying angle of the arms (cubitus valgus).
      vii. Congenital heart disease (up to 50% of cases)
        (1) Coarctation of the aorta, bicuspid aortic valve.
      viii. Primary ovarian failure ("streak ovaries")
        (1) Most common genetic cause of primary amenorrhea.
        (2) Decreased estrogen levels; elevated follicle-stimulating hormone (FSH) and luteinizing hormone (LH) concentrations.

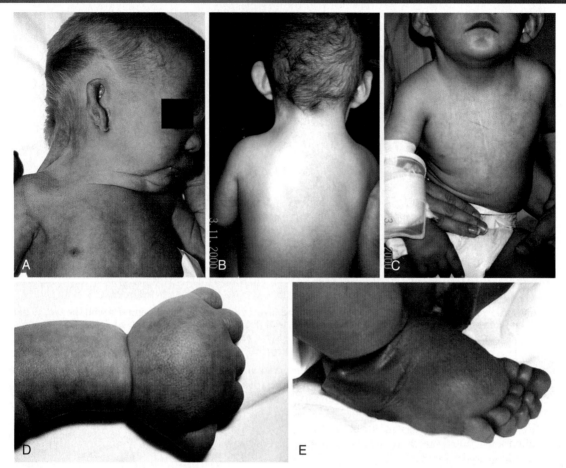

6.6: Turner syndrome. (A) Webbed neck with low hairline, shield chest with widespread nipples, abnormal ears, and micrognathia. (B) Low-set posterior hairline and protruding ears. (C) Mild webbing of the neck and small, widely spaced nipples. Note the midline scar from prior cardiac surgery. (D and E) Prominent lymphedema of the hands and feet. *(From Madan-Khetarpal S, Arnold G: Genetic disorders and dysmorphic conditions. In Zitelli BJ, McIntire SC, Nowalk AJ, editors: Zitelli and Davis' atlas of pediatric physical diagnosis, ed 6, Philadelphia, 2012, Elsevier, Fig. 1.25.)*

2. Klinefelter syndrome (47, XXY)
    a. 47, XXY male; most commonly due to meiotic nondisjunction of the X chromosome during gametogenesis.
    b. Most common congenital abnormality causing primary hypogonadism (1 in 1000 live male births).
    c. Clinical and laboratory findings are those of hypogonadism.
        i. Often initially recognized during puberty with failure of normal testicular growth, incomplete virilization (e.g., reduced facial and pubic hair), and gynecomastia.
        ii. Eunuchoid body habitus with disproportionately long legs.
        iii. Low serum total and free testosterone.
        iv. Elevated FSH and LH concentrations.
III. **Other Patterns of Inheritance**
    A. **Multifactorial (complex) inheritance**
        1. Disorders arising as a result of complex interactions between genetic and environmental factors.
            a. For example, coronary heart disease is associated with various genetic mutations in conjunction with environmental factors (e.g., smoking and diet).
    B. **Mitochondrial DNA disorders**
        1. Overview
            a. Rare disorders caused by mutations in mitochondrial DNA.
            b. Mitochondrial genome is inherited from the mother.
                i. Affected females transmit the mutant gene to all of her children.
                ii. Affected males do not transmit the mutant gene.
            c. Mitochondrial DNA code for enzymes involved in oxidative phosphorylation reactions.
                i. Tissues highly dependent on oxidative phosphorylation (e.g., skeletal muscle, cardiac muscle, liver, kidneys, and central nervous system) are most affected.

2. Leber hereditary optic neuropathy
   a. Characterized by the painless loss of vision, often beginning in the late teens.

C. Genomic imprinting
1. The expression of some traits is highly dependent upon which parent the variant is inherited.
2. Examples include Prader-Willi syndrome and Angelman syndrome.
   a. Caused by deletions involving 15q11-13.
      i. In Prader-Willi syndrome, the deletion is found only on the chromosome 15 inherited from the father (i.e., genomic information at 15q11-13 is derived only from the mother). Manifestations include hypotonia, delayed development, hyperphagia (causing obesity), and mild intellectual disability.
      ii. Angelman syndrome due to deletion of the same region of chromosome 15 inherited from the mother (genomic information at 15q11-13 is derived only from the father). Manifestations include intellectual disability, gait ataxia, and inappropriate laughter.

IV. Disorders of Sex Differentiation
A. Overview
1. Chromosomal sex is determined at fertilization.
   a. XX—female; XY—male.
2. Sex differentiation involves a series of events whereby the sexually indifferent gonads and genitalia progressively acquire male or female characteristics.
   a. Depends on the presence or absence of the Y chromosome, which contains the *SRY* gene.
      i. Sex-determining region of the Y chromosome (*SYR*) gene causes the development of the indifferent gonads into testes.
      ii. Fetal testes then produce anti-Müllerian hormone (AMH) and testosterone, the latter being partially converted to dihydrotestosterone (DHT) by 5α-reductase in peripheral tissues.
      iii. DHT regulates the development of the prostate and external male genitalia.
3. Conversely, in the absence of the Y chromosome, the indifferent gonads become ovaries and the Müllerian ducts develop (into fallopian tubes, uterus, and upper vagina).

B. Androgen insensitivity syndrome
1. Overview
   a. X-linked disorder associated with a loss-of-function mutation in the androgen receptor gene (*AR*).
   b. Patients have male karyotypes (46, XY) and male gonads (i.e., produce androgens and AMH).
      i. Production of AMH by fetal testes causes apoptosis of paramesonephric duct structures (i.e., the fallopian tubes, uterus, and upper vagina do not form).
   c. Despite the presence of androgens, the mutation in the androgen receptor results in a failure of the androgen effect. For this reason, patients may exhibit a completely female phenotype or a male phenotype with undervirilization/infertility.
2. Clinical manifestations
   a. Testes are present within inguinal canal or abdomen; however, the lack of androgen effect causes female body habitus.
   b. If not identified during the newborn period, patients present at puberty with a lack of axillary/pubic hair and primary amenorrhea.
3. Karyotype is essential to differentiate an under-masculinized male from a virilized female.
4. Male karyotype (46, XY); normal serum testosterone and DHT; increased LH.
   a. Despite the presence of androgens, the receptor defect causes a lack of negative feedback on the hypothalamus and pituitary (thus LH is elevated).

V. Congenital Anomalies
A. Definition
1. Defects that are present at birth.
B. Types
1. Agenesis
   a. Complete absence of an organ due to the absence of primordial tissue.
2. Malformation
   a. Disturbance in the morphogenesis (development) of an organ; usually arise during early gestation (first 9 weeks).
3. Deformation
   a. Congenital anomaly caused by extrinsic factors physically impinging upon the developing fetus.
   b. Common to a small degree in relation to the rapid fetal growth at term (called uterine constraint).
   c. Pathologic deformation may be seen with oligohydramnios (reduced amniotic fluid volume).
      i. Amniotic fluid is predominantly composed of fetal urine; therefore any condition that reduces urine production will cause oligohydramnios.
      ii. Oligohydramnios → loss of cushioning effect on the fetus → extrinsic compression with flattening of the face and compression of the skull.
         (1) In the rare situation of bilateral renal agenesis, there is no urine produced and thus no amniotic fluid.
         (2) Constellation of findings, known as Potter's sequence, include the absence of amniotic fluid, marked fetal compression, and severe pulmonary hypoplasia, the latter resulting in death soon after birth.

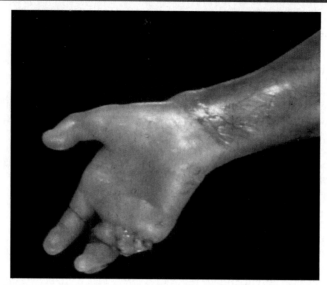

6.7: Amniotic band sequence includes fetal hand deformities. *(From Crum CP, Nucci MR, Lee KR, et al:* Diagnostic gynecologic and obstetric pathology, *ed 2, 2011, Saunders Elsevier, p 1013, Fig. 32.26A.)*

4. Disruption
    a. Defects of organs or body parts due to the destruction of normal fetal tissue.
    b. Etiologies include vascular insufficiency (e.g., thrombosis of placental vasculature) and amniotic bands.
        i. Amniotic bands are fibrous bands that encircle parts of the fetus; complications may include partial amputation of a limb (Fig. 6.7).
5. Aplasia
    a. Defective development of an organ or tissue despite the presence of primordial tissue.
6. Hypoplasia
    a. Incomplete development of an organ or tissue.
7. Atresia
    a. Incomplete formation of a lumen (e.g., duodenal atresia).
VI. **Perinatal and Infant Disorders**
    A. **Stillbirth**
        1. Delivery of a dead fetus at 20 weeks gestation or later.
        2. Etiologies include:
            a. Placental abruption (partial or complete placental detachment due to retroplacental hemorrhage).
            b. Hydrops fetalis (e.g., Rh hemolytic disease of the newborn).
            c. Placental dysfunction.
            d. Congenital infection (e.g., cytomegalovirus, parvovirus, listeria, group B streptococcus; malaria in endemic areas).
    B. **Spontaneous abortion (miscarriage, pregnancy loss)**
        1. Involuntary pregnancy loss before 20 weeks of gestation (or loss of fetus weighing ≤500 g).
        2. Usually presents with bleeding and cramping.
        3. Characterized as being "complete" versus "incomplete."
            a. Complete abortion refers to an empty uterus after documentation of prior intrauterine pregnancy.
            b. Incomplete abortion refers to the presence of residual fetal tissue within the uterus following documentation of fetal demise (associated with increased risk of endometrial infection).
    C. **Sudden infant death syndrome (SIDS)**
        1. Defined as the sudden and unexpected death of an apparently healthy infant under 1 year of age that remains unexplained after a thorough investigation and autopsy.
        2. The most common cause of death between 1 month and 1 year of age.
        3. No single identified cause of SIDS.
            a. Maternal factors include smoking and inadequate prenatal care.
            b. Infant factors include preterm birth, prone sleeping position (babies should be supine), sleeping on a soft surface with pillows/blankets or sleeping in parents' bed.
    D. **Preterm birth**
        1. Birth before 37 weeks of gestation.
        2. Most common cause of neonatal morbidity and mortality.

   3. Risk factors for preterm delivery
      a. Obstetric factors (e.g., preterm premature rupture of membranes, multiple gestation, and infection).
      b. Maternal factors (e.g., substance abuse, tobacco use, extremes of age, and history of preterm delivery).
   4. Complications associated with preterm delivery
      a. Respiratory distress syndrome (secondary to decreased surfactant).
      b. Necrotizing enterocolitis (ischemic necrosis of the bowel).
      c. Germinal matrix hemorrhage (bleeding between the caudate nucleus and the thalamus; may extend into the ventricular system).
      d. Periventricular infarct/leukomalacia (necrosis of white matter, often with dystrophic calcification).
E. **Intrauterine growth retardation (IUGR)**
   1. Defined as a newborn born at less than 10% of predicted weight based on gestational age.
   2. Maternal factors include preeclampsia, poor nutrition, smoking, use of alcohol, or illicit drugs.
   3. Fetal factors include chromosomal disorders, malformations, and congenital infections.
   4. Placental factors include placental abruption and placental infarction.
   5. Ultrasonography is a common initial step in the workup of IUGR.

CHAPTER 7
Environmental Pathology

Chemical Injury, 68
Physical Injury, 69

Radiation Injury, 72

I. Chemical Injury

A. Tobacco

1. Chronic use is associated with multiple detrimental health effects, including:
   a. Atherosclerotic vascular disease
      i. Strokes, myocardial infarction, and abdominal aortic aneurysm.
   b. Cancer
      i. Lung (smoking accounts for ~90% of all lung cancers), esophagus, pancreas, bladder, and others.
   c. Chronic obstructive pulmonary disease
      i. Chronic bronchitis and emphysema.
2. Health effects are primarily to active smokers; however, exposure to second-hand smoke (passive) also increases one's risk.
3. Smokeless tobacco increases one's risk of oral squamous cell carcinoma.
4. Nicotine is strongly addictive and stimulates the release of dopamine and other neurotransmitters that activate the "reward" center of the brain.
   a. Increases respiratory rate, heart rate, and blood pressure.
5. Carcinogens present in cigarette smoke include:
   a. Polycyclic aromatic hydrocarbons, *N*-nitrosamines, aromatic amines, formaldehyde, benzene, and metals (e.g., arsenic, chromium, cadmium, and nickel).

B. Alcohol

1. Alcohol-related disease development is primarily related to the amount and duration of intake; females are at greater risk.
2. Moderate alcohol use is associated with relatively few effects; however, heavy drinking has a variety of detrimental effects.
   a. Definition of "heavy drinking" depends on sex:
      i. Females: more than seven drinks per week or three drinks per occasion.
      ii. Males: more than 14 drinks per week or 4 drinks per occasion.
3. Alcohol absorption and metabolism
   a. Alcohol is absorbed within the stomach (~20%) and the small intestine (~80%).
      i. Blood level of 80 mg/dL (acquired after ~three drinks in most individuals) is a legal definition of intoxication.
      ii. Coma occurs at ~300 mg/dL.
      iii. Chronic drinkers metabolize alcohol more rapidly (i.e., become more tolerant).
   b. Metabolism to acetaldehyde occurs primarily within the liver, via one of three enzyme systems (Fig. 7.1).
      i. The major pathway, involving alcohol dehydrogenase, occurs within the cytoplasm of hepatocytes.
      ii. Cytochrome P450 enzyme and catalase are of lesser importance.
   c. Acetaldehyde is then oxidized by the mitochondrial enzyme acetaldehyde dehydrogenase to acetic acid.
      i. Activity of acetaldehyde dehydrogenase is reduced in some of Asian ethnicity. In these individuals, higher and prolonged levels of acetaldehyde result in clinical manifestations (e.g., facial flushing).
   d. Metabolism of alcohol causes nicotinamide adenine dinucleotide (NAD) to be reduced to NADH.
      i. NAD is required for fatty acid oxidation.
   e. Reduced levels of NAD contribute to the development of hepatic steatosis (fatty liver).
      i. Steatosis, an early pathologic finding associated with alcohol abuse, is reversible with abstention from alcohol.
      ii. Continued ingestion of alcohol, however, can result in worsening liver disease (steatohepatitis [steatosis + inflammation], cirrhosis).

68

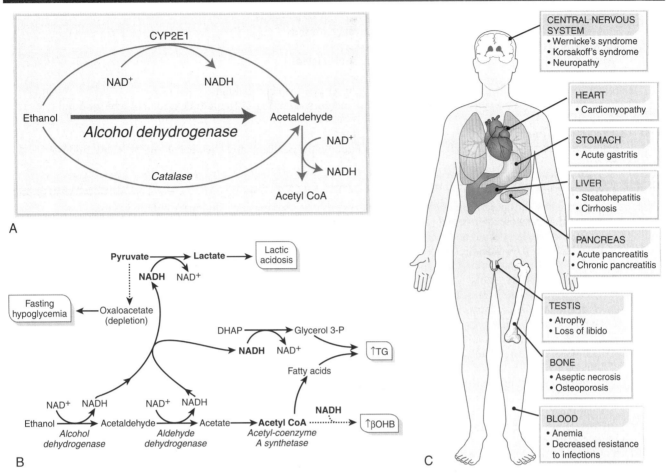

7.1: (A) Three enzymes play a key function in the metabolism of alcohol in liver cells: alcohol dehydrogenase, CYP2E (cytochrome P450 enzyme in the smooth endoplasmic reticulum of the microsomal fraction), and catalase in peroxisomes. Alcohol dehydrogenase is the most important, transforming alcohol into acetaldehyde, which is then oxidized to acetyl coenzyme A (CoA). Nicotine adenine dinucleotide (NAD$^+$) is reduced to NADH in this process, as well as during the action of CYP2E. Acetaldehyde is a toxic metabolite. (B) Laboratory findings that occur in the metabolism of alcohol. Note that the increase in NADH leads to an increased conversion of pyruvate to lactate (causing lactic acidosis with an elevated anion gap). The decrease in pyruvate leads to less oxaloacetate, a substrate for gluconeogenesis. This produces a fasting hypoglycemia. There is an increased conversion of DHAP to glycerol 3-phosphate. Finally, excess acetyl CoA is used to synthesize fatty acids, which, together with the increase in glycerol 3-phosphate, increases triglyceride synthesis (hypertriglyceridemia). (C) Common clinical consequences of chronic alcohol abuse. *β-OHB*, β-Hydroxybutyrate; *DHAP*, dihydroxyacetone phosphate; *NADH*, reduced nicotinamide adenine dinucleotide; steatohepatitis, fatty change; *TG*, triglyceride. (*A and C, From* Pathophysiology, *2009, Saunders Elsevier, pp 75, 77, Figs. 3-9, 3-11, respectively; B, from Pelley JW, Goljan EF:* Rapid review biochemistry, *ed 2, Philadelphia, 2007, Mosby, p 172, Fig. 9-6.*)

    4. Other harmful effects include:
- a. Increased risk of cancers (e.g., oropharynx, larynx, esophagus, and liver).
- b. Acute, as well as chronic, pancreatitis (alcohol is a major cause).
- c. Dilated cardiomyopathy.
- d. Hypertension.
- e. Nutritional deficiencies (e.g., thiamine and folate) and associated complications.
- f. Increased risk of accidents, trauma, and suicide.
- g. Fetal alcohol syndrome
    - i. Prenatal exposure to alcohol can cause a variety of detrimental effects to the fetus, including growth retardation, facial anomalies (small palpebral fissures, indistinct or absent philtrum, flattened nasal bridge, and thin upper lip), and neurologic abnormalities (e.g., microcephaly and developmental disabilities).
    - ii. No amount of alcohol is considered "safe" during pregnancy.

C. Injection drug use
1. Potential for overdose and death due to direct drug effects.
2. In addition, patients are at an increased risk of infectious complications (e.g., hepatitis B, hepatitis C, human immunodeficiency virus, *Staphylococcus aureus* bacteremia).

II. Physical Injury
A. Gunshot wounds
1. Contact wounds are stellate-shaped and contain soot and gunpowder.
2. Intermediate-range wounds exhibit stippling of the skin around the entrance site due to gunpowder burns.

3. Longer range wounds are characterized by an absence of powder burns.
4. Exit wounds are larger and more irregular than entrance wounds.

B. Motor vehicle accidents

1. Major cause of injury-related deaths; frequently alcohol-related.

C. Shaken baby syndrome

1. Injury to a child, usually during infancy, secondary to repeated violent shaking.
2. Characteristics of pathologic findings include retinal hemorrhages (Fig. 7.2), multiple fractures, and subdural hematomas.

D. Thermal injury (burns)

1. Exposure to excessive heat (e.g., fire/flame, hot water, hot objects, steam, and chemicals) causes denaturation of proteins.
2. Classification of burns)
   a. Superficial (first-degree) burns
      i. Limited to the epidermis; heal within a few days without scarring (e.g., sunburn) and are painful.
   b. Partial-thickness (second-degree) burns
      i. Extend into the dermis and painful.
   c. Full-thickness (third-degree) burns
      i. Extend through the skin into subcutaneous tissues and painless due to underlying nerve damage.
      ii. Heals with scarring due to the lack of regenerative adnexal structures; potential for developing squamous cell carcinoma in the burn scar.
3. Complications of severe burns include:
   a. Hypovolemic shock
      i. Disruption of vascular integrity, allowing the leakage of fluid into interstitial spaces.
      ii. Loss of skin barrier allows for increased insensible fluid losses via evaporation.
   b. Infection
      i. Impaired host immune response.
      ii. Loss of skin barrier allows for bacterial invasion and growth.
   c. Hypothermia
      i. Heat lost through damaged skin.

E. Smoke inhalation

1. Results in the inhalation of several injurious chemicals (e.g., carbon monoxide and cyanide).
   a. Carbon monoxide binds to hemoglobin avidly and prevents oxygen delivery to tissues.
   b. Cyanide inhibits an enzyme in the electron transport chain, causing oxidative phosphorylation to cease and death within minutes to hours.

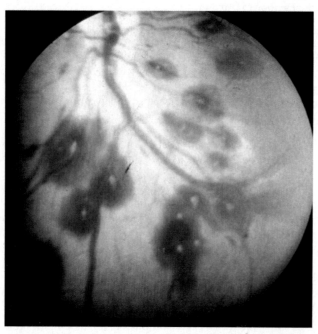

7.2: Multiple retinal hemorrhages in an 8-month-old victim of child abuse. *(Reproduced with permission from Eliott D, Avery R: Nonpenetrating posterior segment trauma. Ophthalmol Clin North Am, 8(4), 1995.)*

TABLE 7.1   Heat Injuries*

TYPES OF INJURY	BODY TEMPERATURE	SKIN	MENTAL STATUS
Heat cramps	37°C (98.6°F)	Moist and cool	Normal
Heat exhaustion	<40°C (<104°F)	Profuse sweating	Normal
Heat stroke	>40°C (>104°F)	Hot and dry (anhidrosis)	Impaired consciousness, CNS dysfunction

CNS, Central nervous system.
*Heat injury is exacerbated by high humidity.

F. Heat injuries (Table 7.1)
   1. Heat cramps
      a. Muscle cramps arising during exercise ("exercise-induced muscle cramps") as a result of fluid and electrolyte losses (not increased ambient temperature).
   2. Heat exhaustion
      a. Constellation of nonspecific symptoms (weakness, malaise, and headache), along with a mildly elevated body temperature.
      b. Brain function, and thus mental status examination, is normal.
      c. Laboratory findings of hemoconcentration (e.g., increased hemoglobin and hematocrit) due to hypovolemia.
   3. Heat stroke
      a. Defined as a markedly elevated body temperature (to >40°C) with associated changes in brain function (mental status changes, delirium, seizures, and coma).
      b. Complications include:
         i. Rhabdomyolysis (elevated creatine kinase and myoglobinuria).
         ii. Acute kidney injury (due to volume depletion and/or myoglobin toxicity) characterized by elevated blood urea nitrogen and serum creatinine levels.
         iii. Disseminated intravascular coagulation (thrombocytopenia, prolonged prothrombin time/partial thromboplastin time, hypofibrinogenemia, and elevated D-dimers).
         iv. Hepatic injury (increases aminotransferase enzymes).
         v. Hypotension (due to fluid losses and cardiac dysfunction).
G. Frostbite
   1. Injury secondary to freezing of tissue (ice crystals cause lysis of cell membranes and cell death).
   2. Superficial involvement (e.g., skin) may result in blistering but eventually heals without tissue loss.
   3. Extension into deeper tissues (muscles, nerves, and tendons) however leads to severe tissue necrosis, necessitating debridement, and/or amputation.
H. Lightning injury
   1. Lightning accounts for ~30 deaths per year in the United States, usually secondary to arrhythmia or respiratory arrest.
I. Electrical injury
   1. Clinical manifestations
      a. Thermal skin burns.
      b. Cardiac arrhythmias (e.g., ventricular fibrillation), potentially fatal.
      c. Rhabdomyolysis (muscle breakdown).
      d. Acute kidney injury (myoglobin-induced tubule injury).
J. Drowning
   1. Respiratory impairment from immersion in a liquid.
   2. May be nonfatal (previously called "near drowning") or fatal.
      a. Common cause of accidental death in the United States.
   3. Pathophysiologic effects
      a. Hypoxemia (secondary to aspiration and/or reflex laryngospasm) with associated complications (e.g., cerebral hypoxia and metabolic acidosis).
      b. Hypothermia.
      c. Aspiration pneumonia.
K. High-altitude illness
   1. Although the concentration of oxygen remains 21% (as at sea level), barometric pressure (P_{atm}) is reduced at altitude.
   2. As illustrated by the alveolar gas equation, patients develop hypoxemia (decreased blood oxygenation):
      a. $PAO_2 = (FiO_2 \times [P_{atm} - PH_2O]) - (PaCO_2/R)$.
      b. Lower barometric pressures at high altitude are therefore associated with lower alveolar oxygenation.
         i. ↓ Partial pressure of alveolar oxygen (PAO_2).
      c. Decreases diffusion of oxygen across the alveolus → hypoxemia (reduced PaO_2) and reduced tissue oxygenation (hypoxia).

      i. Hypoxia stimulates peripheral chemoreceptors in the carotid and aortic bodies to increase the respiratory rate.

        (1) Known as the "hypoxic ventilatory response."

      ii. As ventilation increases, more CO_2 is "blown off" (reduces $PaCO_2$ and causes respiratory alkalosis).

   3. Acute mountain sickness

     a. Usually at elevations above 6500 feet; becoming more likely with an increasing elevation.

     b. Manifestations (e.g., headache, fatigue, lightheadedness, anorexia, nausea and vomiting, and impaired sleep) are usually present within the first 24 hours at altitude, before resolving over 1–2 days.

   4. High-altitude cerebral edema

     a. More likely at elevations above 10,000 feet.

     b. Usually develop symptoms of acute mountain sickness first.

     c. Manifestations include ataxia, lassitude, and mental status changes (e.g., drowsiness, confusion, somnolence, and coma).

     d. Potentially fatal and requires immediate descent and supplemental oxygen.

   5. High-altitude pulmonary edema

     a. More likely at elevations above 10,000 feet.

     b. Characterized by the accumulation of protein-rich fluid within the alveoli (due to breakdown in the alveolar–capillary barrier and pulmonary vasoconstriction).

     c. Presents with cough, dyspnea, tachypnea, and tachycardia.

     d. Imaging shows bilateral diffuse patchy opacities.

     e. Potentially fatal and requires immediate descent and supplemental oxygen.

III. Radiation Injury

A. Ionizing radiation

   1. Medical testing, industrial exposures, and accidental (e.g., nuclear reactor incidents) or intentional (e.g., nuclear weapons) release.

   2. Radiation damages tissues either directly, by damaging DNA, or indirectly via the formation of free radicals.

   3. Tissue susceptibility varies.

     a. Tissues with high cell turnover (hematopoietic precursors within the bone marrow and gastrointestinal mucosa) are very sensitive.

     b. Tissues with low cell turnover (e.g., bone, nervous tissue, muscle, and skin) are more resistant.

   4. Radiation effects in various tissues

     a. Hematopoietic system: lymphopenia (initial change), thrombocytopenia, and hypoplasia of bone marrow.

     b. Vascular system: thrombosis (early), fibrinoid necrosis, and fibrosis (late finding); ultimately ischemic injury.

     c. Gastrointestinal system: diarrhea (acute effect) and bowel obstruction (long-term effect secondary to scarring).

B. Nonionizing radiation injury

   1. Sources include infrared light and visible (UV) light.

   2. Does not penetrate tissue and is easily shielded (e.g., sunscreen and clothing).

   3. Damaging to cells through direct transfer of thermal energy.

   4. Clinical examples include sunburn and corneal burns (photokeratitis).

   5. Long-term complications include skin cancers (basal cell carcinoma, most common; squamous cell carcinoma; malignant melanoma).

I. **Nutrient and Energy Requirements in Humans**
  A. **Recommended dietary allowance**
    1. Average daily dietary intake necessary to meet the nutritional requirements of most individuals; varies with age, gender, and pregnancy.
  B. **Daily energy expenditure**
    1. The total number of kilocalories ("calories") used each day.
    2. Dependent upon physical activity and basal metabolic rate (BMR).
    3. BMR
      a. Controlled by thyroid hormone.
      b. Accounts for 60%–75% of daily energy requirements.
      c. Amount of energy used by the body to support normal physiologic functions (e.g., respiration, temperature maintenance, tissue synthesis, maintenance of ion pumps, etc.).
    4. Factors influencing the BMR:
      a. Body weight
        i. BMR increases as weight increases.
      b. Body composition
        i. Muscle has a higher metabolic activity than adipose tissue; muscular individuals have a higher BMR.
      c. Gender
        i. Males with higher muscle mass than females of similar size and have a higher BMR.
      d. Age
        i. BMR decreases with aging.
      e. Thyroid hormone
        i. Hypothyroidism → decreases BMR.
        ii. Hyperthyroidism → increases BMR.
      f. Fever
        i. Increases resting metabolic rate.
    5. Degree of physical activity
    a. As expected, an increase in physical activity is associated with increased energy expenditure.
II. **Dietary Fuels**
  A. **Carbohydrates**
    1. Glucose
      a. Stored primarily as glycogen in the liver and muscle.
        i. Muscle uses glycogen to support its own energy needs.
        ii. Glucagon stimulates glycogenolysis of hepatic glycogen and used as a source of glucose for the other tissues (e.g., during fasting).
      b. Red blood cells (RBCs) require glucose for energy needs.
        i. Mature RBCs lack mitochondria; glycolysis is used for the generation of adenosine triphosphate (ATP).
      c. Complete oxidation of glucose produces 4 kcal/g.
    2. Digestion of carbohydrates
      a. Amylase (present within saliva and pancreatic secretions) converts polysaccharides (e.g., starch) into disaccharides (e.g., lactose, maltose, and sucrose).

b. Disaccharidases (e.g., lactase, maltase, and sucrase) within the brush border of enterocytes convert disaccharides into monosaccharides (glucose, galactose, and fructose).

    i. Lactase hydrolyzes lactose → galactose + glucose.

    ii. Maltase hydrolyzes maltose → two glucose molecules.

    iii. Sucrase hydrolyzes sucrose → fructose + glucose.

c. Monosaccharides (glucose, galactose, and fructose) are then absorbed via both active and passive processes.

3. Etiologies of carbohydrate malabsorption

    a. Deficiency of amylase.

    b. Deficient disaccharidase enzyme activity

      i. Lactase deficiency

        (1) Inability to metabolize lactose, resulting in bloating, flatulence, and osmotic diarrhea following the ingestion of dairy products.

        (2) Common after childhood in many populations (e.g., Asians, Native Americans, and Blacks).

    c. Disruption of the enterocyte brush border

      i. Viral enteritis (e.g., rotavirus) causes transient disruption of brush border.

    d. Decreased intestinal surface area available for absorption

      i. Celiac disease, tropical sprue.

B. Proteins

1. Role of dietary protein

    a. Provides essential amino acids necessary for protein synthesis.

    b. Provides nitrogen needed for the synthesis of the nonessential amino acids and other nitrogen-containing molecules (e.g., nucleic acids).

    c. Amino acids are also used as substrates for gluconeogenesis.

    d. Complete oxidation of protein produces 4 kcal/g.

2. Digestion of protein

    a. Begins in the stomach as pepsinogen is converted into active pepsin (by gastric acid released from parietal cells).

    b. Pepsin cleaves proteins into smaller polypeptides.

    c. Once the food bolus enters the duodenum, pancreatic proteases (e.g., trypsin) continue the digestive process.

3. Causes of protein malabsorption

    a. Loss of surface area for absorption (e.g., celiac disease).

    b. Loss of pancreatic protease enzymes (e.g., chronic pancreatitis).

C. Fats

1. Role of dietary fats

    a. Energy source: complete oxidation of fat produces 9 kcal/g.

    b. Cell membrane structure and function, hormone precursors, and carriers of fat-soluble vitamins (A, D, E, and K).

2. Digestion of fat

    a. Chewing (mastication), along with mixing in the stomach, breaks down dietary fats into smaller particles thereby increasing the surface area exposed to lipolytic enzymes and bile acids.

    b. Secretin, released as gastric acid enters the duodenum, stimulates the pancreas to secrete bicarbonate into the lumen of the duodenum.

      i. Bicarbonate neutralizes duodenal pH.

      ii. Important because digestive enzymes are inactivated in an acidic environment. Explains why patients with excessive gastric acid (e.g., Zollinger–Ellison syndrome) can develop manifestations of malabsorption (e.g., diarrhea).

    c. Lipolytic enzymes (e.g., lipase and colipase) from the pancreas hydrolyze triglycerides into monoglyceride and two fatty acids.

    d. Absorption of dietary fat occurs primarily within the proximal two-thirds of the jejunum.

    e. Following the absorption into the enterocyte, fatty acids are reformed into triglycerides and cholesterol esters and bound to apoprotein B48 to form chylomicrons.

      i. Apolipoprotein B (ApoB) and microsomal triglyceride transfer protein (MTTP) act together to incorporate triglycerides into chylomicrons.

    f. Chylomicrons cross the basolateral membrane into the intestinal lymphatics before draining into the systemic circulation.

3. Fat malabsorption

    a. Causes loss of fat in the stool (steatorrhea).

    b. Due to disturbance in any of the preceding steps:

      i. Small intestinal disease (e.g., celiac disease).

      ii. Deficient pancreatic enzymes (e.g., chronic pancreatitis).

      iii. Insufficiency of bile acids

        (1) Impaired enterohepatic circulation (e.g., ileal disease and resection).

        (2) Inadequate bile acid synthesis (e.g., liver disease).

        (3) Impaired entry of bile acids into the duodenum (e.g., cholestasis).

iv. Abetalipoproteinemia
  (1) Abetalipoproteinemia is a rare autosomal recessive disorder due to mutations in the *MTTP* gene.
  (2) MTTP catalyzes the transfer of triglycerides to ApoB.
  (3) Impairs absorption of dietary fats; manifests with reduced serum triglycerides, reduced serum cholesterol, and irregularly- shaped RBCs (acanthocytes) due to abnormalities in the membrane.
 c. Complications of fat malabsorption
  i. Fat-soluble vitamin (A, D, E, and K) deficiency.
  ii. Deficiency of essential fatty acids (linoleic acid and linolenic acid) with associated clinical manifestations (e.g., scaly dermatitis and poor wound healing).

III. **Protein–Energy Undernutrition**
 A. **Energy deficit due to deficiency of macronutrients.**
 B. **Severity based on reduction in body mass index (BMI).**
  1. BMI = weight in kilogram per height in square meter.
   a. Normal BMI = 18.5–24.9 kg/m².
 C. **Two major forms are seen in children (Fig. 8.1).**

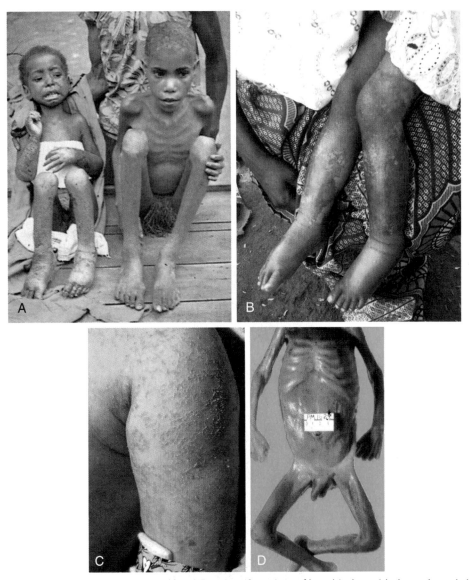

8.1: (A) Kwashiorkor and marasmus. The child on the left exhibits manifestations of kwashiorkor with dependent pitting edema and areas of desquamation on the legs and arms, giving a "flaky paint" appearance. Alternating dark and light areas are noted in the hair. The child on the right has marasmus with "broomstick" extremities due to the loss of muscle and subcutaneous tissue. (B) Pitting edema of the legs in a child with kwashiorkor. (C) Kwashiorkor: "flaky paint" dermatitis. (D) Marasmus. (*A, From Forbes C, Jackson W:* Color atlas and text of clinical medicine, *ed 2, London, 2002, Mosby, p 343, Fig. 7-138; B, from Goldman L, Schafer A: Goldman's Cecil medicine, ed 25, 2016, Saunders Elsevier, p 1435, Fig. 215-2; C, from Katz KA, Mahlberg MH, Honig PJ, et al: Rice nightmare: kwashiorkor in 2 Philadelphia-area infants fed Rice Dream beverage, J Am Acad Dermatol 52(5 Suppl 1):S69–S72, 2005; D, from Stevens A, Lowe J, Scott I: Core pathology, ed 3, 2009, Mosby Elsevier, p 148, Fig. 9-7.*)

1. Kwashiorkor
   a. Characterized by severe protein malnutrition with hypoalbuminemia.
   b. Low levels of albumin are associated with a loss of oncotic pressure, explaining the characteristic finding of bilateral peripheral edema.
   c. Additional manifestations include:
      i.   Marked muscle wasting and retention of fat.
      ii. Patchy depigmentation of the hair and skin ("flaky paint").
      iii. Hepatomegaly (secondary to fatty infiltration).
      iv. Growth retardation.
      v.   Poor prognosis.
2. Marasmus
   a. Disorder of severe caloric deficiency.
   b. Characterized by extreme muscle wasting ("broomstick extremities") and a loss of subcutaneous fat.
   c. Growth retardation.
   d. Better prognosis than kwashiorkor but still relatively high mortality.

IV. **Eating Disorders and Obesity**
   A. **Anorexia nervosa (Fig. 8.2)**
      1. Definition
         a. Eating disorder characterized by a distorted body image, a fear of weight gain, and a relentless pursuit of weight loss (despite being underweight).
      2. Epidemiology
         a. More common in females; onset typically during adolescence.
         b. Coexisting psychologic disorders (e.g., anxiety, depression, and substance abuse) are common.
         c. Increased mortality compared with the general population, commonly related to hypokalemic-induced cardiac dysrhythmia or suicide.
      3. Subtypes
         a. "Restricting" refers to the loss of weight primarily through dieting and/or excessive exercise.
         b. "Binge eating/purging" is characterized by binge eating followed by purging (e.g., self-induced vomiting, misuse of laxatives, enemas, and diuretics) to maintain a low body weight.
      4. Clinical manifestations
         a. Cardiovascular
            i. Structural changes (e.g., myocardial atrophy and fibrosis).
            ii. Functional changes (e.g., bradycardia and arrythmias).

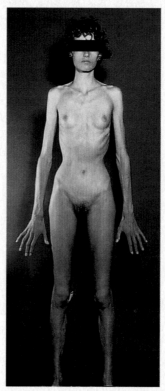

8.2: Anorexia nervosa. Note the loss of muscle and subcutaneous tissue consistent with total calorie deprivation. *(From Forbes C, Jackson W: Color atlas and text of clinical medicine, ed 2, London, 2002, Mosby, p 344, Fig. 7-147.)*

   b. Gynecologic
      i. Decreased gonadotropin-releasing hormone (GnRH) secretion (i.e., hypogonadotropic hypogonadism), causing infertility (anovulation), secondary amenorrhea, and bone demineralization (osteopenia and osteoporosis).
   c. Gastrointestinal
      i. Delayed gastric emptying (gastroparesis) with early satiety and bloating.
   5. Laboratory findings
      a. Decreased levels of GnRH, follicle-stimulating hormone, luteinizing hormone, and estradiol.
      b. Increased serum growth hormone and cortisol (stress hormones).
B. **Bulimia nervosa**
   1. Definition
      a. Eating disorder characterized by recurrent episodes of binge eating (overeating/drinking) followed by self-induced vomiting.
   2. Epidemiology
      a. More common than anorexia nervosa; predominantly arising during adolescence to early adulthood; more common in females.
   3. Clinical manifestations
      a. Complications related to vomiting include the loss of dental enamel (secondary to gastric acid), hypokalemia, and metabolic alkalosis.
      b. Hematemesis (vomiting blood) due to the tear of the distal esophagus (Mallory–Weiss tear).
      c. Esophageal rupture (Boerhaave syndrome).
   4. Laboratory findings
      a. Hypokalemia (often associated with cardiac arrhythmias, a common cause of death), hypochloremia, and metabolic alkalosis.
C. **Obesity**
   1. Definition
      a. Excess body weight; defined by a BMI $\geq 30\,kg/m^2$.
   2. Epidemiology
      a. Extremely common (over 35% of adults in the United States).
      b. Increased prevalence with aging to ~60 years after which weight tends to level off or decline.
      c. Increasing prevalence in children; correlates with an increased risk of obesity during adulthood.
      d. Major preventable cause of death and disability.
   3. Etiology
      a. Ingestion of excess calories, often in relation to one or more environmental factors (e.g., sugar-sweetened beverages, physical inactivity, and/or psychosocial stress).
      b. Rarely, obesity may be associated with an underlying disease state.
         i. Cushing syndrome (excess cortisol; either endogenous or exogenous).
         ii. Hypothyroidism (reduced BMR).
         iii. Brain lesions (e.g., trauma and inflammatory processes) particularly involving the ventromedial or paraventricular regions of the hypothalamus or the amygdala, may be associated with hyperphagia (excessive ingestion of food) and the development of obesity.
   4. Clinical findings associated with obesity (Table 8.1).
V. **Vitamins**

> **25-Hydroxyvitamin D (25-hydroxycholecalciferol)**
> Major circulating form of vitamin D with a long half-life.
> Used as a measure of vitamin D status.

A. **Overview (Fig. 8.3)**
   1. Vitamins are organic compounds required in small amounts from the diet.
   2. Absorption of fat-soluble vitamins is dependent upon fat absorption in the small bowel.
      a. Reason why those with impaired fat absorption (e.g., chronic pancreatitis and bile salt deficiency) may develop a deficiency of fat-soluble vitamins.
   3. Toxicity
      a. Fat-soluble vitamins are stored in adipose tissue and thus may be toxic in excess doses.
      b. Water-soluble vitamins are not stored; excess doses are excreted by kidneys.
B. **Fat-soluble vitamins**
   1. Vitamin A
      a. Functions
         i. Important for rhodopsin (photoreceptor pigment in retina).
         ii. Differentiation and maintenance of epithelial tissues.
      b. Deficiency
         i. Rare in the United States.
         ii. Etiologies: inadequate intake, fat malabsorption, and liver disease.

TABLE 8.1   Clinical Findings Associated With Obesity

CLINICAL FINDINGS	COMMENTS
Cancer	Increased incidence of estrogen-related cancers (e.g., endometrial and breast) due to aromatase enzyme in adipose (converts androgens to estrogens).
Cholelithiasis	Increased incidence of cholecystitis and cholesterol stones (bile is supersaturated with cholesterol).
Diabetes mellitus, type 2	Increased adipose downregulates insulin receptor synthesis and causes hyperinsulinemia. Weight reduction upregulates insulin receptor synthesis.
Hepatomegaly	Hepatic steatosis (fatty change); risk of progression (nonalcoholic steatohepatitis).
Hypertension	Hyperinsulinemia increases sodium retention (mineralocorticoid effect), increasing plasma volume and blood pressure. Complications include left ventricular hypertrophy and stroke.
Hypertriglyceridemia	Decreases high-density lipoprotein, increasing risk of coronary artery disease.
Increased low-density lipoprotein levels	Low-density lipoprotein predisposes to coronary artery disease.
Obstructive sleep apnea	Excess adipose tissue of upper airway contributes to the development; associated with respiratory acidosis (retention of CO_2) and hypoxemia ($\downarrow$ arterial PO_2). Hypoxemia and respiratory acidosis cause vasoconstriction of pulmonary vascular smooth muscle → pulmonary hypertension. Once pulmonary hypertension develops, the right ventricle becomes hypertrophied. The combination of pulmonary hypertension and right ventricular hypertrophy is called cor pulmonale.
Osteoarthritis	Degenerative arthritis occurs in weight-bearing joints (e.g., femoral heads).

CO_2, Carbon dioxide; PO_2, oxygen partial pressure.

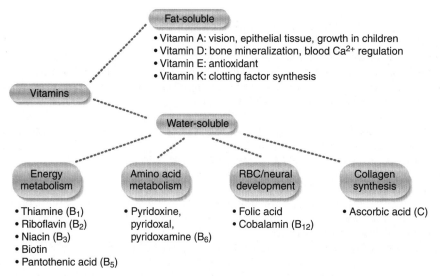

8.3: Classification and functions of the vitamins. Water-soluble vitamins are usually cofactors in key biochemical reactions, whereas fat-soluble vitamins are involved in the growth and development of tissue (vitamin A), neutralization of free radicals (vitamin E), bone mineralization and maintenance of serum calcium (vitamin D), and hemostasis (vitamin K). *Ca²⁺*, Calcium ion; *RBC*, red blood cell. *(From Pelley J, Goljan E: Rapid review biochemistry, ed 3, Philadelphia, 2011, Mosby Elsevier, p 40, Fig. 4-2.)*

    c. Toxicity
       i. Stored in the liver, toxicity possible in those who ingest the liver of polar bears, whales, and shark or with the excessive use as medicinal agent (e.g., isotretinoin in the treatment of acne).
  2. Vitamin D
    a. Most endogenous vitamin D is derived from the photoconversion of 7-dehydrocholesterol in the skin to 25-hydroxyvitamin D in the liver and then to 1,25-dihydroxyvitamin D in the kidneys (Fig. 8.4).
       i. 1,25-Dihydroxyvitamin D (calcitriol)
          (1) Most active form of vitamin D.
          (2) Short half-life precludes its use as a measure of vitamin D levels.
    b. Levels of 1,25-hydroxyvitamin D are controlled by serum levels of calcium and phosphorus.
       i. Hypocalcemia and/or hypophosphatemia trigger the release of parathyroid hormone (PTH) from the parathyroid glands.
       ii. PTH stimulates 1-α-hydroxylase enzyme (kidney) to increase the synthesis of calcitriol, the most active form of vitamin D.

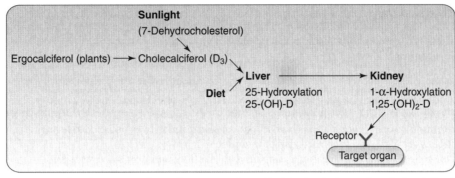

8.4: Vitamin D metabolism. Most vitamin D comes from photoconversion of 7-dehydrocholesterol to cholecalciferol (vitamin D3).

    iii. Granulomatous processes (e.g., sarcoidosis) can cause hypervitaminosis D (due to 1-α-hydroxylase enzyme present within macrophages of granulomata).
  c. As with all fat-soluble vitamins, the absorption of dietary vitamin D is dependent upon intact fat absorption (see Vitamin A discussion).
  d. Functions of vitamin D (calcitriol)
    i. Maintenance of serum calcium and phosphate
      (1) Calcitriol increases calcium and phosphate absorption from the small bowel; increases renal reabsorption of calcium.
      (2) Calcium and phosphate are required for the mineralization of epiphyseal cartilage and osteoid matrix in bone formation.
  e. Vitamin D deficiency
    i. Etiologies include inadequate dietary intake, fat malabsorption, lack of adequate sunlight exposure, liver disease (impaired 25-hydroxylation), and renal disease (impaired 1-α-hydroxylation).
    ii. Manifestations of vitamin D deficiency are those of reduced intestinal absorption of calcium and phosphorous.
    iii. Chronic deficiency → hypocalcemia and hypophosphatemia → bone demineralization.
      (1) Osteomalacia (adults) and rickets (children).
  f. Vitamin D toxicity
    i. Can occur following the ingestion of excess exogenous vitamin D or increased endogenous synthesis (e.g., sarcoidosis).
3. Vitamin E
  a. Functions
    i. Alpha-tocopherol (a major active form of vitamin E) functions as a free radical scavenger (i.e., antioxidant).
    ii. Protects against lipid peroxidation of cell membranes.
  b. Vitamin E deficiency
    i. Fat malabsorption (e.g., chronic pancreatitis)
    ii. Cholestatic liver disease (insufficient bile salts for fat emulsification)
    iii. Reduced enterohepatic recirculation of bile salts (e.g., resection or disease of terminal ileum).
4. Vitamin K
  a. Sources of vitamin K include:
    i. Gut bacterial synthesis of vitamin K (major source); endogenously synthesized vitamin K is activated by the liver microsomal enzyme epoxide reductase.
    ii. Green vegetables (e.g., spinach and broccoli).
  b. Function
    i. Vitamin K is an important cofactor for the γ-carboxylation of glutamate residues within vitamin K-dependent clotting factors (II, VII, IX, and X) as well as anticoagulant factors (proteins C and S).
    ii. γ-Carboxylation allows for calcium binding and clot formation.
  c. Causes of vitamin K deficiency
    i. Use of broad-spectrum antibiotics (eradicates colonic bacteria that synthesize vitamin K).
    ii. Newborns
      (1) Bowel is sterile at birth; therefore newborns are vitamin K deficient for the first week of life.
      (2) Intramuscular vitamin K given at birth to prevent bleeding.
    iii. Decreased epoxide reductase activity
      (1) Liver disease.
      (2) Coumarin anticoagulants (warfarin)
        (a) Rat poison often contains warfarin, explaining the potentially life-threatening bleeding complications associated with the ingestion of rat poison. Treated by vitamin K injection (or fresh frozen plasma when actively bleeding).

    iv. Fat malabsorption

        (1) Like all fat-soluble vitamins, fat maldigestion (e.g., chronic pancreatitis) or malabsorption (e.g., celiac disease) can potentially result in a deficiency of vitamin K.

C. Water-soluble vitamins

  1. Thiamine (vitamin B1)

    a. Sources of thiamine

      i. Common sources include yeast, legumes, brown rice, and cereals made from whole grains.

        (1) Processing of white cereals or rice ("polished" rice) removes thiamine → reason thiamine deficiency is most commonly seen in populations whose diet consists primarily of polished rice or milled white cereals.

      ii. Alcoholics are also at an increased risk of thiamine deficiency.

        (1) Due to inadequate dietary intake, impaired absorption, and decreased storage.

    b. Metabolic function

      i. Thiamine is a cofactor for several enzymes involved in energy metabolism.

    c. Deficiency (known as beriberi)

      i. Populations at risk include chronic alcoholics and those with previous bariatric surgery.

      ii. "Dry" beriberi refers to a symmetrical distal sensorimotor peripheral neuropathy.

      iii. "Wet" beriberi refers to cardiac manifestations (e.g., cardiomegaly, cardiomyopathy, and heart failure).

    d. Wernicke–Korsakoff

      i. Wernicke encephalopathy

        (1) Acute triad of gait ataxia, confusion, and ophthalmoplegia (oculomotor dysfunction).

        (2) Classically seen in alcoholics given intravenous glucose solutions prior to thiamine supplementation.

        (3) Associated with atrophy of the mamillary bodies.

      ii. Korsakoff syndrome

        (1) Refers to chronic neurologic changes, usually a long-term complication of Wernicke encephalopathy; characterized by memory loss and confabulation.

  2. Riboflavin (vitamin B2)

    a. Function

      i. Essential component of coenzymes involved in various metabolic pathways (e.g., energy production and fat metabolism).

    b. Sources

      i. Dairy products, meats, fish, vegetables, and fortified food products.

    c. Deficiency

      i. Uncommon; most likely in anorexia nervosa, malabsorption syndromes.

  3. Niacin (vitamin B3, nicotinic acid)

    a. Function

      i. Required for oxidation–reduction reactions.

        (1) Component of nicotinamide adenine dinucleotide (NAD) and nicotinamide adenine dinucleotide phosphate (NADP).

    b. Sources

      i. Both plant and animal foods are good sources, also endogenous synthesis from tryptophan.

    c. Deficiency (pellagra)

      i. The "4 Ds": dermatitis, diarrhea, dementia, and death.

      ii. Causes of deficiency

        (1) In the United States, primarily seen in alcoholics or anorexia nervosa.

        (2) Malabsorption (e.g., bariatric surgery and malabsorptive disorders) may be contributory.

        (3) Corn-based diets have poor niacin bioavailability (a major cause of niacin deficiency in some regions of the world).

        (4) Carcinoid syndrome (tryptophan diverted to the production of serotonin instead of niacin).

        (5) Hartnup disease

          (a) Inherited disorder associated with impaired tryptophan absorption (less available for the endogenous synthesis of niacin).

  4. Pyridoxine (vitamin B6)

    a. Pyridoxine converted within the liver to the active pyridoxine 5-phosphate.

    b. Functions in various biochemical pathways including gluconeogenesis, conversion of tryptophan to niacin, heme synthesis, and neurotransmitter synthesis.

    c. Mild deficiency is well tolerated; therefore symptomatic deficiency is rare, etiologies include severe malnutrition and chronic use of isoniazid (treatment of tuberculosis).

    d. Clinical manifestations of deficiency include:

      i. Weakness and sensory ataxia due to a peripheral axonal neuropathy, seizures, seborrheic dermatitis, and microcytic anemia.

  5. Vitamin B12 (cobalamin) and folic acid are discussed in Chapter 12.

6. Biotin
   a. Functions as a cofactor in carboxylase reactions.
   b. Found in organ meats, eggs, fish, seeds, and nuts.
   c. Deficiency is rare, historically associated with long-term total parenteral nutrition (TPN) (before routine biotin supplementation was begun).
      i. Excessive ingestion of raw egg whites (contains avidin that binds to biotin, preventing its absorption).
7. Ascorbic acid (vitamin C)
   a. Functions in several biochemical reactions, including:
      i. Collagen synthesis (hydroxylation reactions of proline and lysine residues within collagen).
   b. Sources include citrus fruits, tomatoes, strawberries, and spinach.
   c. Deficiency (scurvy)
      i. Rare in the United States; primarily in alcoholics, older adults.
      ii. Impaired collagen synthesis → defective wound healing, defective tooth formation, and impaired function of osteoblasts and fibroblasts.
      iii. Manifestations include follicular hyperkeratosis and perifollicular hemorrhage, with petechiae and coiled hairs; ecchymoses, bleeding gums (Fig. 8.5).
   d. Toxicity
      i. Excessive vitamin C may cause false negative stool guaiac test result, increased risk of oxalate kidney stones.

VI. **Trace Elements (Micronutrients Required in the Normal Diet)**
   A. Zinc
      1. Zinc is involved in the maintenance of protein structure and enzymatic reactions.
      2. Dietary sources include meat, eggs, and seafood.
      3. Deficiency
         a. Malnutrition and malabsorption syndromes (e.g., following gastric bypass surgery) and increased urinary losses (e.g., diuretics).
         b. Acrodermatitis enteropathica is a rare autosomal recessive disorder of impaired zinc absorption.
      4. Manifestations of deficiency
         a. Diarrhea, dermatitis, growth retardation, and impaired immune function.

   B. Copper
      1. Copper is present in a variety of vegetables and meats.
      2. Important for the function of numerous enzymes, including those involved in the defense of oxidative injury, neurotransmitter synthesis, collagen cross-linking, clotting, and melanin production.
      3. Causes of deficiency include:
         a. Chronic diarrhea or other malabsorptive disorders (e.g., celiac disease and following gastric bypass surgery).
         b. Dialysis (peritoneal or hemodialysis).
         c. Menkes disease (a rare inherited disorder of impaired copper absorption).
      4. Copper excess (Wilson disease—see Chapter 19).

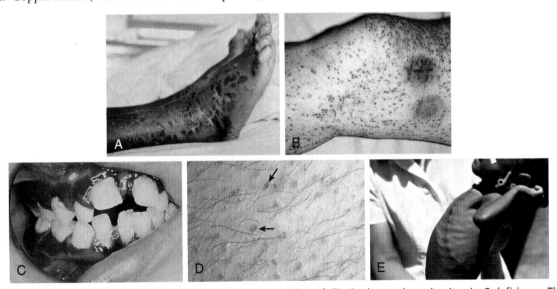

8.5: (A) Pellagra. Note the areas of irregular hyperpigmented skin. (B) Perifollicular hemorrhage in vitamin C deficiency. The areas of hemorrhage surround hair follicles. (C) Gums showing the effects of scurvy. The swelling, inflammation, and bleeding of the gingival papillae are prominent. (D) Corkscrew hairs in vitamin C deficiency. Note the coiled hairs lying within plugged follicles. (E) Scorbutic rosary in vitamin C deficiency (excess osteoid). *(A and C, From Morgan SL, Weinsier RL: Fundamentals of clinical nutrition, ed 2, St. Louis, 1998, Mosby; B, from Callen JP, Palier AS, Creer KE, Swinyer LJ: Color atlas of dermatology, ed 2, Philadelphia, 2000, Saunders; D, from Savin JA, Hunter JAA, Hepburn NC: Diagnosis in color: skin signs in clinical medicine, London, 1997, Mosby-Wolfe, p 85, Fig. 3-8; E, courtesy of Dr. JD Maclean, McGill Centre for Tropical Diseases, Montreal; from Kliegman RM: Nelson textbook of pediatrics, ed 20, 2016, Elsevier, p 329, Fig. 50-1.)*

  C. **Iodine**
    1. Iodine is used to synthesize thyroid hormone.
    2. Present in fish and seafood.
    3. Many countries, including the United States, fortify table salt with iodine; deficiency is therefore rare.
    4. Deficiency results in reduced thyroid hormone (T3 and T4) levels; clinically recognizable as an enlarged thyroid (goiter) secondary to chronic stimulation by thyroid-stimulating hormone.
  D. **Chromium**
    1. Functions as a coenzyme in reactions involving insulin (facilitates the binding of glucose to adipose and muscle glucose transport units).
    2. Deficiency is most often secondary to malnutrition.
    3. Less commonly seen in those receiving TPN without supplementation.
  E. **Selenium**
    1. Present in seafood, liver, kidney, and other meats.
    2. Functions as a component of glutathione peroxidase, which produces reduced glutathione (an antioxidant) and for the iodo-thyronine deiodinase in the production of thyroid hormone.
    3. Deficiency is most often associated with TPN.
  F. **Fluoride**
    1. Useful in the prevention of dental caries.
    2. Added to community water supplies (fluoridation).
    3. Excessive ingestion (e.g., fluoride supplements) or occupational exposure can lead to fluoride toxicity.
      a. Dental fluorosis results in discoloration of the teeth.
      b. Skeletal fluorosis leads to bone fragility with increased fracture risk.
VII. **Dietary Fiber**
  A. **Fiber is the portion of plants that cannot be digested.**
  B. **Soluble fiber (dissolves in water)**
    1. Present in oatmeal, nuts, beans, lentils, and fruits (e.g., apples and blueberries).
    2. May help to lower blood glucose and cholesterol.
  C. **Insoluble fiber (does not dissolve in water)**
    1. Present in wheat products (e.g., whole wheat bread), brown rice, legumes, carrots, cucumber, and tomatoes.
    2. Promotes regular bowel movements.
      a. By preventing constipation, insoluble fiber can protect against diverticulosis.
      b. Binds to potential carcinogens for excretion in the stool, may help to reduce the risk of colorectal carcinoma.
VIII. **Special Diets**
  A. **Dietary Approach to Stop Hypertension (DASH) diet**
    1. Low-salt, low-fat diet with emphasis on fruit and vegetables.
    2. Found to decrease blood pressure more than salt reduction alone.
  B. **"Mediterranean" diet**
    1. No strict definition, generally associated with high dietary intake of fruits, vegetables, whole grains, beans, nuts, seeds, fish, and poultry but little red meat.
    2. Alcohol in moderation is allowed.
    3. Associated with decreased stroke risk and lower overall mortality.
  C. **Low-salt diet**
    1. Dietary salt (sodium chloride) should generally be limited; especially in those with hypertension, heart failure, or kidney disease.

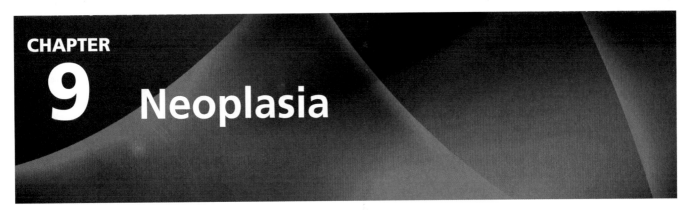

I. **Nomenclature**
   A. **Neoplasia**
      1. New cell growth (benign or malignant).
   B. **Benign tumors**
      1. Neoplasia in which the proliferating cells do not invade or spread to other sites.
   C. **Malignant tumors**
      1. Neoplasia in which the proliferating cells have the ability to invade and spread to other sites (an important criterion of malignancy).
   D. **Tumor of epithelial tissue**
      1. Tumors that arise from surface epithelium (e.g., squamous, glandular, and urothelial), may be either benign or malignant.
   E. **Tumors of connective tissue**
      1. May be either benign or malignant, for example:
         a. Lipoma is a benign tumor of adipocytes.
         b. Liposarcoma is a malignant tumor of adipocytes.
         c. Chondroma is a benign tumor of chondrocytes (cartilage).
         d. Chondrosarcoma is a malignant tumor of chondrocytes.
         e. Leiomyoma is a benign tumor of smooth muscle cells.
         f. Leiomyosarcoma is a malignant tumor of smooth muscle cells.
   F. **Teratoma**
      1. Tumors derived from more than one germ layer (ectoderm, endoderm, and/or mesoderm), may be benign or malignant (Fig. 9.1).
      2. Most common site of origin is the ovary; however, teratomas may also arise from the testis or other sites, usually near the midline (e.g., pineal gland and anterior mediastinum).
   G. **Carcinoma**
      1. Malignancy of epithelial tissue (e.g., squamous cell carcinoma, adenocarcinoma, and urothelial carcinoma).
      2. Primary sites for the development of squamous cell carcinoma (tumor of squamous epithelial cells) include:
         a. Oropharynx, larynx, upper/middle esophagus, lung, cervix, penis, and skin.
         b. Histology of squamous cell carcinoma reveals keratin pearls (stain bright red with hematoxylin–eosin [H&E] stain) and/or intercellular bridge formation (Fig. 9.2).
      3. Primary sites for the development of adenocarcinoma (tumor of glandular epithelium) include:
         a. Lung, distal esophagus to rectum, pancreas, liver, breast, endometrium, ovaries, kidneys, and prostate.
         b. Histologically, adenocarcinoma is characterized by the presence of glands (Fig. 9.3), often containing mucin.
            i. Mucin may be highlighted with the use of periodic acid-Schiff or Alcian blue stain.
      4. Primary sites for urothelial carcinoma include:
         a. Urinary bladder, ureter, and renal pelvis.
   H. **Sarcomas**
      1. Malignant tumors of connective tissue (mesoderm origin).
      2. Examples include those arising in bone (osteosarcoma), cartilage (chondrosarcoma), or skeletal muscle (rhabdomyosarcoma).
   I. **Hamartoma**
      1. Neoplastic growth of cells indigenous to a particular site but in a disorganized fashion.
      2. Examples include pulmonary hamartoma and Peutz-Jeghers polyp.

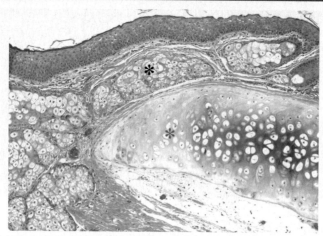

9.1: Teratoma of the ovary. Note squamous epithelium (epithelial origin), sebaceous glands (black asterisk - endodermal origin), and cartilage (red asterisk - mesodermal origin). *(From Clement PB, Young RH: Atlas of gynecologic surgical pathology, ed 3, 2014, Saunders Elsevier, p 420, Fig. 15.29.)*

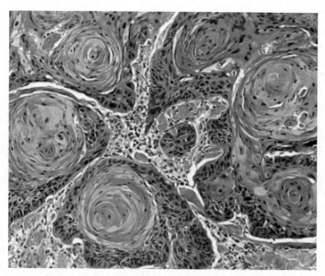

9.2: Invasive squamous cell carcinoma. Note the bright pink "swirls" of keratin (keratin "pearl"). *(From Diagnostic histopathology of tumors, ed 5, Copyright © 2021 by Elsevier, Fig. 23.42.)*

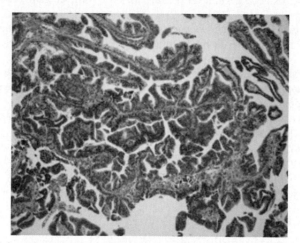

9.3: Adenocarcinoma. Note the glandular growth pattern. *(From Diagnostic histopathology of tumors, ed 5, Copyright © 2021 by Elsevier, Fig. 12C.63.)*

J. Choristoma (heterotopic rest)

1. Refer to nonneoplastic tissue located at a site in which it is not normally present (e.g., pancreatic tissue in the wall of the stomach).

II. Properties of Benign and Malignant Tumors

A. Benign tumors usually resemble parent tissue (i.e., are well differentiated) and do not have the ability to invade or spread to distant sites.
  1. Examples include lipoma and tubular adenoma.

B. Malignant tumors may range from well to poorly differentiated.
  1. Well differentiated (low grade) describes tumors where the histologic appearance is similar to that of the parent tissue.
  2. Poorly differentiated (high grade) refers to tumors in which the histologic appearance does not closely resemble the parent tissue and often requires special techniques to determine the tissue type.
  3. Moderately differentiated (intermediate grade) refers to tumors whose cells exhibit histologic features intermediate between those of low- and high-grade tumors.

C. Cytologic features of malignancy
  1. Pleomorphism
     a. Cells vary in size and shape from one another.
  2. Loss of cell-to-cell cohesion
     a. Diffuse gastric carcinoma and invasive lobular carcinoma of the breast are two examples. In both tumors, the loss of intercellular adhesion molecules (E-cadherins) causes a loss of intercellular adhesion (tumor cells infiltrate as single cells).
  3. Nuclear abnormalities
     a. Nuclei within malignant cells are often larger, irregular, and hyperchromatic (darker), often with large irregular nucleoli.
     b. Increase in nuclear size explains the increase in the nuclear to cytoplasmic (N:C) ratio.
  4. Mitosis
     a. Often increased; abnormal mitotic figures may be seen (Fig. 9.4).

D. Neoplasms develop from a single precursor cell (i.e., they are monoclonal).
  1. Normal tissue is polyclonal.

E. Lymphatic metastasis
  1. Lymphatic spread to regional lymph nodes is a typical finding with most carcinomas.
     a. Breast cancer → axillary lymph nodes.
     b. Papillary carcinoma of thyroid → cervical lymph nodes.
     c. Lung carcinoma → hilar lymph nodes.
  2. Pathogenesis is as follows:
     a. Tumor cells invade lymphatic channels and embolize to the draining lymph node via the afferent lymphatic.
     b. Within the node, tumor cells first invade the subcapsular sinus (the first location of metastatic disease within the node).
     c. Continued growth of the tumor results in partial to complete replacement of the nodal parenchyma.
     d. Tumor cells then invade the efferent lymphatic channel, allowing for spread to additional lymph nodes.
     e. Eventually, if left unchecked, tumor cells gain access to vascular channels and disseminate throughout the body.

F. Hematogenous metastasis
  1. Penetration of the basement membrane (collagenase) allows tumor cells to become invasive and spread into surrounding tissue.
  2. If/when tumor cells enter the vascular system, they travel downstream (embolize) and lodge within another tissue.

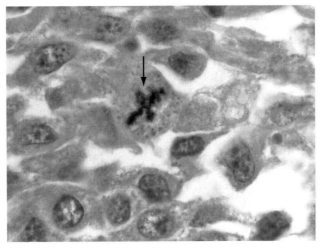

9.4: Abnormal mitotic figure (H&E). This micrograph of a malignant tumor of the skin contains an abnormal mitotic figure (*arrow*). Such abnormalities are frequently seen in malignant tumors and are virtually never found in normal tissues and benign tumors. *(From Young B, O'Dowd G, Woodford P: Wheater's functional histology: a colour text and atlas, ed 6, 2014, Churchill Livingstone Elsevier, p 44, Fig. 2.9.)*

a. To access nutrients (e.g., glucose and oxygen), a blood supply is required (Fig. 9.5).
    b. Angiogenic factors (e.g., vascular endothelial growth factor) are required to form new blood vessels.
3. Sarcomas characteristically spread hematogenously without involving the lymph nodes (unlike carcinoma).
    a. Commonly metastasize to the lungs.
4. Malignant cells that enter the portal vein (e.g., colon cancer) first metastasize to the liver, whereas those that enter the vena cava (e.g., breast cancer) metastasize to the lungs first.
    a. Both carcinomas and sarcomas can disseminate hematogenously, carcinomas just typically invade lymphatics first.
        i. Exceptions include follicular carcinoma of the thyroid, renal cell carcinoma, and choriocarcinoma (all commonly spread through the bloodstream).
G. **Direct tumor implantation (seeding)**
    1. Refers to tumor spread via exfoliation of malignant cells from the tumor surface.

Sloughing of tumor cells is followed by the implantation and growth on and within adjacent tissues or body cavities (pleural, pericardial, or peritoneal).

- Ovarian carcinoma commonly seeds the peritoneal cavity causing omental and peritoneal implants.
- Peripherally located lung tumors may seed the pleura causing malignant pleural effusions (diagnosis can often be made on cytologic examination of effusion fluid).
- Medulloblastoma, a malignant brain tumor within cerebellum, commonly exfoliates malignant cells into the cerebrospinal fluid, thereby seeding the subarachnoid space (called "drop metastasis").

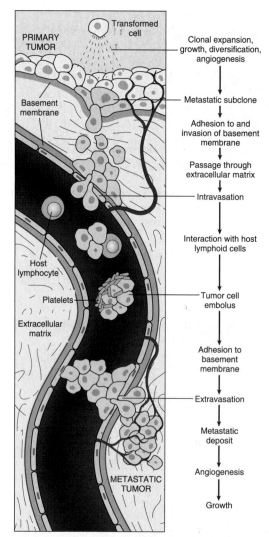

9.5: Sequential steps involved in the hematogenous spread of cancer from a primary to a distant site. To invade from the primary site, cancer cells must lose their cell-to-cell adhesion molecules and then gain the ability to move through the tissue. This occurs as the cells first adhere to, and then degrade the basement membrane, pass through the extracellular matrix, and penetrate the vascular wall of a capillary. Tumor cells that survive in circulation, lodge within the capillary endothelium of a distant organ (e.g., lung) and begin to grow at the new site (metastasis). (*From Kumar V, Fausto N, Abbas A, Aster J: Robbins and Cotran pathologic basis of disease, ed 8, Philadelphia, 2010, Saunders Elsevier, p 298, Fig. 7.36.*)

H. Bone metastasis
1. Vertebral column is a common site for bony metastasis.
2. Carcinomas of the breast, lung, and prostate commonly metastasize to bone.
   a. Batson paravertebral venous plexus is responsible for the predilection of bone metastases to the vertebrae.
3. Osteoblastic metastasis (bone formation within metastatic foci).
   a. Due to the activation of osteoblasts by cytokines released from tumor cells.
   b. Tumors that produce osteoblastic metastasis include prostate cancer (most common) and breast cancer.
   c. Osteoblastic metastasis may be accompanied by an elevated serum alkaline phosphatase (released by osteoblasts).
   d. See radiodensity on imaging.
4. Osteolytic metastases (metastatic foci characterized by bone breakdown).
   a. Due to the activation of osteoclasts by substances (e.g., prostaglandin E_2 and interleukin-1 [IL-1]) released from tumor cells.
   b. Tumors that commonly produce lytic bone metastases include lung cancer, renal cell carcinoma, and multiple myeloma.
   c. May present with pathologic fractures and/or hypercalcemia (with extensive osteolysis).
I. Common metastatic sites/primary tumor
1. Lymph nodes (e.g., metastatic breast/lung cancer, most common).
   a. Most common overall site for metastasis.
2. Lungs (e.g., metastatic breast cancer, the most common cause).
3. Liver (e.g., metastatic colorectal cancer, the most common cause).
4. Bone (e.g., metastatic breast cancer, the most common cause).
5. Brain (e.g., metastatic lung cancer, the most common cause).

III. Cancer Epidemiology
A. Malignancy is the second most common cause of death in the United States (behind heart disease).
B. Various external factors (e.g., tobacco, alcohol, chemicals, radiation, and microbial pathogens).
1. Tobacco, particularly from smoking cigarettes, is a major cause of cancer.
C. Internal factors include hormones, immune status, inheritance, and age.
1. Increasing age is an important risk factor for the development of cancer; majority arise after the age of 55 years.
D. Racial and ethnic differences affect cancer incidence.
1. African Americans at the greatest risk of prostate cancer.
2. Fair-skinned individuals are more likely to develop skin cancer (lack of the protective effect of melanin against ultraviolet light).
E. Cancer incidence by age and sex
1. Children
   a. Malignant neoplasms are the leading cause of disease-related (noninjury) mortality among children 1–14 years of age.
   b. Top three malignancies in children, in decreasing order:
      i. Leukemia (acute lymphoblastic leukemia, most common).
      ii. Central nervous system tumors (e.g., medulloblastoma).
      iii. Neuroblastoma (a malignant tumor of postganglionic sympathetic neurons).
   c. Other malignancies that are more common in children include:
      i. Embryonal rhabdomyosarcoma (malignancy of skeletal muscle).
      ii. Wilms tumor (a malignant tumor of the kidney; derived from the metanephric blastema).
      iii. Retinoblastoma (a malignant tumor of eye).
      iv. Osteosarcoma (a tumor of osteoblasts).
      v. Ewing sarcoma (neuroectodermal malignancy of bone).
2. Adults
   a. Epithelial tumors (e.g., lung, colon, and breast) are far more common in adults.
   b. Top three noncutaneous cancers in males (decreasing order):
      i. Prostate, lung/bronchus, and colorectal.
   c. Top three noncutaneous cancers in females (decreasing order):
      i. Breast, lung/bronchus, and colorectal.
   d. Cancer-related mortality (in descending order):
      i. Males: lung/bronchus, prostate, and colorectal.
      ii. Females: lung/bronchus, breast, and colorectal.
F. Cancer and heredity
1. Inherited predisposition to cancer accounts for ~5% of all cancers.
G. Specific risk factors
1. Nasopharyngeal carcinoma: Epstein–Barr virus (EBV).
2. Squamous cell carcinoma of the oropharynx and esophagus (alcohol and smoking).
3. Hepatocellular carcinoma (hepatitis B virus [HBV], hepatitis C virus [HCV], and aflatoxin).
4. Burkitt lymphoma, endemic type (EBV).
5. Kaposi sarcoma (human herpesvirus 8 [HHV-8]).

H. Tumor prevention
1. Lifestyle modification
   a. Cessation of smoking cigarettes (most important)
      i. Decreases the risk of multiple malignancies.
   b. Increased dietary fiber/decreased saturated fat
      i. Decreases the risk of colorectal cancer.
   c. Reduction of alcohol intake.
   d. Weight loss
      i. Recall that adipose tissue contains an enzyme (aromatase) that converts androgens into estrogens.
      ii. Elevated estrogen levels are associated with an increased risk of breast and endometrial cancer.
   e. Sunscreen
      i. Decreases the risk of developing skin cancer.
   f. Immunization
      i. HBV immunization → decreases the risk of hepatocellular carcinoma due to HBV-induced cirrhosis.
      ii. Human papillomavirus (HPV) immunization → decreases the risk of squamous cell carcinoma of the cervix, penis, and oropharynx.
I. Screening procedures to detect cancer
1. Cervical Papanicolaou (Pap) smears
   a. Decrease the risk of cervical cancer.
2. Colonoscopy
   a. Detects and removes precancerous polyps, thereby decreasing the risk of colorectal carcinoma.
3. Mammography
   a. Detects nonpalpable breast masses.
4. Prostate-specific antigen (PSA)
   a. More sensitive than specific for the diagnosis of prostate cancer (may also be elevated in prostatic hyperplasia and prostatitis).
J. Treatment of underlying disease processes may secondarily decrease cancer risk.
1. Treatment of *Helicobacter pylori* infection decreases the risk of developing malignant lymphoma of the stomach.
2. Treatment of gastroesophageal reflux disease (GERD) decreases the risk of developing esophageal adenocarcinoma
   a. GERD → Barrett esophagus (a potential precursor of esophageal adenocarcinoma).

IV. Carcinogenesis
A. Overview of carcinogenesis
1. Cancer is a multistep process involving gene mutations, telomerase activation, angiogenesis, invasion, and metastasis.
2. Types of gene mutations producing cancer
   a. Point mutations (the most common mutation).
   b. Balanced translocations.
   c. Insertion of a viral genome (insertional mutagenesis).
   d. Other mutations, such as deletion, gene amplification (multiple copies of a gene), and overexpression (increased gene transcription; results in the production of excess protein product).
B. Classes of genes commonly involved mutated in malignancy include:
1. Proto-oncogenes
   a. Normal genes that regulate cell growth and repair.
   b. Mutated forms, known as an oncogene, have lost the ability to regulate cell growth.
   c. An important feature of oncogenes is that a single altered copy allows for unregulated growth.
   d. Oncogenes that are often mutated in human cancers include *KRAS*, *BRAF*, and *ERB-B2* (*HER-2*).
2. Tumor suppressor genes
   a. Regulate gene transcription and DNA repair.
   b. Mutated tumor suppressor genes have lost this ability; cell is no longer able to pause replication to allow for DNA repair (allows for unregulated cell growth).
   c. As opposed to proto-oncogenes, both copies of a tumor suppressor gene must be mutated to cause malignancy.
   d. Tumor suppressor genes commonly mutated in human cancers include *TP53*, *CDKN2A*, and *CDKN2B*.

TP53 is the most commonly mutated gene in human cancer.

3. Antiapoptosis genes
   a. Apoptosis ("programmed cell death") can be induced by a variety of signals (e.g., irreparable DNA damage).
      i. Causes a loss of cell before it can become malignant.
   b. B-cell lymphoma gene 2 (*BCL2*) proteins are antiapoptotic.
      i. Overexpression of these genes prevent apoptosis of irreversibly damaged cells (allows mutated cells to survive).
   c. Chromosomal translocations involving *BCL2* [t(14;18)] cause overexpression of BCL2 (important in the pathogenesis of follicular lymphoma).

4. DNA repair genes
   a. Mismatch repair genes produce proteins that correct errors in nucleotide pairing.
   b. Mutations involving DNA repair genes allow cells with nonlethal damage to proliferate (thereby increasing one's risk of cancer).
   c. Lynch syndrome is characterized by a loss of DNA mismatch repair; causes "hereditary nonpolyposis colorectal carcinoma" and other malignancies.

Xeroderma pigmentosa

Caused by inherited defects in nucleotide excision repair genes.
Affected individuals are at a markedly increased risk (~1000-fold) of skin cancer due to an inability to correct for sunlight-induced (UV radiation) cross-linking of pyrimidine residues.

V. **Carcinogenic Agents**
   A. **Infection**
      1. Oncogenic viruses
         a. HBV: hepatocellular carcinoma.
         b. HCV: hepatocellular carcinoma.
         c. HHV-8: Kaposi sarcoma.
         d. HPV: Cervical cancer and anal cancer.
         e. EBV: Hodgkin lymphoma, Burkitt lymphoma, and nasopharyngeal carcinoma.
         f. Human T-lymphotropic virus 1 (HTLV-1): Adult T-cell leukemia/lymphoma.
      2. *Helicobacter pylori*
         a. Bacterium that infects the stomach; increases the risk of gastric adenocarcinoma and gastric lymphoma.
      3. Parasites
         a. *Schistosoma haematobium* is associated with the development of squamous cell carcinoma of the bladder.
         b. Liver flukes (*Clonorchis*, *Opisthorchis*, and *Fasciola*) are associated with an increased risk of cholangiocarcinoma (cancer of bile ducts).
   B. **Radiation**
      1. Induces free radical injury.
      2. Radiation-induced malignancies include leukemia, thyroid cancer, and others.
   C. **Chemical carcinogens**
      1. Aflatoxin (hepatocellular carcinoma).
      2. Aromatic amines (bladder cancer).
      3. Arsenic (angiosarcoma of liver and squamous cell carcinoma of skin).
      4. Asbestos (lung cancer and mesothelioma).
      5. Benzene (acute lymphoblastic leukemia).
      6. Cigarette smoke, multiple carcinogens including arsenic, cadmium, chromium, nickel, and nitrosamines (lung, larynx, pancreas, bladder, and others)
      7. Vinyl chloride (angiosarcoma of liver)
   D. **Physical injury**
      1. Squamous cell carcinoma may develop in third-degree burn scars or at the orifices of chronically draining sinus tracts (e.g., chronic osteomyelitis).
VI. **Tumor Staging**
   A. **Tumor stage is the most important prognostic factor (more important than histologic grade).**
   B. **Tumor, nodes, metastasis (TNM) stage**
      1. T refers to tumor size and extent of growth.
      2. N refers to the presence or absence of nodal involvement by tumor.
      3. M refers to the presence or absence of extranodal metastases (e.g., liver and lung).
VII. **Cancer Effects on the Host**
   A. **Cachexia (wasting)**
      1. Generalized catabolic reaction with anorexia, muscle wasting, loss of subcutaneous fat, and fatigue.
      2. Due to the release of various cytokines (e.g., tumor necrosis factor) by host.
   B. **Anemia**
      1. Anemia of chronic disease is most common (increased hepcidin, see Chapter 12).
      2. Iron-deficiency anemia in some cases (e.g., colorectal carcinoma with associated gastrointestinal blood loss).
      3. Macrocytic anemia due to folate deficiency
         a. More likely with rapidly growing tumors (e.g., leukemia) that consume folate stores during replication.
      4. Autoimmune hemolytic anemia
         a. Particularly with certain hematologic malignancies (e.g., chronic lymphocytic leukemia).

5. Myelophthisic anemia
   a. Anemia secondary to the replacement of bone marrow by malignant cells and/or fibrous tissue.
   b. The presence of teardrop-shaped red blood cells is a clue.

C. **Increased risk of thrombosis (hypercoagulable effect of malignancy)**
   1. May be associated with increased coagulants and/or release of procoagulants (especially common with pancreatic carcinoma).
   2. Disseminated intravascular coagulation may occur, due to the release of tissue thromboplastin (thromboplastin activates the coagulation system—as seen with acute promyelocytic leukemia (APL).

D. **Fever**
   1. Due to infection and/or release of pyrogens (IL-1).
   2. Infections are a common cause of death in those with cancer.

E. **Paraneoplastic syndromes**
   1. Distant effects of a tumor unrelated to metastatic disease.
   2. May be the first evidence of malignancy.
   3. Ectopic release of hormones from tumor.
      a. Adrenocorticotropic hormone released from small-cell lung cancer—causing Cushing syndrome.
      b. Antidiuretic hormone (ADH) released from small-cell carcinoma of the lung—causing the syndrome of inappropriate ADH (SIADH).
         i. Clue is severe hyponatremia (e.g., serum sodium < 120 mEq/L)
      c. Parathyroid hormone-related peptide released from squamous cell carcinoma of the lung—causing hypercalcemia.
   4. Tumor-related neurologic manifestations
      a. Encephalitis due to antibodies against the N-methyl-D-aspartate receptor (ovarian teratoma).
      b. Myasthenia gravis due to antibodies against the acetylcholine receptor at the neuromuscular junction (thymoma).
      c. Lambert–Eaton myasthenic syndrome due to antibodies against the presynaptic P/Q type voltage-gated calcium channel (small-cell lung cancer).
      d. Opsoclonus-myoclonus syndrome
         i. Hypotonia, ataxia; associated with neuroblastoma.
   5. Tumor-related skin changes

Tumor markers

Tumor markers are used to follow the course of therapy.
- Alpha-fetoprotein (AFP)—hepatocellular carcinoma, yolk sac tumor
- Cancer antigen 19-9 (CA 19-9)—pancreatic adenocarcinoma
- CA-125—ovarian surface epithelial tumors (e.g., serous carcinoma)
- Prostate-specific antigen (PSA)—prostatic adenocarcinoma
- Carcinoembryonic antigen (CEA)—colorectal carcinoma

      a. Acanthosis nigricans (gastric carcinoma).
      b. Sudden eruption of multiple seborrheic keratosis; known as the sign of Leser-Trélat (gastric carcinoma).

I. **Lipoprotein Disorders**
   A. **Overview**
      1. Cholesterol and triglycerides are insoluble in water and therefore must bind with proteins, called apoproteins, to form lipoproteins.
      2. Lipoproteins have a central core of cholesterol esters and triglycerides surrounded by free cholesterol, phospholipids, and apolipoproteins (Fig. 10.1).
         a. Polar groups of the surface molecules face outward, thereby making the lipoproteins water soluble and able to circulate in the bloodstream.
      3. Apolipoproteins also act as ligands for lipoprotein receptors to regulate lipoprotein metabolism.
   B. **Lipoprotein composition**
      1. Chylomicrons (CMs)
         a. Least dense lipoprotein comprised mostly of triglycerides.
         b. Transport diet-derived triglycerides in circulation; absent during fasting.
      2. Very-low-density lipoprotein (VLDL)
         a. Secreted by the liver and carries endogenous triglycerides in circulation.
         b. Calculated by dividing serum triglyceride by 5 (TG/5).
      3. Intermediate-density lipoprotein (IDL)
         a. Product of VLDL catabolism.
      4. Low-density lipoprotein (LDL)
         a. Delivers cholesterol to the periphery ("bad" cholesterol).
      5. High-density lipoprotein (HDL)
         a. Involved in reverse cholesterol transport ("good" cholesterol).
   C. **Exogenous lipoprotein pathway (Fig. 10.2)**
      1. Enterocytes (epithelial lining cells of the small intestine) absorb dietary monoglycerides and fatty acids.
      2. Dietary lipids are then recombined, along with apolipoprotein B (ApoB-48), to create a nascent (newly formed) CM.
      3. Nascent CMs are absorbed into intestinal lymphatics, drain into the thoracic duct, and empty into the bloodstream.
      4. Once in circulation, HDL transfers apoprotein C-II (ApoC-II) and apoprotein E (ApoE) to the nascent CM to form a "mature" CM.
      5. Mature CMs circulate to muscle and adipose tissue where ApoC-II interacts with an enzyme attached to the luminal surface of endothelial cells (lipoprotein lipase).
         a. Activation of lipoprotein lipase requires insulin.
      6. Lipoprotein lipase releases free fatty acids (FFAs) from the CM. FFAs are used by muscle for energy or stored within the adipose tissue.
         a. Residual particle, known as a "CM remnant," has ApoE on the surface.
         b. ApoE interacts with the hepatic LDL receptor (allows for the uptake of the CM remnant).
   D. **Endogenous lipoprotein pathway (Fig. 10.3)**
      1. With the liver, fatty acids are recombined with ApoB-100, to form VLDL, and secreted into circulation.
      2. Using the same process as described for CMs, VLDL circulates to muscle and adipose tissue where lipoprotein lipase releases FFAs to form IDL.
         a. IDL is cleaved to form LDL and then taken up by the liver and other tissues (via receptor-mediated uptake).

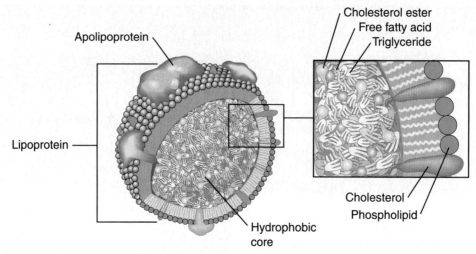

10.1: Lipoprotein structure. Lipoproteins are spherical particles with a hydrophobic core and an amphiphilic surface. The surface consists of a single layer of phospholipids. This surface layer also contains proteins (making it soluble in the water phase of plasma) and free cholesterol. The hydrophobic core mainly contains triglycerides and cholesterol esters. *(From McPherson, R, Pincus, M:* Henry's clinical diagnosis and management by laboratory methods, *ed 21, Philadelphia, 2007, Saunders, p 227, Fig. 17.1.)*

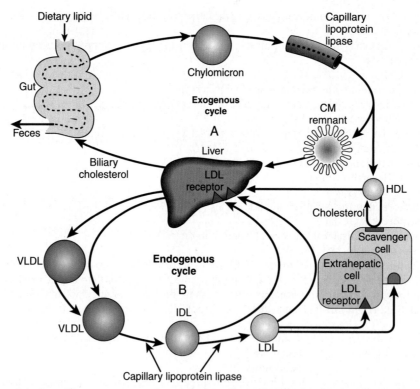

10.2: Schematic of lipid metabolism. The exogenous cycle on the top shows chylomicron (CM) synthesis from enterocytes in the small bowel. CMs that are synthesized in the small intestine enter the circulation. Capillary lipoprotein lipase hydrolyzes triglyceride in the CM releasing fatty acids and glycerol (not shown) and produces a CM remnant that is removed by the liver. The endogenous cycle on the bottom shows the liver synthesizing very-low-density lipoprotein (VLDL). VLDL enters the circulation, where capillary lipoprotein lipase hydrolyzes the triglyceride into fatty acids and glycerol (not shown) eventually producing intermediate-density lipoprotein (IDL), a remnant of VLDL. IDL is taken up by the liver, or continues to be hydrolyzed, becoming low-density lipoprotein (LDL). LDL is the primary carrier of cholesterol (CH). Most extrahepatic cells have receptors for LDL because they all need CH for cell membrane synthesis or, in some cases, for hormone synthesis (e.g., vitamin D and adrenal cortex hormones). Some of the CH returns to the liver and some goes to scavenger cells. CH released from scavenger cells is bound to high-density lipoprotein (HDL) to produce HDL-CH. HDL transports the CH to the liver, where it is used to synthesize bile salts and acids. *(Modified from Gaw A, Murphy MJ, Srivastava R, et al:* Clinical biochemistry: an illustrated colour text, *ed 5, 2013, Churchill Livingstone Elsevier, p 133, Fig. 66.2.)*

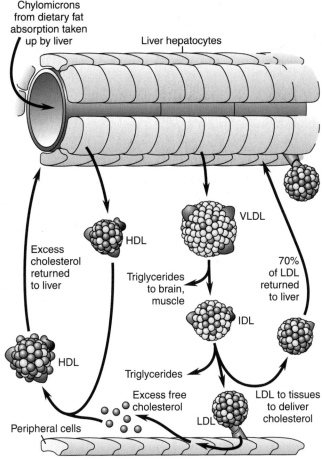

Chylomicrons
from dietary fat
absorption taken
up by liver

Liver hepatocytes

VLDL

HDL

Excess
cholesterol
returned
to liver

70%
of LDL
returned
to liver

Triglycerides
to brain,
muscle

IDL

HDL

Triglycerides

Excess free
cholesterol

LDL to tissues
to deliver
cholesterol

LDL

Peripheral cells

10.3: Schematic of lipoprotein metabolism in the body. Chylomicrons from dietary fat absorption are taken up by the liver and resynthesized into high-density lipoprotein (HDL) and very-low-density lipoprotein (VLDL). HDL circulates to the peripheral tissues and takes up excess cholesterol for transport back to the liver. Triglycerides are removed for tissue use from VLDL, which becomes intermediate-density lipoprotein (IDL). Additional triglyceride removal leads to the formation of low-density lipoprotein (LDL). LDL is absorbed by peripheral tissues to obtain cholesterol. About 70% of the circulating LDL returns to the liver. *(From Copstead LE, Banasik JL: Pathophysiology, ed 5, 2013, Saunders Elsevier, p 380, Fig. 18.2.)*

E. **Triglycerides**
1. CMs (carrying exogenous triglyceride) and VLDL (carrying endogenous triglyceride) transport most of the triglyceride in circulation.
   a. Normal serum triglyceride <150 mg/dL.
2. Elevated triglyceride levels (hypertriglyceridemia)
   a. An increase in CMs and/or VLDL will cause hypertriglyceridemia.
   b. Cutaneous manifestations of hypertriglyceridemia include eruptive xanthomas (Fig. 10.4D).
   c. Markedly elevated serum triglycerides (>1000 mg/dL) may cause the patient's plasma to appear "milky."
      i. "Lipemia retinalis" on the funduscopic examination (Fig. 10.4E); not seen with hypercholesterolemia.
3. Standing plasma test
   a. Can be used to determine which fraction (CM, VLDL, or both) accounts for the elevation in serum triglycerides.
   b. An aliquot of the patient's plasma is placed in a refrigerator overnight. The next morning, the specimen tube is evaluated.
      i. The presence of a creamy layer on top indicates hyperchylomicronemia (because CMs are the least dense lipoprotein and therefore float on the surface).
      ii. Conversely, elevated levels of VLDL cause the serum to be turbid.
      iii. The presence of both a creamy layer on top and a turbid plasma indicates that both fractions are elevated.
F. **LDL**
1. Comprised predominantly of cholesterol, a primary vehicle for cholesterol transport in circulation.
   a. Recall that LDL is derived from the hydrolysis of IDL.
2. LDL removed from circulation using LDL receptors in peripheral tissues (primarily liver).
3. An increase in serum LDL is associated with an increased risk of developing atherosclerotic vascular disease (e.g., coronary heart disease and peripheral arterial disease [PAD]).

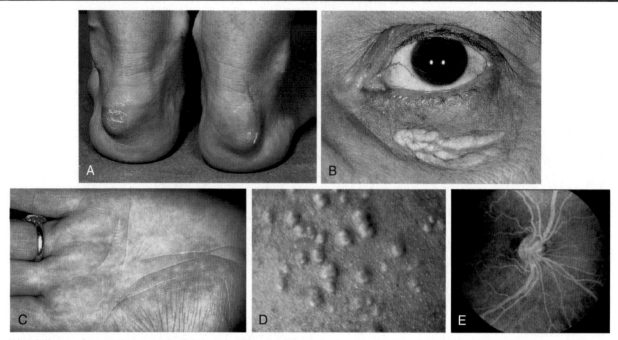

10.4: (A) Achilles tendon xanthoma. Note the slightly yellow nodular lesions at the distal end of the Achilles tendon. (B) Xanthelasma. Note the yellow, raised lesions on the lower left eyelid. (C) Palmar xanthomas. Note the yellow macules on the palm that are accentuated in the creases. (D) Eruptive xanthomas. Note the numerous small yellow papules distributed over the skin. (E) Lipemia retinalis. Note the milk-like retinal vessels. *(A, Courtesy Lant AF, MD, and Dequeker J, MD, London; B, From Yanoff M, Duker J: Ophthalmology, ed 3, St. Louis, 2009, Mosby, Fig. 12.9-18; C, Courtesy Marsden RA, MD, St. George's Hospital, London; D, E, from Melmed S, Polonsky KS, Larsen PR, Kronenberg HM: Williams textbook of endocrinology, ed 12, 2011, Saunders Elsevier, p 1651, Fig. 37.17G, B, respectively.)*

      a. The most common dermatologic manifestation of hypercholesterolemia (LDL) is xanthomas (firm, nontender cutaneous deposits of cholesteryl ester-enriched foam cells); Fig. 10.4A–C.
    4. Calculated LDL = total cholesterol − HDL − (TG/5).
      a. CMs, carrying dietary lipids, take hours to clear after a meal.
        i. For this reason, patients must fast for 8–12 hours before the measurement of serum triglycerides. Otherwise, the remaining CMs will falsely elevate the patient's triglyceride (and render a falsely low calculated LDL level).
    5. Functions of cholesterol
      a. Major component of cell membranes.
      b. Synthesis of steroid hormones and bile salts.
    6. Serum LDL level
      a. Optimal level: <100 mg/dL.
      b. As levels rise, there is a proportionate increase in the risk of developing atherosclerotic vascular disease.
  G. HDL
    1. Functions in "reverse cholesterol transport" whereby cholesterol from the periphery is returned to the liver for removal from circulation.
    2. Elevated HDL levels are associated with a decreased risk for the development of atherosclerotic vascular disease (e.g., coronary heart disease).
      a. Factors that increase HDL include niacin, exercise, and moderate alcohol intake.
    3. HDL also has a function in the transfer of apoproteins (e.g., ApoE, ApoC-II) between lipoprotein fractions.
    4. Optimal HDL levels are >60 g/dL, suboptimal when <40 mg/dL.
II. Arteriosclerosis
  A. Definition
    1. General term used to refer to the process of arterial "hardening" whereby the vessel walls thicken and lose elasticity.
  B. Subtypes
    1. Mönckeberg medial sclerosis
      a. Calcification within the wall of muscular arteries.
      b. Age-related phenomenon: not clinically significant as it does not encroach upon the vascular lumen.
    2. Atherosclerosis
      a. Most important subtype, prevalence increases with age.
      b. Affects large- (elastic) and medium-sized (muscular) arteries.
      c. Appear as raised yellow plaques that encroach upon vessel lumina.
      d. Risk factors for the development of atherosclerosis include:
        i. Increasing age
        ii. Hypertension (HTN)

iii. Diabetes mellitus (DM)
iv. Smoking
v. Dyslipidemia (↑ LDL and ↓ HDL)
e. Pathogenesis (in sequence):
    i. Endothelial injury/dysfunction
        (1) Occurs in association with turbulent nonlaminar blood flow.
        (2) Reason that branch points (e.g., carotid bifurcation) are commonly affected.
    ii. LDL infiltrates the intima (Fig. 10.5).
    iii. Monocytes adhere to and enter the intima (becoming macrophages).
    iv. Endothelial and inflammatory cells release various cytokines (e.g., interleukin-1), triggering an influx of macrophages and T cells.
    v. Phagocytosis of LDL by macrophages to form "foam" cells; collections of foam cells appear as "fatty streaks" (the first grossly recognizable finding of atherosclerosis).
    vi. Smooth muscle cells are recruited to the site as well, eventually contributing to the formation of an atherosclerotic plaque.
    vii. As a late event, the plaque undergoes calcification as well.
    viii. In summary, an atherosclerotic plaque is comprised of smooth muscle cells, macrophages, T cells, lipids, and extracellular matrix (e.g., collagen and elastic fibers).
        (1) Necrotic core of the plaque is comprised of lipids.
        (2) Overlying fibrous cap is comprised of smooth muscle cells and collagen.
f. Common sites of atherosclerosis
    i. Abdominal aorta (below renal arteries)
    ii. Iliac arteries
    iii. Coronary arteries
    iv. Popliteal arteries
    v. Internal carotid arteries
g. Complications of atherosclerosis include:
    i. Gradual narrowing of vessel lumen (due to the expansion of atherosclerotic plaque); causes ischemia of involved tissues (Fig. 10.6).

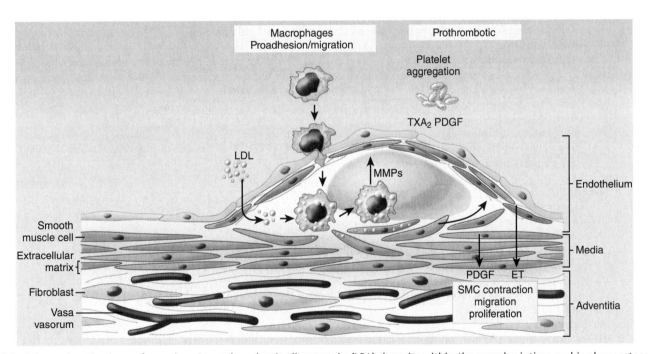

10.5: Atherosclerotic plaque formation. Excess low-density lipoprotein (LDL) deposits within the vascular intima and is phagocytosed by macrophages to form "foam cells." Subsequently, the macrophages release numerous cytokines including matrix metalloproteinases (MMPs). Platelets release thromboxane A2 (TXA2) and platelet-derived growth factor (PDGF) as well as inflammatory cytokines that attract macrophages and produce endothelial cell dysfunction (not shown). Smooth muscle cells (SMCs) contract (endothelin [ET]), proliferate (undergo hyperplasia), and migrate beneath endothelial cells. The yellow material beneath the endothelium represents necrotic debris. In later stages, matrix components produce collagen, proteoglycans, and elastin forming the mature fibrous plaque, the primary lesion of atherosclerosis. *(Modified from Goldman L, Ausiello D: Cecil's medicine, ed 23, Philadelphia, 2008, Saunders Elsevier, p 473, Fig. 69.1B.)*

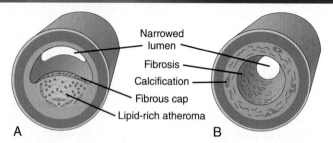

10.6: Atheroma of coronary arteries. (A) A soft atheroma consists of a semiliquid, lipid-rich core covered on the luminal side by a thin fibrous cap. (B) A hard atheroma consists of fibrous tissue, which is prone to calcification. It narrows the lumen and prevents normal dilatation of the artery. *(From* Pathophysiology, *2009, Saunders Elsevier, p 125, Fig. 4.36.)*

        (1) PAD (atherosclerosis of peripheral arteries) causes claudication (cramping pain in the buttock, thigh, and calf with ambulation) and poor wound healing with the risk of tissue necrosis (gangrene).

        (2) On examination, the affected limb exhibits reduced skin temperature, decreased hair growth on dorsum of the toes, diminished pedal pulses, and bruits over femoral and/or popliteal arteries.

        (3) Diagnosis of PAD

           (a) Ankle-brachial index

           Ratio < 0.9 is consistent with PAD.

           (b) Angiography

           (c) Ultrasonography

    ii. Plaque rupture

        (1) Rupture of the plaque's fibrous cap exposes procoagulant substances within the plaque. This is followed by the formation of an overlying platelet thrombus, which causes either partial or complete vascular occlusion and the acute onset of ischemia downstream (a major cause of an acute myocardial infarction).

    iii. Vascular weakness

        (1) Atherosclerotic thickening of the intima increases the distance that oxygen must diffuse to reach the deeper layers of the media.

        (2) Results in ischemia and weakness of the vessel wall; increased risk of aneurysm formation (discussed later).

    iv. Embolization

        (1) Fragments of atherosclerotic plaque ("atheroemboli") may break off and travel downstream causing an acute vascular occlusion.

        (2) Manifests with pain, pallor, paresthesia, paralysis, and pulselessness.

  3. Arteriolosclerosis

    a. Hyaline arteriolosclerosis

      i. Thickening of arteriole with associated luminal narrowing.

      ii. Due to the leakage of plasma components across the endothelium.

      iii. Risk factors include HTN and DM.

    b. Hyperplastic arteriolosclerosis

      i. Form of arteriolar narrowing seen in association with severe HTN.

      ii. Due to the duplication of basement membrane and hyperplasia of smooth muscle cells ("onion skinning").

      iii. Commonly involves renal arterioles (Fig. 10.7).

III. Aneurysms

  A. Definition

    1. Localized abnormal area of vascular dilation.

  B. Types

    1. Saccular aneurysm

      a. Aneurysm in which only a portion of the wall is dilated.

      b. "Berry" aneurysms, usually located around the circle of Willis at the base of the brain, is an example.

    2. Fusiform aneurysm

      a. Aneurysm in which there is circumferential dilation of the vessel, an example being abdominal aortic aneurysms (AAAs).

  C. Pathogenesis

    1. Weakness of the vascular wall in association with inherited (e.g., Ehlers–Danlos syndrome and Marfan syndrome) or acquired (atherosclerosis, HTN, and infection) conditions.

  D. AAA

    1. Usually arise below the renal arteries.

    2. Typically a disease of older males (>60 years), particularly in smokers.

    3. Weakening of the vessel wall, usually in association with atherosclerosis, results in a localized area of dilation (aneurysm).

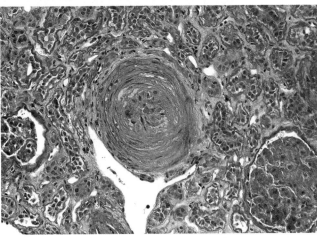

10.7: Hyperplastic arteriolosclerosis. Hyperplasia of the smooth muscle within small arteries and arterioles causes marked luminal narrowing, associated with severe hypertension. *(From Rosai and Ackerman's surgical pathology, ed 11, Copyright © 2018 by Elsevier, Fig. 23.90.)*

    4. Clinical manifestations
      a. Often asymptomatic; may have pulsatile abdominal mass.
      b. Portions of the plaque may embolize downstream resulting in ischemia of the distal extremities.
      c. Rupture is the most severe complication; characteristically associated with the sudden onset of abdominal or flank pain and hypotension.
        i. Aneurysm diameter is the greatest predictor of rupture.
        ii. Aneurysm diameter of ≥5.5 cm is associated with the highest risk.
E. Popliteal artery aneurysm
    1. Presents as a pulsatile mass behind the knee.
F. Mycotic aneurysm
    1. Weakening of vessel secondary to an infection.
G. Berry (saccular) aneurysm of cerebral arteries
    1. Typically located at the base of the brain around the circle of Willis.
    2. Most common site is the junction between the anterior cerebral and anterior communicating arteries.
    3. Thought to be a developmental abnormality (the absence of smooth muscle and intimal elastic lamina) in conjunction with HTN.
    4. More common in females, as well as certain inherited disorders (e.g., Marfan syndrome and autosomal dominant polycystic kidney disease).
    5. Rupture causes subarachnoid hemorrhage ("worst headache ever").
    6. Use of cocaine increases the risk of rupture.
H. Syphilitic aneurysm
    1. Complication of tertiary syphilis.
    2. Thought secondary to immune-mediated narrowing of vasa vasorum (endarteritis obliterans) resulting in ischemia and dilation of the vessel.
      a. Characteristically affects the ascending aorta (causing an aneurysm) and the aortic valve ring (causing aortic regurgitation).
    3. Grossly, see irregular intimal wrinkling ("tree barking") due to inflammation and scarring.

IV. Aortic Dissection
A. Definition
    1. Tear within the intima of the aorta, followed by the flow of blood into the wall causing the layer to "dissect" (split) as blood flows through the media of the aorta.
B. Epidemiology
    1. More common in males (4:1).
    2. Risk factors include increasing age (50+ years), HTN, and structural abnormalities of the aortic wall (e.g., Marfan syndrome and Ehlers–Danlos syndrome).
C. Pathogenesis
    1. First is a tear in the aortic intima (usually occurs within 10 cm of the aortic valve).
    2. Next, the high pressure of arterial blood flow causes the layers of the wall to split (dissect) as blood flows through the wall (forming a "false" lumen).
      a. Blood may dissect proximally and/or distally for a variable distance (Fig. 10.8).
      b. Potential for aortic rupture or myocardial ischemia from extension into the coronary arteries.
      c. Compression of the "true" lumen by the "false" lumen results in ischemic injury, potentially affecting aortic branch vessels.

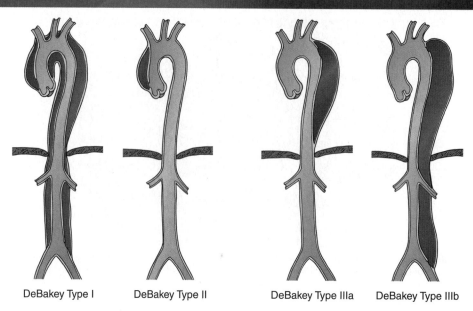

DeBakey Type I DeBakey Type II DeBakey Type IIIa DeBakey Type IIIb

Stanford Type A Stanford Type B

10.8: Diagram showing various patterns of aortic dissection. *(From* Rutherford's vascular surgery and endovascular therapy, *ed 9, Copyright © 2019 by Elsevier, Fig. 81.1.)*

D. Clinical manifestations
1. Acute onset of severe sharp pain in the anterior chest (may radiate into the back), acute aortic insufficiency possible.
2. Chest X-ray shows a widening of the aortic root.
3. Loss of pulse in upper extremities.
    a. Due to compression of the subclavian artery by the false lumen (blood within the wall).
4. Potential for rupture into the pericardial sac (causing cardiac tamponade).

V. Disorders of the Venous System
A. Varicose veins (Fig. 10.9)
1. Abnormally dilated, elongated, tortuous, and subcutaneous veins (≥3 mm in diameter).
2. Risk factors include prolonged standing, advanced age, pregnancy, and venous thrombosis.
3. Due to incompetence of venous valves with the subsequent retrograde flow of blood from the deep veins into superficial (subcutaneous) veins.

B. Venous thromboses
1. Venous thrombi are associated with stasis of blood flow (e.g., prolonged immobilization and postoperative state), often in association with an inherited thrombophilia (e.g., deficiencies of antithrombin, protein C, and protein S).
2. Most often originate within deep veins of the lower extremity (thus the term "deep venous thrombosis" [DVT]), particularly the calf region.
    a. Venous thrombi rarely arise within other veins (e.g., portal vein, hepatic vein, and cerebral veins).
3. DVT
    a. Acute manifestations
        i. Swelling of the affected leg relative to the other leg (>3 cm difference in circumference), pain, and erythema.
        ii. Pain on dorsiflexion of the foot (Homans sign).
        iii. Pitting edema (secondary to an increased hydrostatic pressure behind the venous obstruction).
    b. Chronic manifestations
        i. Stasis dermatitis
            (1) Erythematous and eczematous areas of discoloration, particularly of lower medial leg and ankle.
            (2) Due to increased venous pressure behind the obstructing venous thrombosis with associated extravasation of fluid (causing edema) and red blood cells into the skin (causing skin discoloration).
4. Superficial thrombophlebitis (inflammation of a clotted vein)
    a. Phlebitis refers to the inflammation of a vein; thrombosis is the presence of clot within the vein.
    b. Risk factors
        i. Intravenous cannulation.
        ii. Varicose veins.
        iii. Malignancy (classically adenocarcinoma of the pancreas; known as "Trousseau syndrome").
    c. Clinical manifestations
        i. Pain and tenderness to palpation along the course of the inflamed superficial vein.

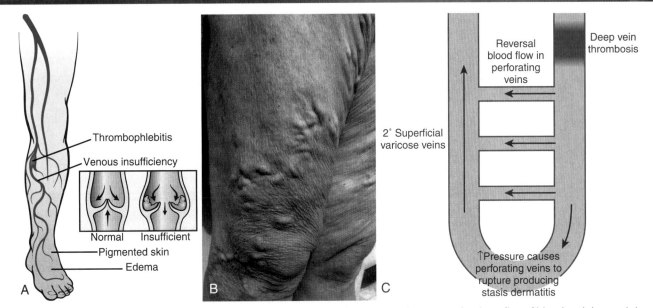

10.9: (A) Varicose veins of the calf. The inset shows venous valvular insufficiency, which accounts for the reflux of blood and the serpiginous dilation of the veins. Complications are also depicted, including thrombophlebitis (inflammation of the vein), pigmented skin from rupture of perforating branches around the malleolus (called stasis dermatitis), and edema due to increased hydrostatic pressure in the venous system. (B) Note the marked bilateral superficial varicosities on the lower extremity. The veins in the thighs are distended and tortuous. (C) Secondary superficial varicose veins from a deep vein thrombosis. Increased pressure behind the thrombus reverses blood flow through the perforating branches (damages the valves) and increases pressure in the superficial vessels, causing dilation. Increased pressure around the medial malleolus of the ankles ruptures the vessels and causes stasis dermatitis. *(A, From* Pathology for the health professions, *ed 4, 2012, Saunders Elsevier, p 158, Fig. 7.32; B, from Swartz MH:* Textbook of physical diagnosis: history and examination, *ed 7, 2014, Saunders Elsevier, p 397, Fig. 12.7.)*

    C. Superior vena cava (SVC) syndrome
        1. Definition
           a. Clinical manifestations are associated with obstruction of the SVC.
        2. Pathogenesis
           a. Extrinsic compression, or direct tumor invasion, of the SVC (most commonly a primary lung cancer).
        3. Clinical manifestations
           a. Edema and purple discoloration of the face, neck, and shoulders.
           b. Headache, confusion, and visual changes.
VI. Thoracic Outlet Syndrome
    A. Anatomy
        1. Thoracic outlet is bounded by the spinal column, the first ribs, and the clavicle.
        2. Structures that pass through the thoracic outlet include the brachial plexus, subclavian vein, and subclavian artery.
    B. Definition
        1. Thoracic outlet syndrome refers to clinical manifestations that arise when one or more of these neurovascular structures are compressed as they pass through the thoracic outlet.
    C. Etiologies
        1. Cervical rib, tight anterior scalene muscles, or positional changes in the neck and arms, particularly in muscular individuals.
    D. Clinical manifestations
        1. Symptoms are often exacerbated by sustained use of hands, especially when elevated (e.g., overhead lifting and brushing hair).
        2. Vascular signs (e.g., arm "falls asleep" while the person is sleeping).
        3. Nerve root signs (e.g., numbness and paresthesia [tingling]).
        4. Positive Adson test: diminished to absent radial pulse when a patient has the neck hyperextended, the arm extended, and looking to the side of the outstretched arm.
VII. Lymphatic Disorders
    A. Overview
        1. Lymphatics return excess fluid and proteins from interstitial spaces to the bloodstream.
        2. Thin-walled; predisposed to involvement by infection or tumor.
    B. Lymphangitis
        1. Inflammation of lymphatic vessel; usually following cutaneous inoculation of the microorganism (most commonly *Streptococcus pyogenes*).

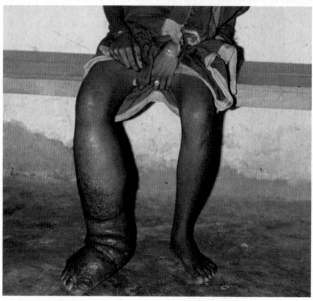

10.10: Elephantiasis (lymphedema) of the right leg due to filariasis (*Wuchereria bancrofti*). *(From Cohen J, Powderly W, Opal S:* Infectious diseases, *ed 3, Philadelphia, 2010, Elsevier, Fig. 115.1a.)*

    2. Following entry into the lymphatics, the invading organism then travels toward the draining lymph node causing red, tender streaks on the skin.

    3. Nodular lymphangitis is a form of lymphadenitis characterized by the development of tender subcutaneous nodules; usually in association with *Sporothrix schenckii* (sporotrichosis).

C. Lymphedema

    1. Definition

      a. Collection of lymphatic fluid within an interstitial tissue or body cavity.

    2. Epidemiology

      a. Rare in the United States; usually a complication of radical mastectomy and axillary lymphadenectomy, with or without associated radiation.

      b. Worldwide, the most common cause is filariasis (Fig. 10.10).

    3. Clinical manifestations

      a. Swelling of the affected limb with a feeling of "heaviness" or "tightness."

D. Chylothorax

    1. Definition

      a. The presence of chyle in the pleural space.

      b. Chyle is the fluid absorbed from the intestines that drains via the thoracic duct into the bloodstream at the junction of the left subclavian and jugular veins.

      c. Appears "milky" due to the presence of CMs (high triglyceride content).

    2. Etiology

      a. Damage to the thoracic duct (e.g., tumor and trauma).

VIII. Vasculitis

A. Definition

    1. Inflammation of the vessel wall; may be either infectious or noninfectious.

    2. Depending upon the entity, the various vasculitides involve specific blood vessels.

      a. Some primarily involve small vessels (arterioles, venules, and capillaries), whereas others tend to affect medium-sized muscular arteries, larger elastic arteries, or a combination of the above.

    3. Clinical manifestations depend upon the specific vascular bed(s) affected.

B. Mechanisms underlying noninfectious vasculitis

    1. Immune complex deposition

      a. Characteristic of the following:

        i. Systemic lupus erythematosus (various immune complex deposits).

        ii. Drug reactions (e.g., penicillin)

        iii. Hepatitis (HBsAg—anti-HBsAg antibody).

    2. Antineutrophil cytoplasmic antibodies (ANCAs)

      a. ANCAs are antibodies against various components within the neutrophil cytoplasm.

      b. Antiproteinase-3 (PR3-ANCA, previously c-ANCA)

        i. Associated with granulomatosis with polyangiitis (GPA).

    c. Antimyeloperoxidase (MPO-ANCA, previously p-ANCA)
      i.   Associated with microscopic polyangiitis.
  3. Antiendothelial cell antibodies and T-cell-mediated immune reactions sometimes involved as well.

Giant cell (temporal) arteritis

- Most common form of systemic vasculitis in adults.
- A disease of older adulthood (mean age 67 years).
- Classified as a large vessel vasculitis; however, often involves muscular arteries, particularly those in the head (e.g., temporal, ophthalmic, occipital, and vertebral).
- Manifestations
  - Blurred vision, potential for permanent blindness
    - Due to the involvement of the ophthalmic artery.
    - Reason that suspected cases must be treated emergently.
  - Headache
    - Due to involvement of the temporal artery.
    - On examination, may have tenderness and nodular thickening of the temporal artery.
  - Jaw claudication
    - Pain with prolonged chewing, due to claudication of muscles of mastication.
  - Polymyalgia rheumatica
    - Present in ~50% of patients.
    - Manifestations, which present relatively acutely (over days), include aching pain and stiffness in the shoulders/upper arms, neck, and hips, as well as marked morning stiffness and decreased ability to dress, brush hair, etc.
- Laboratory findings
  - Elevated erythrocyte sedimentation rate (ESR) and C-reactive protein (CRP).
- Diagnosis
  - Usually biopsy of the temporal artery (see giant cells within the wall).
- Treatment
  - Steroids.

C. **Takayasu arteritis**
    1. Rare, systemic, and inflammatory vasculitis of unknown etiology affecting the aorta and its major branches.
    2. Female to male ratio (8:1); usually presenting between 10 and 40 years.
    3. Known as "pulseless disease" due to claudication and decreased pulsation of one or both brachial arteries.
      a. Characterized by a systolic blood pressure (SBP) difference of greater than 10 mm Hg between the arms.
    4. Laboratory findings include elevated ESR and CRP.

D. **Kawasaki disease**
    1. Acute illness of early childhood.
    2. Characteristically affects small- to medium-sized arteries (e.g., coronary), risk of coronary artery aneurysms, and death.
      a. Use echocardiography to diagnose.
    3. Diagnosis requires a fever of at least a duration of 5 days plus other manifestations:
      a. Desquamative skin rash of feet and hands.
      b. "Strawberry" tongue.
      c. Bilateral conjunctivitis.
      d. Unilateral cervical lymphadenopathy.
    4. Treatment: Intravenous immunoglobulin and aspirin.

E. **Polyarteritis nodosa**
    1. Vasculitis of medium-sized muscular arteries; risk of rupture and/or ischemia.
    2. Usually presents in the fifth to the sixth decade; more commonly males (4:1).
    3. Affects skin, central and/or peripheral nervous system, gastrointestinal (GI) tract, and kidneys (spares the lungs).
      a. HTN and renal failure are major sequelae.
    4. Associated with hepatitis B virus infection in many cases.
    5. Histology reveals destruction of the vessel wall by inflammatory cells.

F. **Granulomatosis with polyangiitis (GPA)**
    1. Previously known as Wegener granulomatosis, GPA more commonly affects older adults.
    2. Associated with a necrotizing vasculitis; primarily involving the upper and lower respiratory tract as well as the kidneys.
      a. Causes chronic sinusitis, nasopharyngeal ulcerations; collapse of nasal bridge ("saddle nose" deformity).
      b. Bilateral pneumonitis (nodules and cavitary lesions).
      c. Renal disease (rapidly progressive glomerulonephritis).
    3. Antibodies against proteinase 3 (Anti-PR3) with positive cytoplasmic (C-ANCA) staining on immunofluorescence are seen in most cases.

G. **Eosinophilic granulomatosis with polyangiitis (EGPA)**
   1. Formerly known as Churg–Strauss syndrome.
   2. Small vessel necrotizing vasculitis of unknown etiology.
   3. Associated with antineutrophilic cytoplasmic antibodies, particularly MPO-ANCA, in many cases.
   4. Classic findings of asthma, allergic rhinitis, and eosinophilia.
      a. Pain, numbness, and weakness (due to peripheral neuropathy) are common.
   5. Histology shows granulomas and eosinophilic infiltration of involved tissues.
H. **IgA vasculitis (Henoch–Schonlein purpura)**
   1. Immunoglobulin A (IgA)-mediated vasculitis involving small vessels of the skin, GI tract, kidneys, and joints.
   2. Usually seen in children (the most common systemic vasculitis of childhood).
   3. Presents with rash of lower legs (palpable purpura), abdominal pain, hematuria, and joint pain.
I. **Thromboangiitis obliterans (Buerger disease)**
   1. Inflammatory disease of small- to medium-sized vessels within the extremities; causes vascular occlusion and ischemia of affected tissues (ulceration and gangrene).
   2. Only seen in association with the use of tobacco; smoking cessation required to stop disease progression.
   3. Most common in males; typically, 20–45 years of age.
IX. **Vascular Tumors and Tumor-Like Conditions**
   A. **Port wine stain**
      1. Congenital vascular malformations (commonly known as a birthmark); characterized by progressive vascular dilatation of preexisting blood vessels (i.e., not a neoplastic process).
      2. Often involves the face (Fig. 10.11).
      3. Associated with somatic activating mutation in the *GNAQ* gene.
      4. May arise in association with ipsilateral cerebral or meningeal vascular lesions (Sturge–Weber syndrome).
   B. **Infantile hemangioma**
      1. Benign tumors of endothelial cells.
      2. Characteristically arise within a few weeks of birth and then rapidly enlarge over months; spontaneous regression over a few years.
   C. **Pyogenic granuloma**
      1. Benign vascular tumor of the skin and/or mucosal surfaces (e.g., gingiva, lips, and fingers). Fig. 10.12.
      2. Comprised of lobules of capillary-sided vessels ("lobular capillary hemangioma").
      3. Usually arise in children or young adults; sometimes seen on the gingiva in pregnant women ("granuloma gravidarum").
      4. Circumscribed exophytic friable lesions (may bleed); treatment is surgical resection.

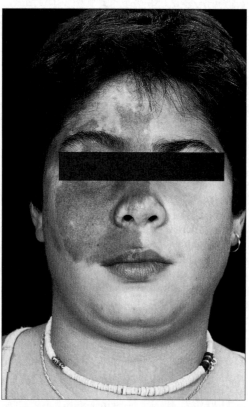

10.11: Port wine stain in a patient with Sturge–Weber syndrome. *(By courtesy of Atherton D, MD, Institute of Dermatology and Children's Hospital at Great Ormond Street, London, UK.)*

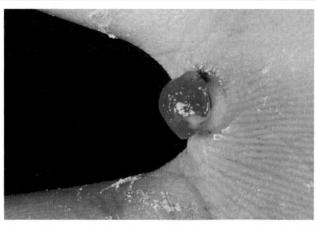

10.12: Pyogenic granuloma. Bright red, raised, hemorrhagic, friable papule that developed rapidly following the minor trauma to the area. *(From Zitelli B, McIntire S, Nowalk A:* Zitelli and Davis' atlas of pediatric physical diagnosis, *ed 6, 2012, Saunders Elsevier, p 351, Fig. 8.111B.)*

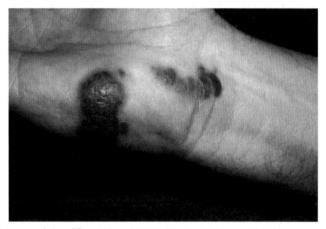

10.13: Kaposi sarcoma. *(From* Andrews' diseases of the skin, *ed 13, © 2020, Elsevier I, Figure 19.61.)*

    D. **Cavernous hemangioma**
       1. Benign tumor comprised of widely dilated vessels; tend to involve deeper structures (c.g., liver); do not regress spontaneously.
    E. **Kaposi sarcoma**
       1. Low-grade malignant tumor of endothelial cells.
       2. Manifests as purple-red lesions of the skin and/or mucous membranes (Fig. 10.13).
       3. Due to reactivation of latent human herpes virus 8; more common in those with impaired T-cell function (e.g., human immunodeficiency virus and transplantation).
    F. **Angiosarcoma**
       1. Rare, highly aggressive malignancy of endothelial cells.
         a. Most commonly develops in the skin of the head and neck.
         b. Usually in older individuals; no sex predilection.
       2. Risk factors
         a. Radiation (e.g., following mastectomy).
         b. Lymphedema ("lymphangiosarcoma").
         c. Various exposures (e.g., thorium dioxide, vinyl chloride, and arsenic) increase one's risk of developing angiosarcoma in the liver.
X. **Hypertension**
    A. **Definition**
       1. Elevated arterial blood pressure (BP).
    B. **Staging**
       1. Normal BP: systolic <120 mm Hg and diastolic <80 mm Hg.
       2. Elevated BP: systolic 120–129 mm Hg and diastolic <80 mm Hg.

3. HTN
   a. Stage 1—systolic 130–139 mm Hg or diastolic 80–89 mm Hg.
   b. Stage 2—systolic ≥140 mm Hg or diastolic ≥90 mm Hg.
C. **Epidemiology**
   1. Primary (formerly "essential") HTN accounts for ~90% of cases.
   2. Remaining 10% represent "secondary" HTN.
   3. In the United States, ~30% of the adult population is hypertensive.
D. **Hemodynamics of BP:**
   1. Mean arterial pressure (MAP) is the average arterial pressure throughout one cardiac cycle.
      a. MAP is the product of cardiac output (CO) and systemic vascular resistance (SVR) (MAP = CO × SVR).
      b. An increase in the CO, the SVR, or both will increase MAP.
   2. MAP can be calculated from routine BP readings.
      a. MAP = DBP + 1/3(SBP − DBP)
   3. SBP, the pressure in the arteries during ventricular systole, correlates with stroke volume (SV) and the compliance of the aorta.
      a. SV
         i. Volume of blood pumped out of the left ventricle during each cardiac contraction.
         ii. Equals the difference between end-diastolic volume (EDV) and end-systolic volume (ESV).
            (1) SV = EDV − ESV
         iii. SV is dependent upon three variables.
            (1) Preload (i.e., EDV).
            (2) Afterload (resistance against which the left ventricle must pump against).
            (3) Cardiac contractility.
      b. Compliance of aorta
         i. Refers to the ability of the aorta to expand during systole.
            (1) Aortic compliance decreases with aging (less elastic tissue within the wall of aorta).
      c. SBP increases with any of the following:
         i. Increased preload.
         ii. Increased cardiac contractility.
         iii. Decreased aortic compliance (e.g., aging).
      d. SBP decreases with any of the following:
         i. Decreased preload (e.g., hypovolemic shock).
         ii. Decreased cardiac contractility (e.g., following myocardial infarction and cardiogenic shock).
         iii. Increased afterload (e.g., severe aortic stenosis).
   4. Diastolic blood pressure (DBP), the BP when the heart is at rest (i.e., during diastole), is primarily dependent upon the state of contraction (tonicity) of the peripheral resistance arterioles and blood viscosity.
      a. DBP increases with any of the following:
         i. Vasoconstriction of peripheral resistance arterioles.
         ii. Increased blood viscosity (e.g., increased red cell mass; polycythemia vera, see Chapter 13).
      b. DBP decreases with any of the following:
         i. Vasodilation of peripheral resistance arterioles (e.g., septic shock and anaphylactic shock).
         ii. Decreased blood viscosity (e.g., severe anemia).
   5. Role of sodium in HTN
      a. Excess sodium increases plasma volume and SV.
         i. An increase in SV leads to an increase in the CO (CO = HR × SV) and thus MAP (MAP = CO × SVR).
E. **Complications of HTN**
   1. Stroke (both ischemic and hemorrhagic).
   2. Renal disease (HTN is second only to DM as a cause of end-stage renal disease).
   3. Cardiovascular disease (e.g., myocardial infarction, left ventricular hypertrophy, heart failure, atherosclerotic vascular disease, aortic dissection, and atrial fibrillation).
   4. Retinopathy.
F. **Primary HTN**
   1. Definition
      a. Elevated BP with unknown underlying secondary cause.
   2. Risk factors
      a. Advancing age (especially for SBP, see above discussion).
      b. Obesity.
      c. Family history.
      d. Race (African American).
      e. High sodium diet.
      f. Excess alcohol.
      g. Lack of physical exercise.

G. Secondary HTN
 1. Accounts for 10%–15% of all cases of HTN.
 2. Major etiologies include primary aldosteronism and renovascular disease.
 3. Primary aldosteronism
    a. Pathologically elevated levels of aldosterone may occur in association with:
       i. Bilateral adrenal hyperplasia
       ii. Adrenal adenoma
       iii. Adrenal carcinoma (rare)
    b. Aldosterone increases the reabsorption of sodium at the distal convoluted tubule (thereby increasing blood volume and BP as described above).
    c. Sodium reabsorption is accompanied by the secretion of potassium in exchange for sodium (risk of hypokalemia).
    d. Characterized by elevated aldosterone, low plasma renin.
 4. Renovascular HTN
    a. Renal artery stenosis
       i. Most common cause of renovascular HTN; usually in older males.
       ii. Due to atherosclerotic narrowing of the renal artery.
          (1) See discrete area of narrowing within the proximal renal artery on angiography.
       iii. Reduction in renal blood flow activates the renin-angiotensin-aldosterone system (RAAS).
       iv. Aldosterone increases sodium reabsorption and blood volume, as discussed above.
       v. Angiotensin II has a direct vasoconstrictive effect (increasing SVR).
       vi. Characterized by elevated plasma aldosterone and renin.
    b. Fibromuscular dysplasia of renal artery
       i. Idiopathic narrowing of muscular arteries (e.g., renal arteries); may be bilateral.
       ii. More common in females, usually younger (<50 years).
       iii. Causes a "string of beads" appearance on angiography within the midportion of the affected renal artery.
       iv. Reduces renal blood flow and activates the RAAS (plasma aldosterone and renin levels are both elevated).

H. Severe HTN (hypertensive crises)
 1. Defined as markedly elevated BP (no set number, some use $\geq 180/120$ mm Hg) with or without target organ dysfunction.
    a. Hypertensive urgency describes a situation in which the elevated BP is not accompanied by progressive target organ dysfunction.
    b. Hypertensive emergency describes a situation in which the elevated BP is accompanied by evidence of acute ongoing end-organ damage.
       i. Examples of acute end-organ damage include:
          (1) Hypertensive encephalopathy
          (2) Stroke
          (3) Myocardial ischemia/infarction
          (4) Aortic dissection
          (5) Acute renal failure/insufficiency
          (6) Retinopathy
          (7) Microangiopathic hemolytic anemia
       ii. In hypertensive emergencies, the BP should be lowered within minutes to an hour to halt the ongoing end-organ injury.

I. **Overview of Normal Anatomy**
   A. **Cardiac conduction (Fig. 11.1).**
   B. **Blood supply to the heart muscle (Fig. 11.2)**
      1. Left anterior descending (LAD) coronary artery
         a. Supplies blood to the anterior LV, the anterior two-thirds of the interventricular septum, and the apex of the heart.
      2. Left circumflex coronary artery
         a. Supplies blood to the lateral wall of the LV.
      3. Right coronary artery (RCA)
         a. Supplies blood primarily to the right atrium (RA) and right ventricle (RV); branches also supply the sinoatrial node, the atrioventricular node, and the posterior one-third of the interventricular septum.
      4. Collateral circulation
         a. Collaterals are anastomotic connections between arteries; either through the growth and expansion of preexisting arterioles or through the local production of angiogenic factors such as vascular endothelial growth factor released in response to chronic hypoxia (chronic myocardial ischemia).
         b. Collateral flow is important because it may decrease, or even prevent, myocardial infarction.
      5. Myocardial perfusion occurs during diastole.
         a. As the ventricles contract, the myocardial vasculature undergoes compression. For this reason, the majority of perfusion occurs during diastole.
           i. Useful to consider in patients with tachycardia, as the heart rate increases, there is less time in diastole and thus less time for perfusion to occur.
           ii. The subendocardial region of the heart is the most susceptible to ischemia because this region receives the least blood flow (recall that blood flows from the epicardial surface toward the endocardium).

II. **Ventricular Hypertrophy**
   A. **Definition**
      1. Increase in ventricular mass due to an increase in the number and/or size of sarcomeres within cardiac myocytes; occurs as a compensatory response to increased pressure and/or volume load imposed on the ventricular wall.
   B. **Pathogenesis**
      1. Sustained pressure and/or volume overload on the heart increases wall stress and alters gene expression.
      2. Increased pressure load (afterload)
         a. Afterload is the pressure against which the ventricle must contract to eject blood.
         b. With increasing afterload, the wall thickens (see Fig. 2.11).
         c. Etiologies of left ventricular hypertrophy (LVH) include systemic hypertension (most common) and aortic stenosis.
         d. Etiologies of right ventricular hypertrophy (RVH) include pulmonary hypertension (PH) and pulmonic stenosis.
   C. **Negative consequences of ventricular hypertrophy**
      1. Increased myocardial oxygen demand (increasing the risk of angina).
      2. Reduced compliance (the ability of heart muscle to stretch is reduced); potential for heart failure (HF).

III. **Heart Failure**
   A. **Definition**
      1. HF is a clinical syndrome characterized by failure of the heart to maintain cardiac output under normal filling pressures.
   B. **Epidemiology**
      1. Increased incidence and prevalence with aging.

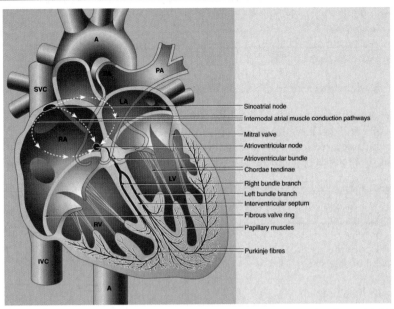

11.1: The conducting system of the heart. The initial impulse originates spontaneously in the sinoatrial (SA) node, located in the right atrium near the entry of the superior vena cava (SVC). The impulse rate is controlled by the autonomic nervous system. The impulse then passes through the atria (causing them to contract) before reaching the atrioventricular (AV) node. From the AV node, the impulse is carried along the bundle of His, before dividing into right and left bundle branches that then become Purkinje fibers. *(From* Wheater's *functional histology, ed 6, 2014, Fig. 8.5.)*

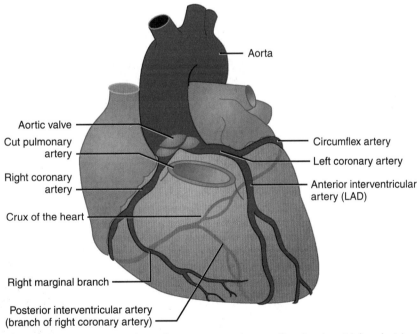

11.2: Coronary arterial vasculature, anterior view. The right coronary artery supplies the sinoatrial and atrioventricular nodes and most often the inferior aspect of the heart; the left coronary artery divides into the left anterior descending and the circumflex arteries. *LAD, Left anterior descending artery. (From Bogart BI, Ort FH:* Elsevier's integrated anatomy and embryology, *2007, Mosby Elsevier, p 56, Fig. 4-22.)*

C. Classification
1. HF with reduced ejection fraction (EF) (systolic dysfunction)
    a. Characterized by an EF of ≤40%.
        i. EF = stroke volume divided by left ventricular end-diastolic volume (SV/LVEDV).
        ii. Normal EF ~ 55%–70%.
2. HF with preserved EF (diastolic dysfunction)
    a. EF is within the normal range; however, diastolic filling is impaired (i.e., stiff myocardium with reduced compliance).
D. Left- versus right-sided HF
1. Etiologies of predominantly left-sided heart failure (LHF) include systemic hypertension, mitral or aortic valve dysfunction, and/or left ventricular infarction.

2. Etiologies of predominantly right-sided heart failure (RHF) include PH, pulmonic or tricuspid valve dysfunction, and/or right ventricular infarction.
3. LHF and RHF may each occur separately or concurrently (known as biventricular failure).
   a. LHF is the most common cause of RHF.

E. LHF

1. Clinical syndrome developing when the LV fails to pump adequate blood into the systemic circulation to meet metabolic demands.
   a. Blood backs up behind the failing LV into the pulmonary circulation, resulting in an increase in the intravascular hydrostatic pressure and the development of pulmonary edema.
   b. Etiologic factors include a reduction in contractility (e.g., myocardial ischemia, myocarditis, and dilated cardiomyopathy); valvular dysfunction (e.g., mitral and aortic); decreased wall compliance (e.g., LVH secondary to systemic hypertension).
2. Pathologic findings in LHF
   a. Lungs are heavy and congested; exude pink frothy fluid (edema) on sectioning.
   b. Histologic examination reveals pink-staining fluid within alveoli (Fig. 11.3A), and alveolar macrophages containing hemosiderin ("HF cells").
      i. Iron is derived from the breakdown of red cells that leaked into alveoli; appreciated as blue granules within macrophages (Prussian blue stain).
3. Clinical manifestations
   a. Dyspnea (difficulty breathing)
      i. In most patients, dyspnea occurs only with exertion. In advanced stages, patients may develop dyspnea at rest; primarily as a result of pulmonary congestion and edema (interstitial and/or intra-alveolar fluid).
         (1) Fluid within the lungs decreases compliance and increases the work of breathing.
   b. Orthopnea
      i. Dyspnea occurring in the recumbent position. Recumbency reduces the effect of gravity, allowing fluid to reenter the vascular space thereby increasing preload.
         (1) The failing heart cannot handle the extra volume; pulmonary edema (and difficulty breathing) develops.

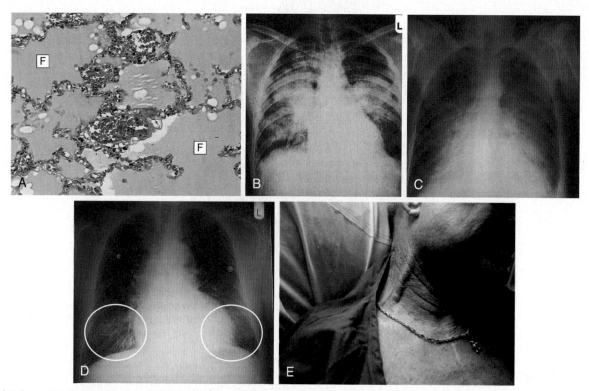

11.3: (A) Pulmonary edema. The pink fluid "F" fills the alveoli. (B and C) Chest radiograph showing pulmonary edema. Note the fluffy alveolar infiltrates ("bat-wing" or "angel wing" configuration) throughout both lung fields. (D) Kerley B lines (septal edema; circles) in both lower lobes in a patient with pulmonary edema. (E) Jugular venous distention in a patient with right-sided heart failure. *(A, From Stevens A, Lowe J, Scott I: Core pathology, ed 3, 2009, Mosby Elsevier, p 172, Fig. 10.33; B, from Walker BR, Colledge NR, Ralston SH, Penman ID: Davidson's principles and practice of medicine, ed 22, St. Louis, 2014, Churchill Livingstone Elsevier, p 482, Fig. 17.11; C, from Ashar BH, Miller RG, Sisso SD: The Johns Hopkins internal medicine board review, ed 4, St. Louis, 2012, Elsevier, p 53, Fig. 6-3A. Taken from Haslett C, Chilvers ER: Davidson's principles and practice of medicine, ed 19, Philadelphia, 2003, Churchill Livingstone, Fig. 12.22A; D, from Forbes CD, Jackson WF: Color atlas and text of clinical medicine, ed 3, St. Louis, 2003, Mosby, p 223, Fig. 5.97; E, from http://courses.cvcc.vccs.edu/ WisemcmDljug.)*

   ii. Relieved by standing, sitting, or sleeping propped on pillows. These measures reduce venous return and thus preload.
      (1) Severity graded by the number of pillows that cause symptomatic relief (e.g., three-pillow orthopnea is worse than one-pillow orthopnea).
   c. Paroxysmal nocturnal dyspnea
      i. Similar pathophysiology as orthopnea but less common, usually only occurring in severe HF.
      ii. Characterized by awakening after a couple of hours of sleep with severe breathlessness (feeling of suffocation).
      iii. Relieved by sitting up; however, compared with orthopnea, the resolution is much slower.
   d. Wheezing
      i. Due to narrowing of small airways by peribronchiolar edema fluid ("cardiac asthma").
   e. Fatigue and weakness
      i. Reduced perfusion of skeletal muscles.
   f. Bibasilar inspiratory crackles
      i. Opening of edematous alveoli by the inflow of air during inspiration.
   g. Apical S3 and S4 heart sounds
      i. S3 due to blood entering a volume-overloaded ventricle (elevated left ventricular end-diastolic pressure [LVEDP]).
      ii. S4 due to blood entering a noncompliant "stiff" ventricle.
   h. Mitral regurgitation (MR)
      i. Due to the stretching of support structures around the mitral valve (MV) in conjunction with dilated LV (elevated LVEDV).
      ii. Apical holosystolic murmur; resolves with the treatment of HF.
   i. Chest radiograph of LHF
      i. Congestion in the upper lobes (early finding).
      ii. Perihilar congestion ("bat-wing configuration"), Fig. 11.3B.
      iii. Fluffy ("ground glass") alveolar infiltrates (Fig. 11.3C).
      iv. Kerley B lines (septal edema, Fig. 11.3D).
      v. Air bronchogram (air in small airways surrounded by fluid).
   j. Serum B-type natriuretic peptide (BNP) is increased.
      i. BNP is a cardiac neurohormone secreted by volume-overloaded "stretched" ventricles.
      ii. Used to diagnose HF (equivocal cases) and monitor the effectiveness of therapy and prognosis.
         (1) Normal BNP excludes HF.
         (2) Elevated BNP despite therapy is a poor prognostic sign.
F. RHF
   1. Characterized by impaired function of the RV with a buildup of blood behind the failing ventricle (systemic venous congestion).
   2. Etiologies include:
   a. LHF (a major cause of RHF).
      i. With LHF, congestion of pulmonary vasculature increases workload (afterload) on the RV.
   b. Decreased right ventricular contractility
      i. Myocardial infarction involving the RV.
   c. Decreased right ventricular compliance (i.e., stiff ventricle), impairs diastolic filling.
      i. Restrictive cardiomyopathy and RVH
   d. Increased RV preload
      i. Tricuspid regurgitation (TR) and pulmonic regurgitation.
   2. Clinical and laboratory findings
   a. Jugular venous distention (Fig. 11.3E)
      i. Reflects increased blood in the venous system behind the failing RV.
   b. Hepatomegaly
      i. Right upper quadrant pain/tenderness; due to backup of venous blood into the liver (hepatic congestion).
      ii. Causes expansion of hepatic sinusoids and central venules; potential for centrilobular necrosis (necrosis of zone III hepatocytes).
      iii. Aminotransferase enzyme (aspartate aminotransferase and alanine aminotransferase) elevation due to hepatocyte injury.
   c. Ascites
      i. Elevated hydrostatic pressure within the portal vein causes the extravasation of fluid into the peritoneal cavity (ascites).
   d. Hepatojugular reflux
      i. Exam maneuver is which compression of the liver causes distention of jugular veins.
   e. Dependent pitting edema
      i. Secondary to increased venous hydrostatic pressure, particularly in dependent regions due to the added effect of gravity.
   f. Tricuspid valve regurgitation
      i. Right ventricular dilation causes stretching of the support structures around the tricuspid valve, preventing adequate closure.
      ii. Holosystolic murmur, right mid-sternal border. Resolves with the treatment of HF.

IV. **Ischemic Heart Disease**
   A. **Definition**
      1. Cardiac injury and dysfunction occurring when there is an imbalance between myocardial oxygen demand and supply.
      2. Typically, due to reduced coronary blood flow (i.e., coronary heart disease [CHD]).
         a. Myocardial oxygen extraction is near-maximal at rest; therefore any increase in oxygen demand must be met by an increase in myocardial oxygen supply (i.e., blood flow).
   B. **Epidemiology**
      1. The major cause of death in the United States and worldwide.
      2. Incidence peaks in men after the age of 60 years and in women after 70 years.
   C. **Risk factors**
      1. Age (the most important risk factor).
      2. Family history of ischemic heart disease (IHD) (particularly if early onset).
      3. Dyslipidemia
         a. Elevated low-density lipoprotein.
         b. Low high-density lipoprotein.
      4. Smoking.
      5. Hypertension (HTN).
      6. Diabetes mellitus.
   D. **Clinical manifestations**
      1. Stable angina
         a. Chest pain due to inadequate myocardial oxygenation, usually secondary to a reduction in myocardial oxygen supply in conjunction with increased myocardial oxygen demand (Fig. 11.4).
            i. Atherosclerotic narrowing (>50% stenosis) of one or more coronary arteries.
            ii. Precipitants include exercise, cold weather, and emotional stress.
         b. Manifestations
            i. Retrosternal chest pain ("pressure" or "heaviness"); duration of 2–10 minutes.
            ii. Precipitated by exertion (e.g., exercise and climbing stairs); relieved by rest and/or nitroglycerin.
            iii. Pain may radiate into the left inner arm, shoulder, or jaw.
            iv. Electrocardiography (ECG) shows ST-segment depression >1 mm.
      2. Vasospastic (variant, Prinzmetal) angina
         a. Vasospasm of coronary artery with associated myocardial ischemia and associated manifestations.
         b. Often occurs at rest; patients do not necessarily have coexisting coronary artery disease (although they often do).
         c. Vasospasm is thought related to an imbalance between vagal and sympathetic tone (often occurs at night when vagal tone is higher).
         d. Causes transmural ischemia (ECG reveals ST-segment elevation).
      3. Unstable angina
         a. Refers to angina that is worsening, occurring with minimal exertion, or at rest. No biochemical or ECG evidence of infarction.
         b. Due to coronary atherosclerosis with overlying thrombus causing partial occlusion of lumen.
         c. Risk of progression to acute myocardial infarction (AMI).
      4. Chronic IHD
         a. Refers to the manifestations of chronic myocardial ischemia (i.e., HF and dilated cardiomyopathy).
      5. AMI
         a. Episode of myocardial ischemia of sufficient severity and duration to cause necrosis of cardiac myocytes.
            i. Region of necrosis depends upon the affected vessel (Fig. 11.5).
         b. Decreased coronary blood flow usually follows acute thrombosis of a ruptured atherosclerotic coronary plaque.
            i. Thromboxane A_2 (TXA_2) has platelet aggregating and vasoconstricting properties (synthesis inhibited by aspirin).
         c. Less common causes of myocardial infarction include:
            i. Vasculitis of coronary artery (e.g., Kawasaki disease).
            ii. Global hypoperfusion (shock).
            iii. Coronary artery embolus or vasospasm.
         d. Classification of AMI
            i. ST elevation myocardial infarction (STEMI)
               (1) Transmural (full thickness) infarct, usually secondary to an occlusive coronary artery thrombosis.
               (2) Elevation of cardiac biomarkers (e.g., troponin).
               (3) New Q wave formation on ECG.
            ii. Non-ST elevation myocardial infarction (NSTEMI)
               (1) Infarct of the subendocardial region of the heart.
               (2) Elevation of cardiac biomarkers (e.g., troponin).
               (3) Absence of Q waves; high risk of reinfarction.

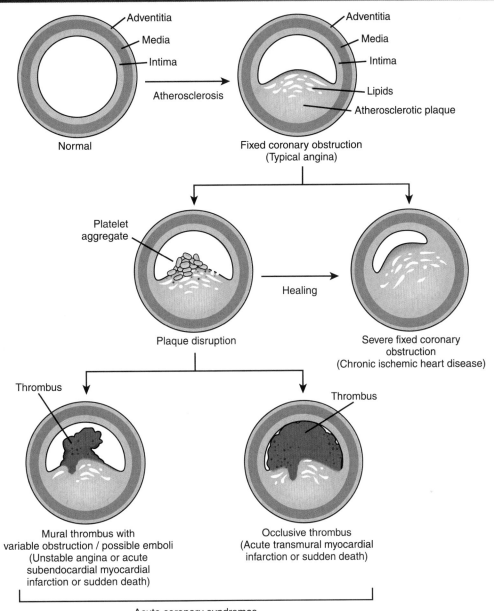

11.4: Sequential progression of coronary atherosclerosis beginning with a stable chronic plaque responsible for typical angina and leading to the various acute coronary syndromes. *(From Ashar BH, Miller RG, Sisso SD:* The Johns Hopkins internal medicine board review, *ed 4, St. Louis, 2012, Elsevier, p 30, Fig. 4-1. Modified and redrawn from Schoen FJ:* Interventional and surgical cardiovascular pathology: clinical correlations and basic principles, *Philadelphia, 1989, WB Saunders, p 63, and from Zipes DP, Libby P, Bonow RO, Braunwald E, editors:* Braunwald's heart disease: a textbook of cardiovascular medicine, *ed 7, Philadelphia, 2005, WB Saunders, Fig. 12-12.)*

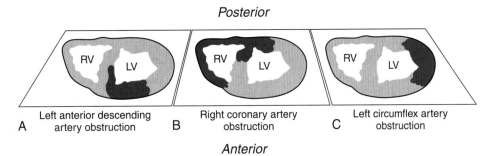

11.5: (A) The distribution of an infarction involving the left anterior descending coronary artery. (B) The distribution of an infarction involving the distribution of the right coronary artery. (C) The distribution of an infarction involving the distribution of the left circumflex coronary artery. *LV,* Left ventricle; *RV,* right ventricle. *(Modified from Damjanov I:* Pathology for the health-related professions, *ed 2, Philadelphia, 2000, Saunders, p 154, Fig. 7-15.)*

 e. Ischemia/reperfusion injury in AMI

  i. Reperfusion may occur spontaneously or, more commonly, following medical intervention (e.g., percutaneous coronary intervention or fibrinolytic therapy).

  ii. Restoration of blood flow allows for cellular recovery of reversibly damaged myocytes; however, further injury can arise following the formation of reactive oxygen species ("reperfusion injury").

 f. Gross changes in AMI (vary by time since infarct)

  i. First 12 hours, no gross changes.

  ii. By 24 hours, the infarct becomes dark (due to hemorrhage).

  iii. By 1–3 days, the infarct center becomes tan to yellow with the surrounding area of hyperemia.

  iv. Between 3 and 7 days, the border remains hyperemic with progressive softening of the center.

  v. By 7–10 days, the infarct becomes bright yellow.

  vi. Over weeks to months, the infarct becomes gray to white due to the formation of a dense fibrous scar.

 g. Microscopic findings in AMI (also vary by time since infarct)

  i. During the first 12 hours, only minimal changes (wavy fibers).

  ii. By 12–24 hours, changes begin to become more prominent with early coagulation necrosis (cytoplasm becomes more eosinophilic [pink], nuclei begin to fade). Early neutrophilic infiltrate at the periphery of the infarct.

  iii. Between 1 and 3 days, coagulation necrosis becomes increasingly evident (more widespread eosinophilia and fading of nuclei); neutrophilic infiltrate becomes widespread.

  iv. Between 3 and 7 days, neutrophils are replaced by macrophages; phagocytosis of dead cellular debris causes tissue weakening (risk of rupture).

  v. By 7–10 days, widespread phagocytosis of dead cells; granulation tissue forms at the periphery of the infarct.

  vi. Over weeks to months, dense scar tissue is formed.

 h. Complications of myocardial infarction

  i. Ventricular arrhythmias (e.g., tachycardia and fibrillation); common early cause of death.

  ii. Cardiogenic shock.

  iii. HF.

  iv. Myocardial rupture

   (1) Most likely within the first 2 weeks postinfarction (before scarring leads to increased tensile strength).

   (2) Free wall rupture

    (a) Usually due to the infarct of the LV; causes hemopericardium and cardiac tamponade.

   (3) Posteromedial papillary muscle rupture

    (a) Due to thrombosis of the RCA (only blood supply to posteromedial papillary muscle).

    (b) Causes acute MR and LHF.

   (4) Rupture of interventricular septum (most common site of rupture)

    (a) Causes ventricular septal defect (VSD) with left-to-right shunting (LV → RV). Results in RV overload and RHF.

    (b) Increased (step-up) SaO_2 within RV.

  v. Pericarditis with or without effusion

   (1) Most likely within the first week after the infarct.

   (2) Characterized by the presence of pleuritic chest pain that is relieved by leaning forward and a friction rub on auscultation.

  vi. Ventricular aneurysm

   (1) Late finding (weeks after myocardial infarction); characterized by a precordial bulge.

   (2) Stasis of blood within aneurysm is associated with an increased risk of thrombus formation and the potential for embolization to distant sites.

 i. Laboratory diagnosis of AMI

  i. Serial testing for cardiac troponins I (cTnI) and T (cTnT).

   (1) First appear within 3–12 hours, peak at 24 hours, and return to baseline within 7–10 days.

   (2) Gold standard for the diagnosis of an AMI.

   (3) May also be used to diagnose reinfarction. If suspected, measure cTnI and then repeat 3–6 hours later. If the second troponin has increased by ≥20%, then reinfarction is likely.

 j. ECG findings in STEMI (Fig. 11.6) include inverted T waves, elevated ST segments, and Q waves.

6. Sudden cardiac arrest/death

 a. Definition

  i. Sudden cardiac arrest refers to the sudden cessation of cardiac activity. A patient becomes unresponsive with cessation of breathing and circulation.

  ii. Sudden cardiac death (SCD) refers to a patient death within 1 hour of symptom onset; often secondary to ventricular arrhythmia.

 b. Causes of SCD include:

  i. CHD

   (1) Major factor (~70% cases); may be the first manifestation of CHD.

  ii. Electrolyte abnormalities (e.g., hypokalemia or hyperkalemia).

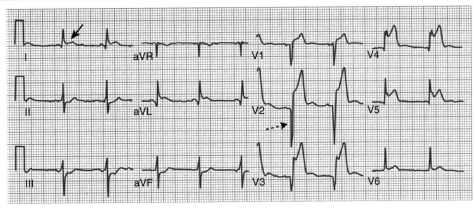

11.6: Electrocardiogram showing an acute anterior myocardial infarction. There is ST-segment elevation in lead 1 (*solid arrow*), aVL, and V1 to V6. Q waves (*interrupted arrow*) are present in leads V1–V4. *(From Goldman L, Ausiello D: Cecil's textbook of medicine, ed 23, Philadelphia, 2008, Saunders Elsevier, p 502, Fig. 72-1.)*

    iii. Illicit drugs (e.g., cocaine).
    iv. Acidemia (metabolic or respiratory).
    v. Cardiomyopathy (e.g., hypertrophic).
    vi. Conduction defects (long QT syndrome).

Acute myocardial infarction

- May or may not have precipitating trigger (e.g., strenuous exercise, emotional stress).
- More common in the morning hours (increased levels of catecholamines, cortisol).
- Clinical manifestations include the sudden onset of severe, crushing retrosternal chest pain; often described as "pressure" or "heaviness" ("like an elephant sitting on chest"). Discomfort may radiate into the left arm, neck, or jaw.
- Pain tends to last longer than 30 minutes; not relieved by rest or nitroglycerin.
- Anxiety (feeling of "impending doom"), shortness of breath, nausea, vomiting, diaphoresis, and/or palpitations may accompany the discomfort.
- Asymptomatic (i.e., "silent MI") in ~20% of cases; especially older adults and diabetics (due to autonomic neuropathy, a common finding in diabetics).

Postcardiac injury pericarditis (Dressler syndrome)

- Pericarditis arising after a latent period (1–8 weeks) following a myocardial infarction (or other cardiac injury).
- Due to anti-myocardial antibodies (type II hypersensitivity reaction [HSR]).

V. **Congenital Heart Disease**
   A. **Overview**
     1. Congenital heart disease refers to any defect involving the heart and/or large arteries and veins that is present at birth.
   B. **Fetal circulation**
     1. Oxygenation of blood occurs in the placenta and then returns to the fetus via the umbilical vein.
       a. About half of the blood passes through the ductus venosus into the inferior vena cava (IVC), bypassing the liver.
       b. Remainder of blood within the umbilical vein flows into the liver, before draining through the hepatic veins into the IVC.
     2. Blood in the IVC then returns to the RA.
       a. Majority of the blood returning through the IVC passes into the left atrium via the foramen ovale.
       b. Remainder of blood within the RA flows across the tricuspid valve, into the RV, and into the pulmonary artery (PA) before being diverted through the ductus arteriosus into the aorta (bypassing the lungs).
     3. Prior to birth
       a. Pulmonary vascular resistance is high (vasoconstriction).
       b. Systemic vascular resistance is low (low resistance in the placenta).
       c. Foramen ovale and ductus arteriosus are both patent (allow oxygenated blood returning from the placenta to bypass the lungs).
     4. After birth
       a. The ductus arteriosus and the foramen ovale both close, causing blood to flow through the PA for oxygenation in the lungs.

- Present in up to 25% of the population; usually, not clinically significant.
- Due to failure of the septum primum and septum secundum to fuse postnatally.

C. **Left-to-right shunts**
  1. Characterized by the flow of oxygenated blood from a left-sided heart chamber (SaO_2 95%) into, and mixing with, poorly oxygenated blood (SaO_2 75%) within a right-sided heart chamber.
  2. Manifestations include:
     a. Increased oxygen saturation ("step-up"); from 75% to 80% or more, within affected right heart chambers.
     b. Volume overload on the right heart.
     c. Increased blood flow and pressures within the pulmonary circulation; eventually, causing RVH secondary to the chronic pressure overload on the RV.
        i. If/when pressures on the right exceed those on the left, there is a reversal of the shunt ("Eisenmenger syndrome"), and patients become cyanotic as poorly oxygenated blood is diverted into the systemic circulation.
  3. VSD
     a. Most common congenital heart defect (~40% of cases).
     b. Blood flows from the high pressure of the LV into the low-pressure RV (Fig. 11.7A).
     c. Results in volume overload, as well as increased oxygenation, within the RV and PA.
  4. Atrial septal defect (ASD)
     a. Defect in the atrial septum; accounts for 10% of all congenital heart defects.
     b. Most common congenital heart defect in adults (because often not identified during childhood).
     c. Blood flows from the high-pressure left atrium into the low-pressure RA (Fig. 11.7B).
     d. Results in volume overload, and a "step-up" in oxygenation within the RA, RV, and PA.
     e. Risk of paradoxical embolism (the passage of venous clot through the ASD into the systemic circulation).
  5. Patent ductus arteriosus (PDA)
     a. Refers to the persistence of an open communication between the PA and the aorta (i.e., the ductus arteriosus remains patent).
        i. Usually closes after birth due to reduced pulmonary pressures and declining levels of prostaglandin E2.
     b. Left-to-right shunting of blood from the high-pressure aorta through the ductus into the lower pressure of the PA (Fig. 11.7C).
     c. Oxygen levels in PA are increased.
     d. Continuous harsh "machinery" murmur is heard throughout systole and diastole.
     e. If/when pressures within the pulmonary circulation exceed those within the aorta, the shunt reverses and poorly oxygenated blood from the PA enters the aorta through the PDA.
        i. "Differential cyanosis" refers to pink upper body and cyanotic lower body; a result of the ductus being distal to the aortic arch vessels (the upper body receives oxygenated blood and is therefore pink, while the lower body receives poorly oxygenated blood and is therefore cyanotic).
     f. NSAIDs (e.g., indomethacin) sometimes given to stimulate closure of the ductus (decrease prostaglandin levels via inhibition of cyclooxygenase).
D. **Right-to-left shunts**
  1. Commonly referred to as "cyanotic congenital heart disease" because patients may present early in life with cyanosis.
  2. Right-to-left shunts allow poorly oxygenated blood (O_2 saturation of around 75%) to be shunted into and mixed with the well-oxygenated blood (O_2 saturation of ~95%) in a left heart chamber.
  3. The net result is a reduction in oxygenation ("step-down") from 95% to 80% or less in affected chambers or vessels.
     a. With small shunts, the SaO_2 remains >85% (cyanosis does not occur).
     b. With large shunts, oxygen levels are even lower (cyanosis occurs).
  4. Tetralogy of Fallot
     a. Most common right-to-left shunt (~5% of all congenital diseases).
     b. Refers to the presence of a VSD, infundibular pulmonic stenosis, RVH, and overriding aorta (Fig. 11.7D).
     c. The degree of stenosis across the pulmonic valve correlates with the presence/absence of cyanosis.
     d. With severe stenosis, increased right-to-left shunting through the VSD makes cyanosis more likely.
     e. Radiograph shows a "boot-shaped" heart (indicative of RVH).
     f. Tet spells (hypoxic spells)
        i. Caused by a sudden increase in hypoxemia and cyanosis related to crying and feeding.
        ii. Squatting (or compression of legs against the chest) increases peripheral vascular resistance, transiently diminishes the severity of the shunt, and cyanosis resolves.
  5. Transposition of the great arteries
     a. Embryologic defect due to abnormal formation of the truncal and aortopulmonary septa (Fig. 11.7E).
        i. Aorta arises from the RV.
        ii. PA arises from the LV.

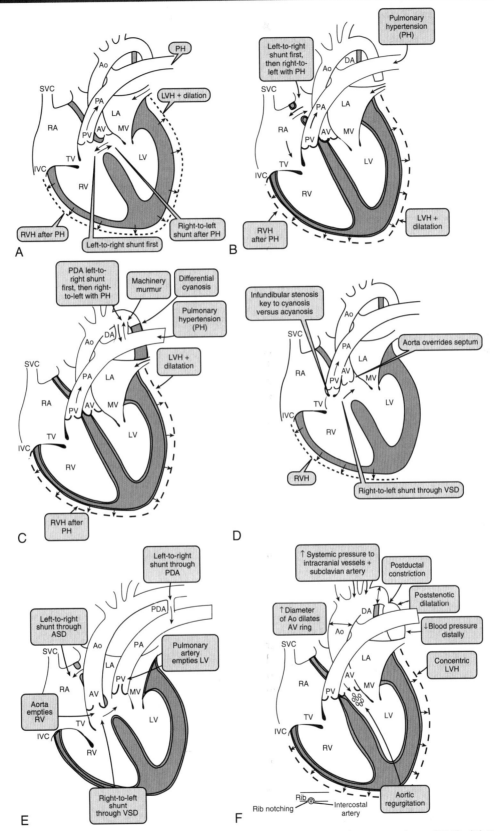

11.7: (A) Ventricular septal defect (VSD). (B) Atrial septal defect (ASD). (C) Patent ductus arteriosus (PDA). (D) Tetralogy of Fallot. (E) Complete transposition of the great vessels. (F) Postductal coarctation. *Ao*, Aorta; *AV*, aortic valve; *DA*, ductus arteriosus; *IVC*, inferior vena cava; *LA*, left atrium; *LV*, left ventricle; *LVH*, left ventricular hypertrophy; *MV*, mitral valve; *PA*, pulmonary artery; *PH*, pulmonary hypertension; *PV*, pulmonary valve; *RA*, right atrium; *RV*, right ventricle; *RVH*, right ventricular hypertrophy; *SVC*, superior vena cava; *TV*, tricuspid valve. *(A–F, From Goljan EF: Star series: pathology, Philadelphia, 1998, Saunders.)*

b. Incompatible with life unless there is communication between the two parallel circuits to allow blood flow to the lungs for oxygenation.
   i. Examples of "protective" shunts include patent foramen ovale, ASD, VSD, and/or PDA.
6. Total anomalous pulmonary venous return
   a. Pulmonary veins do not return to the left atrium but rather empty oxygenated blood into the systemic venous system (e.g., RA, superior vena cava, and IVC).
7. Truncus arteriosus
   a. Aorta and PA share a common trunk with intermixing of blood.
8. Tricuspid atresia
   a. Valve orifice fails to develop.
E. **Coarctation of the aorta**
   1. Narrowing of the aorta just distal to the origin of the left subclavian artery; often described as being preductal, postductal, or juxtaductal, depending upon its location relative to the ligamentum arteriosum.
      a. Preductal refers to coarctation of the aorta between the left subclavian artery and the ductus arteriosus (which usually remains patent); often presents in childhood.
      b. Postductal (Fig. 11.7F) refers to coarctation of the aorta distal to the ligamentum arteriosum (usually presents later in life).
      c. Juxtaductal refers to coarctation by the ligamentum arteriosum.
   2. Clinical manifestations
      a. Increased blood flow and pressure proximal to the coarctation through aortic branch vessels.
         i. Proximal to the coarctation (i.e., head, upper extremities), there is an increase in blood flow and pressure.
         ii. Distal to the coarctation (lower extremities), blood flow and pressure are decreased.
            (1) Typically, >10 mm Hg pressure differential between upper and lower extremities.
      b. Systemic hypertension
         i. Narrowing of the aorta reduces renal blood flow, causing prolonged activation of the renin–angiotensin–aldosterone system.
      c. Development of collateral circulation
         i. Collaterals develop between the intercostal arteries above and below the constriction (Fig. 11.8).
         ii. Increased blood pressures proximal to the coarctation are transmitted from the aorta into the subclavian, internal thoracic, and intercostal arteries.
         iii. Chest radiograph shows rib notching on the undersurface of the ribs (increased blood flow through intercostal arteries wear away the bone, producing rib notching).
F. **Long QT syndrome**
   1. Inherited disorder of myocardial repolarization characterized by prolongation of the QT interval on the ECG and increased risk of life-threatening ventricular arrhythmias.
      a. Torsades de pointes (a specific type of polymorphic ventricular tachycardia) most common.
   2. The most common mutations affect potassium or sodium channels.
      a. LQT1 (a mutation in the potassium channel gene—*KCNQ1*).
         i. Arrhythmias often triggered by swimming and diving.
      b. LQT2 (a mutation in the potassium channel gene—*KCNH2*).
         i. Auditory triggers and postpartum period.
      c. LQT3 (a mutation in a sodium channel gene—*SCN5A*).
         i. Arrhythmias commonly arise during sleep.
   3. Accompanied by sensorineural hearing loss in some cases (Jervell–Lange-Nielsen syndrome).

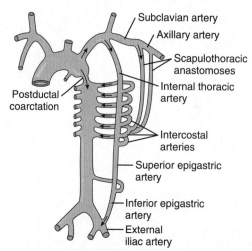

11.8: Postductal coarctation and collateral circulation. (*From Moore A, Roy W: Rapid review gross and developmental anatomy, ed 3, Philadelphia, 2010, Mosby Elsevier, p 49, Fig. 2.29.*)

VI. Acquired Valvular Heart Disease

A. Rheumatic fever (RF)

1. Definition
   a. Acute, noninfectious, inflammatory sequela to a group A β-hemolytic streptococcal (*Streptococcus pyogenes*) pharyngitis.
   b. Presents with joint, skin, subcutaneous, neurologic, and cardiac symptoms a few weeks after the infection.

2. Acute RF
   a. Usually occurs in children between 5 and 15 years of age.
   b. Develops over 1–5 weeks (average, 20 days) after a group A streptococcal (GAS) (*S. pyogenes*) pharyngitis.
      i. Once the patient develops manifestations of RF, pharyngeal cultures are usually negative (reason to do serology).
   c. Pathogenesis of acute RF (Fig. 11.9)
      i. Antibody-mediated disease (Type II HSR) following a GAS infection of the pharynx.
      ii. Host immune response against the organism cross-reacts against similar proteins in human tissue ("molecular mimicry").
      iii. Immune response may be against the endocardium, myocardium, pericardium, and/or other tissues (e.g., joints and skin).
   d. Clinical manifestations of acute RF
      i. Migratory polyarthritis (~75% of cases)
         (1) Most common initial presentation of acute RF.
         (2) Arthritis involves the large joints (knees), ankles, and wrists.
         (3) No permanent joint damage.
      ii. Inflammation of the heart (carditis); ~35% of cases
         (1) Most serious complication of acute RF.
         (2) May involve any portion of the heart
            (a) Pericardium, myocardium, and/or endocardium.
         (3) HF is the most common cause of death in acute RF.
         (4) "Aschoff bodies" are a postmortem histologic finding in the heart (Fig. 11.10) characterized by a central area of fibrinoid necrosis surrounded by Anitschkow cells (activated macrophages).
         (5) Valvular involvement
            (a) Sterile, verrucous vegetations develop along the lines of valve closure.
            (b) MV is nearly always involved, whereas the aortic valve is often affected as well; however, right-sided valves are rarely affected.
      iii. Subcutaneous nodules
         (1) Seen in ~10% of cases; located on the extensor surfaces of forearms.
      iv. Erythema marginatum
         (1) Seen in ~10% of cases.
         (2) Presents as C-shaped areas of erythema around normal-appearing skin.
      v. Sydenham chorea
         (1) A late manifestation seen in ~10% of cases; characterized by reversible rapid, involuntary movements.
   e. Diagnosis of acute RF (Jones criteria)
      i. Two or more major manifestations or one major and two minor manifestations.
      ii. Major criteria include:
         (1) Polyarthritis (joint swelling).
         (2) Carditis.
         (3) Subcutaneous nodules.
         (4) Erythema marginatum.
         (5) Sydenham chorea.
      iii. Minor criteria include a history of acute RF, arthralgia, fever, and increased acute-phase reactants.
      iv. Throat culture/rapid strep antigen test are often negative by the time that RF presents (do serology).
      v. The best method to detect a recent streptococcal infection is through serology (looking for the presence of antistreptococcal antibodies, particularly if titers are increasing).
         (1) Antistreptolysin O (ASO).
         (2) AntiDNAase B (use if ASO negative).

3. Chronic rheumatic heart disease
   a. Potential complication of acute RF; presents decades later (i.e., middle age).
   b. Due to chronic low-grade inflammation and damage to heart valves (most commonly affects MV); may present with either regurgitation or stenosis.

B. Mitral stenosis

1. Definition
   a. Narrowing (stenosis) of the mitral orifice; usually a complication of chronic rheumatic heart disease.

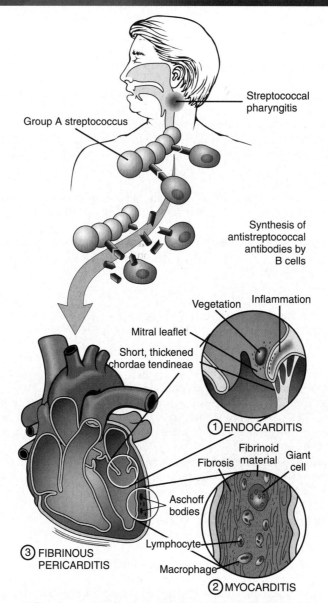

11.9: Pathogenesis of rheumatic fever. After streptococcal pharyngitis ("strep throat"), the host immune response directed against the streptococci cross-reacts against the heart and several other organs, most notably the joints, skin, and central nervous system. In the heart, it causes endocarditis, myocarditis, and pericarditis. (From Damjanov I: Pathology for the health professions, ed 4, 2012, Saunders Elsevier, p 150, Fig. 7-23.)

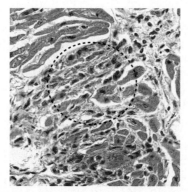

11.10: The Aschoff nodule in rheumatic fever is composed of an area of degenerate collagen surrounded by activated histiocytic cells (interrupted circle) and lymphoid cells. These lesions stimulate fibroblast proliferation and lead to scarring. (From Stevens A, Lowe J, Scott I: Core pathology, ed 3, 2009, Mosby Elsevier, p 187, Fig. 10.59.)

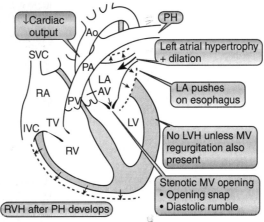

11.11: Mitral stenosis. *Ao*, Aorta; *AV*, aortic valve; *IVC*, inferior vena cava; *LA*, left atrium; *LV*, left ventricle; *LVH*, left ventricular hypertrophy; *MV*, mitral valve; *PA*, pulmonary artery; *PH*, pulmonary hypertension; *PV*, pulmonary valve; *RA*, right atrium; *RV*, right ventricle; *RVH*, right ventricular hypertrophy; *SVC*, superior vena cava. *(From Goljan EF: Star series: pathology, Philadelphia, 1998, Saunders.)*

2. Pathophysiology
   a. Stenosis of the MV → elevated left atrial (LA) pressure → LA dilation (Fig. 11.11).
   b. Atrial distention → ↑ risk of atrial fibrillation
      i. Risk of cardiac thromboemboli.
   c. Being the most posterior heart chamber, LA enlargement can cause compressive effects (e.g., dysphagia due to compression of the esophagus).
   d. Transmission of the elevated LA pressures "upstream" into the pulmonary circulation (i.e., PH) can, over time, cause RVH and RHF.
3. Examination findings
   a. Opening snap followed by an apical early to mid-diastolic murmur.
      i. Elevated LA pressures cause the fibrotic MV to "snap" open.
      ii. Subsequent murmur occurs as blood flows across the stenotic valve.
4. Diagnosis
   a. Echocardiography.

C. Mitral regurgitation (MR)
1. Incompetence of the MV; allows blood to flow back into the left atrium during ventricular systole (Fig. 11.12A, B).
2. Etiologies
   a. Mitral valve prolapse
      i. Myxomatous degeneration of valve leaflet; bulging of leaflet into left atrium during systole.
   b. Papillary muscle rupture/dysfunction
      i. Posteromedial papillary muscle is more vulnerable to ischemia because it is only supplied by the posterior descending artery.
      ii. Anterolateral papillary muscle is less susceptible because of the dual blood supply from the LAD and circumflex arteries.
   c. Left ventricular distention
      i. Due to the stretching of valvular support structures ("functional" regurgitation) secondary to volume overload (e.g., HF); resolves with the treatment of HF.
   d. Perforation of valve leaflets, ruptured chordae tendineae (e.g., infective endocarditis).
   e. Rheumatic heart disease.
3. Pathophysiology
   a. Retrograde systolic flow of blood from the LV into the left atrium.
   b. Acute MR
      i. Etiologies include sudden rupture of papillary muscle or chordae tendineae.
      ii. LA volume and pressure are suddenly increased, resulting in acute pulmonary vascular congestion and edema.
      iii. Variably decreased cardiac output (potential for cardiogenic shock).
   c. Chronic MR
      i. MR that develops more slowly is accompanied by compensatory dilation of the left atrium (thus LA pressures are not as elevated).
      ii. If not corrected, patients eventually develop PH and associated complications (e.g., RVH and HF).
4. Clinical manifestations
   a. Cough and crackles (due to pulmonary edema).
   b. Fatigue and dyspnea on exertion (due to reduced forward cardiac output).
   c. Palpitations (due to atrial fibrillation, a common occurrence).
   d. "Blowing" apical holosystolic murmur.

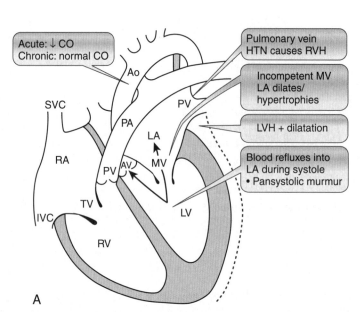

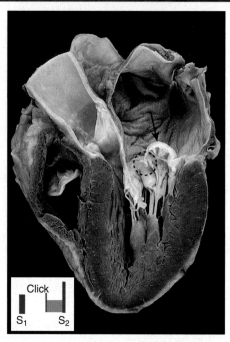

11.12 (A) Mitral regurgitation. In systole, there is retrograde blood flow into the left atrium (LA), causing it to dilate and hypertrophy. The increased pressure in the LA is transmitted back into the pulmonary circulation (pulmonary hypertension) and the right ventricle (RV), causing concentric right ventricular hypertrophy. Pulmonary congestion and edema are common findings. The cardiac output is decreased in acute mitral valve (MV) regurgitation but is normal in chronic MV regurgitation. (B) MV prolapse. The arrow shows prolapse of the posterior mitral leaflet into the LA. The interrupted circle shows rupture of one of the chordae tendineae, which produced mitral regurgitation. *Ao,* Aorta; *AV,* aortic valve; *CO,* cardiac output; *HTN,* hypertension; *IVC,* inferior vena cava; *LV,* left ventricle; *LVH,* left ventricular hypertrophy; *PA,* pulmonary artery; *PH,* pulmonary hypertension; *PV,* pulmonary valve; *RA,* right atrium; *RVH,* right ventricular hypertrophy; *SVC,* superior vena cava; *TV,* tricuspid valve. *(A, From Goljan EF:* Star series: pathology. *Philadelphia, 1998, Saunders; B, from Kumar V, Fausto N, Abbas A:* Robbins and Cotran pathologic basis of disease, *ed 7, Philadelphia, 2004, Saunders, p 592, Fig. 12-23.)*

5. Diagnosis
   a. Echocardiography.
D. Aortic stenosis
   1. Obstruction of blood flow across the aortic valve.
   2. Etiologies
      a. Degenerative changes with calcification
         i. Normal aortic valve has three leaflets (i.e., is tricuspid).
         ii. Bicuspid aortic valves, which are present in ~1%–2% of the population, undergo more rapid degeneration and are therefore more likely to become stenotic.
      b. Congenital stenosis (major cause in children).
      c. Chronic rheumatic heart disease.
   3. Pathophysiology
      a. Fibrosis and calcification of the aortic valve causes narrowing and obstruction of the left ventricular outflow tract (LVOT).
      b. LV must generate high pressure to push blood across the narrowed orifice.
      c. Higher pressure load on the LV leads to the development of LVH (with associated clinical manifestations and complications).
   4. Clinical manifestations
      a. Develop when the orifice is <1 cm² (normal aortic orifice 3 cm²).
      b. Initially, cardiac output remains normal at rest (i.e., long asymptomatic period).
      c. With exertion, however, the cardiac output often fails to increase appropriately; patients develop exercise-induced symptoms. Once symptoms arise, patients have a limited life expectancy with increased risk of sudden death and therefore require valve replacement.
         i. Dyspnea.
         ii. Syncope (inadequate blood flow to the brain).
         iii. Angina (inadequate blood flow to coronary arteries).
      d. Harsh crescendo–decrescendo systolic ejection murmur heard best at the right second intercostal space with radiation into the neck.
      e. Diminished A2 component of S2
      f. S4 (blood entering noncompliant stiff LV).
      g. LVH

       i. Evidence of LVH on ECG (Sokolow and Lyon criteria): amplitude of S wave in lead V1 + amplitude of R wave in V5 or V6 (whichever is the tallest) ≥ 35 mm.

    h. Hemolytic anemia

       i. Due to mechanical disruption of red cells striking the stenotic valve (intravascular hemolysis).

       ii. Peripheral smear shows fragmented red cells (schistocytes).

       iii. Hemoglobinuria (hemoglobin in the urine) may occur and causes urine to appear pink.

  5. Diagnosis

    a. Echocardiography.

E. Aortic regurgitation

  1. Definition

    a. Retrograde flow of blood from the aorta into the LV during diastole.

    b. Due to incompetence of the aortic valve and/or abnormality of the valvular support structures.

  2. Etiologies

    a. Infectious endocarditis.

    b. Chronic rheumatic heart disease.

    c. Abnormalities of ascending aorta (aortic root dilation and Marfan syndrome).

  3. Pathophysiology

    a. Incompetence of aortic valve → retrograde flow of blood back into the LV during diastole.

       i. Acute AR: LVEDP is markedly increased; cardiac output and systolic blood pressure (SBP) are reduced.

       ii. Chronic AR: compensatory left ventricular dilation allows for increased SV and SBP, whereas the diastolic blood pressure (DBP) is decreased as blood regurgitates back into the LV during diastole.

        (1) Increased pulse pressure (difference between SBP and DBP); volume overload on LV.

  4. Clinical manifestations

    a. "Blowing" decrescendo early diastolic murmur heard best at left edge of sternum.

    b. Widened pulse pressure (see earlier) with bounding pulses ("water-hammer pulse"), head nodding with each heartbeat.

  5. Diagnosis

    a. Echocardiography.

F. Tricuspid regurgitation (TR)

  1. Incompetence of tricuspid valve with retrograde systolic flow of blood into RA.

  2. Etiologies

    a. RHF (the most common cause)

       i. Distention of RV → stretching of support structures around tricuspid valve (impairs closure). Resolves with the treatment of HF.

    b. Structural abnormalities of the leaflets and chordae

       i. Examples: infective endocarditis and carcinoid heart disease (see later).

  3. Pathophysiology

    a. Retrograde flow into RA → right atrial dilation and backup of blood into the venous system.

  4. Clinical manifestations

    a. Peripheral edema, ascites, jugular venous distention, hepatomegaly (i.e., findings of RHF).

    b. High-pitched pansystolic murmur; increased intensity on inspiration.

       i. During inspiration, venous return to the right side of the heart increases (increasing murmur intensity of right-sided lesions).

  5. Diagnosis

    a. Echocardiography.

G. Pulmonic stenosis

  1. Impaired flow of blood from RV across narrowed right ventricular outflow tract.

    a. Uncommon, often congenital defect; may arise secondary to carcinoid heart disease.

  2. Clinical manifestations

    a. RVH (increased pressure load on the RV).

  3. Diagnosis

    a. Echocardiography.

H. Pulmonary regurgitation

  1. Incompetence of pulmonic valve, results in early diastolic flow from the PA into the RV (causing volume overload of the RV).

  2. Clinical manifestations

    a. Diastolic murmur, increased intensity with inspiration.

  3. Diagnosis

    a. Echocardiography.

I. Carcinoid heart disease

  1. Release of bioactive compounds (e.g., serotonin) from a carcinoid tumor directly into the systemic circulation (usually from metastatic tumor within the liver).

  2. Causes plaque-like fibrotic thickening of right-sided heart valves resulting in TR and/or pulmonic stenosis.

J. Infective endocarditis (IE)
1. Definition
   a. Microbial infection of the heart valve or mural endocardium.
2. Risk factors
   a. Increasing age, male sex, and poor dentition.
   b. Structural valvular defect (e.g., degenerative or congenital defects).
   c. Acquired valvular defect (e.g., catheterization and prosthetic valve).
   d. Injection of intravenous (IV) drugs.
3. Pathophysiology
   a. Endocardial injury (e.g., turbulent blood flow) → fibrin clot forms over the defect → seeding of the clot by bacteria.
      i. Organisms (e.g., bacteria and fungi) adhere to the clot (or directly invade the valve leaflet in some cases).
   b. The host immune response, in conjunction with continued growth of the organism, cause "vegetations" to form.
      i. Vegetations are comprised of bacteria, platelets, fibrin, and leukocytes.
   c. Ultimately, endocardial surfaces (e.g., valve leaflets and chordae) are damaged.
   d. Endocardial injury may be associated with regurgitant blood flow.
   e. Potential for the embolization of vegetation material (see later discussion).
   f. IE is more common on the left side of the heart (i.e., mitral and/or aortic valve) due to the higher pressures.
      i. Right-sided heart valves are normally spared (notable exception being those who inject IV drugs).
4. Microbiology
   a. *Staphylococcus aureus*
      i. Overall, the most common etiologic agent.
      ii. Also, the most common agent in those with the history of injection drug use.
   b. Viridans group *Streptococcus* (following oral surgery).
   c. *Streptococcus gallolyticus* (*bovis*) if present suggests colonic ulceration (e.g., ulcerative colitis and colon cancer).
   d. Fungal endocarditis (more likely in those who inject IV drugs).
5. Clinical manifestations (Fig. 11.13)
   a. Acute versus subacute
      i. Acute endocarditis

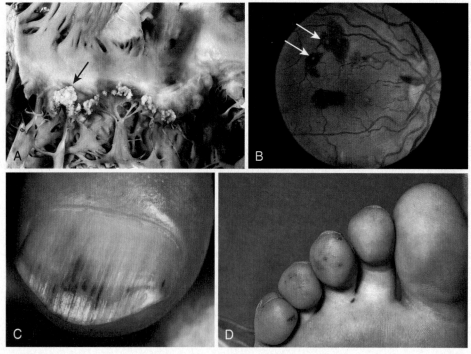

11.13: (A) Acute bacterial endocarditis. Large, friable, and irregular vegetation (*arrow*) is present on the margin of the mitral valve. Smaller vegetations are present along the line of closure of the valve. (B) Roth spots. Note the areas of hemorrhage with white dots in the center (*white arrows*). (C) Splinter hemorrhages in the nail bed. Note the longitudinal red hemorrhages in the nail bed. These represent areas of microembolization. (D) Osler nodes on the pads of the toes. These represent areas of microembolization of vegetation material and are usually painful. (*A, From Pathology: a color atlas, St. Louis, 2000, Mosby, p 11, Fig. 1-16; B, from Bouloux, P: Self-assessment picture tests medicine, Vol 1, London, 1997, Mosby-Wolfe, p 63, Fig. 125; C, from Swartz MH: Textbook of physical diagnosis, ed 5, Philadelphia, 2006, Saunders Elsevier, p 747, Fig. 8-10; D, from Bouloux P: Self-assessment picture tests medicine, Vol 3, London, 1997, Mosby-Wolfe, p 45, Fig. 89.*)

                (1) Characterized by abrupt onset and rapid progressive destruction of valve leaflets.
                (2) Most commonly caused by *S. aureus*.
                (3) Highly virulent organisms may involve previously normal valve leaflets.
            ii. Subacute endocarditis
                (1) More indolent infection, involving previously damaged valve.
                (2) Commonly secondary to streptococci.
        b. Fever (90% of cases).
        c. Roth spots (retinal hemorrhage with pale center).
        d. Splinter hemorrhages (linear subungual hemorrhage).
        e. Janeway lesions (painless areas of hemorrhage on palms and soles).
        f. Osler nodes (small tender nodules on the pads of the fingers or toes).
        g. Septic emboli (embolization of vegetation).
            i. Emboli commonly involve the brain, kidney, spleen, and heart (although essentially any tissue may be affected).
            ii. Complications include tissue infarction (e.g., stroke), metastatic abscess (e.g., cerebral abscess), or inflammation of artery (arteritis) with the subsequent formation of mycotic aneurysm.
        h. Heart murmurs (regurgitant types); may change in intensity with progressive destruction of the leaflets and support structures.
            i. Regurgitation may be secondary to the failure of leaflet coaptation, leaflet perforation, and/or rupture of chordae.
        i. Neutrophilic leukocytosis.
    6. Diagnosis
        a. Blood cultures (preferably before antibiotics).
        b. Transthoracic echocardiography (TTE) or transesophageal echocardiography (TEE) (to detect valvular vegetations).
            i. TTE is usually performed first (less invasive).
            ii. TEE is more sensitive and may identify lesions missed by TTE.
  K. Nonbacterial thrombotic endocarditis (marantic endocarditis)
    1. Sterile, nondestructive platelet thrombi; most often associated with an underlying malignancy or systemic lupus erythematosus (SLE) ("Libman–Sacks" endocarditis).
    2. Pathogenesis unclear; endothelial injury secondary to circulating cytokines is thought to trigger platelet and fibrin deposition.
    3. Lack of inflammatory reaction make these lesions prone to embolization (causing infarction at distant site).
VII. Myocardial and Pericardial Disorders
  A. Myocarditis
    1. Definition
        a. Inflammation of the myocardium; either infectious or noninfectious.
    2. Epidemiology
        a. May arise at any age, most common in young adulthood.
        b. More common in males (who also have a worse prognosis).
    3. Etiologies include:
        a. Viruses (e.g., coxsackievirus, adenovirus, parvovirus, and SARS-CoV-2).
            i. Most common cause of myocarditis; due to the immune response.
        b. Parasitic (e.g., *Trypanosoma cruzi*)
            i. *T. cruzi* causes Chagas disease (mostly Central/South America).
        c. Immune-mediated disorders (e.g., acute RF, SLE, rheumatoid arthritis, Kawasaki disease, and others).
    4. Pathology
        a. Lymphocytic infiltrate with focal necrosis is characteristic histologic finding in viral myocarditis (Fig. 11.14).
    5. Clinical manifestations
        a. Variable depending on the degree of involvement; ranges from subclinical disease to HF, arrhythmias, and sudden death.
    6. Diagnosis
        a. Echocardiography, cardiac catheterization, and endocardial biopsy.
  B. Pericarditis
    1. Definition
        a. Inflammation of the pericardium.
    2. Etiology
        a. Viral (e.g., coxsackievirus and echovirus).
        b. Metabolic disorders (e.g., uremia and hypothyroidism).
        c. Radiation.
        d. Systemic autoimmune disorders (e.g., SLE).

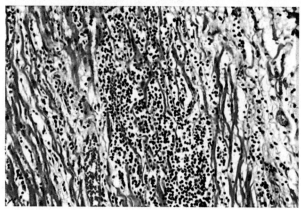

11.14: Myocardial biopsy specimen showing myocarditis. Note the lymphocytic infiltrate. *(From Marx JA, Hockberger RS, Walls RM: Rosen's emergency medicine concepts and clinical practice, ed 8, St. Louis, 2014, Elsevier Saunders, p 1099, Fig. 82-4.)*

 3. Pathology
   a. Fibrinous exudate on pericardium; due to increased vascular permeability with deposition of a fibrin-rich exudate.
   b. Pericardial effusion (fluid in the pericardial sac).
   c. Postinflammatory scarring, risk of constrictive pericarditis (see later).
 4. Clinical manifestations
   a. Pleuritic chest pain (relieved when leaning forward).
   b. Pericardial friction rub (does not disappear on breath holding; differentiates pericardial friction rub from a pleural friction rub).
   c. New widespread ST-segment elevation on ECG.
C. Pericardial effusion
 1. Definition
   a. Excessive fluid (or blood) within the pericardial sac.
   b. May be seen in association with acute pericarditis, following trauma (e.g., gunshot wound to chest), or tumor involvement of pericardium (e.g., breast cancer and lung cancer).
 2. Clinical manifestations
   a. Muffled heart sounds
     i. Fluid around heart obscures heart sounds.
   b. Cardiac tamponade
     i. Compression of the heart by pericardial fluid impairs cardiac filling, causing
       (1) Elevated jugular venous pressure (JVP).
       (2) Hypotension (secondary to decreased SV and cardiac output).
     ii. Life-threatening, requires immediate drainage of the fluid (pericardiocentesis).
     iii. Pulsus paradoxus
       (1) Refers to an abnormally large decrease in SBP of >10 mm Hg on inspiration.
       (2) Due to the displacement of interventricular septum into the LV as more blood returns to the right side of heart during inspiration. Normally, the LV can accommodate for this phenomenon. In situations (e.g., tamponade and constrictive pericarditis) in which the LV cannot compensate, the left ventricular SV, and thus SBP, are reduced.
 3. Diagnosis
   a. Echocardiography.
   b. Chest radiograph shows a "water bottle" configuration.
D. Constrictive pericarditis
 1. Definition
   a. Thickening of the pericardium, with or without calcification, resulting in impaired cardiac filling; a potential complication of essentially any pericardial disease process.
 2. Clinical manifestations
   a. Elevated JVP.
   b. Kussmaul sign (the lack of an inspiratory decline in JVP).
   c. Pulsus paradoxus.
 3. Imaging
   a. May reveal calcification of parietal pericardium.

VIII. Cardiomyopathy
  A. Definition
    1. Broadly defined as the disease of heart muscle.
    2. Typically, used to refer to myocardial disease occurring in the absence of an underlying process (e.g., CHD, HTN, and valvular disease) that would explain the myocardial dysfunction.
  B. Dilated cardiomyopathy
    1. Definition
      a. Spectrum of heterogeneous myocardial disorders characterized by dilation and impaired contraction of the LV or both ventricles.
        i. Dilated cardiomyopathy presenting with an associated arrhythmia (i.e., atrial fibrillation, ventricular tachycardia) is known as "arrhythmogenic cardiomyopathy."
    2. Epidemiology
      a. May present at any age; most common between 20 and 60 years.
    3. Genetic and acquired etiologies
      a. Up to 50% have an evidence of familial disease (usually autosomal dominant inheritance).
        i. The major genetic mutation involves *TTN* (gene that encodes for the sarcomere protein titin).
        ii. Duchenne and Becker muscular dystrophy (both X-linked recessive) are additional inherited causes of cardiomyopathy.
      b. Acquired etiologies include:
        i. Alcohol abuse.
        ii. Drugs (e.g., doxorubicin and trastuzumab).
        iii. Autoimmune disorders.
        iv. Pregnancy (postpartum cardiomyopathy).
    4. Pathophysiology
      a. Ventricular dilation with generalized decrease in contractility.
    5. Clinical manifestations
      a. Manifests with signs and symptoms characteristic of HF (fatigue, dyspnea, edema, etc.).
      b. Chest X-ray shows global enlargement of the heart.
      c. Ventricular arrhythmias (potentially fatal).
  C. Hypertrophic cardiomyopathy
    1. Definition
      a. Disease of the heart characterized by unexplained LVH in the absence of abnormal loading condition (e.g., systemic hypertension or aortic stenosis).
    2. Pathogenesis
      a. Autosomal dominant with variable penetrance.
      b. Mutation involve sarcomere contractile protein genes (e.g., cardiac myosin-binding protein C and β-myosin heavy chain).
    3. Pathology
      a. Hypertrophy of the myocardium often disproportionately affects the interventricular septum.
      b. Histology shows chaotic disorganized myofibers ("myofiber disarray").
      c. May be associated with obstruction of the LVOT as the MV encounters the thickened interventricular septum during systole (called "systolic anterior motion of the MV") → causes a reduction in cardiac output.
      d. Obstruction of the LVOT is exacerbated by maneuvers that reduce preload (chamber size), decrease afterload, or increase LV contractility (e.g., exercise).
        i. Explains why exercise (possibly in conjunction with decreased preload) is a common trigger for the development of symptoms.
    4. Clinical manifestations
      a. Fatigue, dyspnea, chest pain, and syncope (reduced cardiac output).
      b. Harsh crescendo–decrescendo systolic murmur (due to LVOT obstruction)
        i. Murmur intensity increases (obstruction worsens) with decreased preload (e.g., abrupt standing and Valsalva maneuver).
        ii. Murmur intensity decreases (obstruction lessens) with increased preload (recumbency and passive leg raising).
      c. Angina, syncope, or sudden death from ventricular tachycardia or fibrillation (especially with exercise as noted above).
    5. Diagnosis/screening
      a. Echocardiography.
  D. Restrictive cardiomyopathy
    1. Definition
      a. Variety of conditions, all of which are characterized by an excessively stiff myocardium and impaired diastolic filling.

2. Etiologies
   a. Cardiac amyloidosis—the deposition of amyloid within the myocardium (the most common cause, usually immunoglobulin light chains—AL amyloid).
   b. Cardiac sarcoidosis.
   c. Myocardial fibrosis (following mediastinal radiation).
   d. Endocardial fibroelastosis (children).
   e. Storage diseases of heart (e.g., hereditary hemochromatosis)
      i. Iron overload can cause restrictive cardiomyopathy but is more likely to present as a dilated cardiomyopathy.
   f. Familial (mutations in cardiac sarcomere protein genes, particularly troponin I and β-myosin heavy chain).
3. Pathophysiology
   a. Decrease in ventricular compliance → impaired cardiac filling (diastolic dysfunction).
4. Clinical manifestations
   a. Progressive HF (fatigue, weakness, peripheral edema, ascites, dyspnea on exertion, etc.).
   b. Elevated JVP.
   c. Failure of inspiratory decrease in the jugular venous pulse (Kussmaul sign).
5. Diagnosis
   a. Echocardiography, cardiac catheterization, and endocardial biopsy (select cases).

IX. **Tumors of the Heart**
   A. **Cardiac myxoma**
      1. Benign mesenchymal tumor of the heart.
      2. Most common primary cardiac tumor in adults.
      3. Most arise from the left atrium.
         a. If pedunculated, may obstruct the MV ("ball-valve" effect) with auscultation of a "tumor plop" early in diastole.
      4. Tumor fragments may embolize into the systemic circulation causing infarcts (e.g., strokes).
      5. Rarely seen as a component of Carney complex, an autosomal dominant disorder characterized by myxomas, pigmented mucocutaneous lesions, and endocrine tumors (e.g., pituitary adenoma and thyroid adenoma).
   B. **Rhabdomyoma**
      1. Usually in children, strong association with tuberous sclerosis.
      2. Spontaneous regression typical.

I. **Erythropoiesis**
  A. **Production of red blood cells (RBCs)**
    1. Occurs in the bone marrow (BM) in response to erythropoietin (EPO), a growth factor produced in the kidneys (primarily) and liver.
      a. Major stimulus for EPO release is renal hypoxia.
      b. Renal hypoxia activates hypoxia-inducible factor, a transcription factor that enhances the production of EPO.
  B. **EPO stimulates the proliferation and differentiation of marrow erythroid precursor cells (Fig. 12.1).**
    1. In early gestation, the production of blood cells (hematopoiesis) occurs in the mesenchyme of the yolk sac.
    2. In mid-gestation, hematopoiesis occurs in the liver and spleen.
    3. By the third trimester, hematopoiesis has localized to the BM.
  C. **RBCs**
    1. Overview
      a. RBCs have a diameter of 6–8 μm and a biconcave shape (increases flexibility).
      b. Cell membrane contains various cytoskeletal proteins (e.g., spectrin, ankyrin, band 3, and band 4.2).
      c. Cytoplasm contains hemoglobin (Hb) and glycolytic enzymes.
      d. Mature RBCs lack a nucleus, mitochondria, and human leukocyte antigens.
      e. The absence of mitochondria leaves the red cell dependent upon glycolysis.
    2. Biochemistry of red cells (Fig. 12.2)
      a. Embden–Meyerhof pathway (glycolysis)

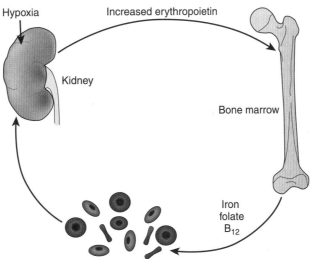

12.1: Regulation of red blood cell production. *(Adapted from Hoffman R, Heidrick E, Benz E, et al: Hematology: basic principles and practice, ed 4, Philadelphia, 2005, Churchill Livingstone, Fig. 29-2.)*

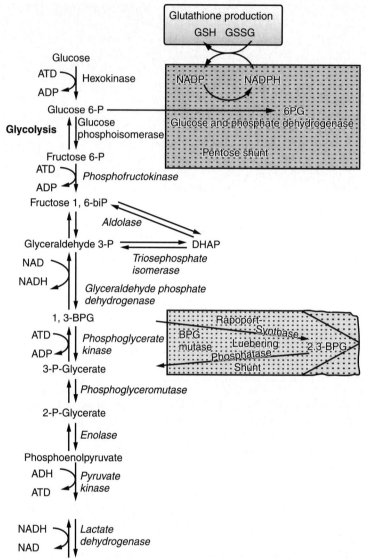

12.2: Red blood cell metabolism. Glycolysis, pentose shunt (*shaded area*), and Rapoport–Luebering shunt (*shaded area*). *1,3-BPG*, 1,3-Bisphosphoglycerate; *2,3-BPG*, 2,3-bisphosphoglycerate; *6PG*, 6-phosphogluconate; *ADP*, adenosine diphosphate; *ATP*, adenosine triphosphate; *DHAP*, dihydroxyacetone phosphate; *GAPD*, glyceraldehyde phosphate dehydrogenase; *GSH*, reduced glutathione; *GSSG*, oxidized glutathione; *NAD⁺*, nicotinamide adenine dinucleotide; *NADP⁺*, oxidized form of nicotinamide adenine dinucleotide phosphate; *NADPH*, reduced form of nicotinamide adenine dinucleotide phosphate. *(From* Hematology: basic principles and practice, *ed 7. Copyright © 2018 by Elsevier, Figure 44.1.)*

     i. Source of adenosine triphosphate (ATP), necessary for the maintenance of ion pumps and cellular structure.

     ii. Enzyme deficiencies within the pathway (e.g., pyruvate kinase [PK] and hexokinase) → decreased ATP generation → increased susceptibility to hemolysis.

  b. Pentose phosphate pathway (hexose monophosphate shunt)

     i. Primary source of the reduced form of nicotinamide adenine dinucleotide phosphate (NADPH) (required for the reduction of oxidized glutathione).

     ii. Glucose-6-phosphate dehydrogenase (G6PD) is the initial and rate-limiting enzyme (converts glucose-6-phosphate to 6-phosphogluconolactone).

     iii. Inherited G6PD deficiency renders red cells more susceptible to hemolysis, particularly in association with oxidant stress (e.g., infection, ketoacidosis, and/or ingestion of certain drugs/fava beans).

  c. Methemoglobin reductase pathway

     i. Normal Hb contains iron in the ferrous (Fe^{2+}) state.

     ii. Oxidation of heme iron to the ferric (Fe^{3+}) state forms methemoglobin.

     iii. Methemoglobin does not bind to oxygen and must be reduced back to Hb (Fe^{2+}).

       (1) Catalyzed by the cytochrome b5 methemoglobin reductase system.

        iv. Increased levels of methemoglobin (methemoglobinemia) can be seen in association with the use of various medications (e.g., local anesthetics, nitrates/nitrites, and sulfonamides) or as an inherited condition (usually a quantitative or qualitative deficiency of cytochrome b5 reductase).

        v. Manifestations, which depend upon the level of methemoglobin, include cyanosis, weakness, dizziness, coma, and death.

        vi. Clue to diagnosis: chocolate brown appearance to blood.

    d. Rapoport–Luebering shunt

        i. Bisphosphoglycerate mutase converts 1,3-bisphosphoglycerate (1,3-BPG) to 2,3-bisphosphoglycerate (2,3-BPG).

        ii. 2,3-BPG facilitates the release of oxygen to the surrounding tissues (i.e., shifts the oxygen dissociation curve to the right).

  3. Red cell lifespan

    a. Normal red cells live for ~120 days in circulation.

    b. Senescent red cells are phagocytosed by splenic macrophages and degraded into various components.

        i. Amino acids and iron are recycled.

        ii. Heme → biliverdin → bilirubin.

          (1) Explains why increased red cell breakdown (i.e., hemolysis) causes hyperbilirubinemia and jaundice.

D. Measurement of red cell production (reticulocyte count)

  1. Reticulocytes represent newly released immature red cells.

    a. Reticulocytes are identified via supravital staining (highlights residual RNA that remains for approximately the first 24 hours after entry into circulation).

    b. Enumeration of reticulocytes used to evaluate the production of RBCs (Fig. 12.3).

  2. Reticulocytes should comprise about 1% of all red cells in circulation (to replace normal red cell senescence).

    a. In anemic states, the number of reticulocytes should rise to compensate for the deficit.

  3. Reticulocyte production index ("reticulocyte count")

    a. Useful evaluation of the BM response to anemia.

    b. To calculate, first determine the number of reticulocytes, as a percentage of all circulating red cells (i.e., reticulocyte percentage).

    c. In anemia, this count must be corrected to prevent an overestimation as follows:

        i. Reticulocyte percentage is multiplied by the patient's hematocrit (Hct) divided by 45 (reticulocyte percentage × [Hct/45]).

          (1) The denominator "45" represents a normal Hct.

        ii. In addition, because red cells are released from the BM at an earlier stage of development in those with anemia, a second correction is performed if there are polychromatophilic red cells (early red cell precursors) on the peripheral smear (usually simply divide the reticulocyte percentage, as described above, by 2).

    d. Example

        i. Consider a patient who has a Hct of 30%. If 6% of his/her red cells are reticulocytes, then the initial correction results in a reticulocyte count of 4% (6 × [30/45]).

        ii. To account for the increased maturation time, the initial "correction" of 4% is divided by 2 to give a "reticulocyte production index" of 2%. In other words, twice as many reticulocytes are entering the blood per day as in a normal individual (2% instead of 1%).

  4. In anemia, patients can normally increase RBC production by two to three times the normal rate within 1 week (or more if there is a parenteral supply of iron).

    a. Failure of the BM to increase red cell production within 1–2 weeks implies impaired erythropoiesis.

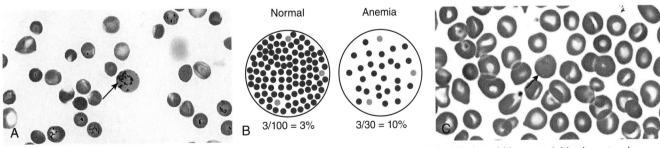

12.3: (A) Peripheral blood reticulocytes with a methylene blue stain. Red blood cells (RBCs) with thread-like material in the cytosol represent residual RNA (*arrow*). The patient has a hemolytic anemia; therefore the number of reticulocytes is increased. (B) Correction of the reticulocyte count for the degree of anemia. On the left side of the image, the normal reticulocyte count is 3% when three reticulocytes (*pale blue RBCs*) are expressed as a percentage of 100 RBCs in the microscopic field. However, the same three reticulocytes account for 10% of the RBCs in a patient with anemia, who has only 30 RBCs in the microscopic field. (C) Polychromasia. The arrow indicates a blue discolored RBC without a central area of pallor. These are more immature erythroid precursors that require anywhere from 2 to 3 days to mature. (*A, From Naeim F:* Atlas of bone marrow and blood pathology, *Philadelphia, 2001, Saunders, p 12, Fig. 1-15B; B, from Goljan EF, Sloka KI:* Rapid review laboratory testing in clinical medicine, *Philadelphia, 2008, Mosby Elsevier, p 146, Fig. 5-3; C, from Naeim F:* Atlas of bone marrow and blood pathology, *Philadelphia, 2001, Saunders, Fig. 1-15A.*)

In anemia, reticulocyte production should increase 2- to 3-fold
(i.e., reticulocyte production index of > 2%; some authors use 3%)
If, however, the corrected reticulocyte count is less than expected (i.e., < 2%–3%), then the bone marrow response is inadequate (called "ineffective" erythropoiesis), and one must consider a nutrient deficiency (e.g., iron, folate, B12) or primary bone marrow disorder (e.g., aplastic anemia, see later).

   E. **Extramedullary hematopoiesis (EMH)**
       1. Definition
           a. Hematopoiesis occurring outside the BM; most commonly in the liver and spleen.
       2. Etiologies
           a. Intrinsic disease of the BM (e.g., replacement of marrow by a metastatic tumor).
           b. Compensatory response to chronic severe anemia (e.g., chronic hemolytic disorders).
   F. **Erythroid hyperplasia**
       1. Definition
           a. Increased numbers of erythroid precursors within the BM.
           b. Not the same as EMH which refers to the production of hematopoietic cells (RBCs, white blood cells [WBCs], and platelets) *outside* the marrow cavity.
       2. Clinical manifestations
           a. Bony changes (Fig. 12.4); "hair-on-end" appearance as seen on X-ray imaging of the skull and enlargement of facial bones.
II. **Complete Blood Count (CBC)**
   A. **Definition**
       1. Laboratory test that provides information about circulating blood cells.
           a. RBCs, WBCs, and platelets.
   B. **RBC indices**
       1. Hb—the amount of Hb in grams per deciliter (dL) of whole blood.
       2. Hct—red cells as a percentage of blood volume.
       3. Erythrocyte count—number of erythrocytes per microliter (µL) of blood.
       4. Mean corpuscular volume (MCV)
           a. MCV—a measure of the average red cell volume (normal 80–100 fL).
           b. Useful in the classification of anemia
               i. Microcytic (MCV < 80 fL)
               ii. Normocytic (MCV 80–100 fL)
               iii. Macrocytic (MCV > 100 fL)
       5. Mean corpuscular hemoglobin concentration (MCHC)
           a. Measure of Hb concentration in a given volume of red cells.
               i. Decreased MCHC
                   (1) Indicates decreased Hb production.
                   (2) Recognized by an enlarged central area of pallor on the blood smear (called "hypochromasia").

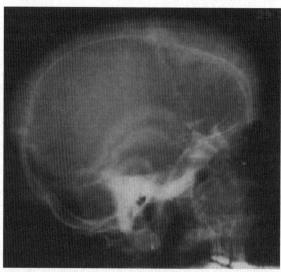

12.4: Lateral radiograph of the skull shows the typical "hair-on-end" appearance, with thinning of the cortical bone and widening of the marrow cavity from accelerated erythropoiesis (e.g., severe hemolysis in sickle cell disease). *(From Bouloux P: Self-assessment picture tests medicine, Vol. 1, London, 1997, Mosby-Wolfe, p 49, Fig. 97.)*

ii. Central area of pallor is normally one-third of the diameter of the RBC.

iii. Increased MCHC

  (1) Characteristic finding in hereditary spherocytosis (HS) in which portions of the red cell membrane are phagocytosed by splenic macrophages. As the red cell membrane is lost, the volume of the cell is reduced (i.e., Hb becomes more concentrated, MCHC is increased).

6. Red cell distribution width (RDW)

  a. Measures variation in red cell size.

  b. Useful if elevated (e.g., iron deficiency); indicates the presence of two cell populations (i.e., microcytic cells and normocytic cells).

C. Leukocyte (WBC) count

1. Number of WBC per volume of blood (normal 4000–11,000/μL of blood).

2. The white cell "differential" provides a measure of each type of leukocyte as a percentage of the total WBC count.

  a. Immature cells (e.g., bands, metamyelocytes, etc.) are included in the differential cell count.

3. Absolute cell count

  a. The percentage of each type of WBC is multiplied by the total WBC count to obtain an "absolute cell count" for each type of leukocyte.

   i. For example, a patient with 30% lymphocytes and a total WBC count of 10,000/μL has an absolute lymphocyte count of 3000 cells/μL (0.30 × 10,000).

  b. When determining an absolute neutrophil count (ANC), add the percentage of neutrophils and bands.

   i. For example, a patient with a total WBC count of 10,000/μL with 55% neutrophils and 5% bands has an ANC of 6000/μL (0.60 × 10,000).

D. Platelet count

1. Number of platelets per microliter of blood (normal 150,000–400,000/μL).

2. Platelets are derived from cytoplasmic budding of megakaryocytes.

3. Unlike mature RBCs, platelets exhibit human leukocyte antigens on their membranes.

III. Laboratory Studies in the Evaluation of Anemia

A. Iron studies (Fig. 12.5)

1. Serum ferritin

  a. Unbound ("free") iron is toxic (impairs cellular metabolism and forms free radicals).

  b. For this reason, iron must be either bound to transferrin (for transport in circulation) or stored (as ferritin or hemosiderin).

   i. Ferritin is a water-soluble storage form of iron.

   ii. Hemosiderin is a water-insoluble storage form derived from the lysosomal breakdown of ferritin. On microscopic examination, hemosiderin has a refractile, golden brown appearance on routine H&E-stained sections (appears blue with use of a Prussian blue stain).

  c. Serum ferritin levels reflect total body iron stores; used as a clinical marker of iron status (i.e., iron deficiency is characterized by a reduction in serum ferritin).

  d. Conversely, serum ferritin levels may be increased in those with various inflammatory states (e.g., rheumatoid arthritis, malignancy, infective endocarditis).

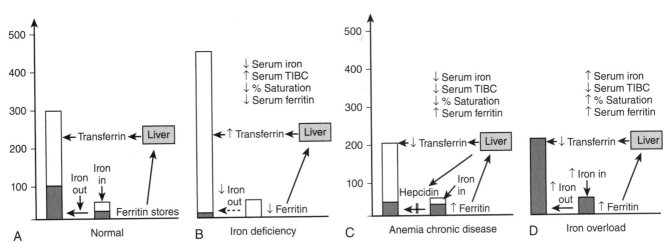

12.5: Iron studies (normal) (A) and in iron deficiency (B), anemia of chronic disease (C), and iron overload (D). The column represents transferrin, the iron-binding protein. The small box represents ferritin within bone marrow macrophages. In health, a roughly equal amount of iron enters and leaves the macrophages. Iron entering the macrophages is derived largely from the recycling of iron from senescent red blood cells. The amount of ferritin in the macrophages has a negative feedback with hepatic transferrin synthesis (decreased ferritin stores stimulates hepatic synthesis of transferrin and vice versa). Refer to the text for discussion of the anemias. *TIBC,* Total iron-binding capacity.

i. Recall that interleukin-6 (IL-6) stimulates the liver to produce various acute-phase reactants, including ferritin and hepcidin, the latter explaining anemia of chronic disease (ACD) (see later).

ii. Ferritin is also increased in iron overload states.

e. Summary

i. Serum ferritin is decreased in iron deficiency.

ii. Serum ferritin is increased in iron overload states (e.g., hereditary hemochromatosis) as well as in chronic inflammation/disease states.

2. Serum iron

a. Serum iron represents iron bound to transferrin.

b. Transferrin is synthesized in the liver and functions as a carrier of iron.

c. Iron deficiency and ACD are both characterized by a decrease in serum iron.

d. Iron overload states (e.g., hemochromatosis) are characterized by an increase in serum iron.

3. Serum total iron-binding capacity (TIBC)

a. TIBC is a measure of transferrin concentration.

i. ↓ TIBC = ↓ transferrin; ↑ TIBC = ↑ transferrin.

b. Transferrin delivers iron to erythroid precursors in the BM.

c. Iron bound to transferrin is either derived from storage (i.e., BM macrophages) or the diet.

i. Duodenum is the primary site of iron absorption.

d. Transferrin synthesis varies inversely with ferritin stores.

i. As ferritin decreases, hepatic synthesis of transferrin increases.

e. Summary

i. In iron deficiency: ferritin ↓, TIBC ↑.

ii. In iron overload (or ACD): ferritin ↑, TIBC ↓.

4. Iron saturation (%)

a. Percentage of transferrin binding sites occupied by iron.

i. Iron saturation (%) = (serum iron/TIBC) × 100.

ii. Normal iron saturation ~ 33%.

b. Decreased in iron deficiency and ACD.

c. Increased in iron overload states.

5. Hb electrophoresis

a. Useful in the detection of variant Hb molecules (i.e., hemoglobinopathy).

i. Hb variants are separated based on electrophoretic mobility.

ii. Used to identify inherited hemoglobinopathies

(1) Change in globin chain structure (e.g., sickle cell disease).

(2) Abnormal globin chain synthesis (e.g., thalassemia).

b. Types of normal Hb in adults (Fig. 12.6).

i. HbA: 2α- and 2β-globin chains (97% of total Hb).

ii. HbA2: 2α- and 2δ-globin chains (2% of total Hb).

iii. HbF: 2α- and 2γ-globin chains (1% of total Hb).

IV. Anemia

A. Definition

1. Reduction in red cell mass; identified on a CBC by a decrease in the Hb and/or Hct.

B. Anemia may be absolute or relative.

1. Absolute anemia refers to a true decrease in RBC mass.

a. Either secondary to a reduction in red cell production (e.g., nutrient deficiency or aplastic anemia) or increased red cell loss (e.g., hemolysis or hemorrhage).

2. Relative anemia refers to an apparent reduction in RBC mass (i.e., decreased Hct) secondary to an increase in plasma volume (i.e., hemodilution).

C. Anemia is a sign of underlying disease.

1. When identified, the underlying etiology must be identified.

D. Clinical manifestations

1. Fatigue, dyspnea with exertion, pallor of the skin and conjunctivae, rapid bounding pulses, and systolic flow murmurs.

V. Microcytic Anemias

A. Definition

1. Decrease in red cell mass (i.e., anemia) with decreased MCV (<80 fL).

B. Etiologies

1. Iron deficiency (most common)

2. ACD

3. Thalassemia

4. Sideroblastic anemia (some types, least common)

	Pattern				Types of Anemia	Interpretation and Discussion
A.	A_2 2%	S	F 1%	A 97%	None	Normal Hb electrophoresis
B.	A_2 2%	S	F 1%	A 97%	Microcytic	α-Thal trait. Note that the proportion of the Hb types remains the same; however, the patient has a microcytic anemia.
C.	A_2 5%	S	F 2%	A 93%	Microcytic	β-Thal minor. Note that HbA is decreased because β-globin chain synthesis is decreased. There is a corresponding increase in HbA$_2$ and HbF.
D.	A_2 10%	S	F 90%	A	Microcytic	β-Thal major. Note that there is no synthesis of HbA.
E.	A_2 2%	S 45%	F 1%	A 52%	No anemia	Sickle cell trait. Note that there is not enough HbS to cause spontaneous sickling in the peripheral blood.
F.	A_2 2%	S 90%	F 8%	A	Normocytic	Sickle cell disease. Note that there is no HbA. There is enough HbS to cause spontaneous sickling.

12.6: Hemoglobin (Hb) electrophoresis in various hemoglobinopathies. *(From Goljan E, Sloka K: Rapid review laboratory testing in clinical medicine, St. Louis, 2008, Mosby Elsevier, p 159, Fig. 5-12.)*

C. Pathogenesis

1. Hb is comprised of heme (i.e., iron + protoporphyrin) bound to globin chains (Fig. 12.7).
   a. A decrease in any of the three components (iron, protoporphyrin, or globin chains) cause Hb production to decrease and red cells to become smaller than normal (i.e., microcytic).
      i. Decreased iron (iron deficiency and ACD).
      ii. Decreased globin chain synthesis (thalassemia).
      iii. Decreased protoporphyrin synthesis (congenital and acquired types, including lead poisoning, vitamin B6 deficiency), "sideroblastic anemia."
2. Iron metabolism
   a. Iron stores are greater in men, largely due to menstrual and/or pregnancy losses of blood in women.
   b. Iron is derived from the diet, as either heme iron or nonheme iron (Fig. 12.8).
      i. Heme iron, which is present in the Hb and myoglobin of animal sources (e.g., red meat), is more readily absorbed.
      ii. Nonheme iron, which is derived from plants and iron-fortified foods, is less readily absorbed.
   c. Absorbed in the ferrous (Fe^{2+}) state.
      i. Low pH of gastric acid reduces dietary ferric iron to the absorbable ferrous (Fe^{2+}) state.
      ii. Primary site of iron absorption is the duodenum.
      iii. Divalent metal transporter 1 (DMT1) allows iron to move from the gut lumen into the enterocyte.
         (1) Iron may remain stored within the enterocyte (as mucosal ferritin) or be absorbed into circulation.
         (2) Transfer of iron from the enterocyte into circulation is dependent upon ferroportin (a transmembrane protein).

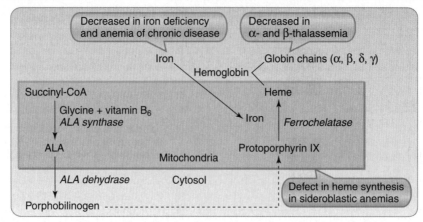

12.7: Pathophysiology of microcytic anemias. Microcytic anemias are all characterized by a reduction in hemoglobin synthesis, from a decrease in the synthesis of either heme or globin chains. *ALA,* Aminolevulinic acid.

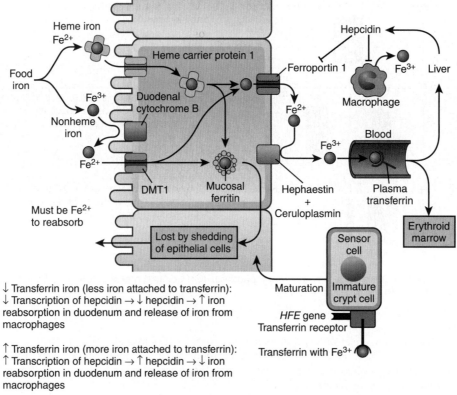

12.8: Iron absorption. The absorption of iron is dependent on total iron stores in the body, which is reflected in the amount of iron that is bound to transferrin. Enterocytes absorb ferrous iron (Fe^{2+}) directly via heme carrier protein 1 or through the divalent metal transporter (DMT1). Absorbed iron is either stored in the cytoplasm as mucosal ferritin or transferred to the ferroportin 1 port, where it is converted to ferric iron (Fe^{3+}) by hephaestin and ceruloplasmin. Plasma transferrin then binds the iron and carries it to erythroid precursors in the bone marrow. The *HFE* gene regulates the production of hepcidin, the "master" iron regulatory hormone. Hepcidin, which is produced in the liver, regulates iron absorption from the diet as well as that released from storage sites. For example, when iron stores are decreased, less transferrin iron binds to the receptor, less hepcidin is produced, and more iron is allowed to enter the circulation and be released from bone marrow macrophages. Conversely, when iron stores are adequate, there is an increased amount of transferrin iron bound to the receptor, more hepcidin is produced, and less iron is allowed to enter the circulation (either from enterocytes or from bone marrow macrophages). *(Modified from Kumar V, Fausto N, Abbas A, Aster J:* Robbins and Cotran pathologic basis of disease, *ed 8, Philadelphia, 2010, Saunders Elsevier, p 661, Fig. 14-22.)*

d. Iron absorption is regulated.
  i. Because there is no physiologic method to dispense with excess iron, iron levels are regulated at the site of absorption (recall that excess iron is toxic via the generation of free radicals).
  ii. Iron (complexed with transferrin) is sensed by receptors on hepatocytes (transferrin receptor protein 1—TfR1).
  iii. Iron binding to the TfR1 receptor causes the hepatocytes to secrete hepcidin (the "master" iron regulatory hormone).
  iv. Hepcidin binds to and degrades ferroportin, thereby trapping iron within cells (enterocytes and macrophages) and preventing its absorption into circulation.
    (1) Recall that hepcidin is an acute-phase reactant released in response to inflammatory cytokines (e.g., IL-6).
    (2) The excess hepcidin causes iron to be "trapped" within BM macrophages, thereby explaining the mechanism underlying ACD.
  v. Summary
    (1) ↓ Body iron → ↓ hepcidin → ↑ iron absorption and ↑ iron release from BM macrophages.
    (2) ↑ Body iron → ↑ hepcidin → ↓ iron absorption and ↓ iron release from BM macrophages.
3. Iron deficiency anemia (IDA)
  a. When inadequate iron is available for normal Hb production, patients develop "IDA."
  b. Epidemiology
    i. Although more prevalent in lower- to moderate-income countries, IDA remains relatively common in the United States, especially among the impoverished.
    ii. Specific groups most at risk include:
      (1) Breastfed infants without iron supplementation (increased iron requirements for growth).
      (2) Toddlers with high intake of cow's milk (low concentration and low bioavailability of iron in cow's milk along with intestinal blood loss induced by exposure to cow's milk protein).
      (3) Women of child-bearing age (iron loss in association with menses and/or pregnancy).
    iii. In adults, major causes of iron deficiency include:
      (1) Chronic blood loss (e.g., heavy menstrual bleeding, gastrointestinal hemorrhage).
      (2) Inadequate intake (strict vegetarians).
      (3) Impaired absorption (e.g., celiac disease or bariatric surgery).
    iv. Summary of causes (Table 12.1)
  c. Pathogenesis
    i. Inadequate levels of iron → decreased heme synthesis → decreased Hb formation → decreased RBC formation.
  d. Laboratory findings (Table 12.2)
    i. Decreased serum ferritin (best indicator).
    ii. Decreased MCV.
    iii. Decreased serum iron.
    iv. Decreased transferrin iron saturation.
    v. Increased TIBC and RDW.

TABLE 12.1   Causes of Iron Deficiency Anemia

CLASSIFICATION	CAUSES	DISCUSSION
Blood loss	Gastrointestinal loss	• Peptic ulcer disease • Hemorrhagic gastropathy • Hookworm infestation • Colon polyps/colorectal cancer • Diverticular bleeding • Ulcerated Meckel diverticulum • Angiodysplasia
Increased utilization	Heavy menstrual bleeding	• Most common cause in women of child-bearing age.
	Pregnancy or lactation	• Increased iron requirements necessitate the use of prenatal vitamins.
	Infants and children	• Iron is required for tissue growth and expansion of blood volume.
Decreased absorption	Celiac disease Postgastric surgery	• Loss of small intestinal villi impairs the absorption of iron and other nutrients. • Gastric resection may result in a loss of acid production (impairs the release of elemental iron from food).
Intravascular hemolysis	Microangiopathic hemolytic anemia	• Intravascular hemolysis produces a loss of hemoglobin in the urine (hemoglobinuria) with the potential for iron deficiency. • Paroxysmal nocturnal hemoglobinuria. Intravascular hemolysis of RBCs caused by complement-mediated destruction of RBCs.

RBC, Red blood cell.

TABLE 12.2   Laboratory Findings in Microcytic Anemias

TEST	IRON DEFICIENCY	ANEMIA OF CHRONIC DISEASE	α-THAL/β-THAL MINOR	LEAD POISONING
MCV	↓	Normal to ↓	↓	↓
Serum iron	↓	↓	Normal	↑
TIBC	↑	↓	Normal	↓
Percent saturation	↓	↓	Normal	↑
Serum ferritin	↓	↑	Normal	↑
RDW	↑	Normal	Normal	Normal
RBC count	↓	↓	↑	↓
Hb electrophoresis	Normal	Normal	α-Thal trait: normal β-Thal trait: ↓HbA, ↑HbA₂/F	—
Ringed sideroblasts	None	None	None	Present
Coarse basophilic stippling	None	None	None	Present

Hb, Hemoglobin; *MCV*, mean corpuscular volume; *RBC*, red blood cell; *RDW*, red blood cell distribution width; *Thal*, thalassemia; *TIBC*, total iron-binding capacity.

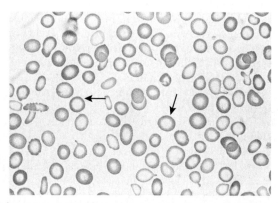

12.9: Peripheral blood smear in iron deficiency anemia. The enlarged central area of pallor in the red blood cells (*arrows*) indicates a decrease in hemoglobin synthesis, a characteristic of the microcytic anemias. The mean corpuscular hemoglobin concentration is decreased. Also note the size variation, which explains the increased RBC distribution width (RDW). *(From Wickramasinghe SE, McCullough J:* Blood and bone marrow pathology, *London, 2003, Churchill Livingstone, Fig. 11-6.)*

    e. Stages of iron deficiency
      i. As iron stores are depleted, serum ferritin and serum iron levels decrease while transferrin levels increase (i.e., increased TIBC).
      ii. All iron studies are abnormal before patients become anemic.
      iii. Eventually, anemia develops when red cell production is inadequate to replace those lost through senescence.
      iv. IDA is initially normocytic, normochromic (i.e., normal red cells, just fewer of them). Eventually becomes microcytic and hypochromic (Fig. 12.9).
    f. Additional findings
      i. BM biopsy (if performed) would show an absence of iron stores (Prussian blue stain used to highlight iron).
      ii. Elevated free erythrocyte protoporphyrin (FEP).
        (1) When iron levels are low, there is less iron available to bind with protoporphyrin to form heme, leaving increased levels of protoporphyrin unbound to iron (i.e., elevated FEP).
      iii. Thrombocytosis (increased platelet count)
        (1) Reactive phenomenon.
      iv. Plummer–Vinson syndrome
        (1) Triad of IDA, esophageal web, and atrophic glossitis.
      v. Spoon-shaped nails (koilonychia)
   4. ACD
    a. Definition
      i. Anemia arising in chronic inflammatory states (e.g., chronic infection, malignancy, and systemic inflammatory disorders).
    b. Epidemiology
      i. Second most common anemia worldwide after iron deficiency.
      ii. Increasing prevalence with age.

iii. Common associations include rheumatoid arthritis, inflammatory bowel disease, and malignancy.
   c. Pathogenesis
      i. Increased production of inflammatory cytokines.
         (1) IL-6 stimulates the liver to produce various acute-phase reactants (e.g., hepcidin). Hepcidin restricts iron trafficking (degrades ferroportin, trapping iron within BM macrophages). Thought to be an evolutionary phenomenon to limit the availability of iron to invading microbial organisms.
         (2) IL-1 reduces erythropoiesis.
         (3) Tumor necrosis factor suppresses GATA1, an essential erythroid transcription factor.
   d. Laboratory findings include:
      i. Normal to decreased MCV.
         (1) Red cells often remain normocytic in those with ACD (may become microcytic in chronic severe inflammatory states).
      ii. Increased serum ferritin (important differentiation from iron deficiency).
      iii. Decreased serum iron, TIBC, and percent iron saturation.
      iv. Elevated FEP
         (1) Less iron available, more protoporphyrin remains "free."
      v. Anemia is usually mild (Hb rarely <8 g/dL).
      vi. BM biopsy (if performed) would show increased iron stores.

D. Thalassemia
   1. Thalassemias are inherited disorders of globin chain production.
      a. Reduced globin chains (alpha, beta) cause an imbalance in the alpha- to beta-chain ratio.
      b. Unpaired globin chains damage the red cell precursors, causing them to die in the BM ("ineffective erythropoiesis") or undergo hemolysis in circulation.
   2. Adult Hb types
      a. HbA is the major adult Hb (~97%).
         i. Contains two α-globin chains and two β-globin chains.
      b. HbF comprises ~1% of the Hb in an adult.
         i. Contains two alpha chains and two gamma chains.
      c. HbA2 comprises ~2% of the Hb in an adult.
         i. Contains two alpha chains and two delta chains.
   3. Thalassemia classification
      a. Alpha-thalassemia
         i. Four genes control α-globin chain synthesis.
            (1) Two genes on each chromosome 16.
            (2) Patients may have loss of one, two, three, or all four genes.
            (3) Severity of the disease varies inversely with the number of residual alpha-chain genes.
         ii. Alpha-thalassemia minima (silent carrier)
            (1) Loss of a single alpha-chain gene (a-/aa).
            (2) Benign carrier state, no anemia.
         iii. Alpha-thalassemia minor
            (1) Due to a loss of two alpha-chain genes.
            (2) When both genes are missing from the same chromosome (i.e., aa/--), then the patient's offspring is at an increased risk of more severe forms of alpha-thalassemia.
               (a) More common in those of Asian descent.
            (3) When there is a loss of one alpha-chain gene from each chromosome 16 (i.e., a-/a-), then the patient's offspring is less likely to have a severe phenotype.
               (a) More common in those of African descent.
            (4) Mild hypochromic, microcytic anemia.
               (a) Laboratory findings
                  • Decreased MCV, Hb, and Hct.
                  • Increased red cell count.
                  • Target cells on blood smear.
                  • Normal RDW, serum ferritin.
                  • Normal Hb electrophoresis
                     (i) Because all variants of Hb require α-globin chains, the Hb electrophoresis is normal (despite the reduction in Hb, the relative proportions of each Hb variant are normal).
                  • In summary: ↓ Hb, ↓ MCV, ↑ RBC count, and normal Hb electrophoresis.
            (5) Alpha-thalassemia minor is a diagnosis of exclusion.
               (a) All other causes of microcytic anemia must be excluded first.
               (b) Clue to the diagnosis: family history of mild microcytic anemia with negative workup (i.e., normal Hb electrophoresis and iron studies).

      iv. HbH disease
        (1) Characterized by a loss of three of the four alpha-chain genes (--/a-).
        (2) Severity of the disease is variable; some become transfusion-dependent.
      v. Hb Barts
        (1) Due to a loss of all four alpha-chain genes (--/--).
        (2) Severe anemia developing in utero (incompatible with life).
  b. Beta-thalassemia
    i. Two β-globin genes (one from each parent). A mutation in one or both of these genes results in decreased to absent β-globin chain production (beta-thalassemia).
    ii. Genotype
      (1) β: normal β-globin gene expression.
      (2) β^+: reduced β-globin gene expression.
      (3) β^0: the complete absence of β-globin gene expression.
    iii. Clinical syndromes vary according to the combination of inherited β-globin genes.
      (1) Beta-thalassemia major
        (a) Transfusion-dependent anemia; due to the inheritance of two beta-thalassemia alleles (e.g., β^0/β^0, β^+/β^+, or β^+/β^0).
      (2) Beta-thalassemia intermedia
        (a) Anemia, but not transfusion-dependent.
        (b) Due to less severe genetic mutations; variable genotype (β^+/β^0 or β^+/β^+).
      (3) Beta-thalassemia minor
        (a) Asymptomatic with mild or no anemia.
        (b) Due to heterozygosity for beta-thalassemia mutation (e.g., β/β^0 or β/β^+).
    iv. Pathogenesis
      (1) Decreased synthesis of β-globin chains.
      (2) Unpaired α-globin chains damage the red cell membrane.
      (3) Damaged erythroid precursors are often removed prior to their release from the BM ("ineffective erythropoiesis").
    v. In an attempt to compensate for severe anemia, patients may develop EMH (causing hepatosplenomegaly) and/or erythroid hyperplasia (causing enlargement of facial bones and "hair-on-end" skull X-ray; Fig. 12.4).
    vi. Blood smear
      (1) Microcytic, hypochromic red cells (i.e., smaller and lightly stained).
      (2) Target cells (RBCs that are thinner than normal with a peripheral rim of Hb and dark central collection of Hb).
        (a) Nonspecific but common finding in thalassemia.
    vii. CBC
      (1) Decreased Hb, Hct, MCV, and MCHC.
      (2) Normal RDW.
      (3) Increased erythrocyte (RBC) count.
    viii. FEP
      (1) Normal (heme synthesis is normal).
    ix. Hb electrophoresis
      (1) Decreased to absent HbA ($2\alpha/2\beta$) due to reduction in β-globin chains.
      (2) Corresponding increase in HbA2 ($2\alpha/2\delta$) and HbF ($2\alpha/2\gamma$).
4. Sideroblastic anemia
  a. Heterogeneous group of inherited and acquired disorders in which anemia is accompanied by the presence of ring sideroblasts in the BM.
    i. Ring sideroblasts are erythroblasts with iron deposits present within the mitochondria.
    ii. Visualized on Prussian blue stain as a perinuclear ring of blue granules (Fig. 12.10).
    iii. Variety of etiologies; all associated with defective heme synthesis.
  b. X-linked sideroblastic anemia
    i. Rare inherited form of sideroblastic anemia, usually due to mutation in *ALAS2* (a gene that encodes for aminolevulinic acid [ALA] synthetase—the first and rate-limiting enzyme of heme synthesis).
  c. Acquired etiologies include:
    i. Vitamin B6 deficiency
      (1) Vitamin B6 (pyridoxine) activated to pyridoxal-5′-phosphate, a cofactor for ALA synthase.
    ii. Isoniazid (INH)
      (1) INH inhibits pyridoxine phosphokinase, an enzyme necessary for the activation of pyridoxine to pyridoxal-5′-phosphate.
    iii. Lead poisoning
      (1) Lead inhibits two enzymes in the heme synthetic pathway (ALA dehydratase and ferrochelatase).

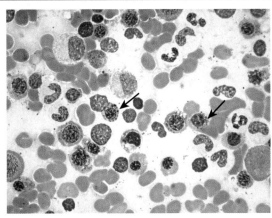

12.10: Ringed sideroblasts in a bone marrow aspirate. Dark blue iron granules around the nucleus of developing normoblasts (*arrows*) represent iron trapped within the mitochondria and indicate a defect in mitochondrial heme synthesis (sideroblastic anemia). *(From Porwitt A, McCullough J, Erber WN: Blood and bone marrow pathology, ed 2, London, 2011, Churchill Livingstone Elsevier, p 402, Fig. 27.8C.)*

      (2) Lead also inhibits an enzyme involved in the degradation of RNA (pyrimidine-5′-nucleotidase), explaining residual ribosomal RNA found in the red cell cytoplasm ("basophilic stippling").
   iv. Myelodysplasia (see Chapter 13).
  d. Pathogenesis
    i. Heme is the end product of porphyrin synthesis.
    ii. Negative feedback with δ-ALA synthase.
      (1) ↑ Heme, ↓ ALA synthase; ↓ heme, ↑ ALA synthase.
    iii. When heme synthesis is impaired, iron remains trapped within the mitochondria of developing erythroid precursors.
      (1) Mitochondria is the site of heme synthesis.
    iv. Results in an iron overload state (iron accumulates within the mitochondria of erythroblasts).
      (1) Visualized as ring sideroblasts on Prussian blue stain of the BM aspirate smear (Fig. 12.10).
      (2) Causes death of erythroblasts (ineffective erythropoiesis).
    v. Laboratory findings
      (1) ↑ Serum iron, iron saturation, ferritin.
      (2) MCV varies.
      (3) ↓TIBC.

VI. Macrocytic Anemias
  A. Definition
    1. Anemia in which the patient's red cells are larger than normal (i.e., they are macrocytic).
  B. Two groups; nonmegaloblastic and megaloblastic.
    1. Nonmegaloblastic macrocytic anemia
      a. Multifactorial (e.g., alcohol abuse, liver disease, hypothyroidism).
    2. Megaloblastic anemia
      a. Macrocytic anemia due to defective DNA synthesis.
      b. Cytoplasmic maturation proceeds normally; however, impaired nuclear maturation causes "nuclear cytoplasmic disassociation."
      c. Etiologies include folate and/or vitamin B12 deficiency.
      d. Biochemistry of megaloblastic anemia
        i. Both vitamin B12 and folate are necessary for the synthesis of deoxythymidine monophosphate (dTMP) in the biosynthesis of DNA.
        ii. Impaired DNA synthesis (e.g., B12 or folate deficiency) most prominently affects rapidly dividing cells (e.g., hematopoietic precursors).
        iii. Cells are enlarged with "open" chromatin ("megaloblasts").
        iv. Many of the megaloblastic hematopoietic precursors undergo apoptosis within the marrow, causing pancytopenia (triad of anemia, leukopenia, and thrombocytopenia).
        v. DNA biosynthetic pathway (Fig. 12.11)
          (1) Methionine synthase removes the methyl group (–CH$_3$) from 5-methyl-tetrahydrofolate (methyl-THF) (the circulating form of folate) to produce tetrahydrofolate (THF).
            (a) Methyl group of methyl-B12 is transferred to homocysteine to form methionine.
          (2) Deficiency of vitamin B12 traps folate in the methyl-THF form (called the "methyl-THF trap").
          (3) Deficiency of either folate or vitamin B12 increases plasma homocysteine.
          (4) THF used to synthesize methylenetetrahydrofolate.

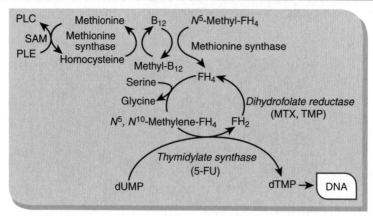

12.11: Vitamin B12 and folic acid in DNA metabolism. See text for discussion. *dTMP*, Deoxythymidine monophosphate; *dUMP*, deoxyuridine monophosphate; *FH2*, dihydrofolate; *FH4*, tetrahydrofolate; *FU*, fluorouracil; *MTX*, methotrexate; *PLC*, phosphatidylcholine, *PLE*, phosphatidylethanol-amine; *SAM*, S-adenosylmethionine; *TMP*, trimethoprim. (*Modified from Pelley J, Goljan FF: Rapid review biochemistry, Philadelphia, 2004, Mosby, Fig. 4-3.*)

      (5) Carbon from the methylene group is transferred to deoxyuridine monophosphate to form dTMP.
        (a) This step, catalyzed by thymidylate synthase, is irreversibly inhibited by 5-fluorouracil.
      (6) Generates dihydrofolate (FH2); reduced to THF by FH2 reductase.
        (a) FH2 reductase is inhibited by methotrexate (MTX) and trimethoprim (TMP).

C. Vitamin B12 (cobalamin)
  1. Water-soluble vitamin only found in animal products (e.g., meat, eggs, and dairy).
  2. Absorption is a complex process (Fig. 12.12)
    a. Requires gastric acid and pepsin for release from food.
      i. Gastric acid produced by parietal cells of the stomach.
    b. Requires R-binder (haptocorrins)
      i. Secreted in the saliva; binds B12 in the stomach to prevent its degradation by gastric acid.
    c. Requires intrinsic factor (IF).
      i. Also produced by gastric parietal cells, required for B12 absorption in the terminal ileum.
    d. Requires pancreatic proteases
      i. Proteases cleave B12 from R-binder (freeing B12 to bind with IF).
    e. Absorption occurs in the ileum.
  3. Causes of vitamin B12 deficiency
    a. Malabsorption
      i. Autoimmune gastritis (pernicious anemia)
        (1) Most common cause.
        (2) Immune-mediated destruction of gastric parietal cells (the cells that produce IF and gastric acid).
        (3) Antiparietal cell and anti-IF antibodies.
        (4) Elevated gastrin (loss of feedback with gastric acid, which is also decreased).
      ii. Total or partial gastrectomy
        (1) Gastric acid (needed to release B12 from food) and IF (needed for B12 absorption) are both produced in the stomach.
      iii. Pancreatic insufficiency
        (1) Pancreatic enzymes necessary to release R-binder from B12.
      iv. Use of dietary cobalamin by bacteria (bacterial overgrowth) or the fish tapeworm (*Diphyllobothrium latum*).
      v. Nitrous oxide
        (1) Inactivates methionine synthase and increases the excretion of cobalamin.
      vi. Resection or disease of terminal ileum
        (1) Crohn disease.
    b. Nutritional deficiency (rare)
      i. Strict vegans, breastfed infants of B12 deficient mother.
      ii. Usually takes years to develop because efficient enterohepatic circulation prevents loss of the vitamin.
  4. Clinical manifestations of vitamin B12 deficiency
    a. Fatigue, weakness, lassitude, etc. (anemia).
    b. Glossitis with smooth tongue (atrophy of the papillae).
    c. Neurologic disease
      i. Subacute combined degeneration (damage to the dorsal and the lateral corticospinal tracts of the spinal cord) is characterized by slowly progressive paresthesia of lower extremities, ataxia (due to loss of proprioception and vibratory sensation), and weakness.
      ii. Altered mental status (irritability, delusions, and paranoia).

Cobalamin absorption and effects

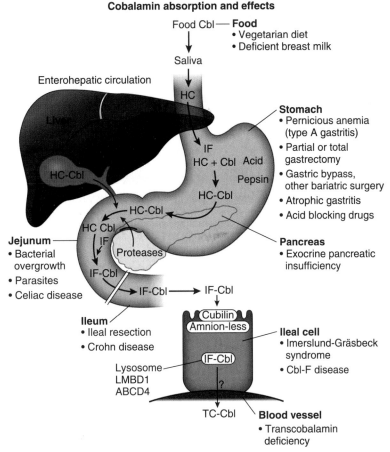

12.12: Absorption of vitamin B12 (cobalamin—Cbl) and associated defects. *ABCD4*, ATP-binding cassette subfamily D member 4 (defect); *Cbl*, cobalamin; *Cbl-F*, cobalamin F (defect); *HC*, haptocorrin (also called R-protein or R-factor); *IF*, intrinsic factor; *LMBD1*, probable lysosomal cobalamin transporter (defect); *TC*, transcobalamin. *(From Young NS, Green SL, High KA, editors:* Clinical hematology, *Philadelphia, PA, 2006, Mosby Elsevier, pp 242–251.)*

5. Laboratory findings
   a. Decreased serum vitamin B12.
   b. Elevated serum homocysteine (not specific, also seen with folate deficiency).
   c. Elevated serum methylmalonic acid (sensitive and specific).
   d. MCV usually markedly increased (>115 fL)—both vitamin B12 and folate deficiency.
   e. Peripheral blood findings include:
      i. Pancytopenia.
      ii. Macro-ovalocytes (enlarged, egg-shaped red cells).
      iii. Hypersegmented neutrophils (Fig. 12.13)
         (1) Characterized by more than five nuclear lobes.
         (2) Due to the disparity between normal cytoplasmic maturation and impaired nuclear maturation.
         (3) Hypersegmentation is highly sensitive and specific for megaloblastic anemia.
   f. BM findings
      i. Megaloblastic nucleated cells with a primitive open (lacy) chromatin pattern.
   g. Schilling test
      i. Historical significance only, no longer performed.
      ii. Oral dose of radiolabeled vitamin B12 given in conjunction with a large parenteral dose of unlabeled vitamin B12, the latter is given to saturate vitamin B12-binding proteins.
      iii. Absorption of the radiolabeled vitamin B12 measured in a 24-hour urine sample.
      iv. Malabsorption is indicated if less B12 is excreted than expected.
      v. Test is then repeated, along with IF. If B12 absorption corrects following the addition of IF, then the diagnosis of pernicious anemia is confirmed.
6. Neurologic manifestations of vitamin B12 are not clearly understood.
   a. Thought that abnormalities in odd-chain fatty acid metabolism may underlie the disorder (Fig. 12.14).

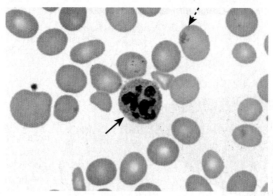

12.13: Peripheral blood in megaloblastic anemia showing a hypersegmented neutrophil (*solid arrow*) with nine lobes. Neutrophils normally have less than five nuclear segments. Hypersegmented neutrophils are excellent markers of folate and vitamin B12 deficiency. Dashed arrow shows an oval-shaped erythrocyte (called macroovalocyte), a second peripheral blood smear finding associated with megaloblastic anemia. (*From Naeim F:* Atlas of bone marrow and blood pathology, *Philadelphia, 2001, WB Saunders, p 180, Fig. 14-10B.*)

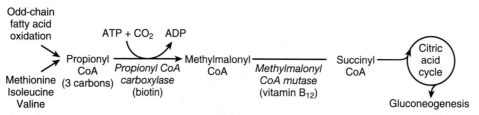

12.14: Odd-chain fatty acid metabolism. *ADP,* Adenosine diphosphate; *ATP,* adenosine triphosphate. (*From Pelley J, Goljan E:* Rapid review biochemistry, *ed 2, Philadelphia, 2007, Mosby, p 117, Fig. 7-4.*)

   i. Methylmalonyl CoA converted to succinyl CoA using the enzyme methylmalonyl CoA mutase (B12 is a cofactor).
   ii. Deficiency of vitamin B12 blocks this step → increased reactants proximal to the block (i.e., propionyl CoA and methylmalonyl CoA and their corresponding acids).

Elevated serum (or urine) methylmalonic acid is an important clue to a diagnosis of B12 deficiency.

   D. Folate
   1. Absorption
      a. Polyglutamate form is present in many plant and animal products (especially dark green vegetables and organ meats).
      b. Conjugase enzyme in the intestines cleaves dietary polyglutamate to monoglutamate (allows for the absorption of folate in the jejunum).
         i. Long-term use of phenytoin, which inhibits the intestinal conjugase enzyme, may lead to folate deficiency.
      c. Following absorption in the jejunum, folate circulates as methyl-THF.
   2. Deficiency
      a. May occur after months of inadequate intake (stores are limited).
      b. Etiologies
         i. Dietary deficiency rare; many foods are fortified; may be seen in certain populations with poor diet (e.g., alcoholics and elderly) or children solely fed goat's milk (lacks folate).
         ii. Malabsorption (e.g., celiac disease and tropical sprue).
         iii. Drugs (e.g., MTX, TMP, and phenytoin)
         iv. Those with disorders with increased cell turnover/proliferation (e.g., chronic hemolysis and pregnancy) have increased folate requirements.
   3. Clinical manifestations
      a. Pancytopenia.
      b. Maternal folate deficiency in early pregnancy increases the risk of neural tube defects in offspring.
   4. Laboratory findings
      a. Megaloblastic changes in the BM.
      b. Pancytopenia.
      c. Hypersegmented neutrophils and macro-ovalocytes on blood smear.
      d. Decreased serum and RBC folate.
      e. Elevated serum homocysteine.
      f. Serum methylmalonic acid is normal (useful in the differentiation from B12 deficiency).

TABLE 12.3   Clinical and Laboratory Findings in Vitamin B$_{12}$ and Folic Acid Deficiencies

LABORATORY AND CLINICAL FINDINGS	PERNICIOUS ANEMIA	OTHER VITAMIN B$_{12}$ DEFICIENCIES	FOLIC ACID DEFICIENCY
Achlorhydria	Present	Absent	Absent
Autoantibodies	Present	Absent	Absent
Chronic atrophic gastritis	Present	Absent	Absent
Gastric carcinoma risk	↑	None	None
Hypersegmented neutrophils	Present	Present	Present
Mean corpuscular volume	↑	↑	↑
Neurologic disease	Present	Present	Absent
Pancytopenia	Present	Present	Present
Plasma homocysteine	↑	↑	↑
Serum gastrin level	↑	Normal	Normal
Serum methylmalonic acid	↑	↑	Normal

  5. Diagnosis
      a. Serum and/or RBC folate.
 E. **Important to distinguish folate from vitamin B12 deficiency.**
      1. Both cause megaloblastic anemia; however, neurologic changes (e.g., subacute combined degeneration of the cord) only seen with vitamin B12 deficiency.
      2. Pharmacologic doses of folic acid correct the hematologic abnormality in both deficiency states; however, neurologic findings will not correct with folic acid.
 F. **Comparison table of vitamin B12 and folic acid deficiency (Table 12.3).**
 G. **Nonmegaloblastic macrocytosis (with or without anemia)**
      1. MCV in nonmegaloblastic macrocytosis is usually only marginally elevated (~105 fL).
      2. Alcohol
          a. Common cause of macrocytosis; mechanism unclear.
          b. Abstinence from alcohol reverses the macrocytosis.
      3. Liver disease
          a. Alters lipid composition of the red cell membrane.
      4. Reticulocytosis
          a. Reticulocytes are larger than mature RBCs; therefore patients with increased reticulocytes (e.g., those recovering from acute blood loss) may have an elevated MCV.
VII. **Normocytic Anemias: Corrected Reticulocyte Count of <3%**
 A. **Acute blood loss**
      1. Bleeding may be external (e.g., gun/knife wounds) or internal (e.g., ruptured aortic aneurysm).
      2. Loss of whole blood (i.e., plasma and red cells) causes Hb and Hct to remain normal initially.
          a. Once the plasma volume is restored, either through fluid replacement or redistribution from extravascular spaces, the Hb/Hct levels decline.
      3. EPO released by the kidneys stimulates erythroid maturation.
          a. Reticulocytosis develops in ~5–7 days.
 B. **Aplastic anemia**
      1. Syndrome of BM failure characterized by pancytopenia and aplasia/hypoplasia of the BM.
          a. Despite the presence of anemia, reticulocyte count is low (production is impaired).
      2. Epidemiology
          a. Rare with no sex preference; often young (15–25 years of age).
      3. Etiologies (Table 12.4)
          a. Identifiable causes include drugs and other environmental exposures (e.g., benzene, insecticides, and antineoplastic agents).
      4. Pathogenesis
          a. Although often considered idiopathic, immune-mediated destruction of multipotent hematopoietic stem cells is thought the most likely mechanism.
      5. Clinical manifestations
          a. Fever and/or recurrent infections due to neutropenia.
          b. Hemorrhage due to thrombocytopenia.
          c. Fatigue and decreased exercise tolerance due to anemia.

TABLE 12.4 Causes of Aplastic Anemia

CLASSIFICATION	EXAMPLES AND DISCUSSION
Idiopathic	• ~50%–70% of cases are idiopathic.
Drugs	• Dose-related causes are usually reversible (e.g., alkylating agents and antimetabolites). • Idiosyncratic reactions are frequently irreversible (e.g., chloramphenicol and phenylbutazone).
Chemical agents	• Toxic chemicals in industry and agriculture (e.g., benzene and insecticides such as DDT and parathion).
Infection	• May involve all hematopoietic cell lines (pancytopenia) or only erythroid cell line (pure RBC aplasia). • Examples—EBV, CMV, parvovirus, and HCV.
Physical agents	• Whole-body ionizing radiation (e.g., nuclear accident).
Miscellaneous	• Thymoma (may be associated with pure RBC aplasia). • Paroxysmal nocturnal hemoglobinuria.

CMV, Cytomegalovirus; *EBV*, Epstein–Barr virus; *HCV*, hepatitis C virus; *RBC*, red blood cell.

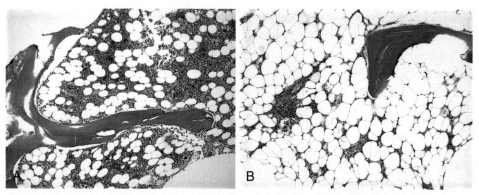

12.15: Bone marrow biopsy with normal hematopoietic cellularity (A) and hypocellularity (B; aplastic anemia). The empty spaces represent the adipose tissue. *(From Goldman L, Schafer A: Goldman's Cecil medicine, ed 25, St. Louis, 2016, Elsevier Saunders, p 1114, Fig. 165-1.)*

    6. Laboratory findings
      a. Pancytopenia.
      b. Decreased reticulocytes (reticulocyte production index < 3).
      c. Hypocellular BM with fat replacement (Fig. 12.15).
C. Pure red cell aplasia (PRCA)
    1. Rare, characterized by an absence of erythroid precursors in the BM.
      a. Due to suppression of an early erythroid precursor or progenitor cell.
      b. Remaining hematopoietic cell lineages are normal.
    2. Primary versus secondary causes
      a. Primary PRCA is due to an autoimmune attack on erythroid precursor cells (idiopathic).
      b. Secondary PRCA is due to a virus (e.g., parvovirus B19), neoplasm (e.g., chronic lymphocytic leukemia, thymoma), or drugs (e.g., phenytoin, azathioprine, sulfonamides).
        i. Parvovirus B19 binds erythroid cells via the "P" red cell antigen, causes direct viral-mediated destruction of proerythroblasts.
D. Anemia in chronic kidney disease
    1. Anemia in those with chronic kidney disease is common, especially advanced stages, is related to reduced levels of EPO and/or increase in inflammatory cytokines (i.e., ACD).
    2. Hematologic findings include:
      a. Normocytic anemia.
      b. Burr cells (i.e., RBCs with undulating membrane) on the blood smear.
      c. Prolonged bleeding time (uremia impairs platelet function, reversible with dialysis).
E. Malignancy
    1. Several possible etiologies, including:
      a. Replacement of marrow by a tumor.
        i. A peripheral blood smear can provide clues to the presence of an infiltrative process of the marrow (e.g., metastatic disease), including:
          (1) Immature granulocytes and nucleated RBCs ("leukoerythroblastosis").
          (2) Teardrop-shaped red cells.
        ii. Anemia secondary to the BM replacement is known as myelophthisic anemia.
      b. Bleeding from a tumor (e.g., colorectal carcinoma).

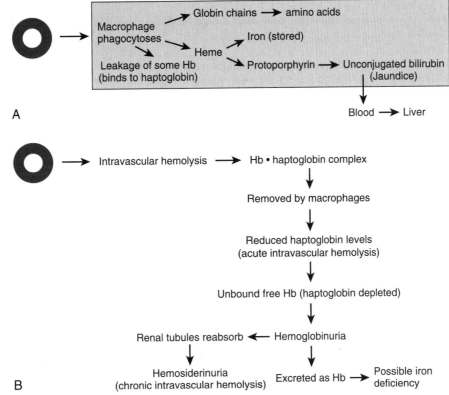

12.16: Extravascular (A) and intravascular (B) hemolysis of red blood cells (RBCs). In extravascular hemolysis, macrophage destruction of RBCs produces unconjugated hyperbilirubinemia and, in some cases, a decrease in serum haptoglobin. In intravascular hemolysis, hemoglobinuria, hemosiderinuria, and a decrease in serum haptoglobin are key findings. *Hb*, Hemoglobin. *(From Goljan EF: Star series: pathology, Philadelphia, 1998, Saunders, Fig. 12-2.)*

  c. Indirect effect of the neoplasm (e.g., autoimmune hemolysis, cytokine-mediated inhibition of erythropoiesis).
  d. Treatment complication (e.g., suppression of erythropoiesis by radiation and/or chemotherapy).

VIII. Normocytic Anemias: Corrected Reticulocyte Count >3%
 A. Hemolytic anemia (premature destruction of red cells).
  1. Normal red cell lifespan is 120 days.
 B. Pathogenesis of hemolytic anemia
  1. "Intrinsic" or "extrinsic" types of hemolytic anemia.
   a. Intrinsic means that the hemolysis is due to an intrinsic defect in the RBC itself (e.g., HS or G6PD deficiency).
   b. Extrinsic means that the hemolysis is due to some factor "extrinsic" to the red cell (e.g., mechanical or immune-mediated destruction).
  2. Mechanisms of RBC hemolysis (Fig. 12.16)
 C. Intravascular hemolysis
  1. Refers to RBC hemolysis occurring within the vasculature.
  2. Etiologies
   a. RBC enzyme deficiency (e.g., PK or hexokinase deficiency) → reduced ATP production → failure of membrane pumps (swelling makes the RBCs prone to hemolysis).
   b. Complement-mediated destruction (e.g., IgM-mediated hemolysis; IgG-mediated in some cases).
   c. Mechanical trauma (e.g., aortic stenosis).
   d. Infections (e.g., malaria or babesiosis).
  3. Laboratory findings
   a. Hemoglobinemia (free Hb in circulation)
   b. Hemoglobinuria (free Hb in urine)
   c. Hemosiderinuria (hemosiderin in urine, due to shedding of proximal renal tubule cells containing iron).
   d. Increased serum lactate dehydrogenase (LDH) (a nonspecific marker of cell breakdown).
   e. Decreased serum haptoglobin
    i. Haptoglobin binds to free Hb in circulation, removed via phagocytosis by hepatic and splenic macrophages.
    ii. During active hemolysis, haptoglobin is consumed faster than it can be produced—the reason for the decline in haptoglobin in those with hemolysis.
    iii. Since haptoglobin is synthesized in the liver, severe hepatic dysfunction is another potential cause of reduced haptoglobin levels.

D. Extravascular hemolysis
1. Hemolysis occurring "outside" the vasculature, that is, phagocytosis of red cells by macrophages (usually within the spleen and/or liver).
2. Etiologies include:
    a. Coating of RBCs with IgG and/or C3b (macrophages have receptors to remove opsonized cells).
    b. Abnormal red cell shape (e.g., spherocytes, sickle cells) or inclusions (e.g., Heinz bodies).
3. Clues to the presence of hemolysis
    a. Increased unconjugated bilirubin (UCB) and jaundice (usually apparent with bilirubin levels >2.5 mg/dL).
        i. UCB is an end product of heme metabolism.
    b. Increased serum LDH—a nonspecific marker of cell breakdown.
    c. Decreased haptoglobin (with severe hemolysis).
E. Hereditary spherocytosis (HS)
1. Pathogenesis
    a. Genetic mutations involving proteins of the RBC membrane and cytoskeleton (e.g., spectrin, ankyrin, band 3, and band 4.2).
        i. Usually inherited in an autosomal dominant fashion.
        ii. Most commonly involves the *ANK1* gene (ankyrin).
    b. Loss of cytoskeletal proteins causes areas of membrane weakness.
    c. Weak areas of the membrane are progressively lost, causing a loss of cell volume (cells become spherical, i.e., they become "spherocytes").
    d. Spherocytes are not as deformable as normal red cells, becoming entrapped and destroyed (in the spleen, liver, and BM).
    e. The net result is variably shortened red cell lifespan.
2. Clinical manifestations
    a. Fatigue, dyspnea on exertion, and other manifestations of anemia.
    b. Jaundice (increased bilirubin deposits in the skin).
    c. Splenomegaly (a major site of red cell breakdown).
    d. Increased risk of cholelithiasis (gallstones)
        i. Dark black pigmented gallstones comprised of calcium bilirubinate.
3. Laboratory findings
    a. Normocytic anemia with spherocytosis (Fig. 12.17).
    b. Increased MCHC.
        i. Unique, an important clue to the diagnosis.
    c. Increased total and UCB (due to increased red cell breakdown).
    d. Increased RBC osmotic fragility
        i. Compared with normal RBCs, spherocytes have a limited ability to expand in hypotonic solutions. For this reason, they lyse at NaCl concentrations higher than would normal biconcave red cells (called "increased osmotic fragility").

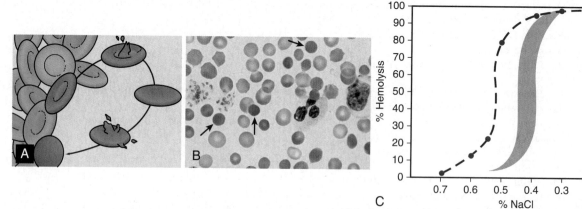

12.17: (A) Schematic showing the formation of microvesicles on the red blood cell (RBC) membrane that occur in those with membrane defects. The removal of the microvesicles via splenic macrophages, eventually leads to the formation of a spherocyte. Spherocytes are not very deformable and are thus phagocytosed and destroyed by splenic macrophages. (B) Peripheral blood with spherocytes in hereditary spherocytosis. Numerous, round, dense RBCs without central areas of pallor represent spherocytes (*arrows*). The mean corpuscular hemoglobin concentration is increased. (C) Osmotic fragility test. Comparison of RBC lysis in severe hereditary spherocytosis (*interrupted line*) and normal blood (*shaded area*). Red cells in HS become more susceptible to osmotic lysis (i.e., exhibit increased osmotic fragility). (*A, From Zitelli B, McIntire S, Nowalk A: Zitelli and Davis' atlas of pediatric physical diagnosis, ed 6, St. Louis, 2012, Saunders Elsevier, p 435, Fig. 11-14; B, from Pathology: a color atlas, St. Louis, 2000, Mosby, p 75, Fig. 5-7; C, from McPherson R, Pincus M: Henry's clinical diagnosis and management by laboratory methods, ed 22, Philadelphia, 2011, Saunders, p 573, Fig. 32-11.*)

F. Hereditary elliptocytosis
1. Pathogenesis
   a. Autosomal dominant disorder in which mutations, usually involving spectrin, lead to weakening of the red cell membrane cytoskeleton.
   b. Elliptical red cells are less mechanically stable (akin to spherocytes) and undergo extravascular hemolysis by macrophages (spleen, liver, and BM; same as HS).
2. Clinical manifestations
   a. Severity varies; some are asymptomatic while others develop severe hemolytic anemia.
   b. Splenomegaly (a major site of red cell trapping/hemolysis).
3. Laboratory findings
   a. Elliptocytes account for >25% of the RBCs in the peripheral blood.
   b. RBC osmotic fragility is increased.

G. Paroxysmal nocturnal hemoglobinuria (PNH)
1. Rare clonal hematopoietic stem cell disorder.
2. May affect either sex and occur at any age (although usually middle age).
3. Due to an acquired mutation in the *PIGA* (phosphatidylinositol glycan anchor, class A) gene.
   a. *PIGA* is responsible for the first step in the synthesis of the glycosylphosphatidylinositol (GPI) anchor to which inhibitors of complement (CD59 and CD55) bind.
   b. Without the anchor, these inhibitors of complement cannot bind, and the red cell becomes susceptible to complement-mediated intravascular hemolysis.
      i. Loss of free Hb in the urine explains the hemoglobinuria.
4. Despite the name, most patients have chronic hemolysis (not just at night).
5. Note that the defect in the GPI-A anchor is associated with complement-mediated lysis of neutrophils and platelets as well (i.e., may cause pancytopenia).
   a. Paradoxically, the lysis of platelets makes the patient more susceptible to thrombosis; believed related to the release of procoagulant substances that contribute to platelet activation.
6. Clinical manifestations
   a. Iron deficiency possible, due to the loss of iron in urine (hemoglobinuria).
   b. Increased incidence of thrombosis (a major cause of death in PNH).
   c. Increased risk of aplastic anemia.
7. Peripheral blood findings
   a. Pancytopenia
      i. Anemia is usually normocytic but may become microcytic if hemoglobinuria results in iron deficiency.
   b. Decreased serum haptoglobin.
   c. Hemoglobinemia.
   d. Hemoglobinuria.
8. Diagnosis
   a. Flow cytometry of peripheral blood sample shows a population of cells lacking GPI-anchored proteins (e.g., CD59 and CD55).

Consider the diagnosis of paroxysmal nocturnal hemoglobinuria in the following scenarios using the acronym CATCH

- **C**ytopenias
- **A**plastic anemia/myelodysplasia
- **T**hrombosis
- **C**oombs-negative hemolysis
- **H**emoglobinuria

H. Sickle cell disease
1. Definition
   a. Inherited group of disorders characterized by the presence of HbS.
2. Pathogenesis
   a. Genetic mutation characterized by the substitution of valine in place of glutamic acid at the sixth position of the β-globin chain to form HbS.
   b. When deoxygenated, HbS forms polymers that distort the red cell membrane, forming "sickled" red cells.
      i. Red cells become dehydrated and rigid.
   c. Although initially reversible upon reoxygenation, sickling eventually becomes irreversible → hemolysis and chronic anemia.
   d. A second major effect of sickle cell disease is vascular occlusion.
      i. Sickled red cells adhere to one another (they become "sticky"), causing microvascular obstruction/ischemic injury (e.g., spleen, bone, and brain).

3. Sickle cell trait (HbAS)
   a. Heterozygosity for the sickle cell (HbS) mutation.
   b. Benign carrier state without anemia.
      i. Levels of HbS are inadequate for spontaneous sickling to occur except in extreme situations.
   c. HbA >50 %, HbS 35%–45%, HbF <2%.
4. Sickle cell anemia (HbSS)
   a. Homozygous inheritance of the HbS mutation.
   b. Nearly all Hb is HbS; small amounts of HbF and HbA2 (no HbA).
      i. Most important factor that determines whether sickling occurs is the level of HbS (>60%).
      ii. HbS polymerization causes cells to become overly rigid and prone to hemolysis (red cell lifespan markedly shortened).
   c. Reticulocytosis (compensation for increased red cell destruction).
   d. Unconjugated hyperbilirubinemia (due to hemolysis).
   e. Elevated serum LDH (from hemolyzed red cells).
   f. Low serum haptoglobin (haptoglobin is consumed as it binds to free Hb).
   g. Peripheral blood smear findings
      i. Sickled red cells (Fig. 12.18A)
      ii. Howell–Jolly bodies represent residual nuclear material in those without a functioning spleen (Fig. 12.18C).
5. Mating of two people with sickle cell trait
   a. 25% chance of having a normal child.
   b. 50% chance of having a child with sickle cell trait.
   c. 25% chance of having a child with sickle cell disease.
6. HbS is protective against *Plasmodium falciparum* malaria.
7. Factors that increase the concentration of deoxyhemoglobin (deoxyHb), and therefore increase the risk of sickling, include:
   a. Acidosis: shifts the oxygen dissociation curve to the right (oxygen is released more freely from RBCs).
   b. Volume depletion: intracellular dehydration causes the concentration of deoxyhemoglobin to increase.
   c. Hypoxemia: decreased PaO_2.
8. HbF prevents sickling.
   a. HbF avidly binds to oxygen (prevents red cell deoxygenation and thus sickling).
      i. Newborns have residual HbF, replaced by HbS over the first several months, explains the onset of symptoms at about 6 months of age.
      ii. Hydroxyurea increases the synthesis of HbF; sometimes used to ameliorate the manifestations of sickle cell disease.
9. Clinical manifestations of sickle cell anemia
   a. Anemia
      i. Hb usually in the 6–9 g/dL range.
   b. Peripheral blood smear
      i. Sickle cell disease: sickled red cells, target cells, nucleated RBCs, and Howell–Jolly bodies.
      ii. Sickle cell trait characterized by normal blood smear.
   c. Acute pain episodes (vaso-occlusive crises)
      i. May either arise spontaneously or follow various stressors (e.g., infection or dehydration).
      ii. Often presents in young children with dactylitis (pain in the fingers and toes) secondary to bone infarction in hands/feet (Fig. 12.18B)
   d. Acute chest syndrome
      i. Acute illness characterized by fever, pulmonary infiltrates on imaging, respiratory difficulties, and hypoxia.
      ii. Precipitating factors include pneumonia and pulmonary infarction.
      iii. May lead to respiratory failure and death.
   e. Avascular necrosis of bones
      i. Ischemic infarction of bone secondary to occlusion of the microvasculature (vaso-occlusion) by sickled red cells.
   f. Autosplenectomy
      i. Spleen is initially enlarged but dysfunctional by age 10–12 months.
      ii. Nuclear remnants (Howell–Jolly bodies) appear in RBCs, indicating a loss of splenic function.
      iii. By young adulthood, repeated episodes of splenic infarction (due to vaso-occlusion) result in splenic fibrosis and a loss of splenic function ("autosplenectomy"); associated with an increased risk of infection by encapsulated bacteria (e.g., *Streptococcus pneumoniae*, *Salmonella* spp.) and the reason for the prophylactic use of penicillin in these patients.
   g. "Aplastic crisis"
      i. Refers to the sudden decrease in erythroid production due to parvovirus B19.
      ii. Parvovirus, which infects erythroid precursors via "P" antigen, causes transient suppression of erythropoiesis (7–10 days).

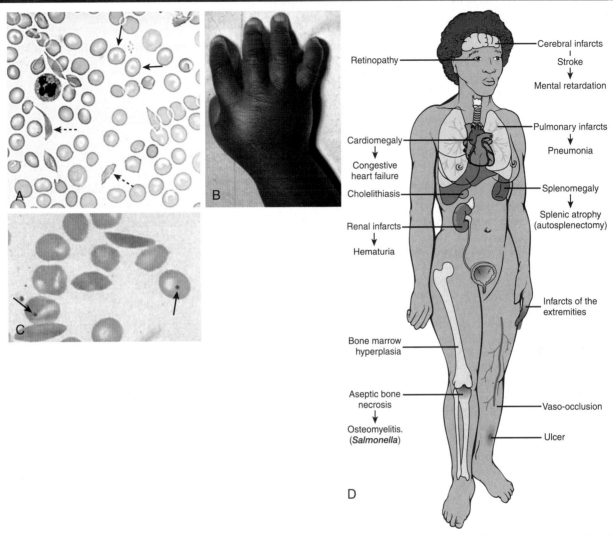

12.18: (A) Peripheral blood with target cells and sickle cells. Sickle cells (*interrupted arrows*) appear as dense, boat-shaped cells, whereas the target cells exhibit a "bull's-eye" appearance (*solid arrows*). Target cells contain excess membrane that bulges in the center of the cell. (B) Sickle cell anemia. This is the hand of young child with painful, swollen fingers (dactylitis) caused by infarction (aseptic necrosis) of the metacarpal bones. This acute syndrome usually arises around the age of 6 months as HbF is replaced by HbS. (C) Peripheral blood with sickle cells and Howell–Jolly (HJ) bodies. The three dense, boat-shaped sickle cells and the two cells containing a single dark, round inclusion (*arrows*) represent nuclear remnants. HJ bodies in sickle cell disease indicate splenic dysfunction. (D) Clinicopathologic findings in sickle cell anemia. The findings are a consequence of infarctions, anemia, hemolysis, and recurrent infections. (*A, From Hoffbrand AV: Color atlas: clinical hematology, ed 3, St. Louis, 2000, Mosby, p 103, Fig. 5-85A; B, from Forbes C, Jackson W: Color atlas and text of clinical medicine, ed 3, London, 2004, Mosby, p 419, Fig. 10.48; C, from Henry JB: Clinical diagnosis and management by laboratory methods, ed 20, Philadelphia, 2001, Saunders, Fig. 26-2A; D, from Pathology for the health professions, ed 4, St. Louis, 2012, Saunders Elsevier, p 208, Fig. 9-10.*)

     iii. In those with a shortened red cell lifespan (e.g., sickle cell anemia and other chronic hemolytic disorders), the transient suppression of hematopoiesis is significant, potentially causing a profound worsening of anemia.

     iv. Clue to the suppression of erythropoiesis is reticulocytopenia.

  h. Sequestration crisis

     i. Potentially life-threatening complication characterized by massive pooling of red cells within the spleen.

       (1) Can cause hypovolemic shock and death.

     ii. As opposed to aplastic crisis, splenic sequestration is characterized by increased reticulocytes.

  i. Cholelithiasis

     i. Chronic hemolysis → chronic hyperbilirubinemia → elevated bilirubin in gallbladder → calcium bilirubinate stones (dark black coloration).

  j. Strokes (vaso-occlusion in the brain).

  k. Leg ulcers (vaso-occlusion in the skin of the legs).

      l. Retinopathy (vaso-occlusion of the retinal artery).

     m. Renal disease

         i. Low oxygen tension of the renal medulla can precipitate sickling (in both sickle cell trait and disease), resulting in vaso-occlusion; ischemic injury within the renal medulla leads to hematuria and loss of ability to concentrate urine (hyposthenuria).

     n. Priapism

         i. Persistent, prolonged, and painful erection.

        ii. Due to impaired venous outflow from the penis.

  10. Diagnosis

     a. Hb analysis

         i. High-performance liquid chromatography, preferred method of diagnosis.

        ii. Hb electrophoresis (cellulose acetate at pH 8.4) separates HbS from other Hb variants (time-consuming and labor-intensive).

     b. Prenatal screening of fetal DNA (identifies specific gene mutation).

  11. Preventive measures in sickle cell disease

     a. Hydroxyurea to increase HbF.

     b. Prophylaxis with penicillin, routine immunizations.

     c. Folic acid supplementation.

         i. Increased folate requirements in those with rapid cell turnover.

  12. Overview of findings in sickle cell disease (Fig. 12.18D).

I. G6PD deficiency

  1. Most common enzymatic disorder of red cells.

  2. X-linked (i.e., male-dominant disease).

  3. Protective against *P. falciparum*; more common in African, Middle Eastern, Mediterranean, and Asian populations.

  4. G6PD, the initial enzyme of the pentose phosphate pathway, is involved in the reduction of nicotinamide adenine dinucleotide phosphate to NADPH.

     a. NADPH is necessary to maintain glutathione in a reduced state (GSH), for protection against oxidant injury.

     b. Deficiency of GSH leads to hemolysis under conditions of increased oxidative stress (e.g., infection, ingestion of fava beans or certain drugs [e.g., primaquine, dapsone, and sulfonamides], and/or acidosis).

  5. Subtypes of G6PD deficiency

     a. Mediterranean variant

         i. Severe enzyme deficiency, severe hemolysis.

     b. A⁻ variant

         i. Most common type in African Americans; associated with less severe enzyme deficiency and thus less severe hemolysis.

  6. Peripheral blood smear

     a. Heinz bodies

         i. Represents denatured globin chains, often attach to the red cell membrane.

        ii. Requires supravital staining with crystal violet (appears purple).

     b. Bite cells

         i. Due to the removal of Heinz bodies by splenic macrophages.

  7. Clinical manifestations

     a. Sudden onset of back pain with hemoglobinuria 2–3 days after exposure to oxidant stress; jaundice possible depending upon the degree of hemolysis.

  8. Laboratory findings

     a. Normocytic anemia with increased reticulocyte count.

     b. Hyperbilirubinemia, elevated LDH.

     c. Bite cells on the blood smear.

     d. Heinz bodies (supravital staining); best screen during active hemolysis.

     e. RBC enzyme analysis (used to confirm the diagnosis but must be performed after resolution of the acute hemolytic episode).

J. Pyruvate kinase (PK) deficiency

  1. Autosomal recessive inherited RBC enzyme disorder resulting in chronic hemolysis.

     a. Second most common RBC enzyme defect but the most common cause of chronic hemolysis from an RBC enzyme deficiency.

         i. The most common enzyme deficiency (G6PD) causes episodic, not chronic hemolysis.

  2. Deficiency of PK results in a lack of ATP for metabolic activity and increased susceptibility to hemolysis.

TABLE 12.5   Classification of Immune Hemolytic Anemias

TYPES OF IMMUNE HEMOLYTIC ANEMIA	EXAMPLES
Autoimmune: Warm antibodies (IgG)	• Primary or idiopathic (no underlying cause) • Secondary (e.g., SLE)
Autoimmune: Cold antibodies (IgM)	• Primary or idiopathic • Secondary • *Mycoplasma pneumoniae* (anti-I antibodies) • Infectious mononucleosis—EBV (anti-I antibodies) • Paroxysmal cold hemoglobinuria (IgG not IgM; hemolysis secondary to bithermal antibody)
Autoimmune: Drug-induced	• **Drug reaction against Rh antigens on the RBC:** Drug alters Rh antigens on RBCs. IgG auto-antibodies are directed against the altered Rh antigen (not the drug). Macrophages recognize and phagocytose the opsonized RBCs (Type II HSR). Hemolysis ceases weeks after cessation of the drug. Direct Coombs is positive. • **Drug-dependent drug absorption:** An IgG antibody is directed against a drug attached to the RBC membrane (e.g., penicillin). Macrophages phagocytose the RBC (extravascular hemolysis). Type II HSR. Direct Coombs test is positive for IgG during the period of drug administration. • **Drug-dependent immune complex:** Drug loosely binds to the RBC membrane. IgM binds to the drug, activates complement, and causes intravascular hemolysis of the RBC. • Type III HSR. Direct Coombs test is positive for C3. There is no direct Coombs test to identify IgM. • **Nonimmunologic protein absorption:** Drug induces changes to the RBC membrane properties, causing them to hemolyze. Associated with prolonged exposure to high-dose cephalosporins. Direct Coombs test result is negative.
Alloimmune	• Hemolytic transfusion reaction (see Chapter 16) • ABO hemolytic disease of newborn (see Chapter 16) • Rh hemolytic disease of newborn (see Chapter 16)

EBV, Epstein-Barr virus; *HSR*, hypersensitivity reaction; *RBC*, red blood cell; *SLE*, systemic lupus erythematosus.

     a. Clinical manifestations are not as severe as would be expected based on the Hb concentration. The reason is that reactants proximal to the enzyme block, including 2,3-BPG, are increased.

     b. Elevated levels of 2,3-BPG allow oxygen to be released to the tissues more readily, thereby helping to offset the effects of anemia.

  3. Clinical manifestations

     a. Chronic hemolytic anemia from birth.

  4. Laboratory findings

     a. Increased reticulocyte count.

     b. Increased total and UCB.

     c. Increased LDH.

     d. Decreased haptoglobin.

     e. Anemia may or may not be present, depends on degree of compensation.

     f. Echinocytes on the peripheral smear (RBCs with thorny projections).

  5. Confirmatory test

     a. Measurement of PK activity in RBCs and/or identification of a pathogenic mutation in the *PKLR* gene (PK in liver and RBCs).

K. Immune hemolytic anemia (IHA)

  1. Definition

     a. Destruction of RBCs associated with the binding of antibodies and/or complement to the RBC surface.

     b. Site of destruction may be either extravascular or intravascular.

  2. Classification of IHAs (Table 12.5)

  3. Autoimmune hemolytic anemia (AIHA)

     a. Autoantibodies against red cell antigens.

     b. Classified into "warm" and "cold" types based on the optimal reactivity temperature.

     c. In warm AIHA, antibody (usually IgG) is most active at normal body temperature. Red cells bound with IgG undergo extravascular hemolysis (i.e., phagocytosed by macrophages in the spleen, liver, and BM) often associated with an underlying condition (e.g., infection or autoimmune disorder).

     d. In cold AIHA, the antibody (usually IgM) is most active at 3°C–4°C and often targets either the "I" or "i" antigen. Called "cold agglutinins" because the autoantibody can cause agglutination of RBCs in cooler regions of the body.

        i. Cryoglobulins are another type of cold-reacting antibody that, unlike the other types, usually do not cause hemolysis. Cryoglobulins may lead to inflammation of the vasculature (vasculitis) and/or vascular occlusion.

Paroxysmal cold hemoglobinuria

- Donath–Landsteiner antibody (usually IgG antibodies against the "P" red cell antigen).
- Rare with a variety of associations, often associated with viral infection in children or malignancy in adults.
- Antibody binds at colder temperatures in periphery, activates complement, and causes intravascular hemolysis.
- Presents within minutes to few hours after cold exposure; sudden onset of fever, chills, and red to brown urine (hemoglobinuria).

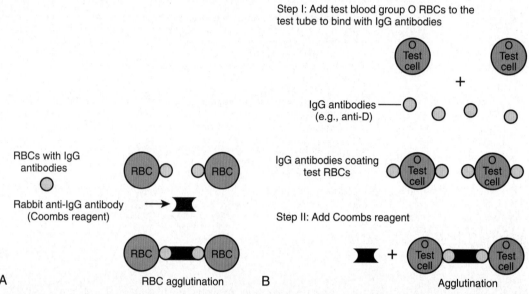

12.19: Schematic of the direct Coombs test (A) and indirect Coombs test (B). In the direct Coombs test (A), red blood cells (RBCs) sensitized with IgG antibodies (or C3b, C3d) are agglutinated when Coombs reagent (anti-IgG antibody) is added to the test tube. (B) In the indirect Coombs test, IgG antibodies (e.g., anti-D) in the serum must first bind to blood group type O test RBCs added to the test tube. Addition of Coombs reagent causes the sensitized type O test RBCs to agglutinate, indicating that IgG antibodies are present in the serum. The specificity of the antibodies (e.g., anti-D IgG antibodies) is determined by other tests performed in the blood bank. *(From Goljan EF: Pathology: Saunders text and review series, Philadelphia, 1998, Saunders, p 289, Fig. 12-11.)*

4. Clinical manifestations of AIHA
   a. Jaundice
      i. More common with extravascular hemolysis because UCB levels tend to be higher.
      ii. In intravascular types of hemolysis, phagocytosis of the haptoglobin–Hb complex often limits the level of UCB to less than that required to cause jaundice.
   b. Hepatosplenomegaly
      i. Due to "work hypertrophy" as the macrophages within the liver and spleen destroy the red cells (extravascular hemolysis).
5. Laboratory findings
   a. Evidence of hemolysis on peripheral blood smear (e.g., spherocytes and/or schistocytes).
   b. Increased reticulocytes (indicative of BM response to anemia).
   c. Positive direct antiglobulin test (DAT)
      i. Also known as a Coombs test; detects the presence of antibodies and/or complement on the red cell surface (Fig. 12.19A).
      ii. Hallmark finding of autoimmune hemolysis.
   d. Positive indirect antiglobulin test
      i. Also known as indirect Coombs test (Fig. 12.19B); detects the presence of antibodies against red cell antigens in the serum.
   e. Unconjugated hyperbilirubinemia (i.e., increased UCB)
      i. Seen with both extravascular and intravascular hemolysis; levels tend to be higher with extravascular hemolysis (see previous discussion).
   f. Hemoglobinuria
      i. Particularly seen with intravascular hemolysis.
   g. Decreased serum haptoglobin.
   h. Anemia (normocytic)
      i. May or may not be present; depends upon the severity of hemolysis and associated marrow response.

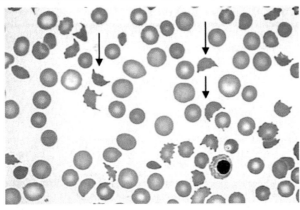

12.20: Microangiopathic hemolytic anemia with schistocytes *(arrows)*. Nucleated cell is a nucleated red blood cell. *(From Carey WD: Cleveland clinic: current clinical medicine, ed 2, St. Louis, 2010, Saunders Elsevier, p 578, Fig. 1.)*

   L. **Macroangiopathic hemolytic anemia**
      1. Definition
         a. Hemolysis secondary to direct mechanical trauma to RBCs.
         b. Usually within the heart (e.g., prosthetic heart valve or stenotic aortic valve).
   M. **Microangiopathic hemolytic anemia**
      1. Definition
         a. Fragmentation of red cells as they attempt to traverse fibrin or platelet thrombi within the microvasculature.
      2. Laboratory findings
         a. Normocytic anemia
            i.   If long standing, may become microcytic due to iron deficiency caused by the loss of iron in urine (hemoglobinuria).
         b. Decreased serum haptoglobin.
         c. Hemoglobinuria.
         d. Hemosiderinuria (hemosiderin in urine; Prussian blue stain positive).
         e. Schistocytes (fragmented RBCs) on blood smear (Fig. 12.20).
   N. **Summary of normocytic anemia (Table 12.6)**

TABLE 12.6 Summary of Normocytic Anemias

ANEMIA	PATHOGENESIS	COMMENTS
Reticulocytosis <3%		
Acute blood loss	• Loss of whole blood	• Initial Hb and Hct normal • Infusion of normal saline uncovers anemia
Early iron deficiency	• Decreased iron stores	• Normocytic before microcytic • Iron studies abnormal (↓ serum ferritin)
Early ACD	• Iron trapped in macrophages by hepcidin	• Normocytic before microcytic • Iron studies abnormal (↑ serum ferritin)
Aplastic anemia	• Suppression/loss of myeloid stem cells	• Pancytopenia • Hypocellular marrow
Chronic kidney disease	• Deficiency of EPO	• Presence of burr cells
Reticulocytosis ≥2%		
Hereditary spherocytosis	• AD disorder • Defect ankyrin or other membrane proteins • Extravascular hemolysis	• Increased osmotic fragility • Treat with splenectomy
Hereditary elliptocytosis	• AD disorder • Defect in spectrin and band 4.1 • Extravascular hemolysis	• Elliptocytes >25%
Paroxysmal nocturnal hemoglobinuria	• Acquired loss of GPI anchor for complement inhibitors (e.g., CD59 and CD55) in myeloid stem cell clone • Complement-mediated destruction of hematopoietic cells cause intravascular hemolysis	• Pancytopenia • Flow cytometry best test • Thrombosis common complication

(Continued)

TABLE 12.6   Summary of Normocytic Anemias—cont'd

ANEMIA	PATHOGENESIS	COMMENTS
Paroxysmal cold hemoglobinuria	• IgG cold antibody with bithermal activity • Attaches to RBCs in cold temperature and fixes complement • Detaches in warm temperature, associated with complement-mediated intravascular hemolysis	
Sickle cell anemia	• AR disorder • Valine substitution for glutamic acid in the β-globin chain • Extravascular hemolysis	• HbAS: HbA, 55%–60%; HbS, 40%–45% • HbSS: HbS, 90%–95%; HbF, 5%–10%; no HbA
G6PD deficiency	• XR disorder • Deficiency of GSH causes oxidant damage and intravascular hemolysis	• Bite cells in peripheral blood • Heinz body preparation: used to screen during active hemolysis • Enzyme assay: confirmatory test when hemolysis subsides
Pyruvate kinase deficiency	• AR disease • ↓ ATP synthesis • Extravascular hemolysis	• ↑ 2,3-BPG shifts oxyhemoglobin dissociation curve to right
Warm AIHA	• IgG with or without C3b • Extravascular hemolysis	• Positive direct Coombs test result • SLE, the most common cause
Cold AIHA	• IgM with C3b • Intravascular hemolysis	• Association with *Mycoplasma pneumoniae*, EBV • Positive direct Coombs test result
Drug-induced immune hemolytic anemia	• Drug hapten: penicillin • Immunocomplex: quinidine • Autoantibody: methyldopa	• Positive direct Coombs test result
Alloimmune hemolytic anemia	• Antibodies against foreign RBC antigens • Extravascular hemolysis	• Hemolytic transfusion reaction • ABO and Rh HDN • Positive direct Coombs test result
Microangiopathic and macroangiopathic hemolytic anemia	• Mechanical destruction of RBCs with the formation of schistocytes • Intravascular hemolysis	• Calcific aortic stenosis most common cause • Other causes TTP and HUS • Chronic hemoglobinuria may cause iron deficiency
Malaria	• Transmitted by female *Anopheles* mosquito • Intravascular hemolysis	• Rupture of RBCs corresponds with fever

ACD, Anemia of chronic disease; *AD*, autosomal dominant; *AIHA*, autoimmune hemolytic anemia; *AR*, autosomal recessive; *ATP*, adenosine triphosphate; *BPG*, bisphosphoglycerate; *DAF*, decay accelerating factor; *EBV*, Epstein–Barr virus; *EPO*, erythropoietin; *G6PD*, glucose-6-phosphate dehydrogenase; *GPI*, glycosylphosphatidylinositol; *GSH*, glutathione; *Hb*, hemoglobin; *HbAS*, sickle cell trait; *HbSS*, homozygous for sickle cell disease; *Hct*, hematocrit; *HUS*, hemolytic uremic syndrome; *RBC*, red blood cell; *Rh HDN*, rhesus hemolytic disease of the newborn; *SLE*, systemic lupus erythematosus; *TTP*, thrombotic thrombocytopenic purpura; *XR*, X-linked recessive.

I. **Benign Qualitative White Blood Cell Disorders**
   A. **Definition**
      1. Abnormalities in the structure and/or function of white blood cells (WBCs).
   B. **Pathogenesis**
      1. Defects in leukocyte structure
         a. Chédiak–Higashi syndrome
            i. Autosomal recessive disorder characterized by impaired lysosomal transport in association with *LYST* gene mutation.
            ii. Blood smear shows giant abnormal azurophilic granules within neutrophils.
            iii. Presents in childhood with recurrent severe bacterial infections (usually *Staphylococcus aureus*), partial oculocutaneous albinism.
            iv. Cranial and peripheral neuropathy (muscle weakness, ataxia, and sensory loss).
      2. Defects in leukocyte function
         a. Leukocyte adhesion deficiency (LAD)
            i. Autosomal recessive defects in leukocyte adhesion.
            ii. Impairs the transmigration of WBC from the circulation into the tissues.
            iii. Neutrophils remain in circulation (explaining the characteristic neutrophilic leukocytosis).
            iv. LAD type 1 is due to a deficiency of CD18, the β2 subunit of integrin (impairs adherence of WBC to the endothelium).
            v. LAD type 2 is due to defective fucosyl transferase necessary to form ligands to bind with selectins (i.e., impairs "rolling" of white cells along the endothelium).
            vi. Manifestations include impaired wound healing, delayed separation of the umbilical cord, and a propensity for the development of recurrent, and potentially life-threatening, bacterial and fungal infections.
            vii. Absence of pus (leukocytes cannot leave the circulation to reach the site of infection).
         b. Phagocytosis defect
            i. Impaired opsonization (X-linked agammaglobulinemia)
               (1) Also known as Bruton agammaglobulinemia.
               (2) Due to mutations in the gene for Bruton's tyrosine kinase (BTK).
               (3) BTK is required for B-cell receptor signaling and is essential for B-cell survival and differentiation.
               (4) T-cell function is normal.
               (5) Physical findings include small or absent tonsils and lymph nodes.
               (6) Patients develop recurrent upper (otitis media and sinusitis) and lower respiratory tract infections, usually in the first year of life.
         c. Microbicidal defect
            i. Chronic granulomatous disease
               (1) Deficient function in the nicotinamide adenine dinucleotide phosphate oxidase.
               (2) Lack of "respiratory burst" (impaired generation of superoxide, hydrogen peroxide, and hypochlorous acid).
               (3) Inability to kill catalase-positive microorganisms (e.g., Aspergillus, S. aureus); persistent infection explains the granulomatous host response.
               (4) Increased risk of developing autoimmune disorders (e.g., inflammatory bowel disease).
            ii. Myeloperoxidase (MPO) deficiency
               (1) Autosomal recessive condition characterized by partial or complete MPO deficiency.

        (2) MPO converts hydrogen peroxide and chloride ions into hypochlorous acid (bleach), a very potent microbicidal agent.

        (3) Often asymptomatic, although patients may develop disseminated *Candida* infections.

C. Benign leukocyte reactions

1. Leukemoid reaction (Fig. 13.1)
   a. Refers to a WBC count of >50,000/μL from a cause other than leukemia; essentially an "exaggerated response" to infection, medication, or other processes.
   b. Consists primarily of mature neutrophils; usually in association with increased bands (called a "bandemia" or "left shift").

2. Leukoerythroblastosis (leukoerythroblastic reaction)
   a. Refers to the presence of both immature white cells (e.g., promyelocytes, myelocytes, and metamyelocytes) and immature red cells (normoblasts and nucleated red blood cells) within the peripheral blood (Fig. 13.2).
   b. Due to the premature release of immature cells from the bone marrow; either as a compensatory response to severe physiologic stress (e.g., acute blood loss or hemolysis) or in association with an infiltrative process of the bone marrow (e.g., metastatic carcinoma or primary myelofibrosis [PM]). A clue to an infiltrative process is the presence of teardrop-shaped red cells.

3. Pelger–Huet anomaly
   a. Benign condition in which most neutrophils have a bilobed, spectacle-shaped nucleus.
   b. Defect of neutrophil segmentation related to mutations in the lamin B receptor (*LBR*) gene.
   c. No effect on neutrophil function or survival.

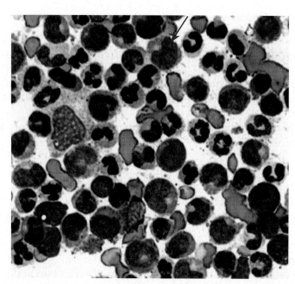

13.1: Neutrophil leukemoid reaction in the peripheral blood. Note the great number of segmented and band neutrophils as well as metamyelocytes (*red arrow*). (*From Goldman L, Schafer A: Goldman's Cecil medicine, ed 25, 2016, Elsevier Saunders, p 1130, Fig. 167.2.*)

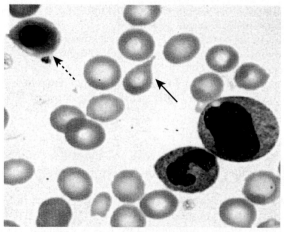

13.2: Leukoerythroblastic reaction. The solid arrow shows a teardrop red blood cell (RBC). Immature myeloid cells are also present, note the nucleated RBC (*interrupted arrow*). (*From Naeim F: Atlas of bone marrow and blood pathology, Philadelphia, 2001, Saunders, p 52, Fig. 4.10B.*)

II. **Benign Quantitative White Blood Cell Disorders**
   A. **Disorders involving neutrophils**
      1. Neutrophils, also known as polymorphonuclear leukocytes, are the most prevalent WBC in circulation (adults).
         a. Comprise ~40%–70% of the total WBC count.
         b. Normal absolute neutrophil count (ANC): >1500 cells/μL.
      2. Neutropenia
         a. Definition
            i. Abnormally low number of neutrophils in circulation (ANC <1500 cells/μL in adults).
               (1) Mild neutropenia: ANC ≥1000 and <1500 cells/μL.
               (2) Moderate neutropenia: ANC ≥500 and <1000 cells/μL.
               (3) Severe neutropenia: ANC <500 cells/μL.
            ii. Neutropenia, especially when severe (ANC < 500 cells/μL), is associated with an increased risk of bacterial infections.
         b. Causes include:
            i. Direct bone marrow suppression (e.g., drugs, chemical toxins, and radiation).
            ii. Splenic sequestration (hypersplenism) in which blood cells become entrapped within an enlarged spleen.
               (1) Splenic enlargement is usually secondary to cirrhosis-induced portal hypertension (see Chapter 19).
            iii. Inherited disorders of production (e.g., Shwachman–Diamond syndrome).
            iv. Immune-mediated destruction (e.g., systemic lupus erythematosus or rheumatoid arthritis).
               (1) Felty syndrome: a triad of rheumatoid arthritis, splenomegaly, and neutropenia.
            v. Decreased production
               (1) B12 or folate deficiency
               (2) Myelodysplastic syndromes (MDS)
               (3) Infiltrative processes of the marrow
               (4) Aplastic anemia
            vi. Nutritional (e.g., starvation).
            vii. Benign ethnic neutropenia (constitutional neutropenia).
               (1) Inherited cause of mild to moderate neutropenia; typically seen in those of African descent. No increased risk of infection. Associated with the Duffy null [Fy(a-b-)] phenotype.
      3. Neutrophilia (neutrophilic leukocytosis)
         a. Definition
            i. Increased number of circulating neutrophils (in adults: >7000 neutrophils/μL).
         b. Causes include:
            i. Acute infectious disorders (e.g., bacterial, fungal, and some viral).
            ii. Drugs (e.g., corticosteroids, growth factors, and catecholamines).
            iii. Tissue necrosis (e.g., burns, trauma, myocardial infarction).
            iv. Physiologic stresses (e.g., strenuous exercise).
            v. Smoking (mechanism unknown).
            vi. Postsplenectomy (loss of neutrophilic entrapment within the spleen; no clinical significance).
         c. Mechanisms of neutrophilia include:
            i. Infection and/or tissue necrosis stimulate the immune system to release interleukins (e.g., IL-6) that stimulate the bone marrow to increase the production and release of neutrophils.
            ii. Catecholamines (e.g., strenuous exercise and epinephrine injection) cause a shift of neutrophils from the marginating to the circulating pool (called "demargination").
   B. **Disorders involving eosinophils**
      1. Eosinophilia
         a. Definition
            i. Absolute eosinophil count of >500 cells/μL.
         b. Mechanisms
            i. IL-5 stimulates the production of eosinophils.
            ii. Eotaxin is chemotactic for eosinophils.
         c. Causes include:
            i. Allergic response (e.g., seasonal allergies and asthma).
            ii. Parasitic (invasive).
            iii. Neoplasms (various; both hematologic and nonhematologic).
            iv. Addison disease (adrenocortical insufficiency).
      2. Eosinopenia
         a. Decreased number of eosinophils in circulation.
         b. Most commonly due to excess glucocorticoids (Cushing syndrome).

C. Disorders involving basophils
1. Basophilia
    a. Defined as an absolute basophil count of >200 cells/μL.
    b. Characteristic finding in myeloproliferative neoplasms (e.g., polycythemia vera [PV] and chronic myelogenous leukemia [CML]).
D. Disorders of monocytes
1. Monocytosis
    a. Defined as an absolute monocyte count of >1000 cells/μL.
    b. May be seen in those recovering from neutropenia or those with indolent infections (e.g., tuberculosis, subacute bacterial endocarditis).
2. Disorders of lymphocytes
    a. Lymphocytosis
        i. Definition
            (1) Absolute lymphocyte count >5000 cells/μL in adults (or >8000 cells/μL in children).
        ii. Causes include:
            (1) Viral infections (e.g., Epstein–Barr virus [EBV] and cytomegalovirus).
            (2) Bacterial infection (e.g., *Bordetella pertussis*).
                (a) Lymphocytosis-promoting factor released from *B. pertussis* impairs the entry of lymphocytes into lymph nodes.
            (3) Neoplasia (e.g., chronic lymphocytic leukemia—CLL).
        iii. "Atypical" lymphocytosis
            (1) Refers to the presence of benign, reactive lymphocytes in the peripheral circulation.
            (2) Characteristic finding in acute infectious mononucleosis (EBV) and other viral infections.
            (3) Atypical lymphocytes are identified by the characteristic appearance on the blood smear (enlarged cytoplasm indented by adjacent red cells, see Fig. 13.3).
        iv. Infectious mononucleosis ("mono")
            (1) Definition
                (a) An acute illness classically characterized by fever, fatigue, pharyngitis, and lymphadenopathy.
                (b) Due to an acute EBV infection.
                (c) Although EBV may be contracted at any age, the characteristic "mononucleosis syndrome" is most likely to occur in those infected as an adolescent or young adult (~15–24 years).
            (2) Viral transmission and dissemination
                (a) Transmission of EBV is primarily through saliva (e.g., kissing).
                (b) Virus infects epithelial cells and B lymphocytes of the oropharynx (EBV enters B lymphocytes via attachment to the CD21 receptor).
                (c) Ultimately, infected B lymphocytes disseminate the virus throughout the body (EBV remains latent within B cells indefinitely).

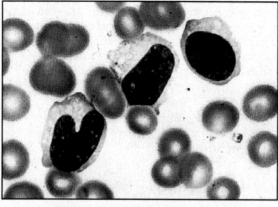

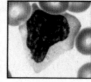
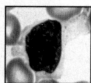

13.3: Peripheral blood with atypical lymphocytes. The lymphocytes are large and have abundant blue-gray cytoplasm. Note indentation of lymphocytes by surrounding red blood cells. (*From Naeim F: Atlas of bone marrow and blood pathology, Philadelphia, 2001, Saunders, p 168, Fig. 13.1.*)

(3) Clinical manifestations (develop after an incubation period of 4–8 weeks).
    (a) Fatigue, pharyngitis, and generalized lymphadenopathy.
    (b) Hepatitis
       • Usually only identified based on elevated levels of aminotransferase enzymes (aspartate aminotransferase and alanine aminotransferase). Clinical manifestations of hepatitis (e.g., jaundice) are much less common.
    (c) Splenomegaly
       • Risk of splenic rupture, patients must avoid contact sports.
    (d) Generalized, erythematous skin rash following treatment with ampicillin or amoxicillin (Fig. 13.4); does not represent a medication allergy.
(4) Laboratory findings
    (a) Lymphocytosis.
    (b) The presence of "atypical" lymphocytes on the blood smear (may account for >20% of the total number of WBCs).
    (c) Positive heterophile antibody test (initial screening test)
       • Heterophile antibodies are antibodies against nonhuman antigens (e.g., horse red cells).
       • Detection of heterophile antibodies is used in diagnostic testing (Monospot test).
       • If the Monospot is negative in a patient suspected of having infectious mononucleosis, either repeat the test in a few days or test for the presence of specific anti-EBV antibodies.
    (d) Specific antibodies against EBV
       • IgM and IgG anti-viral capsid antigen (VCA) antibodies.
       • IgM anti-VCA suggests an acute EBV infection in the appropriate clinical setting.
       • IgG anti-VCA antibodies persist for life; a marker of previous EBV infection.
       • EBV nuclear antigen (EBNA).
       • IgG anti-EBNA appears several weeks after the onset of symptoms and persists for life (if present, excludes acute EBV).

b. Lymphopenia
  i. Definition
    (1) Absolute lymphocyte count of <1500 cells/μL in adults (<3000 cells/μL in children).
  ii. Etiologies
    (1) Viral infections (e.g., human immunodeficiency virus, influenza virus, hepatitis virus, etc.).
    (2) Congenital immunodeficiency disorders (e.g., X-linked agammaglobulinemia).
    (3) Medications (e.g., corticosteroids and cytotoxic chemotherapy).
    (4) Ionizing radiation (lymphocytes are very sensitive to radiation).
    (5) Protein-energy undernutrition.

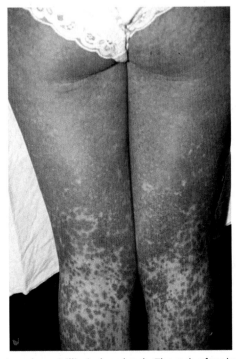

13.4: A patient with infectious mononucleosis and ampicillin-induced rash. The rash often has a violaceous hue and is often accompanied by pruritus. *(Courtesy of Dr. Stephen Gellis.)*

III. Lymphoid Leukemias
A. Acute lymphoblastic leukemia/lymphoblastic lymphoma (ALL/LBL)
1. Definition
   a. ALL/LBL is a malignancy of lymphoblasts (i.e., pre-B or pre-T cells).
   b. Characterized by an accumulation of lymphoblasts within the bone marrow (diagnosis requires that >20% of bone marrow cells be lymphoblasts).
2. Epidemiology
   a. ALL is the most common acute leukemia in children.
   b. ALL is the overall most common malignancy in children.
   c. Most cases (~85%) arise from pre-B cells (i.e., B-cell ALL/LBL); usually in children younger than 5 years of age.
      i. The less common T-cell ALL/LBL often presents as a thymic mass in adolescent males.
   d. Down syndrome associated with increased risk.
3. Diagnosis
   a. Presence of >20% lymphoblasts in the bone marrow (Fig. 13.5).
   b. Differentiation of lymphoblasts (i.e., acute lymphoid leukemia) from myeloblasts (i.e., acute myeloid leukemia) is based on the presence or absence of specific cellular markers as identified using flow cytometry and/or cytochemical stains.
      i. Lymphoblasts (i.e., ALL) are positive for terminal deoxynucleotidyl transferase (TdT) but negative for MPO.
      ii. Myeloblasts (i.e., acute myelogenous leukemia [AML]) have the reverse staining pattern (positive for MPO but negative for Tdt).
4. Pathogenesis
   a. Impaired B- or T-cell maturation and unregulated proliferation.
      i. Due to various cytogenetic and/or molecular abnormalities.
   b. "Crowding out" of normal hematopoietic cells by the malignant cells leads to the development of various cytopenias.
      i. In some instances, the malignant cells proliferate in nonhematopoietic tissues (skin, testes, etc.) as well.
5. Clinical manifestations
   a. Fever/infection (due to neutropenia).
   b. Bleeding, easy bruising, and petechiae (due to thrombocytopenia).
   c. Fatigue, dyspnea, and pallor (due to anemia).
   d. Bone pain (due to expansion of marrow cavity by malignant cells).

B. Chronic lymphocytic leukemia (CLL)
1. CLL is the same disease as small lymphocytic lymphoma (SLL), differing only in presentation.
   a. CLL presents primarily with lymphocytosis, whereas SLL presents primarily with lymphadenopathy (Fig. 13.6A). Distinction not absolute, however.
2. Epidemiology
   a. Most prevalent leukemia in adulthood, usually older (median age at diagnosis ⊠ 70 years).
   b. No known environmental risk factors.
3. Pathogenesis
   a. Pathogenesis is unclear; believed to arise from a premalignant B-cell proliferative disorder (called monoclonal B-cell lymphocytosis).
4. Clinical presentation
   a. Patients are often asymptomatic at the time of diagnosis, being diagnosed incidentally after profound lymphocytosis is discovered on a complete blood count performed for another reason.
   b. Symptoms, when present, are typically nonspecific (e.g., fatigue, weight loss, and anorexia).
   c. Immune abnormalities are common.

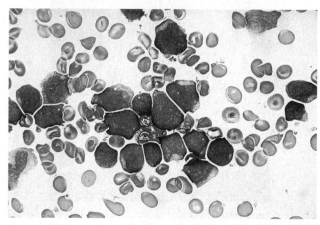

13.5: Lymphoid blasts in a case of acute lymphoblastic leukemia. *(From Underwood's pathology, ed 7, © 2019 Elsevier, Fig. 23.26).*

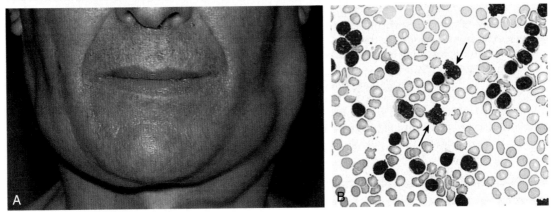

13.6: (A) Chronic lymphocytic leukemia. Note the bilateral cervical lymphadenopathy. (B) Peripheral blood in chronic lymphocytic leukemia. Note the increased number of lymphocytes with dense nuclear chromatin and scant cytoplasmic borders. The lymphocytes are extremely fragile and produce characteristic "smudge" cells (*arrows*) during the preparation of a slide. (*A, From Forbes C, Jackson W: Color atlas and text of clinical medicine, ed 3, London, 2004, Mosby, p 416, Fig. 10.38; B, from Hoffbrand AV: Color atlas: clinical hematology, ed 3, St. Louis, 2000, Mosby, p 179, Fig. 10.11*).

     i. Impaired immunity with an increased risk of infection and secondary malignancies.
     ii. Autoimmune phenomenon (e.g., hemolytic anemia and immune thrombocytopenia).
  5. Diagnosis
    a. Absolute lymphocytosis (absolute lymphocyte count >5000 cells/μL).
     i. "Smudge" cells, which represent fragile malignant cells that are damaged during the preparation of the blood smear, are a clue to the diagnosis (Fig. 13.6B).
    b. Identification of a monoclonal lymphoid population in a peripheral blood sample using flow cytometry.
  6. Prognosis
    a. Variable, often prolonged survival.
    b. Transformation to a more aggressive process, usually diffuse large B-cell lymphoma, occurs in some patients.
     i. Known as Richter syndrome (often a terminal event).
  7. Hairy cell leukemia
    a. Rare B-cell neoplasm seen predominantly in middle-aged White males.
    b. Pathogenesis: activating mutations in *BRAF* in the Mitogen-activated protein kinase (MAPK) signaling cascade.
    c. Indolent tumor with involvement of the splenic red pulp (massive splenomegaly common).
    d. Pancytopenia, secondary to marrow involvement and/or sequestration of cells within the enlarged spleen, is a common finding.
    e. Marrow aspiration may not be possible due to increased fibrosis, resulting in a "dry tap."
    f. Malignant cells ("hairy cells") stain with tartrate-resistant acid phosphatase.
  8. Adult T-cell leukemia/lymphoma
    a. Neoplasm of CD4+ T cells caused by the human T-lymphotropic virus 1 (HTLV-1).
    b. HTLV-1 is endemic in the Caribbean, southern Japan, and areas of Africa.
    c. Transmission via body fluids (e.g., breastfeeding, sharing of needles, and sexual intercourse).
    d. Aggressive course with propensity for lytic bone lesions and hypercalcemia.
    e. Tumor cells exhibit multilobated nuclei ("flower cells").
  9. Mycosis fungoides
    a. Cutaneous T-cell lymphoma of unknown cause; characterized by infiltration of the skin by malignant CD4+ helper T cells.
    b. Skin lesions proceed through phases:
     i. Inflammatory phase → plaque phase → tumor phase.
    c. Tumor cells exhibit marked infoldings of the nuclear membrane ("cerebriform" appearance).
    d. As a late event, tumor cells spread systemically to the lymph nodes and bone marrow.
    e. Sézary syndrome refers to a variant characterized by a generalized exfoliative erythroderma and involvement of the bloodstream by "Sézary" cells (with characteristic cerebriform nuclei).
C. Myeloid disorders
  1. Overview
    a. Three major categories of myeloid neoplasms:
     i. Acute myelogenous leukemia (AML)
     ii. MDS
     iii. Myeloproliferative neoplasms

2. AML
   a. Malignancy of immature myeloid cells (e.g., myeloblasts and promyelocytes); defined by the presence of ≥20% myeloid blasts in the bone marrow.
      i. Auer rods, representing linear collections of azurophilic granules within the cytoplasm of myeloblasts, are a clue to the diagnosis (Fig. 13.7).
   b. Expansion of the clonal (malignant) cell population "crowds out" other hematopoietic precursors resulting in various cytopenias and associated clinical manifestations.
      i. Fatigue and dyspnea (due to anemia).
      ii. Bleeding and easy bruising (due to thrombocytopenia).
      iii. Increased risk of infection (due to neutropenia).
   c. Epidemiology
      i. AML can occur at all ages; however, it is most common in older adults.
      ii. Most common type of acute leukemia in adults.
   d. Risk factors include:
      i. Environmental exposures (chemicals, radiation, and chemotherapeutic agents).
      ii. Genetic abnormalities (e.g., Trisomy 21).
      iii. Underlying hematologic disorders (e.g., aplastic anemia, paroxysmal nocturnal hemoglobinuria, myelodysplasia, and myeloproliferative neoplasms).
   e. Subtypes of AML include:
      i. Acute promyelocytic leukemia
         (1) Block in maturation due to translocation between the long arms of chromosomes 15 and 17 [t(15;17)].
         (2) Retinoic acid receptor alpha (*RARA*) gene on chromosome 17 fused with the promyelocytic leukemia (*PML*) gene on chromosome 15 to create a fusion gene (*PML–RARA*).
         (3) Risk of hemorrhage secondary to acute disseminated intravascular coagulation.
            (a) Prognosis: good with treatment (arsenic trioxide and all-trans retinoic acid).
   f. Diagnosis of AML
      i. Greater than or equal to 20% myeloblasts on bone marrow biopsy.
         (1) Myeloblasts can be differentiated from lymphoblasts by immunophenotyping with flow cytometry or with the use of special stains.
            (a) Myeloblasts are positive for MPO but negative for TdT.
               • Conversely, the lymphoblasts of ALL stain for Tdt but not for MPO.
            (b) Identification of Auer rods is indicative of myeloid differentiation (Fig. 13.7).
3. MDS
   a. Acquired clonal disorders of hematopoietic stem cells.
   b. Characterized by impaired maturation ("dysplastic") and death of hematopoietic precursors prior to their release from the bone marrow ("ineffective hematopoiesis").
      i. Explains the various cytopenias commonly seen in MDS.
   c. Clinical manifestations are those of the various cytopenias.
      i. Fatigue due to anemia, bleeding due to thrombocytopenia, and fever/infection due to neutropenia.
   d. The cause, in most cases, is unknown.
      i. Some follow the use of radiation and/or chemotherapy in the treatment of malignancy ("therapy-related MDS").
   e. Increasing incidence with age, most cases arise after the age of 70 years.
   f. Prognosis depends upon several factors including specific cytogenetic abnormalities, marrow blast percentage, degree of cytopenias, and age of a patient (overall 5-year survival ~ 30%).

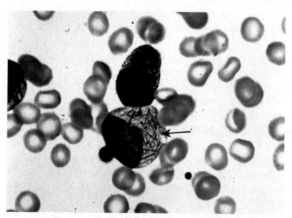

13.7: Peripheral blood in a patient with acute promyelocytic leukemia. Note the promyelocyte containing innumerable Auer rods (*arrow*). *(From Ivan Damjanov MD, PhD, Linder J: Pathology: a color atlas, St. Louis, 2000, Mosby, p 79, Fig. 5.21.)*

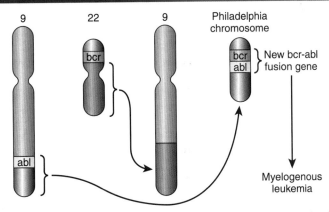

13.8: Balanced translocation between chromosomes 9 and 22 results in the formation of a Philadelphia chromosome. The translocation causes two genes, *ABL* and *BCR*, to become juxtaposed, resulting in a fusion gene. This fusion gene, *BCR–ABL*, is thought to be essential for the development of chronic myelogenous leukemia. *(From Copstead LE, Banasik JL: Pathophysiology, ed 5, 2013, Elsevier Saunders, p 221, Fig. 11.4.)*

4. Myeloproliferative neoplasms
   a. Chronic myelogenous leukemia (CML)
      i. Hematopoietic stem cell disorder due to a reciprocal translocation of the breakpoint cluster region (*BCR*) gene on chromosome 22 with the tyrosine kinase sequence of the Abelson (*ABL*) gene on chromosome 9 (Fig. 13.8).
      ii. Forms abnormal chromosome, called the "Philadelphia chromosome" containing the *BCR–ABL* fusion gene encoding for a protein (BCR–ABL) that exhibits constitutively active tyrosine kinase activity → activates cell signaling pathways.
         (1) Causes myeloid cells of a specific lineage (e.g., neutrophils) to proliferate.
      iii. Usually older adulthood (median age of onset is 67 years) with slight male predominance.
      iv. Exposure to high-dose ionizing radiation is a risk factor.
      v. Laboratories
         (1) Marked leukocytosis (often ≥100,000 WBCs/μL).
         (2) Neutrophils, at all stages of development (i.e., myeloblasts to mature neutrophils).
            (a) Characteristic for these neutrophils to have a low leukocyte alkaline phosphatase (LAP) score; helps to distinguish CML from a reactive leukocytosis in which the LAP score is elevated.
         (3) Basophilia (characteristic finding).
         (4) Normocytic anemia.
         (5) Thrombocytosis in early-stage disease; however, thrombocytopenia arises as the disease progresses.
      vi. Clinical presentation
         (1) Three phases (chronic, accelerated, and blast phase).
            (a) Chronic phase
               • Nonspecific manifestations (e.g., fatigue and left upper quadrant discomfort due to splenomegaly).
            (b) Accelerated phase
               • Occurs as a result of additional cytogenetic abnormalities.
               • Patients suffer from complications secondary to the block in cellular differentiation (e.g., infection due to loss of normally functioning WBCs and bleeding due to thrombocytopenia).
            (c) Blast phase
               • Represents late-stage transformation into an acute leukemia.
               • Because the defect arises in a stem cell, the "blast" phase may proceed as either an acute myeloid leukemia (usually) or an acute lymphoid leukemia.
      vii. Prognosis
         (1) When diagnosed in the chronic phase, treatment with tyrosine kinase inhibitors results in a favorable prognosis.
         (2) Those diagnosed at more advanced stages of the disease have a less favorable prognosis.
   b. Polycythemia vera (PV)
      i. Definition
         (1) PV is characterized by increased bone marrow cellularity in association with marked proliferation of erythroid (primarily) and other cell lineages.
      ii. Pathogenesis
         (1) Mutation in the tyrosine kinase Janus kinase 2 (*JAK2*) gene; renders hematopoietic progenitor cells more sensitive to the effects of growth factors.

iii. Diagnosis
(1) Increase in red cell mass (polycythemia) as evidenced by an elevated hemoglobin (Hb >16.5 g/dL in males, Hb >16.0 g/dL in females).
(2) Characteristic hypercellular bone marrow with increased trilineage hematopoiesis.
(3) Presence of *JAK2* mutation.
(4) Decreased erythropoietin - EPO (considered a minor criterion but important in that this excludes secondary polycythemia, i.e., that associated with hypoxia or an erythropoietin-secreting tumor).
iv. Epidemiology
(1) Usually affects middle-aged to older adults (50–75 years); mean of 60 years.
(2) Male > female.
v. Clinical manifestations
(1) Increased red cell mass (polycythemia).
(a) May be associated with an increased blood viscosity ("hyperviscosity syndrome") characterized by impaired cerebral circulation (e.g., headache, dizziness, and blurred vision with engorged conjunctival and/or retinal vessels), facial plethora, and ruddy complexion.
(2) Increased risk of thrombosis (arterial and venous).
(3) Erythromelalgia (burning sensation and redness of hands and feet).
(4) Aquagenic pruritus (itching after bath or shower) secondary to the overproduction of histamine.
(5) Splenomegaly.
(6) Increased risk of gout and nephrolithiasis secondary to hyperuricemia (secondary to increased cell turnover).
vi. Laboratory findings
(1) Polycythemia
(a) Hemoglobin of >16.5 g/dL males or >16.0 g/dL in females. EPO characteristically low.
(2) Leukocytosis and thrombocytosis are common as well.
c. Essential thrombocythemia (ET)
i. Definition
(1) ET is a clonal stem cell disorder in which the primary effect is marked thrombocytosis (platelet count ≥450,000/μL).
(2) Bone marrow biopsies show increased numbers of large megakaryocytes, singly or in clusters.
(3) Identified mutations include *JAK2* (most common), calreticulin (*CALR*), and the thrombopoietin receptor (*MPL*).
ii. Epidemiology
(1) More common in older adults (median age ~ 65 years).
(2) Female > male (unique; the other myeloproliferative neoplasms are more common in males).
iii. Clinical manifestations
(1) Often asymptomatic; however, some have manifestations like those of PV (e.g., headache, lightheadedness, visual changes, and erythromelalgia).
(2) Increased risk of thrombosis as well as hemorrhage.
d. Primary myelofibrosis (PM)
i. Definition
(1) Myeloproliferative neoplasm characterized by fibrosis of the bone marrow with loss of hematopoiesis, development of various cytopenias, and associated manifestations.
ii. Epidemiology
(1) Least common of the myeloproliferative neoplasms.
(2) Usually affects older adults; male > female.
iii. Clinical manifestations
(1) Decreased hematopoiesis (i.e., fatigue, infection, and bleeding).
(2) Splenomegaly (often prominent) causing abdominal fullness and early satiety.
iv. Laboratory findings
(1) Pancytopenia.
(2) Blood smear shows "teardrop" red cells and leukoerythroblastosis (immature granulocytes and nucleated red cells).
(3) Bone marrow biopsy shows increased fibrous tissue with decreased hematopoietic precursors.
(a) Fibrosis often leads to a "dry tap" (inability to obtain a marrow aspirate).
v. Prognosis
(1) Least favorable prognosis of the myeloproliferative neoplasms.
(2) Increased morbidity and mortality due to hemorrhage, thrombosis, infections, and/or transformation into an acute leukemia.

I. **Lymphadenopathy**
   A. **Definition**
      1. Enlargement of lymph node(s), Fig. 14.1
         a. Normal lymph nodes are typically <1 cm in diameter.
   B. **Etiologies**
      1. Location and extent (localized vs. generalized) are helpful clues to the underlying etiology.
      2. Infection
         a. Overall, the most common cause of lymphadenopathy, especially in children and young adults.
         b. Involved nodes are usually tender; fluctuance suggests abscess.
         c. Bacterial infections characterized by enlargement of nodes draining the site (e.g., axillary adenopathy in a patient with infection of hand).
         d. Systemic viral infections (e.g., Epstein–Barr virus [EBV] and human immunodeficiency virus [HIV]) often cause generalized adenopathy.
      3. Autoimmune disorders
         a. Systemic lupus erythematosus, rheumatoid arthritis (RA), and others.
      4. Malignancy
         a. Lymphadenopathy in middle-aged to older adults is often a sign of malignancy.
         b. Nodes tend to be painless and nonmobile (i.e., fixed to surrounding tissue). Additional clues that suggest malignancy include coexisting weight loss, fever, and night sweats.
         c. Etiologies include:
            i.   Hematologic malignancy (e.g., Hodgkin lymphoma [HL], non-Hodgkin lymphoma [NHL], and leukemia).
            ii. Metastasis (e.g., axillary lymphadenopathy in a female often represents metastatic breast cancer).
         d. Key lymph node groups involved in primary and metastatic cancer.
            i.   Submental lymph nodes: metastatic squamous cell carcinoma arising in the floor of the mouth.
            ii.   Cervical lymph nodes: metastatic head and neck tumors (e.g., thyroid and nasopharynx); HL.
            iii. Left supraclavicular lymph node ("Virchow node") suggests abdominal malignancy (e.g., stomach, gallbladder, pancreas, kidneys, testicles, and ovaries).
            iv.   Right supraclavicular lymph node: metastatic lung or esophageal cancer.
            v.   Axillary lymph nodes: metastatic breast cancer.
            vi.   Epitrochlear lymph nodes: NHL.
            vii. Hilar lymph nodes: metastatic lung cancer.
            viii. Mediastinal lymph nodes: metastatic lung cancer; HL.
            ix.   Inguinal lymph nodes: metastatic squamous cell carcinoma from the vulva or penis.
   C. **Types of reactive lymphadenitis**
      1. Follicular hyperplasia
         a. Due to stimulation of the B-cell compartment of the lymph node.
            i. Unstimulated follicles are known as primary follicles.
            ii. Become a "secondary" follicle when stimulated.

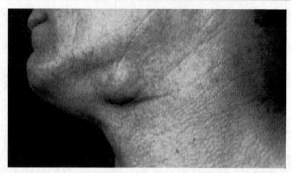

14.1: A patient with an enlarged cervical lymph node. Painful nodes are usually inflammatory, whereas painless nodes are more likely to be malignant. *(From Bouloux P: Self-assessment picture tests: medicine, Vol 1, London, 1997, Mosby-Wolfe, p 41, Fig. 81.)*

b. Histologically characterized by an increase in the number and size of secondary follicles, with variation in shape.
    c. Specific etiologies include early HIV infection, RA, Sjögren syndrome, and toxoplasmosis.
 2. Paracortical hyperplasia
    a. Associated with a T-cell–mediated immune response; characterized by expansion of paracortical regions of lymph nodes.
    b. Viral infections (e.g., EBV and cytomegalovirus) exhibit this pattern.
 3. Sinus histiocytosis
    a. Characterized by the prominence of macrophages within lymphoid sinuses; often found in lymph nodes draining cancers (e.g., axillary nodes in a patient with breast cancer).

II. **Non-Hodgkin Lymphoma**
 A. **Overview**
    1. NHL represents a diverse group of hematologic malignancies in which the malignant clone arises from progenitor B cells, progenitor T cells, mature B cells, or mature T cells.
    2. Presentation and prognosis vary widely; some subtypes present with painless lymphadenopathy that persists for years, whereas other subtypes are very aggressive, causing death within weeks, if untreated.
    3. Some patients develop "B" symptoms.
       a. Fever >38°C (>100.4°F).
       b. Unexplained loss of >10% of body weight over the past 6 months.
       c. Drenching night sweats.
 B. **Diffuse large B-cell lymphoma**
    1. Most common histologic subtype of NHL in the developed world.
    2. Incidence increases with age (median age at presentation 64 years) with slight male predominance.
    3. Cell of origin is a mature B cell.
    4. Presents as a rapidly enlarging mass involving lymph nodes and/or extranodal tissues (e.g., liver, spleen, gastrointestinal [GI] tract, and other tissues).
       a. Extranodal disease is common, seen in a majority of patients at some point during the course of the disease.
    5. Aggressive neoplasm but curable in ~50% of cases.
 C. **Follicular lymphoma**
    1. Second most common histologic subtype of NHL.
    2. Incidence increases with age (median 65 years) with slight male predominance.
    3. Presents with painless lymphadenopathy (involving cervical, axillary, inguinal, and/or femoral regions); extranodal involvement is less common.
    4. Incurable but indolent with prolonged survival.
    5. Tumor cells derived from germinal center B cells.
    6. Pathogenesis
       a. Translocation between chromosomes 14 and 18 [t(14;18)] with juxtaposition of the immunoglobulin heavy chain (*IgH*) gene on chromosome 14 with the *BCL2* gene on chromosome 18.
       b. Leads to overexpression of BCL2 (an antiapoptotic protein) and prolonged cell survival.
 D. **Burkitt lymphoma**
    1. Highly aggressive but often curable neoplasm of mature germinal center B cells.
    2. Usually seen in children or young adults.
    3. Three settings:
       a. Endemic Burkitt: occurs in children, usually equatorial Africa; involvement of jaw bones; strong EBV association.
       b. Sporadic Burkitt: the most common type in the United States; usually presents in children as abdominal mass.
       c. Immunodeficiency-associated Burkitt: usually HIV+ patients.

4. Pathogenesis
   a. MYC overexpression is a consistent feature of Burkitt lymphoma. MYC activates the expression of many genes that are involved in cell growth, including the so-called Warburg effect (aerobic glycolysis).
      i. Most commonly involves translocation of the *MYC* gene on chromosome 8 with the *IgH* gene on chromosome 14 [t(8;14)].
   b. Warburg effect refers to the process where cells use glucose to provide metabolic intermediates necessary for the synthesis of cellular components (allows for rapid cell growth).
5. Histology
   a. "Starry-sky" appearance (macrophages containing necrotic cellular debris [the "stars"] within a background of hyperchromatic tumor cells [the "sky"]).

E. **Mantle cell lymphoma**
1. Uncommon form of NHL; usually seen in older adults.
2. Male > female; White > Black.
3. Malignant cells derived from pregerminal center B cells of the mantle zone.
4. Pathogenesis involves the chromosomal translocation, t(11;14) (q13;q32).
   a. Juxtaposition of *CCND1* gene, encoding cyclin D1, and the *IgH* gene → overexpression of cyclin D1 → cellular proliferation.
5. Presents with painless lymphadenopathy, sometimes with extranodal disease as well (spleen, bone marrow, and GI tract).
6. Moderately aggressive but prolonged survival (~10 years) often possible with treatment.

F. **Marginal zone lymphoma**
1. Indolent tumors, often arising secondary to chronic immune stimulation.
2. Commonly arises within the stomach in association with long-standing *Helicobacter pylori* infection.
   a. Infection stimulates the mucosa-associated lymphoid tissue (MALT), thus the common name of "MALToma" for these tumors.
   b. Other sites of involvement include the thyroid and salivary glands.
3. Lesions may resolve following the treatment of inciting agent (e.g., eradication of *H. pylori* may lead to resolution of those arising within the stomach).

III. **Hodgkin Lymphoma**
A. **Definition**
1. Hematologic neoplasm of germinal center B cells in which the malignant cells (called Reed–Sternberg or RS cells) are surrounded by variable mixtures of mature, nonneoplastic inflammatory cells.
   a. Cytokines (e.g., interleukin-5 [IL-5] and IL-10) and chemokines secreted by the RS cells account for the surrounding inflammatory cells.

B. **Epidemiology**
1. Accounts for ~10% of all lymphomas; overall, more common in males.
   a. Exception: nodular sclerosing subtype (equally common in females; the most common subtype overall).
2. Bimodal age distribution
   a. Early peak in late adolescence/young adulthood (15–34 years).
   b. Second peak in older adults (>50 years).

C. **Pathology**
1. Required for the diagnosis is the presence of RS cells.
   a. RS cells are the malignant cell of HL.
   b. Commonly positive for EBV.
   c. Most RS cells are positive for CD15 and CD30; the exception being the uncommon "nodular lymphocyte predominant" subtype.
   d. "Classic" RS cells are characterized by at least two prominent eosinophilic nucleoli in separate nuclear lobes ("owl's eyes" appearance; Fig. 14.2).
2. Subtypes of HL are based on histologic and immunophenotypic features of the RS cells.
   a. Nodular sclerosing
      i. Most common subtype with an excellent prognosis.
      ii. Usually presents in adolescence (male = female); often with cervical and/or mediastinal lymphadenopathy.
      iii. RS cells are CD15+ and CD30+.
   b. Mixed cellularity
      i. Second most common subtype; good prognosis.
      ii. Usually older adults; males > females.
      iii. RS cells are CD15+ and CD30+.
   c. Lymphocyte-rich
      i. Male > female, older adults; good prognosis.
      ii. RS cells are CD15+ and CD30+.

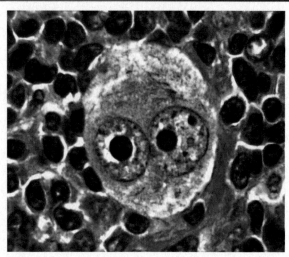

14.2: Classic Reed–Sternberg (RS) cell with two mirror image nuclei, each with a prominent red nucleolus. *(Courtesy of Dr. Fabio Facchetti, Brescia, Italy.)*

   d. Lymphocyte depleted
      i. Less favorable prognosis; usually presenting at an advanced stage.
      ii. RS cells are CD15+ and CD30+.
   e. Nodular lymphocyte predominant
      i. Uncommon "nonclassical" subtype in which the RS cells are CD20+, CD15−, and CD30−.
      ii. Good prognosis.
D. **Clinical manifestations**
   1. HL initially involves localized groups of lymph nodes (commonly cervical, supraclavicular, and anterior mediastinal).
      a. Mediastinal mass in a young person is often HL.
   2. Lymphadenopathy
      a. Although lymphadenopathy is painless, involved nodes become painful following the ingestion of alcohol.
   3. "B" symptoms (fever, weight loss of >10%, and drenching night sweats).
   4. Cough, chest pain, and shortness of breath (suggest mediastinal nodal involvement).
E. **Prognosis**
   1. Dependent upon the clinical stage (more important than histologic subtype); often curable.
   2. Poor prognostic factors include age >45 years, male sex, high stage, and abnormal blood counts (marked leukocytosis and lymphopenia).

Staging of Hodgkin lymphoma (Ann Arbor classification)

- Stage I: Involvement of a single lymph node region (Fig. 14.3).
- Stage II: Involvement of two or more lymph node regions on the same side of the diaphragm.
- Stage III: Involvement of lymph node regions on both sides of the diaphragm and/or localized involvement of an extra-lymphatic organ.
- Stage IV: Diffuse involvement of one or more extra-lymphatic organs.

F. **Important clinical differences from NHL**
   1. HL tends to involve a single lymph node group (e.g., cervical) before spreading in a predictable contiguous fashion to nearby lymph nodes.
   2. HL is less likely to involve extranodal tissues (until late in the disease course) or to involve mesenteric nodes or Waldeyer ring.
IV. **Langerhans Cell Histiocytosis**
   A. **Definition**
      1. Rare disorder characterized by the proliferation of cells that resemble specialized dendritic cells of the skin and mucosa known as Langerhans cells.
         a. Tumor cells are now known to be derived from bone marrow myeloid progenitor cells rather than the Langerhans cell.
      2. Neoplastic cells can involve nearly any organ (e.g., skin, lymph nodes, lungs, liver, spleen, central nervous system, and bone marrow).

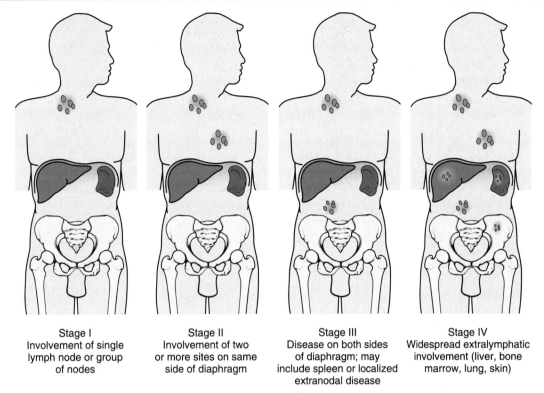

Stage I	Stage II	Stage III	Stage IV
Involvement of single lymph node or group of nodes	Involvement of two or more sites on same side of diaphragm	Disease on both sides of diaphragm; may include spleen or localized extranodal disease	Widespread extralymphatic involvement (liver, bone marrow, lung, skin)

14.3: Staging of Hodgkin lymphoma. *(From Damjanov 1: Pathology for the health professions, ed 4, Philadelphia, 2012, Saunders Elsevier, p 219, Fig. 9-21.)*

B. Clinical presentation
1. Depends on organ involvement; most commonly presents with one or more osteolytic bone lesions (e.g., skull, femur, rib, and vertebra).

C. Pathology
1. Neoplastic cells are positive for CD1a and S-100, and contain Birbeck granules (tennis racket appearance on electron microscopy).

V. Plasma Cell Dyscrasias

A. Definition
1. Neoplastic plasma cell proliferation, usually associated with the production of a monoclonal immunoglobulin (known as the "M protein").

B. Epidemiology
1. Older adults (most cases arise in those >65 years).
2. More common in African Americans.

C. Pathology
1. Increased numbers of plasma cells in the bone marrow ($\geq$10% of cells).
2. Free light chains (κ or λ) in the urine ("Bence Jones protein").

D. Diagnosis
1. Serum protein electrophoresis (SPE)
   a. Shows monoclonal spike (M protein); Fig. 14.4.
2. Serum immunofixation
   a. Used to characterize the M protein (heavy and light chain subclass).
3. Urine protein electrophoresis
   a. Identifies the presence of free light chains in the urine (known as "Bence Jones protein").
4. Free light chain assay
   a. Provides a measure of the amount of "free" kappa or lambda light immunoglobulin chains in the serum.

E. Classification of plasma cell disorders
1. Monoclonal gammopathy of undetermined significance (MGUS)
   a. Most common plasma cell disorder.
   b. Refers to the presence of a monoclonal immunoglobulin in low concentration (<3 g/dL) and without clinical manifestations.

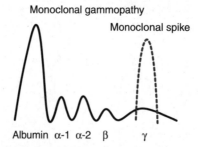

14.4: Serum protein electrophoresis showing a schematic of a monoclonal gammopathy. *(From Goljan EF, Sloka KI: Rapid review laboratory testing in clinical medicine, Philadelphia, 2008, Mosby Elsevier, p 284, Fig. 9-1C.)*

     c. Relatively common with increasing age (especially over 50 years).
     d. Approximately 1% annual progression to myeloma.
  2. Multiple myeloma (MM)
     a. Definition
        i. Monoclonal plasma cell neoplasm of the bone marrow usually associated with the production of a monoclonal immunoglobulin.
     b. Clinical manifestations
        i. Pathologic fractures/bone pain
           (1) Myeloma cells produce an inhibitor of osteoblast differentiation (DKK1) and release MIP1α, an activator of osteoclasts. Net effect is an imbalance between osteoclasts and osteoblasts and the development of lytic bone lesions (Fig. 14.5).
       ii. Anemia
           (1) Causes fatigue, pallor, and decreased exercise tolerance.
           (2) Due to marrow replacement by clonal plasma cell population and/or decreased erythropoietin (secondary to renal disease).
           (3) Peripheral blood smear shows red cells aggregating in a linear fashion (Rouleaux) analogous to a "stack of coins."
       iii. Radiculopathy
           (1) Nerve compression can occur due to the mass effect of the neoplastic plasma cells and/or secondary to vertebral compression fractures.
       iv. Recurrent infection
           (1) MM suppresses normal immune function and decreased functioning immunoglobulins.
       v. Hypercalcemia
           (1) Calcium released from lytic bone lesions.
       vi. Renal insufficiency
           (1) Mechanisms of renal insufficiency in myeloma include nephrocalcinosis (deposition of calcium in the kidney parenchyma/tubules secondary to increased calcium excretion) and deposition of free light chains (Bence Jones protein) in renal tubules. Free light chains are toxic to the tubules, known as "myeloma kidney."
     c. Diagnosis
        i. Bone marrow biopsy/aspirate
           (1) Malignant plasma cells comprise ≥10% of cells in the marrow.
       ii. SPE
           (1) Serum M protein is >3 g/dL ("M spike").
           (2) IgG (70% of cases) > IgA (20%) > pure light chain myeloma (5%–10% of cases).
           (3) Rarely, myeloma may be nonsecretory (i.e., no monoclonal protein produced).
       iii. Urine protein electrophoresis
           (1) Shows filtered light chains (Bence Jones protein) in many cases.
       iv. Skeletal survey (computed tomography, magnetic resonance imaging, and positron emission tomography)
           (1) "Punched out" lytic bone lesions (Fig. 14.5).
           (2) Vertebrae are the most common sites of bone involvement; other sites include the ribs, skull, femur, and pelvis.
     d. Prognosis
        i. Survival varies widely depending upon cytogenetic abnormalities and tumor cell burden, often several years.

VI. Spleen
  A. Splenic functions
    1. Filtration of blood by macrophages → removal of senescent red cells, bacteria, and other organisms.
    2. Antigen trapping and presentation → antibody production.
    3. Reservoir of blood cells (one-third of peripheral blood platelets normally stored within the spleen).
    4. Site of extramedullary hematopoiesis (normal during fetal development and abnormal after birth).

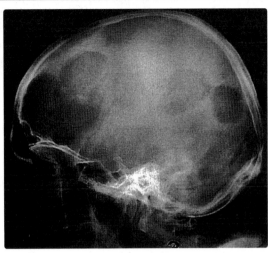

14.5: Skull with numerous osteolytic "punched out" lesions in a patient with multiple myeloma. *(From Gaw A, Murphy MJ, Srivastava R, Cowan RA, O'Reilly Denis St J: Clinical biochemistry: an illustrated colour text, ed 5, St. Louis, 2013, Churchill Livingstone Elsevier, p 53, Fig. 26.4.)*

B. **Splenomegaly**
1. Definition
   a. Enlargement of the spleen.
2. Etiologies
   a. Immune reaction against blood-borne infections ("work hypertrophy").
   b. Splenic congestion (usually secondary to portal hypertension in association with hepatic cirrhosis).
3. Clinical manifestations
   a. Left upper quadrant (LUQ) pain
      i. Stretching of splenic capsule.
   b. Early satiety
      i. Due to compression of stomach by an enlarged spleen.
   c. Peripheral blood cytopenias ("hypersplenism" and "splenic sequestration")
      i. Due to enhanced trapping of cells within the spleen, causes anemia, thrombocytopenia, and neutropenia, alone or in combination.

C. **Splenic dysfunction/splenectomy**
1. Predisposition to infection by encapsulated bacteria
   a. *Streptococcus pneumoniae, Haemophilus influenzae, Salmonella* spp., *Neisseria meningitidis*, and others.
   b. Immunization prior to splenectomy helps to prevent infectious complications.
2. Thrombocytosis
   a. Normally, one-third of peripheral platelets stored within the spleen. Following splenectomy, these platelets remain in circulation (accounting for the increased number).
3. Presence of Howell–Jolly bodies (nuclear remnants) on the peripheral blood smear.
   a. When functioning, splenic macrophages remove Howell–Jolly bodies from circulating red cells.

15 Disorders of Hemostasis

I. Hemostasis

A. Overview

1. Hemostasis is a physiologic process characterized by the formation of a thrombus (blood clot) to limit the loss of blood following injury to the endothelium (e.g., trauma).
2. Involves an interaction between endothelial cells, platelets, and clotting factors.

B. Platelets

1. Anucleate cells derived from cytoplasmic budding of megakaryocytes in the bone marrow.
2. Expected lifespan of ~10 days in circulation; approximately one-third are stored in the spleen (normal count is 150,000–400,000/μL).

C. Clotting factors

1. Extrinsic pathway: factor VII.
2. Intrinsic pathway: factors XII, XI, IX, and VIII.
3. Common pathway: factors X, V, II (prothrombin), and I (fibrinogen).
4. All are produced by the liver (except factor VIII, which is synthesized by endothelial cells).

D. "Primary" hemostasis

1. Refers to the formation of the platelet "plug" at the site of endothelial injury.
2. Injury to blood vessels (damaged endothelium) exposes subendothelial collagen.
3. von Willebrand factor (vWF)
   a. Glycoprotein (Gp) present in blood plasma, the subendothelial matrix, endothelial cells (Weibel–Palade bodies), and platelets (α-granules).
   b. Serves as a link between subendothelial collagen and the platelet (Fig. 15.1).
   c. vWF binds to platelets via the platelet GpIb receptor (platelet "adhesion").
   d. vWF also functions as a carrier protein for FVIII in circulation (VIII:vWF).
      i. Protects factor VIII from proteolysis; severe deficiency of vWF can therefore be associated with decreased factor VIII levels.
4. Platelet adherence is followed by platelet activation and the release of various factors (e.g., adenosine diphosphate [ADP] and thromboxane A2).
5. Results in the activation of a second platelet receptor (GpIIb/IIIa).
   a. GpIIb/IIIa acts as a fibrinogen receptor and is the link between aggregating platelets (i.e., formation of the platelet plug).
   b. Conversion of fibrinogen into fibrin (a more stable molecule) occurs in "secondary" hemostasis.

E. Secondary hemostasis

1. Definition
   a. Series of enzymatic reactions (the "coagulation cascade") in which clotting factors are sequentially activated, ultimately resulting in the conversion of fibrinogen into fibrin.
2. "Intrinsic" and "extrinsic" pathways (Fig. 15.2)
   a. "Intrinsic" pathway initiated by contact with negatively charged surfaces.
   b. "Extrinsic" pathway is initiated by the release of tissue factor (TF) from damaged endothelial cells.
   c. These pathways meet to form the "common" pathway.
3. Most important is the release of TF (extrinsic pathway).
   a. TF converts factor VII into the active form (VIIa).
   b. VIIa then activates factors IX and X to form factors IXa and Xa, respectively.

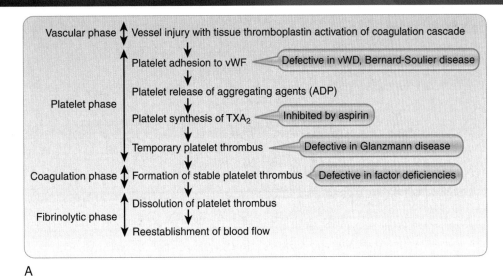

A

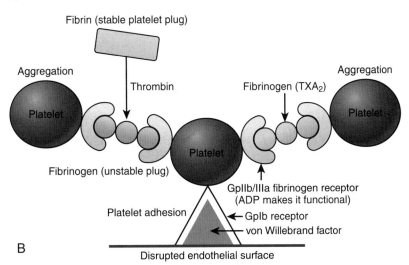

B

15.1: (A) Small-vessel hemostasis response to injury. A vascular phase, platelet phase, coagulation phase, and fibrinolytic phase are involved in small-vessel hemostasis with the formation of a platelet thrombus. (B) Platelet receptors and platelet aggregation. Disruption of the endothelial surface of small vessels exposes von Willebrand factor (vWF). This allows the glycoprotein (Gp) Ib receptor on the platelet to adhere to vWF on the subendothelium ("platelet adhesion"). The platelet releases preformed adenosine diphosphate (ADP) immediately after adhesion. ADP produces conformational changes in the GpIIb/IIIa fibrinogen receptor, rendering it able to bind to fibrinogen molecules. Thromboxane A2 (TXA2) is then synthesized de novo by the platelet. TXA2 enhances fibrinogen attachment to the GpIIb/IIIa receptors on adjacent platelets, causing platelet aggregation and the formation of a temporary platelet thrombus. The platelet thrombus is unstable until thrombin, which is locally produced by the activation of the coagulation system, converts fibrinogen to fibrin. This produces a stable platelet thrombus that stops bleeding from damaged small vessels. *vWD*, von Willebrand disease.

    c. Prothrombin (II) converted to thrombin (IIa).

    d. Thrombin converts fibrinogen into fibrin (the "glue" that binds platelets together).

    e. Cross-linking of fibrin monomers, by activated factor XIII, is the final step in hemostasis (cross-linking stabilizes the clot).

  4. Clotting

    a. Localized to the phospholipid membrane of platelets; requires vitamin K.

    b. Major sources of vitamin K include colonic bacteria (deficient in the newborn) and green leafy vegetables.

      i. Reason why newborns are given vitamin K injection.

    c. Vitamin K is a cofactor for γ-glutamyl carboxylase and necessary for a carboxylation reaction that converts glutamate residues in proteins to γ-carboxyglutamate residues (important for interaction with calcium ions).

      i. Vitamin K is required for the proper function of procoagulant factors II, VII, IX, and X as well as the natural anticoagulants, proteins C and S.

    d. Deficiency of vitamin K inhibits clotting.

      i. Warfarin blocks the vitamin K 2,3-epoxide reductase enzyme necessary for the regeneration of vitamin K (essentially causes the patient to become deficient in activated vitamin K).

      ii. Reversal of warfarin effect

        (1) Vitamin K supplementation.

        (2) In emergent situations (e.g., active bleeding), infuse fresh frozen plasma (FFP) because it contains all of the active clotting factors.

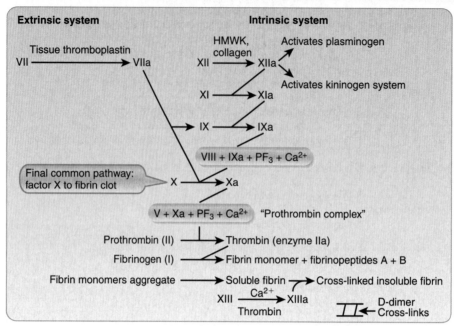

Extrinsic system   **Intrinsic system**

15.2: Coagulation cascade. Both the extrinsic and intrinsic coagulation systems use the final common pathway for the formation of a fibrin clot. *a*, Activated; *HMWK*, high-molecular-weight kininogen; *PF3*, platelet factor 3 (reaction accelerator).

F. Endogenous anticoagulation pathways
1. Overview
   a. Endogenous anticoagulant proteins degrade excess activated clotting factors in circulation to limit clotting to the site of injury.
2. Specific factors
   a. Tissue factor pathway inhibitor
      i. Inhibits factors VIIa and Xa.
   b. Proteins C and S
      i. Protein C, along with protein S as a cofactor, inhibit factors Va and VIIIa.
   c. Antithrombin (AT)
      i. Inhibits thrombin (IIa) and Xa and to a lesser extent VIIa, IXa, XIa, and XIIa.
      ii. AT activity is potentiated by endogenous and exogenous heparins (explaining the use of heparin as an anticoagulant).
   d. Prostaglandin I_2 (prostacyclin)
      i. Synthesized from arachidonic acid by intact endothelial cells.
      ii. Causes vasodilation and inhibits platelet aggregation.

II. Laboratory Testing of Hemostasis
A. Platelet count
1. Quantitative measure of platelet number.
2. Not qualitative, says nothing about platelet function.
B. Prothrombin time (PT)
1. Measures the extrinsic and common pathway (factors VII, X, V, II, and I).
2. Normal PT is 11.0–12.5 seconds (international normalized ratio [INR] of 0.8–1.1).
3. Used to monitor warfarin anticoagulation.
   a. INR standardizes the PT result between laboratories, particularly useful for monitoring warfarin anticoagulation.
C. Activated partial thromboplastin time (aPTT and partial thromboplastin time [PTT])
1. PTT measures the intrinsic and common pathway (XII, prekallikrein, high-molecular-weight kininogen, XI, IX, VIII, X, V, II, and I).
2. Normal PTT is 25–35 seconds.
3. Used to monitor the anticoagulant effect of unfractionated heparin.
D. Bleeding time
1. A measure of primary hemostasis (i.e., time between injury and formation of the platelet plug).
2. No longer routinely performed (difficult to standardize, time-consuming, and does not predict clinical bleeding).
3. Prolonged with any impairment in primary hemostasis (e.g., thrombocytopenia, Bernard–Soulier syndrome, Glanzmann thrombasthenia, and/or von Willebrand disease [vWD]).

E. **Fibrinogen (factor I)**
1. Precursor to fibrin (necessary for stabilization of the platelet clot).
2. Decreased levels of fibrinogen may be seen in:
   a. Disseminated intravascular coagulation (DIC)
      i. DIC is characterized by widespread activation of clotting, results in the consumption of fibrinogen (see later discussion).
   b. Liver disease
      i. Impaired hepatic synthetic capability, as seen in severe liver disease, leads to the decreased production of fibrinogen and other proteins.

F. **Fibrin degradation products (FDPs)/D-dimer**
1. Cleavage of crosslinked fibrin by plasmin forms so-called "FDPs."
   a. The best studied of the FDPs is known as D-dimer.
2. Elevated levels of FDPs/D-dimer indicate a recent episode of intravascular coagulation and fibrinolysis.
   a. When negative, a recent episode of clotting and fibrinolysis will be excluded (i.e., excludes DIC, deep venous thrombosis [DVT], pulmonary embolus, etc.).

III. **Disorders of Bleeding**
A. **Overview**
1. Bleeding disorders ("bleeding diathesis") are conditions of impaired clotting with an associated increased tendency to abnormal bleeding.
2. May affect primary or secondary hemostasis; inherited or acquired.

B. **von Willebrand disease (vWD)**
1. Autosomal dominant disorder associated with a mild bleeding tendency.
   a. Most common inherited bleeding disorder.
2. Due to a quantitative or qualitative deficiency of vWF.
3. Three subtypes include:
   a. Type 1: the most common subtype; characterized by reduced levels of vWF.
   b. Type 2: characterized by dysfunctional vWF.
   c. Type 3: rare; characterized by marked reduction/absence of vWF.
4. Testing
   a. vWF antigen (vWF:Ag) assay
      i. Amount of vWF protein present in the plasma.
      ii. Typically decreased (except in type 2 vWD).
   b. Ristocetin cofactor assay (vWF:RCo)
      i. Measures the ability of vWF to bind to the platelet receptor GPIb.
      ii. Functional test of vWF; decreased in vWD.
   c. Bleeding time
      i. Prolonged in vWD.
   d. PTT
      i. May be prolonged in vWD, due to the degradation of factor VIII in the absence of vWF (a carrier molecule for factor VIII).

C. **Bernard–Soulier syndrome**
1. Autosomal recessive disorder associated with a variable tendency to mucocutaneous bleeding (e.g., bruising, purpura, epistaxis, and gingival bleeding).
2. Due to a deficiency of the platelet membrane GpIb receptor.
   a. Impairs the ability of platelets to bind to subendothelial collagen (impaired platelet adhesion).
3. Laboratory findings
   a. Mild thrombocytopenia (and giant platelets).
   b. Prolonged bleeding time.
   c. Abnormal ristocetin cofactor assay.

D. **Glanzmann thrombasthenia**
1. Autosomal recessive bleeding disorder characterized by a quantitative or qualitative defect in the platelet GpIIb/IIIa receptor.
2. Impairs platelet aggregation, resulting in mucocutaneous bleeding.
3. Laboratory findings
   a. Normal platelet count.
   b. Prolongation of bleeding time.
   c. Abnormal platelet aggregation studies.

E. **Hemophilia A**
1. X-linked recessive disorder; mutation in the *F8* gene resulting in a deficiency of factor VIII.
2. Relatively common; affects approximately 1 in 5000 live male births.
   a. New mutations not uncommon (i.e., may not have a family history).
3. Variable disease severity
   a. Mild hemophilia

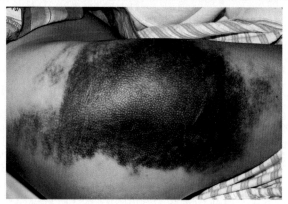

15.3: Extensive deep tissue bleeding in a patient with hemophilia A. *(From Hoffbrand VA: Color atlas of clinical hematology, ed 3, Philadelphia, 2000, Mosby, pp 281–283.)*

      i. Defined as a factor level between 6% and 30% of normal.
      ii. Patients generally only bleed following trauma or surgery (e.g., delayed bleeding after minor procedures such as tooth extraction).
    b. Moderate hemophilia
      i. Defined as a factor activity level between 1% and 5% of normal.
      ii. Patients usually bleed following minor injury.
    c. Severe hemophilia
      i. Most common, defined as <1% factor activity.
      ii. Usually presents within the first 2 years of life with one or more of the following:
        (1) Bleeding following circumcision.
        (2) Intracerebral hemorrhage during the newborn period.
      iii. Bleeding into joints (hemarthrosis), especially larger weight-bearing joints (e.g., knees), and/or soft tissues (hematoma; Fig. 15.3).
  4. Laboratory findings
    a. Prolonged PTT (corrects when mixed with normal plasma—i.e., mixing study).
    b. Normal PT.
    c. Decreased factor VIII activity and concentration.
  5. Treatment
    a. Recombinant factor VIII infusion.
    b. Desmopressin is a synthetic analog of vasopressin (antidiuretic hormone). May be useful in mild hemophilia A (enhances the release of factor VIII and vWF from storage sites within platelets and endothelial cells).
F. Hemophilia B (Christmas disease)
  1. X-linked recessive; characterized by a mutation in *F9* gene resulting in a deficiency of factor IX.
  2. Clinically indistinguishable from hemophilia A but much less common, affecting approximately 1 in 25,000 live male births.
  3. Laboratory findings
    a. Prolonged PTT (corrects when mixed with normal plasma).
    b. Normal PT.
    c. Decreased factor IX activity and concentration.
  4. Treatment
    a. Recombinant factor IX infusion.
G. Thrombocytopenia (platelet count of less than 150,000/μL).
  1. Overview
    a. Although there are inherited conditions associated with thrombocytopenia (e.g., Bernard–Soulier syndrome and Wiskott–Aldrich syndrome), most are acquired.
    b. Three major etiologic categories:
      i. Increased destruction of platelets (e.g., immune-mediated).
      ii. Decreased production of platelets (e.g., aplastic anemia and other bone marrow disorders).
      iii. Splenic sequestration (i.e., splenomegaly).
  2. Causes of thrombocytopenia (Table 15.1).
  3. Workup
    a. First, confirm that the platelet count is decreased.
      i. Repeat the CBC and/or review a blood smear.
      ii. "Pseudothrombocytopenia" refers to a falsely low platelet count due to platelet clumping. This may occasionally be seen with the use of ethylenediaminetetraacetic acid (EDTA) as an anticoagulant. If platelet clumps are noted on the blood smear, repeat the blood draw using a different anticoagulant (e.g., heparin or sodium citrate).

TABLE 15.1   Disorders Producing Thrombocytopenia

DISEASES	COMMENTS
"Acute" immune thrombocytopenia (ITP)	• The most common cause of thrombocytopenia in children, peaks between 2 and 5 years of age. • IgG antibodies against platelet membrane antigens (e.g., GpIIb–IIIa) are detected in many cases. • Acute onset; often follows the recent viral infection. Resolves spontaneously in most cases, usually within 3 months. • Manifestations include epistaxis (nosebleed), easy bruising, and petechiae. • Secondary causes of ITP include HIV, SLE, thyroid disease, and chronic lymphocytic leukemia.
"Chronic" ITP	• As opposed to children, ITP in adults is much more likely be a chronic recurring disorder. • Same pathogenesis (IgG antibodies against the GpIIb–IIIa fibrinogen receptor on platelets). • Insidious onset and presents with epistaxis, easy bruising, and petechiae.
Neonatal alloimmune thrombocytopenia (NAIT)	• Mother becomes sensitized, via breaches in the placental barrier, to an antigen on fetal platelets that she lacks. In other words, the antigen, usually human platelet antigen 1a (HPA-1a), was inherited from the father. • Following sensitization, the mother forms IgG antibodies against the "foreign" platelet antigen. These antibodies, being IgG, can cross the placenta and destroy fetal platelets.
Posttransfusion purpura	• Due to sensitization to HPA-1a, primarily in multiparous women because they are more likely to have been exposed to fetal blood containing HPA-1a-positive platelets. • Once sensitized, any subsequent transfusions of a blood product containing HPA-1a-positive platelets will result in severe thrombocytopenia 7–10 days after the transfusion. • As opposed to NAIT, both donor platelets and the patient's native HPA-1a-negative platelets are destroyed.
Heparin-induced thrombocytopenia (HIT)	• Two forms of HIT. • Type I HIT is not immune-mediated but is due to the direct effect of heparin causing platelet aggregation. Results in mild thrombocytopenia that spontaneously resolves, even if heparin is continued. • Type II HIT is immune-mediated; believed that heparin induces a conformational change in the platelet factor 4 (PF4) protein to form a new antigen (neoantigen). IgG antibodies then develop against this PF4 neoantigen causing severe thrombocytopenia (due to the removal of IgG-coated platelets by macrophages in the spleen). The primary concern of type II HIT, however, is related to the development of potentially life-threatening venous and arterial thrombosis (thrombi thought secondary to platelet activation and endothelial injury by the HIT antibodies).
Thrombotic thrombocytopenic purpura (TTP)	• Acquired (usually) or genetic deficiency of the von Willebrand factor–cleaving metalloprotease (ADAMTS13); an enzyme that acts to cleave ultra-large multimers of vWF that remain attached to the endothelial surface. The absence of this enzyme allows these ultra-large vWF multimers to accumulate on the endothelial surface, particularly in regions of high shear stress (small arterioles and capillaries). Platelets adhere to the large vWF multimers, become activated and aggregate, forming platelet thrombi (consumption of platelets in the thrombi explains the thrombocytopenia). • Classic clinical pentad of thrombocytopenia, fever, renal failure, microangiopathic hemolytic anemia with schistocytes (damage by platelet thrombi), and CNS deficits. Not all findings are required for the diagnosis. • Most recover with treatment (plasma exchange).
Hemolytic uremic syndrome (HUS)	• HUS is a disease primarily of children, often under the age of 5 years. • Major cause of acute kidney injury in children. • Most cases are caused by Shiga toxin-producing strains of *Escherichia coli* (STEC) (in the United States *E. coli* O157:H7). • Classic triad of findings include thrombocytopenia (used up in forming thrombi), acute renal failure, and microangiopathic hemolytic anemia (schistocytes).

CNS, Central nervous system; *Gp*, glycoprotein; '*PF4*, platelet factor 4; *SLE*, systemic lupus erythematosus; *vWF*, von Willebrand factor.

b. Physical examination can help identify other potential etiologies (e.g., splenomegaly).
c. If the etiology remains unclear, consider performing a bone marrow biopsy to confirm the presence of megakaryocytes.
  i. Presence of megakaryocytes suggests increased platelet destruction (e.g., immune thrombocytopenia).
  ii. Absence or decreased number of megakaryocytes correlates with impaired platelet production (i.e., bone marrow failure).

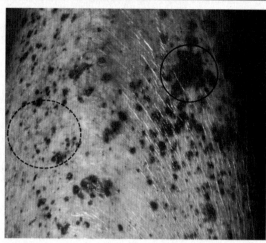

15.4: Petechia (small areas of hemorrhage; *dashed circle*) and ecchymoses (widespread area of hemorrhage; *solid circle*). *(From Walker BR, Colledge NR, Ralston SH, Penman ID: Davidson's principles and practice of medicine, ed 22, St. Louis, 2014, Churchill Livingstone Elsevier, p 1007, Fig. 24.13.)*

 4. Clinical manifestations
    a. Mucocutaneous bleeding (i.e., bleeding into the skin and mucous membranes)
       i. Petechiae (pinpoint areas of hemorrhage into the skin, usually dependent regions of the body) and ecchymosis (Fig. 15.4).
       ii. Easy bruising.
       iii. Epistaxis (nosebleed).
       iv. Gingival hemorrhage.
    b. Risk of spontaneous and potentially life-threatening hemorrhage (e.g., intracranial) with platelet counts of less than 20,000/μL.
 5. Laboratory findings
    a. Thrombocytopenia.
    b. Prolongation of bleeding time.
H. Renal disease (uremia)
 1. Renal failure impairs platelet function and can cause mucocutaneous bleeding (e.g., easy bruising, epistaxis, and gingival hemorrhage).
 2. Laboratories
    a. Prolonged bleeding time.
    b. Normal PT, PTT, and platelet count.
I. Drugs
 1. Variety of medications (e.g., aspirin, warfarin, heparin, and others) can cause bleeding (emphasizes the importance of obtaining a medication history).
J. Factor inhibitors
 1. Factor inhibitors are antibodies that inhibit the activity, or increase the clearance, of a clotting factor.
    a. Usually directed against factor VIII.
 2. Clinical manifestations are like those of factor deficiency states.
 3. Laboratory findings
    a. Increased PT and/or increased PTT, depending upon which factor is inhibited (does not differentiate immune destruction from inherited deficiency).
K. Liver failure/cirrhosis
 1. Liver disease has multiple effects on coagulation, including:
    a. An increased risk of bleeding due to decreased synthesis of coagulation factors.
    b. An increased risk of clotting due to decreased production of endogenous anticoagulants (e.g., AT, proteins C and S).
    c. Decreased synthesis of plasminogen.
    d. Laboratory findings
       i. Prolonged PT and PTT.
       ii. Decreased fibrinogen.
       iii. Increased bleeding time.
    e. Note that many cases of liver disease are associated with cirrhosis-induced portal hypertension which, in turn, leads to splenic enlargement. Thrombocytopenia, due to the sequestration of platelets within the enlarged spleen, can contribute to bleeding in those with liver disease.

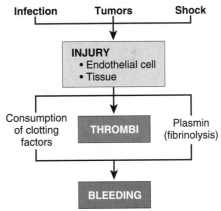

15.5: Disseminated intravascular coagulation. Various diseases contribute to endothelial injury and thus trigger the formation of thrombi in small blood vessels. Once clotting factors are used up, the patients begin to bleed. *(From Ivan Damjanov, MD, PhD: Pathology for the health professions, ed 4, St. Louis, 2012, Saunders Elsevier, p 223, Fig. 9-25.)*

 L. Disseminated intravascular coagulation (DIC)
  1. DIC is characterized by unregulated activation of clotting (Fig. 15.5).
   a. Thrombi form within the microvasculature throughout the body.
   b. Often referred to as a "consumptive coagulopathy" because the clots use up (consume) all remaining clotting factors.
   c. Once clotting factors are used up, the patients then begin to bleed.
  2. Triggers for DIC include:
   a. Sepsis (bacterial, fungal, viral, and parasitic).
   b. Malignancy (e.g., acute promyelocytic leukemia and pancreatic adenocarcinoma).
   c. Trauma (e.g., crush injuries).
   d. Obstetrical complications (e.g., preeclampsia and fetal demise).
   e. Intravascular hemolysis (e.g., acute hemolytic transfusion reaction).
  3. Clinical manifestations
   a. Organ dysfunction secondary to diffuse clotting, including:
    i. Altered mental status and transient neurologic deficits.
    ii. Oliguria or anuria.
    iii. Bowel infarction.
   b. Bleeding
    i. Petechiae and ecchymoses.
    ii. Oozing of blood from wound sites and intravenous lines.
    iii. Bleeding into the lungs or central nervous system (can be life-threatening).
   c. Anemia
    i. Secondary to mechanical trauma of RBCs by fibrin thrombi (i.e., intravascular hemolysis).
  4. Laboratory findings
   a. Prolonged PT and PTT.
   b. Decreased fibrinogen.
   c. Thrombocytopenia.
   d. Increased bleeding time.
   e. Presence of FDPs and D-dimers (negative D-dimer excludes DIC).
   f. Fragmented red cells ("schistocytes") on the blood smear (red cells are broken up as they attempt to traverse the fibrin thrombi in circulation).
  5. Treatment
   a. Most important treatment is a correction of the underlying cause.
   b. For serious bleeding episodes, transfusion of platelet and FFP.
IV. Fibrinolytic Disorders
 A. Once healing of an injured vessel is complete, lysis of the clot occurs (called fibrinolysis) as plasmin degrades fibrin into FDPs.
  1. Plasmin requires activation; via tissue-type plasminogen activator (tPA) or urinary-type plasminogen activator (uPA).
   a. tPA is synthesized and released by endothelial cells.
   b. uPA is produced by monocytes, macrophages, and urinary epithelium.
  2. Fibrinolysis is regulated by:
   a. Plasminogen activator inhibitor (PAI)—an inhibitor of tPA.
   b. Alpha-2-antiplasmin—an inhibitor of plasmin.

TABLE 15.2   Laboratory Findings in Common Hemostasis Disorders

DISORDERS	PLATELET COUNT	BLEEDING TIME	PT	PTT
Thrombocytopenia	↓	↑	Normal	Normal
von Willebrand disease	Normal	↑	Normal	↑
Hemophilia A	Normal	Normal	Normal	↑
Disseminated intravascular coagulation	↓	↑	↑	↑
Aspirin or NSAIDs	Normal	↑	Normal	Normal
Warfarin or heparin	Normal	Normal	↑	↑

NSAID, Nonsteroidal antiinflammatory drug; *PT,* prothrombin time; *PTT,* partial thromboplastin time.

B. **Hyperfibrinolytic states**
   1. Congenital deficiency of a fibrinolytic regulatory protein (e.g., PAI and alpha-2-antiplasmin).
   2. Cardiopulmonary bypass.
   3. Heat stroke.
   4. Thrombolytic therapy.

C. **Laboratory findings in common hemostasis disorders (Table 15.2).**

V. **Disorders of Thrombosis (Hypercoagulable States)**

A. **Acquired hypercoagulable states**
   1. Antiphospholipid syndrome (APS)
      a. Antiphospholipid antibodies (aPLs) refer to a heterogeneous group of autoantibodies, each directed against proteins that bind phospholipid.
      b. Three types of aPLs have been characterized:
         i. Anticardiolipin antibodies.
         ii. Lupus anticoagulants.
         iii. Anti-β2-glycoprotein-I (anti-β2-GPI) antibodies.
      c. APS refers to an autoimmune disorder characterized by the pathologic formation of thromboemboli (venous or arterial) due to the presence of aPLs.
      d. May occur as a primary disease or in association with a systemic autoimmune condition, usually systemic lupus erythematosus.
      e. Pathogenesis
         i. Unclear, may be due to the direct procoagulant effect of antibodies on endothelial cells.
      f. Clinical findings
         i. Venous and/or arterial thrombosis
            (1) Venous thrombi, which are more common, usually arise within deep leg veins causing DVT; risk of pulmonary emboli.
            (2) Arterial thrombi usually involve the cerebral vasculature and therefore may cause a stroke.
         ii. Recurrent pregnancy loss (due to placental thrombosis).
      g. Laboratory findings
         i. Anticardiolipin antibodies (IgG and IgM).
         ii. Anti-β2-GPI antibodies (IgG and IgM).
         iii. Lupus anticoagulant testing
            (1) Prolongation of the PTT that does not correct with a mixing study but does following the addition of excess phospholipid.
   2. Alterations in blood flow (stasis)
      a. Immobility (e.g., hospitalized patients and long car/plane trips).
   3. Malignancy
      a. Various mechanisms (release of procoagulant substances from tumor [e.g., pancreatic adenocarcinoma], patient immobility, indwelling IV lines, and treatment effect).
   4. Pregnancy
      a. Obstruction of venous return by the gravid uterus.
      b. Increased circulating levels of procoagulant proteins (e.g., factor VIII, fibrinogen, and vWF).
      c. Reduced circulating levels of protein S (thereby suppressing natural anticoagulant pathways).

Mixing study

- Used to differentiate a factor deficiency from a factor inhibitor.
- In a mixing study, the patient's plasma is mixed in a 1:1 ratio with normal plasma and then the abnormal coagulation test (PT or PTT) is repeated.
- If the test corrects → factor deficiency.
- If the test does not correct → factor inhibitor.

B. **Inherited hypercoagulable states**
1. Factor V Leiden
   a. Autosomal dominant disorder due to a mutation in the *F5* gene.
      i. Leads to the production of an abnormal factor V which resists degradation by activated protein C ("activated protein C resistance").
   b. Increased risk of venous thrombosis
      i. Most common inherited thrombophilia, more common in the White population.
      ii. Heterozygotes: 5- to 10-fold increased risk of thrombosis.
      iii. Homozygotes: 50- to 100-fold increased risk of thrombosis.
2. Prothrombin G20210A mutation
   a. Second most common inherited thrombophilia, also more common in the White population.
   b. Autosomal dominant; substitution of adenine (A) for guanine (G) at position 20210 of the prothrombin gene.
   c. Increases levels of prothrombin in circulation; risk of thrombosis increased threefold.
3. AT deficiency
   a. Inherited (or acquired) deficiency of AT.
   b. AT inhibits several factors (e.g., thrombin [factor IIa], factor Xa, and other factors).
      i. A deficiency of AT allows these factors to remain active thereby placing the patient at increased risk of clotting.
   c. AT function is enhanced by heparin and heparin-like molecules.
      i. A clue to the diagnosis is heparin resistance (PTT not appropriately prolonged following heparin therapy). Heparin is ineffective because there is little to no AT to enhance.
4. Proteins C and S deficiency
   a. Protein C, using protein S as a cofactor, inhibits factors Va and VIIIa.
      i. Deficiency leads to the increased risk of thromboses (venous primarily), warfarin-induced skin necrosis (due to vascular occlusion resulting from the transient hypercoagulable state).

CHAPTER 16 Immunohematology Disorders

I. Blood Group Antigens

A. Overview

1. Red blood cells (RBCs) contain surface antigens comprised of sugars and/or proteins (glycoproteins).
2. Specific antigens vary between individuals.
3. A blood group refers to a collection of one or more antigens controlled by one or more closely linked genes.
   a. ABO and Rh blood groups are among the most important.

B. Alloantibody versus autoantibody

1. Alloimmunization refers to the development of a host immune response (alloantibody) against an antigen not normally present in an individual.
   a. Exposure to the "foreign" antigen may occur through transfusion, pregnancy, or transplantation.
   b. Alloantibody → antibody against "foreign" antigen.
2. Autoantibodies are antibodies against self-RBC antigens.
   a. For example, *Mycoplasma pneumoniae* infection often causes patients to develop IgM autoantibodies against the "I" red cell antigen. Many of these patients will develop very mild, often subclinical, hemolysis.
   b. Autoantibody → antibody against self-antigen.

II. ABO Blood Group System

A. Definition

1. ABO blood group refers to the O, A, and B red cell antigens (Fig. 16.1).
2. The ABO blood group is unique in that patients develop "naturally occurring" alloantibodies (called "isohemagglutinins") against antigens absent in the individual.
   a. "Naturally occurring" because they do not require previous exposure of blood products containing the antigen.
   b. Appear by 4–6 months, most likely following environmental exposure to bacteria with a similar structure as the missing "A" and/or "B" antigen (molecular mimicry).

B. Blood group "O"

1. Most common blood group, characterized by an absence of both the "A" and the "B" antigen.
2. Antibodies against "A" and "B" are present (i.e., anti-A IgM and anti-B IgM). For unknown reasons, most blood group O individuals also have IgG antibodies (i.e., anti-A IgG and anti-B IgG).
   a. Important because IgG can cross the placenta (see later discussion of ABO hemolytic disease of the newborn [HDN]).

C. Blood group A

1. Second most common blood group.
2. Characterized by the presence of the "A" antigen on the surface of RBCs and naturally occurring anti-B IgM antibodies.
3. For unknown reasons, blood group "A" individuals have an increased incidence of gastric carcinoma.

Summary of ABO blood group

- Type O blood (neither "A" nor "B" antigen present; antibodies against both).
- Type A blood (the presence of the "A" antigen; antibody against "B").
- Type B blood (the presence of the "B" antigen; antibody against "A").
- Type AB blood (both "A" and "B" antigens present; neither antibody present).

	Group A	Group B	Group AB	Group O
Red blood cell type	Type A	Type B	Type AB	Type O
Antibodies present	Anti-B	Anti-A	None	Anti-A and Anti-B
Antigens present	A antigen	B antigen	A and B antigen	None

16.1: ABO blood group antigens and antibodies. The various ABO blood group antigens are produced by the addition of different sugars through the inheritance of different glycosyltransferases. Individuals who express a particular blood group antigen are tolerant to that antigen but produce "naturally occurring" antibodies against the other ABO blood group antigens. *(From Abbas AK, Lichtman AH, Pillai S: Cellular and molecular immunology, ed 8, Philadelphia, 2015, Saunders Elsevier, p 378, Fig. 17-13B.)*

	Forward Type		Back Type	
Blood group	Anti-A	Anti-B	A RBCs	B RBCs
O	−	−	+	+
A	+	−	−	+
B	−	+	+	−
AB	+	+	−	−

16.2: Forward and back typing to identify ABO blood groups. Forward type identifies the blood group antigen by reacting test anti-A and anti-B antibodies against patient red blood cells (RBCs). Back typing identifies the natural antibodies in the patient's serum by reacting test blood group A RBCs and B RBCs against the patient's serum. Refer to the text for discussion of the blood groups and their natural antibodies.

D. Blood group B
  1. Third most common blood group.
  2. Characterized by the presence of the "B" antigen on the surface of RBCs and naturally occurring anti-A IgM antibodies.
E. Blood group AB
  1. Least common of the ABO blood groups.
  2. Both "A" and "B" antigens are present on the surface of RBCs, neither anti-A nor anti-B antibodies.
F. Determination of ABO type in the laboratory (Fig. 16.2).
  1. Forward typing
    a. Identifies an individual's blood group antigens.
    b. Determined by placing an individual's RBCs into separate test tubes containing anti-A or anti-B test serum.
    c. The presence of a particular antigen causes clumping of RBCs when added to the tube containing antibody against that antigen. For example:
      i. If an agglutination reaction occurs in the tube containing anti-A, but not in the tube containing anti-B, then the individual is blood group A.
      ii. If an agglutination reaction occurs in the tube containing anti-B, but not in the tube containing anti-A, then the individual is blood group B.
      iii. If agglutination occurs with both anti-A and anti-B test sera, the patient has both antigens (i.e., blood group AB).
      iv. If agglutination does not occur with either anti-A or anti-B test sera, then the individual has neither antigen (i.e., blood group O).
  2. Backward typing
    a. Method of identifying what natural antibody is present in an individual's serum. Determined by placing a sample of an individual's serum into test tubes that contain either A, B, or O test RBCs.
    b. If the serum agglutinates "B" RBCs but not "A" RBCs, then the individual is blood group A (due to anti-B antibodies).
    c. If the serum agglutinates "A" RBCs but not "B" RBCs, then the individual is blood group B (due to anti-A antibodies).
    d. If the serum does not agglutinate either "A" or "B" RBCs, the individual is blood group AB (neither antibody present).

TABLE 16.1 ABO Genotypes and Serum Reactivity

GENOTYPE	PHENOTYPE IN RBCS	REACTION WITH ANTI-A	REACTION WITH ANTI-B	ANTIBODIES IN SERUM
OO	O	−	−	Anti-A and Anti-B
AA or AO	A	+	−	Anti-B
BB or BO	B	−	+	Anti-A
AB	AB	+	+	Neither

e. If the serum agglutinates both "A" and "B" RBCs, the individual is blood group O (because both anti-A and anti-B antibodies are present).
   3. Codominant inheritance
      a. The "A" and "B" alleles are codominant, meaning that the inheritance of each is expressed.
         i. For example, inheritance of the "A" allele from one parent and the "B" allele from the other parent results in an "AB" blood type.
      b. Each is dominant over the "O" blood type.
         i. For example, inheritance of "A" allele from one parent and "O" from the other parent results in an "A" blood type.
         ii. Those with blood type "O" must have received the "O" allele from each parent.
   G. **Summary of ABO genotypes and serum reactivity (Table 16.1).**
III. **Rh and Non-Rh Antigen Systems**
   A. **Rh antigen system has three adjoining gene loci coding for the D antigen (there is no d antigen), the C and c antigens, and the E and e antigens.**
      1. The absence of "D" antigen is designated "d" even though the antigen does not exist.
   B. **Rh positive status refers to the presence of the "D" antigen; approximately 85% of the population is positive for the "D" antigen.**
      1. Those who lack the "D" antigen are said to be "Rh negative."
   C. **Clinically important non-Rh antigens**
      1. Duffy (Fy) antigens
         a. The Fy red cell antigen acts as the receptor for *Plasmodium vivax*; individuals who lack the Fy antigen are therefore resistant to infection by *P. vivax*.
         b. Majority of African Americans lack the Fy antigen (thought to be an evolutionary phenomenon to protect against *P. vivax* malaria).
      2. "P" antigen
         a. Site of parvovirus B19 attachment; reason parvoviral infections involve erythroid cells.
         b. Autoantibodies against the "P" red cells antigen are often the cause of paroxysmal cold hemoglobinuria, an uncommon form of autoimmune hemolysis.
      3. "I" and "i" antigen systems
         a. Infection may lead to the development of IgM antibodies against the "I" or "i" antigen; potential for immune-mediated hemolysis, cold agglutinins.
            i. Epstein–Barr virus → anti-i IgM antibodies.
            ii. *M. pneumoniae* → anti-I IgM antibodies.
IV. **Blood Transfusion Therapy**
   A. **Pretransfusion testing of donor blood**
      1. ABO and Rh (D) antigen typing.
      2. Antibody screening
         a. Indirect antiglobulin test screens for the presence of "atypical" antibodies (i.e., antibodies against antigens other than "A" and "B" of the ABO blood group).
      3. Infectious disease testing
         a. Donor blood is screened for the presence of various infectious agents, including hepatitis B virus, hepatitis C virus, human immunodeficiency virus, human T lymphotropic virus, West Nile virus, Zika virus, *Treponema pallidum* (cause of syphilis), and *Trypanosoma cruzi* (cause of Chagas disease).
   B. **Pretransfusion screening of recipient**
      1. ABO and Rh (D) antigen typing.
      2. Antibody screen.
      3. Crossmatch
         a. Mixture of donor red cells with the patient's serum (mimics the transfusion).
         b. The lack of agglutination or hemolysis in the test sample indicates a compatible crossmatch (i.e., no apparent antibodies in the patient's serum against RBC antigens in the donor unit).
         c. Compatible crossmatch indicates that the transfusion should be compatible (i.e., no hemolysis) but does not guarantee that the recipient will not develop "atypical" antibodies (i.e., against antigens on donor red cells), a transfusion reaction, or an infectious complication.

Universal donor

- Type "O" red cells have neither the "A" nor "B" red cell antigen and will therefore not trigger an acute hemolytic transfusion reaction. For this reason, type "O" blood can be transfused into any patient in emergent situations where the patient requires the transfusion before the crossmatch can be performed.
- In nonemergent situations, patients should still receive type-specific red cells.

Universal recipient

- Patients with type "AB" red cells have both the "A" and "B" antigens and therefore lack naturally occurring antibodies against either antigen. For this reason, type "AB" individuals may receive a transfusion of any blood group.
- As a rule, patients with type AB blood should still receive type AB blood if available.

C. **Transfusion-associated graft-versus-host disease.**
   1. Occurs when a T-cell immunodeficient patient receives a blood product containing immunologically competent lymphocytes.
   2. The recipient's T cells would normally kill any lymphocytes within the transfused product (which contain "foreign" human leukocyte antigens).
   3. In situations where the recipient is either immunologically incompetent or does not recognize the donor lymphocytes as being "foreign," then donor lymphocytes survive, proliferate, and engraft within the recipient.
      a. Causes a variety of manifestations, including pancytopenia and death of the patient.
   4. Prevented by irradiating the blood unit prior to transfusion (radiation kills lymphocytes within the unit).
   5. Situations in which this is required include intrauterine transfusion, transfusion from close relatives, and those with T-cell immunodeficiency states.
D. **Blood component therapy (Table 16.2).**
E. **Transfusion reactions**
   1. Allergic transfusion reactions
      a. Definition
         i. Type I IgE-mediated hypersensitivity reaction (HSR) against proteins (allergens) present in the donor plasma.
            (1) Initial exposure to allergen → formation of IgE antibodies against the allergen → binding of the antibody to mast cells.
            (2) Upon reexposure, the allergen crosslinks IgE antibodies on mast cells causing degranulation and the release of preformed mediators (e.g., histamine and serotonin).
      b. Clinical manifestations
         i. Urticaria with pruritus, wheezing; mild cases are treated with antihistamines.
         ii. Potential for anaphylaxis (especially IgA deficiency states).
   2. Nonhemolytic febrile transfusion reaction
      a. Most common of all transfusion reactions; manifests with fever, chills, and rigors.
      b. Due to the release of cytokines from white blood cells present in the transfused product; prevent with prestorage leukoreduction (removal of white cells).

TABLE 16.2 Blood Components

COMPONENTS	DISCUSSION
Packed RBCs	Purpose: increase oxygen carrying capacity. Each unit of packed RBCs should raise the Hb by 1 g/dL (Hct by 3%). Lack of the expected increase suggests either continued blood loss, or that the patient is suffering hemolysis (e.g., delayed hemolytic transfusion reaction).
Platelets	Purpose: stop medically significant bleeding related to quantitative (i.e., thrombocytopenia) or qualitative platelet defects (e.g., aspirin). Each single donor platelet unit should raise the platelet count by 5000–10,000 cells/mm³. If the count does not increase as expected, then they are likely either being consumed (e.g., DIC) or destroyed (immune thrombocytopenia).
Fresh frozen plasma (FFP)	Purpose: treatment of multiple coagulation deficiencies (e.g., DIC or cirrhosis) or treatment of warfarin overdose if the patient is bleeding. Contains all active coagulation factors.
Cryoprecipitate	Purpose: treatment of coagulation factor deficiencies involving fibrinogen or factor VIII (e.g., DIC). Cryoprecipitate contains fibrinogen, factor VIII, and factor XIII. Desmopressin acetate is used instead of cryoprecipitate in the treatment of mild hemophilia A or vWD.

DIC, Disseminated intravascular coagulation; *Hb*, hemoglobin; *Hct*, hematocrit; *RBC*, red blood cell; *vWD*, von Willebrand disease.

3. Acute hemolytic transfusion reaction
   a. Usually due to ABO blood group incompatibility.
      i. Example: Patient with type "B" blood receives type "A" red cells. In this case, anti-A IgM in the recipient attaches to the "A" antigen on donor red cells and activates complement causing acute intravascular hemolysis with hemoglobinemia, hemoglobinuria, and decreased haptoglobin (type II HSR).
   b. Nearly always a result of a clerical error.
   c. Direct antiglobulin (Coombs) test will be positive (indicating the presence of antibodies attached to the patient's red cells).
   d. Potential complications include acute renal failure and bleeding (due to disseminated intravascular coagulation).
4. Delayed hemolytic transfusion reaction
   a. Most frequently caused by an IgG antibody in the recipient's blood reacting against an antigen on donor red cells that is "foreign" to the recipient.
   b. Splenic macrophages bind to, and subsequently destroy, donor red cells coated by the antibody (type II HSR).
      i. Hemolysis results in the release of bilirubin (unconjugated bilirubin [UCB] is the end product of heme degradation); for this reason, jaundice is common.
   c. Seen in those with previous exposure to "foreign" blood antigens (i.e., history of blood transfusion and/or pregnancy).
      i. In this case, the pretransfusion antibody screen can be negative because antibody levels had waned.
      ii. Reexposure to the foreign antigen in the transfused unit caused an anamnestic immune response with the increased production of antibodies against the foreign antigen.
   d. Results in extravascular hemolysis as opsonized "foreign" red cells are removed by macrophages in the spleen and liver.
   e. Typically occurs between days 2 and 14 after the transfusion.
   f. Manifestations include:
      i. Reduced hemoglobin.
      ii. Elevated UCB (often with jaundice).
      iii. Positive direct antiglobulin test.
5. Transfusion-associated circulatory overload (TACO)
   a. Refers to cardiogenic pulmonary edema that develops as a result of a transfusion.
   b. Manifestations include:
      i. Respiratory distress.
      ii. Tachycardia.
      iii. Tachypnea.
      iv. Decreased oxygen saturation.
      v. Jugular venous distension.
   c. Treatment includes the use of supplemental oxygen and diuretics.
6. Transfusion-related acute lung injury (TRALI)
   a. Dyspnea, tachypnea, and hypoxia following the infusion of blood products in the absence of underlying lung disease or circulatory overload.
   b. Mechanism is unclear; characterized by increased pulmonary vascular permeability (i.e., noncardiogenic pulmonary edema).
   c. Potentially fatal, estimated mortality rate of 5%–8%.

V. **Hemolytic Disease of the Newborn**
   A. **Definition**
      1. Hemolysis of fetal red cells following the transplacental passage of maternal IgG antibodies against an antigen present on fetal red cells.
      2. Results in varying degrees of extravascular hemolysis and jaundice in the newborn.
   B. **ABO HDN**
      1. Definition
         a. Hemolysis of fetal/newborn red cells secondary to the passage of IgG maternal antibodies against either the "A" or "B" antigen on fetal RBCs (Fig. 16-3A).
         b. Occurs in type "A" or "B" newborns of type "O" mothers.
            i. Recall that some individuals with type "O" blood have IgG (as well as IgM) antibodies against the "A" and "B" red cell antigens.
      2. Epidemiology
         a. Most common type of HDN; present in ~20%–25% of all pregnancies.
         b. Only significant in a small percentage of cases because of poor fetal expression of "A" and "B" antigens.
      3. Pathogenesis
         a. Passage of anti-A IgG and/or anti-B IgG antibodies across the placenta into the fetal circulation.
         b. Maternal antibodies attach to fetal blood group "A" or "B" red cells.
         c. Splenic macrophages in the fetus engulf antibody-coated RBCs, thereby causing extravascular hemolysis (usually mild).
         d. Hemolysis causes unconjugated hyperbilirubinemia (metabolized by the placenta).

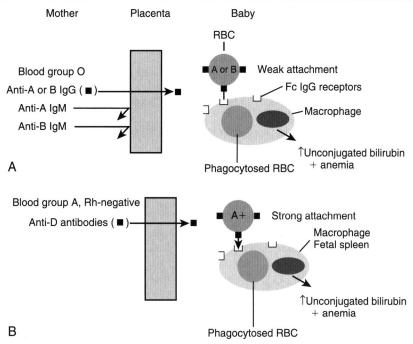

16.3: (A) ABO hemolytic disease of the newborn (HDN). The mother has blood group O, and the baby has blood group A or B. Anti-A and/or anti-B IgG from the mother cross the placenta and attach to fetal blood group A or B red blood cells (RBCs). Sensitized RBCs are phagocytosed and destroyed by splenic macrophages (MPs), producing anemia and unconjugated hyperbilirubinemia. (B) Rh HDN. The mother is Rh negative, and the baby is Rh positive. Mother with anti-D IgG antibodies (i.e., previously sensitized against the "D" antigen). IgG anti-D cross the placenta, attach to fetal Rh (D antigen) positive RBCs, and destroy them, causing anemia and unconjugated hyperbilirubinemia in the child. *(From Goljan EF: Star series: pathology, Philadelphia, 1998, Saunders, Fig. 14-1.)*

  e. ABO HDN may affect the firstborn or any future pregnancy in which an ABO incompatibility exists. There is no natural protection against developing ABO hemolytic disease.
 4. Clinical and laboratory findings
  a. Jaundice is not present at birth due to the placental metabolism of bilirubin prior to delivery. However, jaundice may develop within the first 24 hours of life because the newborn's conjugating enzyme (glucuronosyltransferase) is not well developed.
   i. Most common cause of jaundice during the first day of life.
  b. Anemia may occur if hemolysis is severe.
  c. Weakly positive direct antiglobulin (Coombs) test on cord red cells (due to maternal anti-A and/or anti-B IgG antibodies coating fetal RBCs).
 5. Complications
  a. Severe hemolytic anemia requiring exchange transfusion.
  b. Risk of bilirubin-induced neurologic damage (kernicterus).
   i. Risk is less than with Rh HDN.
    (1) Most anti-A and anti-B antibodies are IgM, which cannot cross the placenta.
    (2) Anti-A and/or anti-B antibodies that cross the placenta do not bind to complement on fetal red cells.
    (3) Most of the anti-A and anti-B antibodies bind to "A" and "B" antigens present in other tissues.
    (4) Relatively few "A" and "B" antigen sites on fetal red cells.
 6. Treatment
  a. Jaundice is treated with phototherapy (discussed later).
  b. Exchange transfusion is sometimes indicated.
C. Rh HDN
 1. Definition
  a. Hemolysis of Rh (D) antigen positive fetal red cells by IgG anti-D maternal antibodies (Fig. 16-3B).
  b. Only occurs in Rh (D) negative women who have been previously sensitized against the "D" antigen, either during a prior pregnancy (does not occur in the first pregnancy) or transfusion.
 2. Epidemiology
  a. Uncommon due to the administration of Rh immune globulin to Rh-negative women (see later).
 3. Pathogenesis
  a. Rh (D antigen) negative mother with Rh (D antigen) positive fetus (in whom the "D" antigen would have been inherited from the father).

    b. Exposure of the Rh-negative mother to Rh-positive fetal RBCs may occur following a fetomaternal hemorrhage (where fetal red cells cross into mother's circulation).

      i. Fetomaternal hemorrhage can occur at the time of delivery, abortion, and other procedures.

    c. Exposure to the "D" antigen results in the development of anti-D IgG antibodies (sensitized for life).

    d. Subsequent Rh-incompatible pregnancies are at risk of a severe Rh HDN (due to anti-D IgG antibodies that cross the placenta and tightly bind to fetal Rh-positive RBCs).

    e. Sensitized fetal RBCs are then removed by macrophages of the reticuloendothelial system (particularly in the spleen).

    f. May result in severe anemia with unconjugated hyperbilirubinemia (once the placenta metabolism of UCB is overwhelmed).

    g. Prolonged hemolysis stimulates extramedullary hematopoiesis in the fetal liver and spleen, potentially causing hepatosplenomegaly.

4. Clinical manifestations

    a. Hydrops fetalis (the most serious complication of Rh HDN)

      i. Hydrops refers to an abnormal collection of fluid.

      ii. Characterized by peripheral edema, ascites, and pleural effusions.

      iii. Due to cardiac and hepatic dysfunction.

        (1)Hepatic dysfunction → decreased albumin synthesis → decreased intravascular oncotic pressure.

        (2) Severe anemia → high-output cardiac failure → increased hydrostatic pressures within pulmonary and peripheral venous circulation → edema/ascites.

    b. Jaundice

      i. Develops shortly after birth; refers to the yellow discoloration of the skin due to the buildup of UCB.

      ii. Note that the levels of UCB are much higher with Rh HDN than is seen with ABO HDN. For this reason, the child is at an increased risk of developing bilirubin-induced neurologic damage (kernicterus).

      iii. UCB, being lipid-soluble, is more likely to cross the blood–brain barrier than the lipid-insoluble conjugated bilirubin.

      iv. Bilirubin is neurotoxic, binds to lipids in the brain, and imparts a yellow discoloration (called kernicterus, Fig. 16.4).

5. Laboratory findings in fetus/newborn

    a. Anemia (more severe than ABO HDN).

    b. Reticulocytosis and nucleated RBCs (indicating accelerated erythropoiesis).

    c. Elevated cord blood bilirubin (due to hemolysis of fetal red cells).

    d. Strongly positive direct and indirect Coombs tests on fetal blood.

6. Treatment

    a. Intrauterine transfusion (in severe cases).

    b. Phototherapy

      i. Photoisomerization of UCB to a nontoxic water-soluble dipyrrole (called lumirubin) which is excreted in the bile or urine.

D. Prevention of Rh immunization.

1. Concurrent ABO incompatibility protects the mother against Rh immunization.

    a. Reason is that fetal red cells would be removed from maternal circulation by anti-A or anti-B IgM antibodies before the mom's immune system became sensitized against the D antigen.

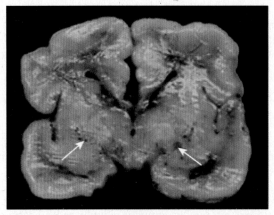

16.4: Cross-section of the brain of a newborn with kernicterus. Arrows depict yellow bilirubin pigment deposited in the basal ganglia. Bilirubin is toxic to neurons and produces long-term neurologic sequelae. *(From Kumar V, Fausto N, Abbas A:* Robbins and Cotran pathologic basis of disease, *ed 7, Philadelphia, 2004, Saunders.)*

2. Administration of Rh immune globulin (anti-D antibodies)
   a. Given during the 28th week of pregnancy; lasts 3 months (until the end of pregnancy).
   b. Following delivery, if the baby is Rh (D antigen) positive, then a second dose of Rh immune globulin is given within 72 hours of birth.
   c. Anti-D immune globulin binds to the D antigen on fetal red cells and "masks" the antigen sites and/or causes the destruction of fetal RBCs prior to sensitization against the D antigen.
   d. If the mom has already become sensitized (i.e., already has anti-D antibodies), then there is no indication for Rh immune globulin (purpose is to prevent sensitization).
E. **Summary of hemolytic disease of newborn (Table 16.3).**

TABLE 16.3 **Comparison of Rh Hemolytic Disease of the Newborn and ABO Hemolytic Disease of the Newborn**

CHARACTERISTICS	RH HEMOLYTIC DISEASE OF NEWBORN	ABO HEMOLYTIC DISEASE OF NEWBORN
Incidence	Uncommon	Common
Blood group association	The mother can be any blood group.	The mother must be group O, and the baby must be group A or B.
Rh association	The mother must be Rh (D antigen) negative, and the baby must be Rh (D antigen) positive.	ABO HDN is protective against Rh sensitization with the exception of an O Rh-positive baby.
Anemia at birth	Frequent and often severe	Usually mild or no anemia. Severe anemia uncommon
Jaundice first 24 h	Frequent; moderate to severe	Mild
Hepatosplenomegaly	Common. Sign of extramedullary hematopoiesis (EMH)	Uncommon
First pregnancy	If the mother is Rh negative and has Rh-positive baby, the baby is not affected, but the mother is at risk of developing anti-D antibodies (prevented by Rh immune globulin).	The baby can be affected if the mother has blood group O and the baby has blood group A or B.
Later pregnancies	If the mother has anti-D and the baby is Rh positive, the baby is at risk for Rh HDN.	Each pregnancy is at risk for ABO HDN if the mother has blood group O.
Direct Coombs test on cord blood	Strongly positive	Weakly positive
Indirect Coombs test on cord blood	Positive	Usually positive
Spherocytes in the peripheral blood	Not present (RBCs fully phagocytosed)	Present (part of the RBC membrane is removed by macrophages)

EMH, Extramedullary hematopoiesis; HDN, hemolytic disease of the newborn; RBC, red blood cell.

I. Disorders of the Upper Airways

A. Choanal atresia

1. Congenital condition in which there is no opening between the posterior nasal cavity and the nasopharynx (i.e., the posterior nasal airway is obstructed by bone, soft tissue, or both).
2. Etiology unknown, often associated with additional congenital anomalies.
3. More common in females; unilateral in two-thirds of cases.
4. If bilateral, patients develop worsening cyanosis with feeding but improve with crying (patients are obligatory mouth breathers).

B. Nasal polyps

1. Nonneoplastic soft tissue masses of the nasal cavity and paranasal sinuses; comprised of edematous mucosa, hyperplastic mucus glands, and inflammation (Fig. 17.1).
   a. Develop as a response to chronic inflammation.
2. In adults, often associated with allergic rhinitis (IgE-mediated).
   a. Nasal smear shows numerous eosinophils.
   b. Triad: asthma, nasal polyps, and aspirin sensitivity.
3. In children, most commonly associated with cystic fibrosis (CF).

C. Obstructive sleep apnea

1. Definition
   a. Episodic spells of apnea or hypopnea during sleep accompanied by respiratory effort-related arousal.
   b. Due to collapse of the upper airway at either the level of the soft palate (i.e., nasopharynx) or the level of the tongue (i.e., oropharynx).
2. Epidemiology
   a. Common disorder affecting approximately 15% of adults, especially those who are obese.
   b. Less common in children, often in association with tonsillar and adenoidal hypertrophy.
3. Pathogenesis
   a. Relaxation and collapse of the upper airway during sleep; related to anatomic (e.g., enlarged tongue and excessive adiposity) and/or neuromuscular (decreased stimulatory output to respiratory muscles) factors.
4. Clinical manifestations
   a. Loud snoring, periodic apneic spells followed by gasps and snorting for air.
   b. Respiratory effort results in partial awakenings/impaired sleep quality leading to morning headaches and daytime sleepiness.
   c. During spells of absent (apnea) or decreased respiration (hypopnea), patients develop hypoxemia and hypercarbia.
5. Complications
   a. Hypertension.
   b. Increased risk of myocardial infarction and stroke.
   c. Increased risk of accidents (secondary to daytime sleepiness and inattentiveness).
6. Diagnosis
   a. Sleep study (polysomnography) is gold-standard diagnostic test.
      i. Used to document apneic spells during sleep.

D. Sinusitis

1. Definition
   a. Inflammation of the paranasal sinuses.

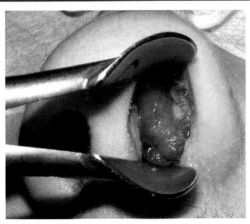

17.1: Nasal polyp. Note the gray-white mass in the left nasal cavity. *(From Swartz MH: Textbook of physical diagnosis, ed 5, Philadelphia, 2006, Saunders Elsevier, p 312, Fig. 11.24.)*

    b. Usually also involves nasal mucosa (thus some use the term "rhinosinusitis").
2. Epidemiology
    a. More common in females, usually mid to older adulthood.
    b. Risk factors include older age, smoking, changes in atmospheric pressure (e.g., scuba diving), asthma, and allergies.
3. Pathogenesis
    a. Impaired drainage of sinus ostia (from paranasal sinus into nasal cavity) leads to the accumulation of secretions within the paranasal sinuses.
      i. Environment favorable for the growth of pathogenic organisms.
    b. Contributing factors include allergic, nonallergic, and viral insults.
      i. Viral upper respiratory infection (most important).
        (1) Commonly rhinovirus, influenza, and parainfluenza.
      ii. Mechanical obstruction (e.g., facial trauma and nasal polyps).
      iii. Thickened secretions (e.g., CF) and impaired mucociliary flow (primary ciliary dyskinesia).
        (1) Kartagener syndrome is a subtype of primary ciliary dyskinesia. Lack of ciliary clearing leads to the retention of secretions and the development of recurrent infections (e.g., sinusitis and pneumonia).
4. Clinical manifestations
    a. Facial pain and pressure overlying involved sinus.
    b. Dental pain (associated with maxillary sinusitis).
    c. Cough from postnasal discharge.
    d. Periorbital cellulitis (extension of infection from the ethmoid sinus).
    e. Risk of cavernous sinus thrombosis with ethmoid sinusitis.
5. Diagnosis
    a. Usually based on clinical manifestations.
    b. Imaging (computed tomography [CT]) only necessary in equivocal cases; shows air-fluid levels and mucosal edema.
E. Nasopharyngeal carcinoma
1. Definition
    a. Malignancy arising from the epithelial cells of the nasopharynx.
2. Epidemiology
    a. Relatively common in parts of Asia (e.g., China), the Middle East, and Northern Africa.
    b. More common in males (3:1).
    c. Peak incidence varies; in high-risk areas, it is more common in the sixth decade of life. May also be seen in adolescents and young adults (especially in low-risk areas such as the United States).
    d. Risk factors (Epstein–Barr virus [EBV] infection, smoking, and genetic predisposition).
3. Pathology
    a. Histologic subtypes
      i. Keratinizing squamous cell carcinoma
        (1) Sporadic type (seen in nonendemic areas).
      ii. Nonkeratinizing carcinoma
        (1) Most common type in endemic areas (e.g., China). Subdivided into differentiated and undifferentiated subtypes.
        (2) Strongly associated with EBV.
        (3) More favorable prognosis than other types.
      iii. Basaloid squamous cell carcinoma
        (1) Rare with poor prognosis.

4. Clinical manifestations
   a. Due to the location in pharyngeal recess, patients often remain asymptomatic until late. Manifestations, once they develop, include recurrent epistaxis, bloody rhinorrhea, and hearing impairment.
   b. Complications include erosion into the skull and cranial nerve palsies (most commonly CN III, IV, V, and VI).
   c. Often metastasizes early (lymph node metastases present at diagnosis in over 75% of cases).
   d. Distant metastases relatively common; involving bone (most commonly), lung, and liver.

F. Laryngeal carcinoma
   1. Definition
      a. Carcinoma involving the larynx (supraglottis, glottis, and subglottis).
   2. Epidemiology
      a. Smoking (the most common cause).
      b. Alcohol (synergistic effect with smoking).
   3. Pathology
      a. Squamous cell carcinoma (Fig. 17.2).
   4. Clinical manifestations
      a. Persistent hoarseness, often in association with painless cervical lymphadenopathy.

II. Atelectasis

A. **Definition**
   1. Loss of lung volume due to the collapse of the airspaces.

B. **Types**
   1. Obstructive (resorptive) atelectasis
      a. Blockage of an airway (e.g., mucus plugs after surgery [common cause], aspiration of foreign material, and centrally located bronchogenic carcinoma) followed by resorption of preexisting air within the airways distal to obstruction.
      b. As intra-alveolar gases are absorbed into circulation, gasless alveoli collapse (i.e., become atelectatic).
      c. May involve all or part of the lung (depends on the site of obstruction).
   2. Nonobstructive atelectasis
      a. Collapse of small airways and alveoli secondary to external compression by air (pneumothorax) or fluid (pleural effusion); surfactant abnormalities.

C. **Clinical manifestations**
   1. Obstructive atelectasis most commonly occurs within the first 24–36 hours after surgery (due to mucus plugging of airways).
   2. Characterized by fever (the most common cause of fever in the first 24–36 hours after surgery) and mild dyspnea.
   3. Examination reveals an absence of breath sounds and dullness to percussion over the involved region.

III. Acute Lung Injury

A. **Pulmonary edema**
   1. Definition
      a. Accumulation of fluid within the alveoli of the lungs.
   2. Etiology
      a. Increased intravascular hydrostatic pressure within pulmonary vasculature.
         i. Most commonly secondary to left-sided heart failure.
         ii. Other etiologies include volume overload and mitral stenosis.

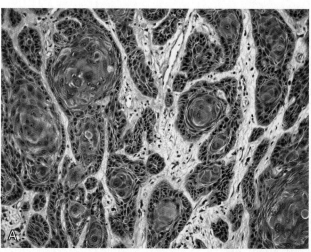

17.2: Well-differentiated invasive squamous cell carcinoma of the larynx. *(From Diagnostic histopathology of tumors, ed 5, Copyright © 2021 by Elsevier, Fig. 4B.10.)*

       iii. Transudate (mostly water, low cellularity).
   b. Decreased oncotic pressure
       i. Etiologies include hypoalbuminemia (e.g., nephrotic syndrome, severe liver disease, and protein-losing enteropathy).
       ii. Transudate.
   c. Microvascular or alveolar injury (e.g., pneumonia and aspiration).
       i. Exudate (the loss of fluid with higher protein and cell content).
  3. Clinical manifestations
   a. Hypoxemia due to impaired alveolar gas exchange (decreased PaO_2, increased $PaCO_2$, and low pH).
   b. Dyspnea due to reduced lung compliance (more difficult to breath).

B. Respiratory distress syndrome (RDS)
  1. Overview
   a. Surfactant, which is produced by Type II pneumocytes, is a complex molecule comprised of various phospholipids.
       i. Surfactant is stored in lamellar bodies.
       ii. Phosphatidylcholine (lecithin) is the major component.
   b. By reducing surface tension, surfactant prevents alveolar collapse on expiration.
   c. Produced in small amounts by the second trimester but only in the later stages of the third trimester are adequate levels produced.
   d. Synthesis is increased by cortisol, thyroxine and decreased by insulin.
  2. Pathogenesis
   a. Decreased surfactant in the fetal lungs.
  3. Risk factors
   a. Preterm delivery (major cause)
       i. Prior to preterm delivery, glucocorticoids are given to increase fetal surfactant production and reduce the risk of developing RDS.
       ii. Those born prior to 28 weeks at the highest risk.
   b. Maternal diabetes
       i. Poorly controlled maternal diabetes mellitus is associated with hyperglycemia in the fetus. Resulting increased levels of fetal insulin impair the production of surfactant.
       ii. Maintaining good glycemic control in the mother will decrease the risk of RDS.
   c. Cesarean delivery (particularly without preceding labor)
       i. Stress of labor and vaginal delivery is associated with a stress-induced release of cortisol (which promotes surfactant production).
  4. Pathology
   a. Widespread atelectasis with massive intrapulmonary shunting (perfusion without ventilation).
   b. Lungs are airless (sink in water).
   c. Leakage of proteins across damaged pulmonary capillaries causes hyaline membrane formation and the impairment of gas exchange (Fig. 17.3).
  5. Clinical manifestations
   a. Respiratory difficulty (e.g., grunting, tachypnea, and intercostal retractions) beginning a few hours after birth; ultimately hypoxemia and cyanosis.
  6. Diagnosis
   a. Chest X-ray shows low lung volume and diffuse reticulogranular ground glass appearance with air bronchograms.
  7. Treatment
   a. Exogenous surfactant, oxygen

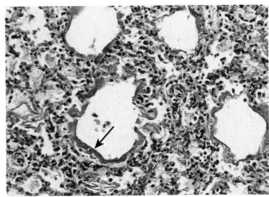

17.3: Neonatal respiratory distress syndrome (RDS). Some of the dilated respiratory bronchioles and alveolar ducts are lined with a fibrin-rich membrane (hyaline membrane) (*arrow*). The subjacent alveoli are collapsed. (*From Damjanov I: Pathology for the health-related professions, ed 2, Philadelphia, 2000, Saunders, p 128, Fig. 5.25.*)

     i. Complications of oxygen therapy, which are now uncommon, include retinopathy of prematurity and broncho-pulmonary dysplasia.

     ii. Oxygen therapy suppresses the release of vascular endothelial growth factor (VEGF) and is associated with a loss of retinal endothelial cells. After the completion of oxygen therapy, the retina returns to being relatively hypoxic, triggering the release of VEGF and neovascularization of the retina ("retinopathy of prematurity").

     iii. Bronchopulmonary dysplasia refers to the disruption of pulmonary development and injury occurring in relation to preterm delivery and the treatment of RDS (i.e., mechanical ventilation and exogenous oxygen therapy).

C. Acute respiratory distress syndrome

1. Definition
   a. Noncardiogenic pulmonary edema occurring in those suffering from various antecedent conditions, including sepsis (most common cause), pneumonia, aspiration, severe trauma, smoke inhalation, acute pancreatitis, etc.
2. Pathogenesis
   a. Initial insult triggers the release of pro-inflammatory cytokines (e.g., tumor necrosis factor [TNF], interleukin-1 [IL-1], and IL-6) and the recruitment of neutrophils to the lungs.
   b. Neutrophils release toxic mediators (e.g., proteases and reactive oxygen species) that damage the capillary endothelium and alveolar epithelium.
      i. Plasma fluid passes through the "leaky" vessels into the pulmonary interstitium and alveoli; impairs gas exchange and decreases lung compliance.
3. Pathology
   a. Three pathologic stages
      i. Exudative stage (the first stage, characterized by edema, acute and chronic inflammation, and proteinaceous fluid—"hyaline membranes").
      ii. Fibroproliferative stage (the second stage, characterized by the resolution of the edema, early fibrosis).
      iii. Fibrotic stage (the final stage, characterized by the obliteration of normal architecture by fibrosis; not everyone proceeds to this stage).
4. Clinical manifestations
   a. Dyspnea, hypoxemia, tachycardia, and tachypnea.
   b. Respiratory alkalosis initially (due to tachypnea); the onset of hypercapnia/respiratory acidosis indicates impending respiratory failure.
   c. Bilateral interstitial infiltrates with alveolar consolidation on imaging.
5. Prognosis
   a. Poor (40%–50% mortality rate).

IV. Pulmonary Infections

A. Pneumonia

1. Definition
   a. Infection of the lung parenchyma; associated with characteristic clinical and radiologic findings.
2. Risk factors
   a. Antecedent viral respiratory tract infection (damages clearance mechanisms and enhances the adherence of bacteria to respiratory epithelium).
   b. Airway obstruction (e.g., bronchogenic carcinoma).
   c. Immunosuppression (e.g., defective antibody production).
   d. Excessive alcohol ingestion (impairs neutrophil mobilization and bacterial killing and suppresses gag reflex).
   e. Smoking (increases pulmonary secretions and damages mucociliary transport).
   f. Advanced age (diminished gag and cough reflexes and impaired immune response).
3. Classification (Fig. 17.4)
   a. Bronchopneumonia
      i. Characterized by patchy areas of consolidation involving one or more lobes, usually involves dependent lung zones.
      ii. Often secondary to aspiration of oropharyngeal contents.
      iii. Neutrophilic exudate, primarily centered around bronchi and bronchioles, with spread to surrounding alveoli.
   b. Lobar pneumonia
      i. Occurs when inhaled organisms reach the subpleural zone of the lung; injury to alveolar walls allows blood and fluid to enter (the entire lobe becomes consolidated).
      ii. Pathologic "stages" of lobar pneumonia
         (1) Stage 1: vascular congestion and alveolar edema with numerous bacteria but few neutrophils.
         (2) Stage 2: the lung develops the consistency of the liver with leakage of RBCs, WBCs, and fibrin into alveoli; known as "red hepatization."
         (3) Stage 3: disintegration of RBCs leads to the deposition of hemosiderin. Appears gray-brown ("gray hepatization").
         (4) Stage 4: resolution of infection with the restoration of the pulmonary architecture. Possibility of developing pulmonary fibrosis and/or pleural adhesions.

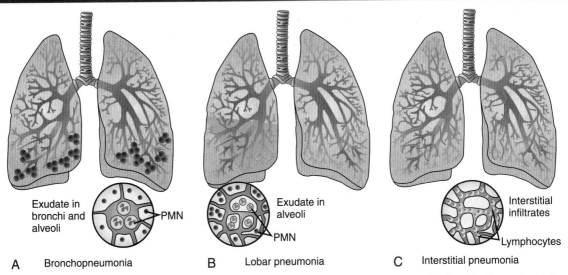

A   Bronchopneumonia   B   Lobar pneumonia   C   Interstitial pneumonia

17.4: Anatomic distribution of various forms of pneumonia. (A) Bronchopneumonia is characterized by focal infiltrates involving peribronchial lobules. (B) Lobar pneumonia involves lobes or large portions of the lungs. (C) Interstitial (atypical) pneumonia usually involves both lungs, which show radiologically visible reticular infiltrates corresponding to thickened alveolar septa. *PMN*, Polymorphonuclear neutrophil. *(From Damjanov I: Pathophysiology, Philadelphia, 2009, Saunders Elsevier, p 171, Fig. 5.23.)*

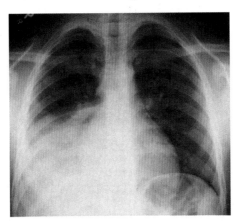

17.5: Posteroanterior radiograph of a right lower lobe pneumococcal pneumonia. Note the alveolar consolidation and the visible border of the right ventricle indicating that the middle lobe is not involved. *(From Kliegman RM, Jenson HB, Behrman RE, Stanton BF: Nelson textbook of pediatrics, ed 18, Philadelphia, 2007, Saunders Elsevier, p 1798, Fig. 397.2A.)*

    c. Atypical pneumonia
       i. Definition
          (1) Pneumonia characterized by typically less severe symptoms; interstitial pulmonary infiltrates on chest X-ray.
          (2) Etiologies include *Mycoplasma pneumoniae* ("walking pneumonia"), *Chlamydia pneumoniae*, *Chlamydia psittaci*, and *Legionella pneumophila*.
  4. Clinical manifestations
    a. Vary depending on the etiologic agent; however, characteristic findings include fever, productive cough, and pleuritic chest pain (i.e., pain worse with inspiration; due to the inflammation of the parietal pleura).
    b. Signs of consolidation
       i. Dullness to percussion.
       ii. Increased vocal tactile fremitus (vibratory sensation when the patient speaks due to increased transmission of sound waves through the area of consolidation).
       iii. Crackles.
    c. Neutrophilic leukocytosis with left shift.
    d. Flecks of blood in sputum ("rusty sputum").
  5. Diagnosis
    a. Chest X-ray is the gold standard (Fig. 17.5).
       i. Findings vary (patchy infiltrates in bronchopneumonia, lobar consolidation in lobar pneumonia, and interstitial infiltrate in interstitial pneumonia).
    b. CT useful in select cases (more sensitive for small areas of consolidation).
  6. Causes of community-acquired pneumonia (Table 17.1).

TABLE 17.1   Summary of Community-Acquired Pneumonia

Neonates	Bacterial • Group B streptococci • *Listeria monocytogenes* • *Chlamydia trachomatis*
Children older than 1 month (viral in up to 70% of cases)	Viral • Respiratory syncytial virus • Parainfluenza • Influenza A and B • Adenovirus • Rhinovirus Bacterial • *Streptococcus pneumoniae* • *Haemophilus influenzae* type b • *Moraxella catarrhalis* • *Mycoplasma pneumoniae* • *Chlamydia pneumoniae*
Adults	Typical bacteria • *S. pneumoniae* • *H. influenzae* • *M. catarrhalis* Atypical bacteria • *Mycoplasma* • *Legionella* spp. Respiratory viruses • Influenza A and B viruses • Severe acute respiratory syndrome coronavirus 2 (SARS-CoV-2) and other coronaviruses • Parainfluenza virus

B. Tuberculosis
  1. Definition
     a. Refers to a chronic pulmonary and systemic disease caused by *Mycobacterium tuberculosis*.
  2. Transmission
     a. *M. tuberculosis* is acquired via the inhalation of aerosolized organisms into alveoli.
     b. Following inhalation, the organisms are phagocytosed by alveolar macrophages.
     c. *M. tuberculosis* begins to replicate within alveolar macrophages.
     d. Activation of innate immunity; Th1 response leads to the production of IFN-γ (activates macrophages and stimulates granulomatous host response to control infection).
     e. Those with impaired immunity (e.g., AIDS and transplant recipients) are at a markedly increased risk of progression to active disease.
  3. Characteristics of *M. tuberculosis*
     a. Strict aerobe, acid-fast (because of mycolic acid in the cell wall).
  4. Screening for tuberculosis
     a. Purified protein derivative (tuberculin skin test)
        i. Intradermal skin test used to screen for *M. tuberculosis*. Does not distinguish infection from active disease.
        ii. Based on the presence of a Type IV (delayed type) hypersensitivity reaction (HSR) against mycobacterial protein antigens.
  5. Primary tuberculosis (Fig. 17.6A).
     a. Refers to the disease in a previously unexposed and therefore unsensitized person.
     b. Organism implants near the pleura within the lower part of the upper lobe or the upper part of the lower lobe.
        i. Forms a small area of inflammation with consolidation known as a "Ghon focus."
        ii. Subsequently, regional lymph nodes become involved.
           (1) Combination of the lung lesion plus involved nodes is known as the "Ghon complex."
        iii. Patients are usually asymptomatic at this point, and infection usually remains isolated within a calcified granuloma.
        iv. If/when host immune response fails to control the initial infection, then the patient develops reactivation of infection (i.e., secondary tuberculosis).
  6. Secondary (reactivation) tuberculosis (Fig. 17.6B)
     a. Refers to the reactivation of primary tuberculosis.
     b. Involves one or both apices of the upper lobes (site of the highest oxygen levels and good for strict aerobes).
     c. Release of pro-inflammatory cytokines and cavitation of tissue.
     d. Clinical findings include fever, night sweats, weight loss, and cough.
     e. Potential for dissemination of the organism

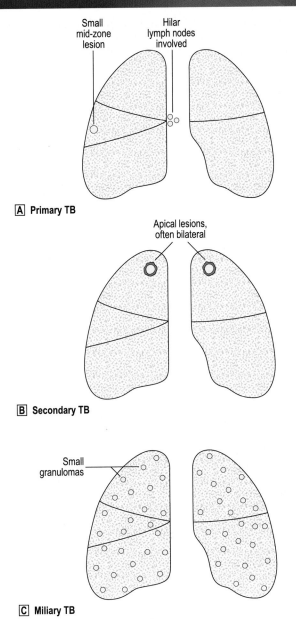

Small
mid-zone
lesion

Hilar
lymph nodes
involved

A Primary TB

Apical lesions,
often bilateral

B Secondary TB

Small
granulomas

C Miliary TB

17.6: Types of pulmonary tuberculosis. *(From Underwood's pathology ed 7, © 2019 Elsevier, Fig. 14.10.)*

      i. "Miliary tuberculosis" (Fig. 17.6C) refers to the hematogenous dissemination of the infection throughout the lungs and/or body.

      ii. Favored sites include the meninges (tuberculous meningitis), kidneys (renal tuberculosis), adrenals (historically a cause of adrenocortical insufficiency), bones (osteomyelitis), and fallopian tubes (salpingitis).

         (1) Involvement of the vertebrae is known as "Pott disease."

   7. Diagnosis

     a. Culture of sputum, bronchoalveolar lavage, and pleural fluid or tissue (e.g., lung biopsy).

     b. Sputum for acid-fast bacilli smear and nucleic acid amplification testing.

     c. Tuberculous pleural effusion is exudative with the predominance of lymphocytes and elevated lactate dehydrogenase.

       i. Although nonspecific, elevated levels of adenosine deaminase within the pleural fluid are characteristic.

C. Pulmonary fungal infections

   1. Contracted via inhalation; cause granulomatous inflammation, usually with central areas of necrosis ("caseous" necrosis).

   2. Of particular concern in immunocompromised patients (risk of invasive disease with systemic spread).

D. Lung abscess

   1. Defined as a localized microbial infection with suppurative inflammation (pus) and necrosis of lung parenchyma.

   2. Aspiration is the most common underlying mechanism by which lung abscesses arise, characteristically in association with abnormalities in swallowing (functional or anatomic).

a. Risk factors include alcoholism, loss of consciousness, seizures, general anesthesia, and head trauma.

b. Often polymicrobial; anaerobes (e.g., *Peptostreptococcus* and *Bacteroides*) common in those with periodontal disease.

3. Hematogenous dissemination (e.g., tricuspid valve endocarditis, and intravenous drug use) is less common (e.g., *Staphylococcus aureus*).

4. Pathology

a. Abscesses vary in size and location, those secondary to aspiration are more likely to occur on the right (more direct airway).

5. Clinical manifestations

a. Fever and productive cough (foul-smelling sputum).

b. Imaging shows cavitation with air-fluid level.

6. Complications

a. Hemoptysis, bronchopleural fistula (connection between lung and pleural cavity), and empyema (collection of pus in pleural space).

V. Vascular Lung Lesions

A. Pulmonary embolism (PE)

1. Definition

a. Sudden obstruction of a portion of the pulmonary artery (PA) vasculature by a thrombus.

b. Thrombi usually arise within the deep veins of the leg (venous thrombi).

2. Risk factors

a. Stasis of blood flow; prolonged immobility, often in association with major trauma or recent surgery (e.g., hip or knee replacement).

b. Hypercoagulable states (e.g., antithrombin deficiency, protein C or S deficiency, factor V Leiden mutation, and prothrombin mutation).

c. Malignancy (e.g., pancreatic cancer).

d. Increasing age, obesity, smoking, and pregnancy.

3. Clinical manifestations

a. Vary depending upon the size of the embolus (Fig. 17.7)

i. Large emboli occlude the proximal portion of the PA ("saddle embolus"); risk of sudden death due to acute right-sided heart failure.

ii. Small emboli occlude small- to medium-sized tributaries of the PA.

b. Potential for pulmonary infarction

i. Blood flow through the bronchial artery (arises from the thoracic aorta) tends to protect against pulmonary infarction; however, those with the decreased flow (e.g., decreased cardiac output) have the potential for developing a pulmonary infarction.

ii. Pulmonary infarctions are wedge-shaped, extend to pleural surface.

c. Clinical manifestations

i. Dyspnea, tachypnea, and pleuritic chest pain.

ii. Syncope and cardiac arrest (severe cases).

iii. May have evidence of deep venous thrombosis (unilateral leg swelling, pain, and erythema).

4. Laboratory findings

a. Respiratory alkalosis ($\downarrow$ arterial $PaCO_2$) and hypoxemia ($\downarrow PaO_2$).

b. Increased D-dimer (not specific; however, a negative result excludes PE).

c. Troponin may be elevated (secondary to acute right ventricular dilation/myocardial injury).

5. Diagnosis

a. Ventilation/perfusion (V/Q) scan low sensitivity and high specificity.

b. CT pulmonary angiogram (CT pulmonary angiography) has good sensitivity and specificity.

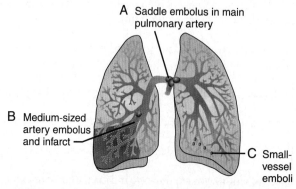

A Saddle embolus in main pulmonary artery

B Medium-sized artery embolus and infarct

C Small-vessel emboli

17.7: Pulmonary embolism. (A) Massive embolism occludes the pulmonary artery or its major branches and may cause death. (B) Medium-sized embolism may cause pulmonary infarcts. (C) Recurrent small emboli may cause pulmonary hypertension due to extensive occlusion of small vessels. *(From Damjanov I: Pathophysiology, Philadelphia, 2009, Saunders Elsevier, p 181, Fig. 5.33.)*

B. **Pulmonary arterial hypertension (PAH)**
  1. Definition
     a. Increased pressure within the pulmonary vasculature (mean PA pressure ≥20 mm Hg at rest).
  2. Classified into five groups
     a. Group 1 (inheritable causes; most common mutation involves bone morphogenic protein receptor 2—*BMPR2*, drugs, and connective tissue disease).
     b. Group 2 (due to left-sided heart disease).
     c. Group 3 (due to chronic lung disorders and hypoxemia).
     d. Group 4 (due to PA obstruction).
     e. Group 5 (due to unidentified mechanisms).
  3. Pathologic findings
     a. Hyperplasia of smooth muscle cells in the pulmonary vasculature.
     b. Atherosclerosis of the main PA (reaction to pressure-induced endothelial injury).
  4. Clinical manifestations
     a. Exertional fatigue and dyspnea (the most common presenting symptom) and chest pain.
     b. Accentuated P2 (high pulmonary pressure causes the pulmonic valve to "slam shut").
     c. Increased jugular venous pressure with accentuated "a" wave (atrial contraction).
     d. Left parasternal heave (a sign of right ventricular hypertrophy—RVH).
        i. Pulmonary hypertension imposes an increased pressure load on the right ventricle leading to the development of RVH.
     e. Right-sided heart failure (cor pulmonale).
        i. Cor pulmonale refers to alterations in the structure and function of the right ventricle from pulmonary hypertension caused by the disease of the lungs (e.g., chronic obstructive pulmonary disease and interstitial lung disease) or pulmonary vasculature (e.g., massive pulmonary embolus).
  5. Diagnosis
     a. Measurement of PA pressures (e.g., right heart catheterization).
     b. Chest X-ray shows enlargement of the main PAs, rapid tapering of the distal vessels, and right ventricular enlargement.
     c. Electrocardiogram shows the right axis deviation with changes reflecting right ventricle strain.
     d. Echocardiography shows right atrial enlargement and right ventricular enlargement.
C. **Antiglomerular basement membrane disease (Goodpasture syndrome)**
  1. Definition
     a. Type of vasculitis affecting the lungs and kidneys.
  2. Pathogenesis
     a. Due to circulating antibodies directed against the noncollagen-1 domain of the alpha-3 chain of Type IV collagen (found in the basement membrane of the lung and kidney).
  3. Clinical presentation
     a. Hemoptysis and hematuria.
VI. **Restrictive Lung Diseases (RLDs)**
  A. **Overview**
    1. Spirometry (Fig. 17.8)
       a. Total lung capacity (TLC): the total amount of air in a fully expanded lung.
       b. Residual volume (RV): the volume of air remaining in the lung after maximal exhalation.
       c. Tidal volume: the volume of air that enters or leaves the lungs during normal quiet respiration.

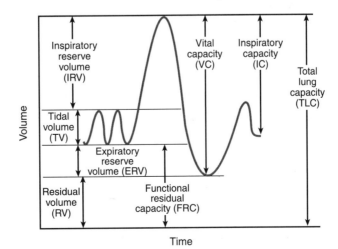

17.8: Spirogram. *(From Pfenninger and Fowler's procedures for primary care, ed 4, Copyright © 2020 by Elsevier, Fig. 81.1.)*

  d. Forced vital capacity (FVC): the total volume of air expelled after a maximal inspiration.
     i. Normal ~ 5 L.
  e. Forced expiratory volume in 1 second (FEV1): the amount of air expelled from the lungs in the first second after a maximal inspiration.
     i. Normal FEV1 is 4 L.
     ii. FEV1/FVC ratio: normally 4/5 or 80%.
  2. RLD
    a. Characterized by limited lung expansion (decrease in TLC), diminished lung compliance (decrease in functional residual capacity), and exertional hypoxemia.
    b. FEV1/FVC ratio normal/increased.
    c. Major etiologies include:
     i. Intrinsic lung disease with scarring (e.g., idiopathic pulmonary fibrosis [IPF] and pneumoconiosis).
     ii. Extrapulmonary disorders characterized by impaired ventilatory movement (e.g., obesity, kyphosis, and neuro-muscular disease).

B. IPF
  1. Definition
    a. Progressive interstitial fibrosis of the lung of unknown etiology.
  2. Epidemiology
    a. Typically presents in those over 60 years, smokers.
  3. Pathogenesis
    a. Unclear, thought to involve repeated cycles of epithelial injury and dysregulated repair.
    b. Patchy interstitial fibrosis (possibly related to elevated levels of transforming growth factor-beta).
    c. Over time, progressive fibrosis causes the lungs to become stiff (i.e., reduced compliance), impairing the ability of the lungs to fill with air.
  4. Clinical and laboratory findings include:
    a. Persistent nonproductive cough and progressively worsening dyspnea on exertion.
    b. Lung volumes and capacities are decreased in proportion (decreased FEV1, decreased FVC, and normal FEV1/FVC ratio).
    c. Limited survival (~3–4 years) without lung transplant.
  5. Diagnosis
    a. High-resolution CT shows peripheral, basilar predominant ground glass opacities associated with honeycombing (cystic changes).

C. Pneumoconioses
  1. Definition
    a. Group of nonneoplastic interstitial lung disorders occurring after the inhalation and deposition of mineral dusts.
  2. Pathogenesis
    a. Inflammation and eventual fibrosis following the inhalation and deposition of inorganic mineral dusts (e.g., coal dust, silica, asbestos, and beryllium).
    b. Particle size determines the site of deposition; those 1–5 μm in diameter are the most injurious because they reach the terminal airways.
  3. Coal workers' pneumoconiosis
    a. Definition
     i. Pneumoconiosis arising as a result of the inhalation of coal dust ("black lung" disease).
    b. Pulmonary manifestations
     i. Anthracosis
      (1) Benign deposits of coal dust within macrophages.
     ii. Simple coal workers' pneumoconiosis
      (1) Small (<1 cm) fibrotic collections of carbon-laden macrophages within the upper lobes and upper portions of the lower lobes.
     iii. Complicated coal workers' pneumoconiosis (progressive massive fibrosis)
      (1) Only occurs in a minority of patients (~10%); characterized by progressively larger nodules of fibrosis, often with central areas of necrosis.
    c. Caplan syndrome may occur (the presence of pneumoconiosis in addition to rheumatoid nodules in the lungs).
  4. Silicosis
    a. Definition
     i. Pneumoconiosis following the inhalation of free crystalline silica (silicon dioxide).
    b. Epidemiology
     i. Most common occupational disease in the world.
      (1) Most often secondary to the inhalation of quartz (crystalline silicone dioxide), a major component of granite, slate, and sandstone.
     ii. Occupational exposure in mining, sandblasting, stone cutting, masonry, and foundry work.

c. Pathophysiology

    i. Inhaled quartz deposits cause the formation of oxygen radicals and the release of inflammatory cytokines (e.g., IL-1 and TNF).

d. Manifestations

    i. Eventual development of fibrous nodules (concentric layers of collagen with or without central cavitation).

    ii. "Eggshell" calcification of hilar lymph nodes (the rim of dystrophic calcification simulates an eggshell).

e. Complications

    i. Silicosis is associated with an increased risk of lung cancer, chronic bronchitis, and tuberculosis (silica impairs the ability of pulmonary macrophages to kill mycobacteria).

5. Asbestos-related disease

  a. Types of asbestos fibers

    i. Serpentine (e.g., chrysotile) fibers are curly and flexible; more likely to deposit in the upper airways allowing for removal by ciliary transport.

    ii. Amphibole (e.g., crocidolite) fibers are more pathogenic (straight and rigid, more likely to follow the flow of air into distal airways).

  b. Sources of asbestos exposure

    i. Various commercial products (automotive brake pads, roofing products, and fireproof clothing), mining of asbestos, destruction of old buildings, and shipbuilding.

  c. Pathology

    i. Asbestos fibers coated with iron and protein (called "asbestos bodies") have a golden, beaded appearance (Fig. 17.9).

  d. Pathogenesis

    i. Analogous to other Pneumoconioses, the engulfment of inhaled asbestos fibers by macrophages is followed by the release of pro-inflammatory and fibrogenic mediators.

  e. Complications

    i. Benign pleural plaques

      (1) Most common manifestation of asbestos.

      (2) Consist of fibrous plaques on parietal pleura and dome of the diaphragm; often calcified.

      (3) Arises decades after exposure, not a precursor to mesothelioma.

    ii. Lung cancer

      (1) Synergistic effect with smoking.

      (2) Most common malignancy associated with asbestos.

      (3) Arises after a long latency period (decades after exposure).

    iii. Malignant mesothelioma

      (1) Tumor of pleural lining cells.

      (2) Toxicity related to the formation of free radicals.

      (3) Tumor encases, and locally invades, subpleural lung tissue.

      (4) Long latency period (decades) after exposure.

6. Berylliosis

  a. Definition

    i. Chronic granulomatous disease of the lung associated with the inhalation of beryllium.

    ii. Beryllium is a metal used in a variety of occupational settings (e.g., defense and aerospace industry, electronics and computer recycling, jewelry making, and dental appliances).

  b. Pathogenesis

    i. Inhalation of beryllium causes a T-lymphocyte cell–mediated delayed hypersensitivity response, granulomatous inflammation within the lung.

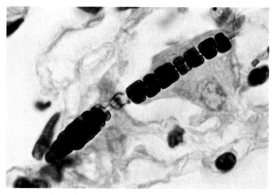

17.9: Asbestos body. The straight, golden-brown, beaded asbestos body represents an asbestos fiber coated by iron and protein. *(From Damjanov I, Linder J: Pathology: a color atlas, St. Louis, 2000, Mosby, p 65, Fig. 4.51B.)*

     c. Clinical manifestations
         i. Dyspnea, cough, weight loss, and fatigue.
         ii. Cor pulmonale (advanced disease).
         iii. Cutaneous nodules (penetration of the skin by beryllium).
     d. Diagnosis
         i. Chest X-rays may show hilar lymphadenopathy or parenchymal abnormalities (e.g., opacities).
         ii. Blood beryllium lymphocyte proliferation test is used to confirm sensitization to beryllium.

D. Sarcoidosis
   1. Definition
     a. Multisystem granulomatous disorder of unknown etiology.
   2. Epidemiology
     a. More common in African Americans.
     b. May present at any age, usually young to middle-aged adults.
   3. Clinical and radiologic findings
     a. Depends upon the site of involvement.
     b. Involvement of the lungs and associated lymph nodes (e.g., hilar and mediastinal) are common; manifests with wdyspnea and cough.
     c. On imaging, enlargement of hilar and mediastinal nodes (called "potato nodes") is apparent. May also have smaller densities throughout the lung parenchyma.
   4. Laboratory findings
     a. Elevated serum angiotensin-converting enzyme (ACE)
         i. ACE produced by the epithelioid cells of the granulomas.
         ii. Elevated serum levels of ACE are noted in many cases; however, poor sensitivity and specificity limit clinical utility.
     b. Hypercalcemia
         i. Macrophages within granulomas contain 1-α-hydroxylase, the enzyme that forms active vitamin D (calcitriol).
     c. Diminished skin test reactivity (anergy).
   5. Pathology
     a. Noncaseating granulomatous inflammation (Fig. 17.10).

E. Hypersensitivity pneumonitis (extrinsic allergic alveolitis)
   1. Definition
     a. Inflammatory interstitial lung disease secondary to an immunologically mediated reaction to one or more inhaled antigens (e.g., bacterial spores, fungi, and animal proteins).
   2. Specific syndromes
     a. Farmer's lung follows exposure to moldy hay containing spores of thermophilic actinomycetes.
     b. Pigeon breeder's lung (bird fancier's disease) follows the inhalation of various bird proteins (feathers and excreta).
     c. Humidifier lung follows the inhalation of thermophilic bacteria present within aerosolized water (e.g., humidifiers).
   3. Pathogenesis
     a. Both humoral and cellular mechanisms thought important with T-cell–mediated delayed-type hypersensitivity playing a key role.
     b. Various inflammatory chemokines and cytokines are released by antigen-presenting cells and lymphocytes.
     c. Reactive oxygen species contribute to the alveolar damage.
   4. Clinical manifestations
     a. Typically arise 4–8 hours after exposure; include malaise, fever, chills, nonproductive cough, and dyspnea.
     b. Symptoms usually resolve within 24–48 hours after removal of the agent only to recur upon reexposure to the antigen.
     c. Potential for the development of the interstitial fibrosis.

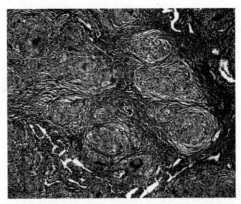

17.10: Sarcoidosis. Note the noncaseating granulomata. *(Modified from Leslie KO, Wick MR: Practical pulmonary pathology: a diagnostic approach, ed 2, Philadelphia, 2011, Elsevier.)*

5. Treatment
   a. Avoidance of provocative antigen(s) to prevent progression of the disease.

VII. Chronic Obstructive Pulmonary Disease
   A. Definition
      1. Chronic lung disorder characterized by fixed airway obstruction causing impaired airflow out of the lungs.
         a. Evidence of impaired flow based on the ratio of FEV1 to FVC of less than 0.7 (FEV1/FVC < 0.7).
      2. Includes chronic bronchitis and emphysema (often both are present).
   B. Epidemiology
      1. Usually middle age to older adults.
      2. Cigarette smoking is a primary underlying risk factor.
      3. Fourth leading cause of death in the United States.
   C. Emphysema
      1. Definition
         a. Pulmonary disorder characterized by permanent enlargement of the airspaces distal to the terminal bronchioles.
      2. Etiologies
         a. Smoking (the most common cause).
         b. α1-Antitrypsin (AAT) deficiency.
      3. Types
         a. Centriacinar emphysema
            i.   Most common form; predominantly associated with smoking.
            ii. Distention of respiratory bronchioles; spares alveoli.
            iii. Preferentially involves the upper lobes.
            iv. Air trapping causes distention of the respiratory bronchioles along with an increase in the RV and TLC.
         b. Panacinar emphysema
            i.   Preferentially involves the lower lobes.
            ii. Destruction of elastic tissue within the entire respiratory unit causing the enlargement of acini from the respiratory bronchiole to the alveolus.
            iii. Type seen with AAT deficiency.
      4. Pathophysiology
         a. Elastic fibers apply radial traction to the outside of small airways, (keeps airways open).
         b. Destruction of this elastic tissue, whether by cigarette smoke-induced inflammation and oxidative stress or excessive protease activity (e.g., AAT deficiency), leads to a loss of the radial traction and decreased recoil. The net effect is to "trap" air within the airspaces distal to the collapsed region of the respiratory unit (Fig. 17.11).
      5. Clinical manifestations
         a. Progressive dyspnea and tachypnea.
         b. Sometimes known as "pink puffers" because they can often maintain oxygenation through pursed lip breathing.
         c. Diminished breath sounds and distant heart sounds due to hyperinflation of the lungs.

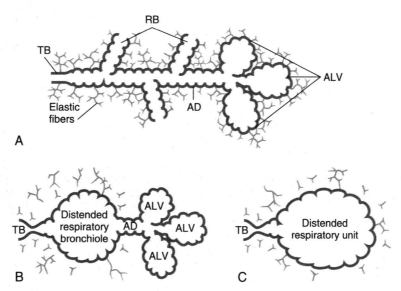

17.11: Types of emphysema. (A) Schematic shows a normal distal airway, including a terminal bronchiole (TB) leading into the respiratory unit consisting of a respiratory bronchiole (RB), alveolar duct (AD), and alveoli (ALV). Elastic fibers apply radial traction to keep these airways open. (B) Centriacinar emphysema is characterized by trapping of air in the respiratory bronchioles. Note how the elastic fibers of the distal TB are destroyed, causing obstruction to airflow. This causes the trapped air to distend the RBs, whose elastic tissue support is destroyed. (C) Panacinar emphysema is characterized by trapping of air in the entire respiratory unit behind the collapsed TB.

6. Imaging
   a. Hyperinflated lungs (i.e., hyperlucent lung fields) with increased anteroposterior (AP) diameter, vertically oriented heart, and flattened diaphragm (Fig. 17.12).
7. Spirometry
   a. FEV1/FVC ratio reduced (<0.7).
8. Arterial blood gas (ABG)
   a. PaO$_2$ is normal initially (decreased late in the disease).
   b. Decreased PaCO$_2$ (tachypnea → respiratory alkalosis).
   c. Decreased bicarbonate (compensatory metabolic acidosis).

D. Chronic bronchitis
1. Definition
   a. Presence of a productive cough for at least 3 months in 2 or more consecutive years.
2. Etiologies
   a. Smoking (most common cause).
   b. CF.
3. Pathogenesis
   a. Excessive sputum production, which is secondary to hyperplasia of mucus cells and bronchiolar inflammation, causes chronic productive cough.
      i. Mucus within airways obstructs airflow.
      ii. In addition, patients often have superimposed upper respiratory tract infection (e.g., virus or bacteria) and/or suffer from the effects of inhaled pollutants/dusts that exacerbate the cough.

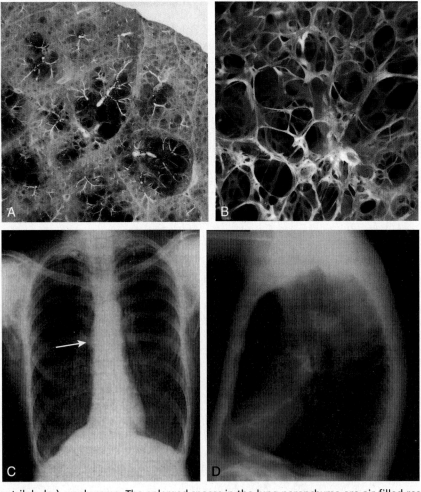

17.12 (A) Centriacinar (centrilobular) emphysema. The enlarged spaces in the lung parenchyma are air-filled respiratory bronchioles that have lost their elastic tissue support. (B) Panacinar emphysema. The enlarged spaces in the lung parenchyma are air-filled respiratory bronchioles, alveolar ducts, and alveoli that have lost their elastic tissue support. (C) Chest radiograph in emphysema showing a vertically oriented heart (*arrow*) and depressed diaphragm. (D) Radiograph of the thorax in a patient with emphysema. There is an increase in lung volume, darkness of the lungs (increased air relative to tissue), and an increase in space between the sternum and the heart. (A and B, *Reproduced by permission of the late Professor B.E. Heard, Brompton, UK; C, from Forbes C, Jackson W: Color atlas and text of clinical medicine, ed 2, London, 2002, Mosby, p 186, Fig. 4.94; D, from Goldman L, Schafer AI: Cecil's medicine, ed 24, Philadelphia, 2012, Saunders Elsevier, p 540, Fig. 88.3B.)*

      b. Mucus plugging of segmental bronchi and proximal bronchioles impairs the flow of air and causes buildup of carbon dioxide (respiratory acidosis).

      c. Histologic findings include both acute (neutrophils) and chronic (lymphocytes, macrophages) inflammation, thickening of bronchiolar wall (edema, smooth muscle cell hyperplasia), peribronchial fibrosis, and increased mucous glands.

          i. Chronic irritation of the respiratory epithelium secondary to smoking eventually leads to the development of squamous metaplasia and the potential for malignant transformation (squamous cell carcinoma).

   4. Clinical manifestations

      a. Productive cough, hypoxemia, and respiratory acidosis (early in the disease).

      b. Cyanosis from reduced oxygen levels ("blue bloaters").

      c. Wheezing and rhonchi.

      d. Increased risk of cor pulmonale.

   5. ABG

      a. Chronic respiratory acidosis with elevated $PaCO_2$, elevated bicarbonate (compensatory metabolic alkalosis), and moderate to severe hypoxemia (decreased PaO_2).

E. Asthma

   1. Definition

      a. Chronic disorder of unknown etiology; classically characterized by recurrent episodes of reversible airway obstruction.

   2. Epidemiology

      a. Common disorder affecting approximately 8% of adults; most cases begin prior to age 25 years.

   3. Pathogenesis

      a. Both genetic and environmental factors.

      b. IgE-mediated (Type I HSR) sensitization to environmental antigens is the most recognized pathway (bronchial hyperreactivity).

          i. Initial exposure to allergen sensitizes the patient; results in the formation of IgE antibodies against the antigen.

          ii. Subsequently, the IgE antibodies bind to mast cells located near airways.

          iii. Upon reexposure, allergen interaction with the bound IgE causes mast cell degranulation (releases histamine and generates pro-inflammatory leukotrienes and prostaglandins).

          iv. The net effect is bronchoconstriction with wheezing, cough, etc.

      c. Cigarette smoke, viral infections (e.g., rhinovirus), exercise, air pollutants (e.g., sulfur dioxide and ozone), and drugs may all trigger an asthmatic attack.

          i. Aspirin and other nonsteroidal antiinflammatory drugs decrease the synthesis of prostaglandins by blocking cyclooxygenase; however, this leaves precursors free to form leukotrienes (bronchoconstrictors).

      d. Th2 cells contribute to the inflammatory cascade by releasing various cytokines, including:

          i. IL-4 (induces B-cell proliferation and stimulates the production of IgE).

          ii. IL-13 (stimulates B-cells/IgE production as well as mucus hypersecretion).

          iii. IL-5 (promotes eosinophil formation and maturation).

   4. Pathology

      a. Histologic changes in bronchi include thickening of the basement membrane, edema, and inflammation (e.g., eosinophils and mast cells).

      b. Sputum may contain Curschmann's spirals (spiral-shaped mucus casts of small airways) and Charcot–Leyden crystals (comprised of granules from eosinophils).

   5. Clinical manifestations

      a. Episodic wheezing, cough, shortness of breath, tachypnea, and the use of accessory muscles of respiration.

   6. Laboratory findings

      a. Respiratory alkalosis (secondary to tachypnea); initial finding

          i. If bronchospasm is not relieved, patients may develop respiratory muscle fatigue and respiratory acidosis.

          ii. Sequence: respiratory alkalosis → normal pH → respiratory acidosis ($\uparrow PaCO_2$, $\downarrow PaO_2$ [hypoxemia]).

             (1) Evolution of pH (from alkalemia → acidemia) necessitates intubation and mechanical ventilation.

      b. FEV1 can be used to determine disease severity.

      c. Eosinophilia common.

F. Bronchiectasis

   1. Definition

      a. Irreversible airway dilation secondary to the destruction of bronchial walls.

   2. Pathogenesis

      a. Airway obstruction (e.g., by mucus in those with CF or foreign bodies) leads to secondary infections (e.g., bacteria) and associated chronic inflammation.

      b. Inflammation eventually damages airways.

          i. Cycle of recurrent infection → inflammation → airway injury → progressive airway distention.

3. Etiologies
   a. Recurrent infections, commonly secondary to airway obstruction
      i. Thickened secretions (e.g., CF).
      ii. Impaired mucus clearance (e.g., ciliary dyskinesia).
      iii. Foreign bodies (children).
4. Pathology
   a. Dilated bronchi and bronchioles containing mucopurulent secretions.
5. Clinical manifestations
   a. Chronic cough with expectoration of foul smelling, sometimes bloody sputum (hemoptysis may be massive).
   b. Cor pulmonale.
6. Radiologic findings
   a. Dilated bronchial markings with extension to lung periphery.

G. **CF**
   1. Definition
      a. Autosomal recessive, multisystem disease associated with dysfunction of the cystic fibrosis transmembrane conductance regulator (CFTR) protein.
   2. Epidemiology
      a. Most common life-limiting inherited disorder among Whites (~1 in 3500 births).
      b. Usually diagnosed during infancy; life expectancy of ~40 years.
   3. Pathogenesis
      a. Caused by mutations in the *CFTR* gene on chromosome 7 (encodes for CFTR protein).
         i. The most common mutation, F508del, results in a deletion of three DNA bases coding for phenylalanine at the 508th amino acid residue.
      b. CFTR malfunction affects ion channels; causing respiratory, biliary, and pancreatic secretions to become excessively viscous and difficult to clear.
         i. Within the lungs, the viscous secretions increase the risk of developing recurrent bacterial infections.
         ii. Within pancreatic ducts, viscous secretions contribute to the development of acute/chronic pancreatitis, malabsorption, and steatorrhea.
         iii. Within bile ducts, impaired drainage of viscous secretions predisposes to the development of secondary biliary cirrhosis.
   4. Clinical manifestations
      a. Respiratory infections (the most common cause of death from CF).
         i. Common pathogens include *Pseudomonas aeruginosa* (most common), *S. aureus*, *Haemophilus influenzae*, *Burkholderia* spp.
         ii. Bronchiectasis common complication.
      b. Nasal polyps, sinusitis
      c. Malabsorption (loss of pancreatic exocrine function) with associated malnutrition and growth impairment.
      d. Infertility, particularly males.
      e. Meconium ileus (bowel obstruction by viscous meconium).
      f. Constipation (chronic straining → rectal prolapse).
      g. Secondary biliary cirrhosis (thickened secretions obstruct bile ductules).
      h. Excess loss of salt (NaCl) in sweat (parents may note salty taste upon kissing the child).

H. **Diagnosis**
   1. Sweat chloride testing, diagnostic criteria:
      a. Sweat chloride >40 mmol/L in infants.
      b. Sweat chloride >60 mmol/L in children and adults.
   2. CFTR mutational analysis.

VIII. **Lung Tumors**
   A. **Lung cancer is the most common cause of cancer mortality (men and women).**
   B. **Incidence increases with age; rare before 40 years.**
   C. **Major risk factor is cigarette smoking (≥80% of cases).**
      1. Cancer risk increases with the quantity and duration of smoking.
      2. Secondhand exposure also increases risk.
   D. **Environmental exposure to radon gas, arsenic, asbestos, and ionizing radiation.**
   E. **Major histologic subtypes of lung carcinoma (Fig. 17.13).**
      1. Adenocarcinoma
         a. Most common histologic type; most common type in nonsmokers.
         b. Tend to present at the periphery of the lung.
         c. Often associated with a gain-of-function mutation in various genes (e.g., *EGFR*, *KRAS*, and *ALK*).
         d. Histology shows variable glandular formation and mucin production (mucin stains are positive).
      2. Squamous cell carcinoma
         a. Centrally located tumors arising from metaplastic squamous epithelial cells.

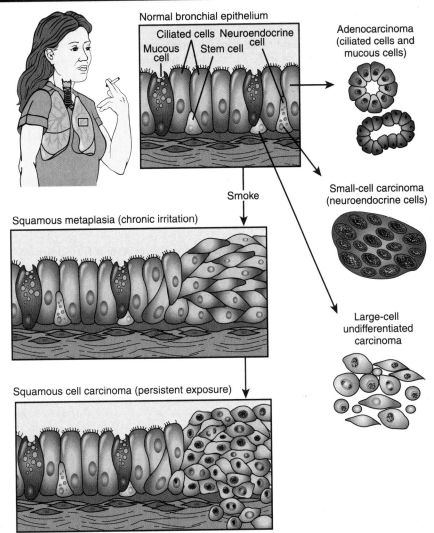

Normal bronchial epithelium

Ciliated cells   Neuroendocrine
                        cell
Mucous   Stem cell
cell

Adenocarcinoma
(ciliated cells and
mucous cells)

Small-cell carcinoma
(neuroendocrine cells)

Large-cell
undifferentiated
carcinoma

Smoke

Squamous metaplasia (chronic irritation)

Squamous cell carcinoma (persistent exposure)

17.13: Bronchogenic carcinoma. Most lung tumors originate from bronchi and are caused by smoking. The columnar epithelium undergoes squamous metaplasia, which can progress to carcinoma in situ and invasive squamous cell carcinoma. Malignant tumors composed of mucous or ciliated cells are classified as adenocarcinomas, whereas those of neuroendocrine cells are classified as small-cell carcinoma. Large-cell undifferentiated carcinomas originate from stem cells. *(From Damjanov I: Pathology for the health professions, ed 4, Philadelphia, 2012, Saunders Elsevier, p 189, Fig. 8.25.)*

      i. Chronic smoking-induced mucosal irritation of airways → squamous metaplasia → dysplasia → squamous carcinoma.
  b. More common in men; highly associated with smoking.
  c. Histology shows intercellular bridges and/or keratin production.
 3. Small-cell carcinoma
  a. Centrally located tumor of neuroendocrine cells.
  b. Highly associated with smoking, rare in nonsmokers.
  c. Histology characterized by small cells with scant cytoplasm, fine "salt and pepper" chromatin, numerous mitoses, and areas of necrosis.
  d. Aggressive tumor with early systemic spread and poor prognosis despite initial sensitivity to chemotherapy and radiation.
  e. Nearly all eventually prove fatal.
 4. Large-cell carcinoma
  a. Nonsmall cell carcinoma without definitive squamous or glandular differentiation.
F. Clinical manifestations
 1. Cough, weight loss, chest pain, dyspnea, and hemoptysis.
 2. May present with manifestations of metastatic tumor (e.g., back pain secondary to vertebral metastasis; headache, seizures, and other neurologic findings secondary to brain metastasis).

G. Complications
1. Pancoast tumor (superior sulcus tumor)
   a. Most commonly secondary to a primary squamous cell carcinoma of the lung.
   b. Tumor at the extreme apex of the lung with invasion of nearby structures (e.g., brachial plexus, subclavian artery, subclavian vein, spinal nerve roots, and paravertebral sympathetic chain).
      i. Involvement of the sympathetic ganglion results in Horner syndrome (ipsilateral ptosis, miosis, and facial anhidrosis).
2. Superior vena cava (SVC) syndrome
   a. Constellation of findings secondary to impaired venous return through the SVC.
   b. Due to any condition that obstructs the flow of blood through the SVC (lung cancer, most common).
   c. Manifestations include facial or neck swelling (exacerbated by lying down or bending).
      i. Purple-red discoloration of head and upper thorax.
   d. Headaches, confusion, or visual changes (due to cerebral edema).
3. Paraneoplastic syndromes
   a. Lambert–Eaton myasthenic syndrome
      i. Antibodies directed against P/Q-type of voltage-gated calcium channels at presynaptic neuromuscular junction impairs the release of acetylcholine.
      ii. The net effect is impaired neuromuscular transmission resulting in muscle weakness.
      iii. Usually associated with small-cell carcinoma.
   b. Ectopic hormone secretion
      i. Cushing syndrome secondary to ectopic ACTH (usually small-cell carcinoma).
      ii. Syndrome of inappropriate ADH due to the ectopic release of ADH (usually by a small-cell carcinoma).
      iii. Hypercalcemia secondary to the release of parathyroid hormone-related peptide (usually squamous cell carcinoma).

H. Diagnosis
1. Imaging, pathologic confirmation.
2. Sputum cytology.
3. Bronchoscopy (transbronchial needle aspiration, bronchioalveolar lavage, and bronchial washings or brushings).
4. CT-guided needle biopsy.

IX. Mediastinal and Pleural Disorders
A. Overview
1. The mediastinum is artificially separated into three compartments.
   a. Anterior mediastinum
      i. Extends from the posterior surface of sternum to the anterior surface of the pericardium and great vessels.
      ii. Contains thymus, adipose tissue, and lymph nodes.
      iii. Neoplasms located within this region include thymoma (see later), teratoma, and lymphoma.
   b. Middle mediastinum
      i. Extends from the posterior aspect of anterior mediastinum to the anterior longitudinal spinal ligament.
      ii. Contains the heart, pericardium, major arteries (ascending and transverse aorta, main pulmonary arteries), as well as the SVC and inferior vena cava, trachea and mainstem bronchi, and associated lymph nodes.
      iii. Neoplasms in this region include lymphoma (Hodgkin and non-Hodgkin).
   c. Posterior mediastinum
      i. Region behind the heart and trachea, includes descending thoracic aorta, esophagus, thoracic duct, and numerous neural structures (e.g., autonomic ganglion and nerves).
      ii. Neoplasms arising within this compartment are primarily of neural origin (neuroblastoma and ganglioneuroma).

B. Mediastinitis
1. Infection of the mediastinum; usually seen as a complication of cardiothoracic surgery.
   a. Less common causes include esophageal perforation, chest trauma, or direct extension of infection from contiguous site (e.g., lung).
2. Usually secondary to Gram-positive organisms
   a. *S. aureus* and *Streptococcus epidermidis*.
   b. Although less common, *Histoplasma capsulatum* may cause extensive fibrosis (chronic fibrosing mediastinitis).
3. Clinical manifestations
   a. Acute mediastinitis: fever, tachycardia, and wound drainage.
   b. Chronic fibrosing mediastinitis may present with complications related to fibrosis of surrounding tissues (e.g., constrictive pericarditis and SVC syndrome).
4. Diagnosis
   a. Imaging studies may show pneumomediastinum and air-fluid levels.
   b. CT useful to assess extent of mediastinal involvement.

C. Thymoma
1. Tumor of thymic epithelial cells; arises within the anterior mediastinum.
2. Usually benign (70% cases); commonly associated with myasthenia gravis.

3. Other associations include pure red cell aplasia, hypogammaglobulinemia, autoimmune disease (e.g., rheumatoid arthritis, systemic lupus erythematosus, and Sjogren syndrome).

D. Pleura
1. Pleural cavity is the potential space between the parietal and visceral pleurae.
    a. The parietal pleura lines the inner chest wall.
    b. The visceral pleura lines the lungs.
2. Forms right and left pleural cavity (separated by the mediastinum).
3. Negative pressure within pleural cavities helps maintain contact between visceral and parietal pleurae.
4. Contains minimal "lubricating" fluid to facilitate sliding of visceral and parietal pleura against one another.

E. Pleural effusion
1. Defined as excessive fluid within the pleural space.
2. Pathogenesis
    a. Alteration in Starling forces
        i. Increased hydrostatic pressure (e.g., heart failure) and/or decreased osmotic pressure (e.g., nephrotic syndrome and cirrhosis).
    b. Increased capillary permeability/impaired lymphatic drainage
        i. Pulmonary infarction, pneumonia, and pleural metastasis.
3. Classification of pleural effusions
    a. Transudates
        i. Protein-poor, cell-poor fluid formed as an ultrafiltrate of plasma.
        ii. Due to an alteration in Starling pressures (e.g., increased hydrostatic pressure and low oncotic pressure).
    b. Exudates
        i. Collection of protein-rich, cell-rich fluid formed secondary to increased vascular permeability (e.g., bacterial pneumonia, tuberculosis, infarction, and metastasis).
        ii. Chylous effusion refers to an exudative pleural effusion comprised of lymph; usually due to injury/obstruction of thoracic duct (tumor and trauma).
            (1) Turbid, milky fluid (due to the presence of chylomicrons).
    c. Laboratory distinction of transudates versus exudates in the pleural fluid (Table 17.2).
4. Clinical and radiologic findings
    a. Dyspnea, nonproductive cough, and chest pain.
    b. Dullness to percussion, diminished breath sounds, egophony ("E" to "A" on auscultation), and pleural friction rub (stops while holding breath as opposed to pericardial rub which persists through breath holding).
    c. Chest imaging shows blunting of the costophrenic angle, air-fluid level (Fig. 17.14).

TABLE 17.2   Pleural Fluid Transudates Versus Exudates

COMPONENTS	TRANSUDATE	EXUDATE
PF protein/serum protein	<0.5	>0.5
PF LDH/serum LDH	<0.6	>0.6
PF LDH	<200 U/L	>200 U/L

LDH, Lactate dehydrogenase; *PF*, pleural fluid.

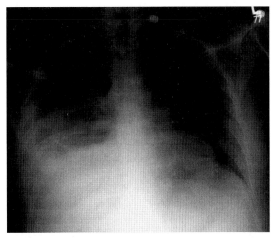

17.14: Frontal chest radiograph showing a right pleural effusion. Note the blunting of the right costophrenic angle and obscuration of the right hemidiaphragm. *(From Pretorius ES, Solomon JA: Radiology secrets, ed 2, Philadelphia, 2006, Mosby, p 539, Fig. 66.2A.)*

F. Pleuritis
1. Definition
   a. Inflammation of the pleura.
2. Background
   a. Visceral pleura (lung surface) is not innervated by pain receptors (nociceptors).
   b. Parietal pleura (chest wall) is innervated; therefore inflammation of the parietal pleura is painful.
3. Etiologies
   a. Infection (viral, bacterial, and fungal).
   b. Autoimmune disorders (e.g., systemic lupus erythematosus).
   c. Pulmonary infarction.
   d. Uremia.
4. Clinical manifestations
   a. Sharp chest pain, particularly on inspiration or with coughing ("pleuritic" chest pain).
   b. Pleural effusion may be present.

G. Pneumothorax
1. Definition
   a. Accumulation of air within the pleural space.
2. Etiologies
   a. Spontaneous
      i. Rupture of an apical subpleural bleb.
      ii. Occurs in the absence of precipitating event.
      iii. Classically seen in tall, thin males between the ages of 10 and 30 years.
      iv. Other risk factors include smoking, family history, and Marfan syndrome.
   b. Nonspontaneous
      i. Precipitating event may include penetrating chest wound, iatrogenic causes (e.g., insertion of central venous lines, mechanical ventilation, and thoracentesis), or barotrauma from scuba diving.
3. Clinical manifestations
   a. Sudden onset of dyspnea and pleuritic chest pain.
   b. Diminished breath sounds, absent tactile or vocal fremitus, and hyperresonance to percussion overlying the pneumothorax.
   c. Upright chest radiography shows white visceral pleural line (pleural edge) and the absence of vessel markings peripheral to the line.

H. Tension pneumothorax
1. Pneumothorax accompanied by the progressive accumulation of air within the pleural cavity. A complication of lung parenchymal tear (e.g., barotrauma) with flap-like tissue "valve" that allows air to enter the pleural cavity on inspiration but then closes on expiration, preventing air from exiting the pleural space.
2. With each successive breath, intrapleural pressures rise causing compression atelectasis.
3. Medical emergency; manifestations include:
   a. Sudden onset of severe dyspnea and pleuritic chest pain.
   b. Hypotension (secondary to interference with venous return).
   c. Deviation of the trachea to the contralateral side.
   d. Depression of the ipsilateral hemidiaphragm.

I. **Oral Cavity, Salivary Gland, and Neck Disorders**
   A. **Oral clefts**
      1. Cleft lip, disfigurement of the upper lip and nose, arises as a result of the failure of medial nasal and maxillary prominences to fuse during early embryologic development.
      2. Cleft palate, an open defect within the palate, occurs when the palatal shelves fail to fuse in the midline during development (Fig. 18.1).
      3. Oral clefts are the most common craniofacial malformation in the newborn.
         a. Native Americans and Alaska natives at the highest risk.
         b. Both cleft lip and palate are present in 50% of cases, more common in males.
         c. Cleft palate alone (~35% of cases); more common in females.
         d. Cleft lip alone (~15% of cases); more common in males.
      4. Complications
         a. Speech and feeding difficulties
         b. Impaired dental development
         c. Recurrent otitis media (related to eustachian tube dysfunction)
         d. Psychosocial effects
      5. Treatment is surgical correction.
   B. **Oral candidiasis (thrush)**
      1. *Candida* infection of the oropharynx (usually *Candida albicans*).
      2. Risk factors for development
         a. Use of broad-spectrum antibiotics, inhaled steroids, dentures, immunosuppression (e.g., cancer, human immunodeficiency virus [HIV]/acquired immunodeficiency syndrome [AIDS], and poorly controlled diabetes).
      3. Manifests with creamy curd-like white plaques on tongue, buccal mucosa, palate, and oropharynx. May be scraped off with tongue depressor, exposing an underlying erythematous, and friable (bleeds easily) mucosa (Fig. 18.2).
   C. **Oral hairy leukoplakia**
      1. Painless, benign white plaque (leukoplakia); typically on the lateral tongue of immunosuppressed patients (e.g., AIDS and transplant patients).
      2. Associated with Epstein–Barr virus infection.
      3. Unlike the lesions of *C. albicans*, cannot be scraped off.
   D. **Kaposi sarcoma**
      1. Low-grade malignant tumor of endothelial cells arising on the palate and other mucocutaneous surfaces.
      2. Caused by human herpesvirus 8; commonly associated with AIDS.
   E. **Aphthous ulcers (aphthous stomatitis; canker sores)**
      1. Most common cause of mouth ulceration, affects approximately one in five individuals.
      2. Localized, shallow, round to oval, and painful oral ulcers (Fig. 18.3).
      3. Often first appear in adolescence or young adulthood, decreasing in frequency with age.
      4. Etiology unclear, likely multifactorial (e.g., genetic predisposition and dysregulated immune response).
      5. Ulcers heal over 1–2 weeks but commonly recur at variable intervals.
   F. **Dental caries**
      1. Tooth decay, secondary to demineralization of dental enamel by acidic by-products from the bacterial fermentation of dietary sugars (primarily *Streptococcus mutans*).

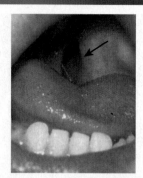

18.1: Cleft palate. Note the defect in the palate (*arrow*). *(From Grieg JD: Color atlas of surgical diagnosis, London, 1996, Mosby-Wolfe, p 68, Fig. 10.7.)*

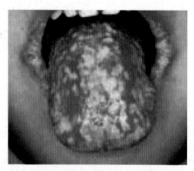

18.2: Oral thrush. Note the extensive white "curd-like" plaque that can be wiped off leaving an erythematous base. *(From Grieg JD: Color atlas of surgical diagnosis, London, 1996, Mosby-Wolfe, p 65, Fig. 10.1.)*

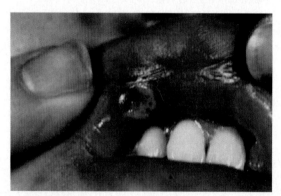

18.3: Aphthous ulcer. Note the ulcerated surface on the lip covered by a shaggy gray exudate. *(From Bouloux P: Self-assessment picture tests: medicine, Vol 1, London, 1997, Mosby-Wolfe, p 35, Fig. 69.)*

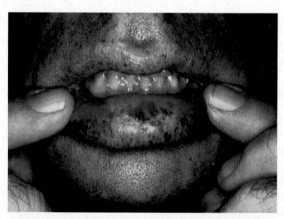

18.4: Peutz–Jeghers syndrome. Note the pigmentation in the lips. Pigmented macules may also be present on the skin (arms, legs, torso, digits, eyelids palate, and tongue). *(From Fitzpatrick JE, Morelli JG: Dermatology secrets plus, ed 4, 2011, Elsevier Mosby, p 131, Fig. 18.4.)*

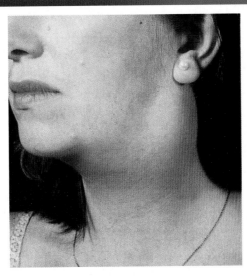

18.5: Branchial cyst. Note the lateral location of the cyst in the neck. *(From Stevens A, Lowe J, Scott I: Core pathology, ed 3, 2009, Mosby Elsevier, p 247, Fig. 12.42.)*

    2. Fluoride makes dental enamel less sensitive to the effects of acid and promotes remineralization; protects against tooth decay.
G. Pigmentary abnormalities of the oral cavity
    1. Peutz–Jeghers syndrome
        a. Rare, autosomal dominant (AD) disorder secondary to mutation in *STK11*, a tumor-suppressor gene.
        b. Triad of mucocutaneous pigmentation of the lips and oral mucosa (Fig. 18.4), hamartomatous polyps of the gastrointestinal (GI) tract, and increased risk of various malignancies (GI, pancreas, and others).
    2. Primary adrenal insufficiency
        a. Usually secondary to autoimmune destruction of the adrenal cortex (Addison disease).
        b. Deficiency of cortisol, with the associated loss of negative feedback on the pituitary, results in an increase in the release of pro-opiomelanocortin (POMC).
            i. POMC is a pituitary prohormone cleaved into adrenocorticotropic hormone (ACTH) and melanocyte-stimulating hormone (MSH).
        c. ↓ Cortisol → ↑ POMC → ↑ ACTH (and ↑ MSH)
            i. MSH stimulates melanocytes to produce more melanin (causing hyperpigmentation of the skin and buccal mucosa).
    3. Lead poisoning
        a. May cause a narrow band of bluish-black pigment along the gingiva.
H. Tooth discoloration
    1. Tetracyclines may permanently discolor developing teeth and are therefore generally avoided in children younger than 8 years of age.
    2. Excess fluoride can cause chalky white mottling of the teeth (called fluorosis).
I. Macroglossia (enlarged tongue)
    1. Associations include hypothyroidism, Down syndrome, acromegaly, systemic amyloidosis, and mucosal neuromas; the latter associated with multiple endocrine neoplasia (MEN) 2B.
J. Atrophic glossitis
    1. Erythematous and smooth tongue, due to atrophy of filiform papillae.
    2. Etiologies include malnutrition, vitamin deficiencies (iron, B12, and folate); presents with pain and burning.
K. Geographic tongue
    1. Recurrent benign inflammatory disorder of unknown etiology; causes map-like white discoloration on the dorsum of the tongue.
    2. Lesions can change in size and location rapidly, thus the alternative name of "benign migratory glossitis."
    3. Usually asymptomatic, some have mild discomfort with burning and food sensitivity.
L. Mucoceles
    1. Benign, soft, fluctuant pink to blue cystic lesion, usually on the lower lip.
    2. Comprised of extravasated mucus from a damaged minor salivary gland or duct, characteristically following trauma (e.g., accidental biting of the lip).
    3. Often resolve spontaneously, recurrences are surgically excised.
M. Oral leukoplakia and erythroplakia
    1. Definitions
        a. Leukoplakia and erythroplakia are clinical terms used to refer to a white or red plaque, respectively.

i. When both findings are present, called leukoerythroplakia.
2. Clinical significance
   a. Leukoplakia or erythroplakia (especially) often indicate the presence of dysplasia and/or cancer (squamous cell car-cinoma), explaining the necessity for biopsy.
3. Risk factors
   a. Alcohol, tobacco (smoking and smokeless), and human papilloma virus (HPV).

N. Lichen planus
1. Chronic inflammatory disorder of the skin and/or mucous membranes mediated by a T-cell lymphocytic reaction to antigens within the surface epithelium.
2. Often has a reticular lacy appearance ("Wickham striae").

O. Odontogenic cysts
1. Epithelial-lined cyst derived from odontogenic epithelium.
2. A specific type, known as a dentigerous cyst, usually presents in third to fourth decade of life, typically in association with an unerupted tooth (e.g., third molar).

P. Ameloblastoma
1. Slow growing but locally invasive benign neoplasm of the jaw.
2. Arises from odontogenic epithelium, commonly near the third molar.
3. Peak incidence in third to fourth decade of life; equally common in males and females.
4. Imaging shows multiloculated radiolucency ("soap bubble-like").
5. Treatment is wide surgical resection.

Q. Squamous cell carcinoma of the oral cavity
1. Most common malignancy of the oral cavity; more common in males.
2. Risk factors
   a. Tobacco (including smokeless tobacco) and alcohol.
   b. HPV (primarily HPV-16), especially in young adults.
   c. Chewing betel (areca) nut (common etiology in Asian countries).
3. Most common sites include:
   a. Base of tongue and tonsillar region (especially in association with HPV).
   b. Lower lip (UV radiation and pipe smoking).
   c. Floor of the mouth and lateral border of the tongue (smokeless tobacco, cigarettes, and alcohol).
4. Regional metastasis to cervical lymph nodes.

R. Sialolithiasis
1. Formation of calculi within a salivary gland or duct; most commonly involving the submandibular gland.
2. Due to stasis of salivary flow in conjunction with duct obstruction.
3. Risk factors
   a. Hypovolemia (e.g., decreased fluid intake and use of diuretics).
   b. Decreased salivary secretions (e.g., use of anticholinergic agents).
   c. Smoking.
4. Presents with pain and swelling of the involved gland, especially after meals (postprandial).

S. Sialadenitis
1. Inflammation of the salivary gland.
2. Etiologies include viral infection (e.g., mumps and HIV), acute bacterial infection (*Staphylococcus aureus*, most common), Sjögren syndrome, and malnutrition.

T. Sjögren syndrome
1. Chronic autoimmune disorder of exocrine glands, particularly affecting salivary and lacrimal glands.
2. Presents with dry eyes and mouth (secondary to diminished lacrimal and salivary secretions, respectively).
   a. Systemic manifestations include generalized malaise, low-grade fever, myalgia, and arthralgia.
3. Antibodies to SSA (anti-Ro) and/or SSB (anti-La) are common but nonspecific.
4. Histology reveals lymphocytic inflammation and glandular atrophy.
   a. Lip biopsy may be used to confirm the diagnosis.

U. Salivary gland tumors
1. Overview
   a. Majority of salivary gland tumors arise within the parotid gland (~80%), most of which (~75%) are benign.
   b. Tumors arising within the other salivary glands (e.g., submandibular, sublingual, and minor) are more likely to be malignant.
   c. Radiation exposure increases the risk (both benign and malignant tumors).
2. Specific tumor types
   a. Pleomorphic adenoma (benign mixed tumor)
      i. Most common benign salivary gland tumor; usually arising within the parotid gland.
      ii. Comprised of an admixture of ductal epithelial cells, myoepithelial cells, and mesenchymal cells.
         (1) Histology reveals epithelial cells within a background of myxomatous tissue (loose connective tissue/mucus) and cartilage.

   iii. Presents as a mobile painless mass.
   iv. Treatment is surgical resection (superficial parotidectomy).
   v. High risk of recurrence if incompletely excised, small risk of malignant transformation (facial nerve palsy is evidence of malignancy).
  b. Warthin tumor (papillary cystadenoma lymphomatosum)
   i. Second most common benign salivary gland tumor.
   ii. More common in males and strongly associated with smoking; arises exclusively within the parotid gland.
   iii. Microscopic examination reveals a double layer of eosinophilic (red) epithelial cells with underlying dense lymphoid infiltrate.
  c. Mucoepidermoid carcinoma
   i. Most common primary malignant salivary gland tumor.
   ii. Usually arises within the parotid gland; less common within other glands (including the minor salivary glands).
   iii. Histologic findings include an admixture of mucin-producing columnar cells, epidermoid (squamous) cells, and polygonal intermediate cells.
   iv. Ranges from low to high grade; prognosis varies accordingly.
  d. Adenoid cystic carcinoma
   i. Slow growing but high-grade malignant salivary gland tumor.
   ii. May arise within either major or minor salivary glands.
   iii. Cells are arranged concentrically around gland-like spaces.
   iv. Growth around nerves (perineural invasion) makes complete surgical resection difficult and thus recurrence is common.

V. Lingual thyroid
1. Refers to the presence of ectopic, but otherwise normal, thyroid tissue at the base of the tongue.
2. Due to the failure of descent during embryologic development.
3. More common in females.
4. May represent the entirety of thyroid tissue.
5. Enlargement can lead to obstructive symptoms (e.g., dysphagia, dyspnea, and dysphonia).

W. Thyroglossal duct cyst
1. Thyroglossal duct becomes obliterated early in embryonic life, but occasionally persists as a cyst within the midline of the neck in close association with the hyoid bone.
2. Due to anomalous migration of thyroid tissue during early gestation.
3. Affects males and females equally.

X. Branchial cleft cyst
1. Congenital anomaly usually presenting in childhood as a lateral neck cyst anterior to the sternocleidomastoid muscle (Fig. 18.5).
2. Due to the incomplete involution of the second branchial cleft.
3. Complications include recurrent infection; treated by surgical excision.

II. Esophageal Disorders
A. Overview of anatomy
1. Upper third of the esophagus contains striated muscle.
2. Middle third has a mixture of both striated and smooth muscle.

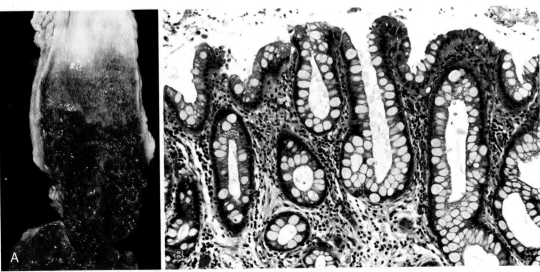

18.6: (A) Gross appearance of reflux esophagitis. Marked hyperemia with focal hemorrhage is present in the area of reflux. (B) Barrett esophagus. This biopsy specimen from the distal esophagus shows intestinal metaplasia with numerous goblet cells replacing squamous epithelium. (A, From Rosai J: Rosai and Ackerman's surgical pathology, ed 9, St. Louis, 2004, Mosby, p 619, Fig. 11.7; B, from Iacobuzio-Donahue CA, Montgomery E, Goldblum JR: Gastrointestinal and liver pathology, ed 2, 2012, Saunders Elsevier, p 44, Fig. 2.12.)

3. Distal third contains smooth muscle.
4. Esophageal lumen is lined by nonkeratinized stratified squamous epithelium.

B. Signs and symptoms of esophageal disease
1. Heartburn (pyrosis)
   a. Burning sensation in the lower chest associated with the reflux of gastric contents into the distal esophagus; tends to worsen with recumbency or with bending.
2. Dysphagia
   a. Refers to difficulty swallowing.
      i. Dysphagia for solid foods alone is characteristic of physical obstruction (e.g., tumor and stricture).
      ii. Dysphagia for solids and liquids is characteristic of disordered motility (e.g., achalasia).

C. Miscellaneous esophageal disorders
1. Tracheoesophageal (TE) fistula
   a. Abnormal connection between the trachea and the esophagus.
   b. The most common type (~84%) consists of esophageal atresia (due to failure of primitive foregut to recanalize) along with a connection (fistula) between the distal esophagus and the trachea (due to failure of lung bud to separate completely from the foregut).
   c. Clinical manifestations include:
      i. Excess amniotic fluid (polyhydramnios); due to inability to swallow, and thus reabsorb, amniotic fluid.
      ii. Abdominal distention (air enters the stomach through fistula between trachea and esophagus).
      iii. Feeding difficulties (food is regurgitated from the blind esophageal loop, risk of aspiration).
   d. TE fistula is often accompanied by other anomalies.
      i. VACTERL (Vertebral anomalies, Anal atresia, Cardiac defects, TE fistula, Renal defects, and Limb defects).

D. Plummer–Vinson syndrome
1. Triad of iron deficiency anemia, dysphagia, and esophageal web (the latter causing dysphagia for solids).
   a. Some also have angular cheilitis and glossitis.
2. Etiology is unknown; however, iron deficiency is thought to be a contributing factor.
3. More common in middle-aged females.
4. Risk factor for the development of squamous cell carcinoma of esophagus and pharynx.

E. Esophageal diverticula
1. Overview
   a. Diverticula represent an "outpouching" of a hollow organ.
   b. "True" diverticula contain all layers of the wall (i.e., mucosa, submucosa, and muscularis propria); "false" diverticula contain only mucosa and submucosa.
   c. Pulsion diverticula arise through areas of weakness.
   d. Traction diverticula are due to extrinsic traction ("pulling effect") on the organ.
2. Zenker diverticulum
   a. Pulsion-type diverticulum occurring between the cricopharyngeal muscle and inferior constrictor muscle (area of weakness is known as Killian triangle).
   b. Clinical manifestations (e.g., halitosis and regurgitation of food) are due to the retention of food within the diverticulum.
   c. Complications include aspiration of retained food, ulceration/bleeding, and squamous cell carcinoma (rare).
3. Traction diverticulum
   a. Diverticulum characteristically arising near the midpoint of the esophagus in association with external traction from an adjacent inflammatory process (e.g., cancer).

F. Hiatal hernia (HH)
1. Herniation of abdominal tissue (usually the stomach) through the esophageal hiatus of the diaphragm.
2. Two types
   a. "Sliding" (the most common type)
      i. Characterized by a "sliding" of the gastroesophageal junction and gastric cardia upward through the hiatus.
      ii. Often asymptomatic; however, larger hernias are associated with an increased risk of gastroesophageal reflux disease (GERD).
   b. Paraesophageal HH (uncommon, ~5% of cases)
      i. Characterized by herniation of the gastric fundus through the hiatus adjacent to the esophagus.
      ii. In addition to GERD, paraesophageal hernias are associated with higher risk of complications (e.g., ulceration, erosions, and ischemia of herniated tissue).

G. GERD
1. Clinical syndrome secondary to the pathologic reflux of gastric acid and bile into the distal esophagus.
2. Prevalence of ~10%–20% in the adult population.
3. Pathogenesis
   a. Incompetence and/or transient relaxation of the lower esophageal sphincter (LES) that allows the reflux of gastric contents into the distal esophagus.

b. Risk factors include HH, pregnancy, alcohol, caffeine, fatty foods, chocolate, obesity, and medications (e.g., calcium channel blockers).

c. *Helicobacter pylori* does not contribute to the development of GERD.

4. Clinical manifestations

   a. Heartburn (retrosternal burning sensation, usually postprandial).

   b. Regurgitation of gastric contents, bitter taste, and halitosis.

5. Complications of chronic GERD

   a. Reflux esophagitis (inflammation of distal esophagus, Fig. 18.6A).

   b. Esophageal ulceration/stricture formation; can cause odynophagia (painful swallowing) and/or dysphagia (difficulty swallowing).

   c. Chronic laryngitis (acid injury to vocal cords).

   d. Dental caries (acid injury to the tooth enamel; also common in bulimia nervosa).

   e. Aspiration pneumonitis/pneumonia.

   f. Barrett esophagus (intestinal metaplasia of distal esophagus, Fig. 18.6B)

      i. Normal esophagus is lined by nonkeratinized stratified squamous epithelium.

      ii. Chronic mucosal irritation secondary to recurrent reflux may, in some cases, cause intestinal metaplasia of the distal esophagus (known as Barrett esophagus).

        (1) Squamous epithelium → columnar epithelium with goblet cells (Barrett esophagus).

      iii. Metaplasia → increased risk of adenocarcinoma of the distal esophagus.

6. Diagnosis of GERD

   a. Usually based on the characteristic clinical history.

   b. If necessary, diagnostic testing includes:

      i. Twenty-four-hour esophageal pH monitoring (abnormally low pH).

      ii. Esophageal endoscopy.

      iii. Manometry (abnormally reduced LES pressure).

H. Infectious esophagitis

1. Infections of the esophagus are more common in immunosuppressed patients (e.g., AIDS, transplant, etc.).

2. Presents with painful swallowing (odynophagia).

3. Pathogens include:

   a. Herpes simplex virus

      i. Endoscopy shows discrete "punched-out" ulcers.

      ii. Biopsies show multinucleated cells with intranuclear inclusions.

   b. Cytomegalovirus

      i. Endoscopy shows shallow serpiginous ulcers.

      ii. Biopsies show large cells with eosinophilic nuclear and cytoplasmic inclusions.

   c. *Candida*

      i. Endoscopy shows yellow-white mucosal plaques.

      ii. Biopsies show fungal yeasts and pseudohyphae (extended yeast forms).

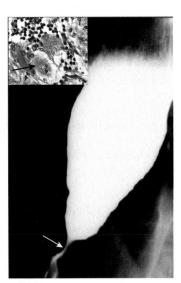

18.7: Barium study of the esophagus in achalasia. Note the dilated esophagus ending in a narrowed esophagogastric junction ("birds-beak" appearance) (*white arrow*). The esophagus proximal to the lower esophageal sphincter is dilated. The inset shows the myenteric plexus with T lymphocytes (*dark cells*) destroying ganglia in the myenteric plexus (*black arrow*). *(From Kliegman R: Nelson textbook of pediatrics, ed 19, Philadelphia, 2011, Elsevier Saunders, p 1265, Fig. 313.1. Inset from Iacobuzio-Donahue CA, Montgomery E, Goldblum JR: Gastrointestinal and liver pathology, ed 2, 2012, Saunders Elsevier, p 13, Fig. 1.18.)*

I. **Medication-induced esophagitis**
1. Pills that lodge within the esophagus may cause direct mucosal injury, usually in association with "dry swallow" (swallowing of pills without fluid).
2. Specific agents (e.g., tetracyclines, nonsteroidal antiinflammatory drugs [NSAIDs], bisphosphonates, ferrous sulfate, and potassium chloride) are particularly injurious.
3. Clinical manifestations include pain on swallowing (odynophagia) and retrosternal pain.

J. **Corrosive esophagitis**
1. Inflammation of the esophagus (esophagitis) secondary to the ingestion of a caustic substance (typically strong acid or alkali), either accidental or in an attempted suicide.
2. Complications include stricture formation, perforation, and squamous cell carcinoma.

K. **Esophageal varices**
1. Dilated submucosal veins of the distal esophagus connecting the portal and systemic circulations.
2. Occur as a complication of portal hypertension, usually in association with cirrhosis.
3. Rupture causes massive hematemesis (vomiting blood), a common cause of death in those with cirrhosis.

L. **Mallory–Weiss syndrome**
1. Longitudinal mucosal tear in the proximal stomach and distal esophagus causing the vomiting of blood (hematemesis).
2. Due to acute increased intragastric and intraabdominal pressures in association with a period of severe vomiting/retching (commonly follows the ingestion of alcohol or in bulimia).

M. **Boerhaave syndrome**
1. "Spontaneous" rupture of the esophagus in association with acutely increased intra-esophageal pressure; characteristically associated with severe vomiting/retching.
2. Presents with the acute onset of severe retrosternal chest pain.
3. Complications
    a. Pneumomediastinum (air in the mediastinum)
        i. Crepitus on palpation of the chest wall and/or crackling sound on auscultation of the chest (Hamman sign).
    b. Pleural effusion (elevated salivary amylase within the pleural fluid).
4. High morbidity and mortality; requires immediate surgical repair.

N. **Achalasia**
1. Esophageal motility disorder characterized by incomplete relaxation of the LES and lack of peristalsis.
    a. Due to degeneration of nitric oxide-producing ganglion cells in the myenteric plexus of the esophageal wall.
    b. Nitric oxide normally allows the LES to relax; the loss of nitric oxide therefore causes LES tone to rise.
2. Epidemiology
    a. Usually presents in the middle age (25–60 years); men and women are equally affected.
    b. Increased risk of developing esophageal cancer, particularly squamous cell carcinoma.
3. Clinical manifestations
    a. Dysphagia for solids and liquids.
    b. Regurgitation of retained material within the esophagus.
    c. Weight loss.
    d. Nocturnal coughing (due to chronic regurgitation).
4. Diagnosis
    a. Manometry reveals incomplete relaxation of the LES and lack of peristalsis.
    b. Barium esophagram shows a dilated esophagus with "bird beak-like" tapering at the distal end (Fig. 18.7).
5. Chagas' disease is an acquired cause of achalasia.
    a. *Trypanosoma cruzi* and associated host immune response destroys ganglion cells within the esophagus and elsewhere.

O. **Diffuse esophageal spasm**
1. Uncommon hypermotility disorder of the esophagus of unknown etiology (thought likely associated with neuronal dysfunction of myenteric plexus).
2. More common in females; manifestations include chest pain and dysphagia for solids and liquids.
3. Barium esophagram reveals a "corkscrew" esophagus.

P. **Esophageal cancer**
1. Overview
    a. Esophageal cancers initially metastasize to regional lymph nodes before spreading to liver, lungs, and bone.
    b. Early manifestations are nonspecific (e.g., weight loss, hematemesis, and nausea). Over time, patients develop dysphagia (initially for solids, later for liquids as well due to progressive luminal narrowing by expanding tumor), indicative of poor prognosis.
    c. Diagnosis: endoscopy with biopsy.
2. Adenocarcinoma
    a. Most common primary esophageal malignancy in the United States, usually arises within the distal esophagus in association with Barrett esophagus.
    b. Risk factors include male sex, increasing age, White race, and long history of gastroesophageal reflux (with Barrett esophagus).

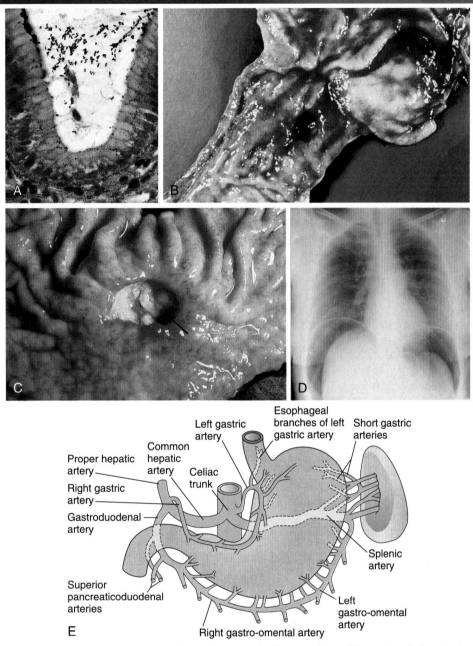

18.8: (A) Silver stain showing *Helicobacter pylori* in the superficial mucus layer. (B) Duodenal ulcer in the first part of the duodenum. (C) Gastric ulcer. Note the sharply delimited peptic ulcer with converging folds of normal gastric mucosa in the upper half. The base of the ulcer contains white necrotic debris, and a bleeding site is note in the right lower quadrant (*black arrow*). (D) Plain abdominal radiograph in a supine patient with a perforated peptic ulcer. Note the presence of air under both diaphragms. (E) Schematic of arterial system in the stomach. The gastroduodenal artery and the left gastric artery are eroded by a duodenal ulcer and gastric ulcer, respectively. *(A, From Kumar V, Fausto N, Abbas A: Robbins and Cotran pathologic basis of disease, ed 7, Philadelphia, 2004, Saunders, p 815, Fig. 17.15; B, from Damjanov I, Linder J: Anderson's pathology, ed 10, St. Louis, 1996, Mosby, p 1680, Fig. 53.21B; C, from Rosai J: Rosai and Ackerman's surgical pathology, ed 10, 2011, Mosby Elsevier, p 621, Fig. 11.30B; D, from Goldman L, Ausiello D: Cecil's textbook of medicine, ed 23, Philadelphia, 2008, Saunders Elsevier, p 1015, Fig. 142.3; E, from Moore A, Roy W: Rapid review gross and developmental anatomy, ed 3, Philadelphia, 2010, Mosby Elsevier, p 73, Fig. 3.15.)*

   3. Squamous cell carcinoma
      a. Most common esophageal malignancy worldwide; the second most common in the United States; more common in African Americans, males.
      b. Most commonly arises within the proximal to mid esophagus, usually in association with smoking and/or alcohol abuse (synergistic effect).
         i. Less common risk factors include achalasia, Plummer–Vinson syndrome, and radiation-induced strictures.

III. Gastric Disorders
   A. Manifestations include:
      1. Hematemesis (vomiting blood), etiologies include:

     a. Peptic ulcer disease (PUD) (the most common cause).

     b. Gastroesophageal varices.

     c. Hemorrhagic gastritis/gastropathy.

  2. Melena (dark, tarry stools)

     a. Usually signifies an upper GI bleed (i.e., proximal to the ligament of Treitz).

     b. Due to the conversion of hemoglobin into hematin (black pigment) by gastric acid.

  3. Vomiting.

B. Infantile hypertrophic pyloric stenosis (IHPS)

  1. characterized by hypertrophy of the gastric pyloric musculature resulting in near-complete obstruction of gastric outlet and forceful (projectile) vomiting.

  2. More common in males (4:1).

  3. Hereditary and environmental factors

     a. Risk factors include family history, maternal smoking during pregnancy, and the use of macrolide antibiotics in the first 2 weeks of life.

     b. Note that pyloric stenosis can also occur in older individuals as a complication of pyloric ulceration/scar formation.

  4. IHPS is not present at birth; most cases appear between 3 and 6 weeks of age.

  5. Clinical findings

     a. Nonbilious projectile vomiting.

     b. Palpable hypertrophied pylorus in the epigastrium ("olive").

     c. Visible hyperperistalsis.

  6. Diagnosis: abdominal ultrasound.

  7. Treatment: surgical (pyloromyotomy).

C. Gastroparesis

  1. Delayed gastric emptying in the absence of mechanical obstruction.

  2. Etiology is often unknown (idiopathic); known associations include:

     a. Diabetes mellitus (autonomic neuropathy).

     b. Medications (e.g., opioid analgesics, calcium channel blockers, and anticholinergics).

     c. Surgical (e.g., injury to vagus nerve).

  3. Clinical manifestations

     a. Early satiety (the feeling of fullness after ingesting only a small amount).

     b. Bloating, nausea, vomiting of undigested food, and upper abdominal pain.

D. Gastritis

  1. Inflammation of the gastric mucosa; may be associated with erosions (partial thickness defect in the mucosa) or ulceration (full thickness defect in the mucosa extending into the submucosa or deeper).

  2. Often classified as "acute" versus "chronic"

     a. Acute gastritis may be used to indicate a short-term disease and/or the presence of neutrophils in the inflammatory infiltrate.

     b. Chronic gastritis may be used to indicate a longer-term disease and/or the presence of chronic inflammatory cells (i.e., lymphocytes, plasma cells, and macrophages) in the inflammatory infiltrate.

  3. Infection (H. pylori)

     a. *H. pylori* infection primarily involves the gastric antrum.

       i. Organisms reside within the superficial gastric mucus layer (Fig. 18.8A).

     b. The major cause of PUD; especially common in areas of poor sanitation and crowded living conditions.

     c. H. pylori is not invasive, instead damages the mucosa via the release of various enzymes (e.g., urease).

       i. Urease hydrolyzes urea into toxic compounds (e.g., ammonium chloride) that directly damage the mucosa.

     d. Host immune response contributes to tissue injury.

     e. Virulence related to the presence of cytotoxin-associated gene A (CagA) and vacuolating cytotoxin (VacA) genes.

     f. Testing for *H. pylori*

       i. Stool antigen assay

         (1) Direct detection of bacterial antigen in stool sample.

         (2) Useful in the diagnosis of acute infection and/or to confirm eradication following treatment.

       ii. Urea breath test

         (1) Based upon the hydrolysis of urea to produce carbon dioxide and ammonia.

         (2) Urea with a radiolabeled carbon is given by mouth. If *H. pylori* is present, urease liberates the labeled CO_2 which is then detected in a breath sample.

         (3) Useful to make the diagnosis of acute infection as well as to confirm eradication following treatment.

       iii. Histologic examination

         (1) Allows direct visualization of the organism from a biopsy of the gastric antrum.

         (2) Useful for diagnosis and/or confirmation of eradication following treatment.

       iv. Biopsy urease test

         (1) Gastric biopsy specimen is placed in a medium-containing urea and a pH reagent. If *H. pylori* is present, urease cleaves urea, liberating ammonia and elevating the pH (pH reagent exhibits a color change).

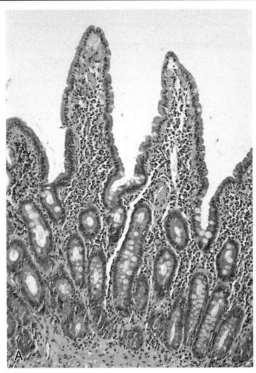
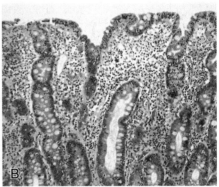

18.9: (A) Normal villus in the small intestine. (B) Celiac disease showing subtotal atrophy of the villi, lengthening of the crypts, and a heavy chronic inflammatory infiltrate in the lamina propria. *(A, From Damjanov I, Linder J: Pathology: a color atlas, St. Louis, 2000, Mosby, p 128, Fig. 7.25B; B, from Damjanov I, Linder J: Pathology: a color atlas, St. Louis, 2000, Mosby, p 128, Fig. 7.25A.)*

    (2) Useful for diagnosis and/or confirmation of eradication following treatment.
   v. Serology (IgG test)
    (1) Questionable accuracy and does not differentiate active from previous infection (i.e., cannot be used to confirm eradication).
   vi. Culture
    (1) Rarely performed (*H. pylori* is difficult to grow).
  g. Clinical manifestations
   i. Epigastric pain, bleeding (iron deficiency possible complication), and ulceration.
  h. Other disease associations with *H. pylori* include:
   i. Gastric adenocarcinoma.
   ii. Low-grade B-cell mucosa-associated lymphoid tissue (MALT) lymphoma (extranodal marginal zone lymphoma).
 4. Autoimmune metaplastic atrophic gastritis
  a. Definition
   i. T-cell-mediated destruction of parietal cells; causes loss of gastric acid and intrinsic factor (IF).
   ii. Although not thought to be pathologic, antibodies against the H+/K+-ATPase (proton pump) and IF are useful diagnostically.
  b. Epidemiology
   i. Relatively common in older adults (~2%).
   ii. More common in women, the median age at diagnosis ⊠60 years.
  c. Sequelae
   i. Pernicious anemia
    (1) Anemia developing as a result of vitamin B12 deficiency in association with inadequate IF (cannot absorb B12 without IF).
   ii. Gastric atrophy
    (1) Loss of gastric glands, often associated with the development of intestinal metaplasia (increasing one's risk of gastric adenocarcinoma).
   iii. Neuroendocrine cell hyperplasia
    (1) Increased risk of well-differentiated neuroendocrine (carcinoid) tumor.
   iv. Hypergastrinemia
    (1) Loss of parietal cells → loss of gastric acid → loss of negative feedback on G cells → hypergastrinemia.
  d. Pathology
   i. Chronic inflammatory infiltrate involving the lamina propria (i.e., chronic gastritis).
   ii. Intestinal metaplasia (similar to Barrett esophagus), a potential precursor to the development of adenocarcinoma.

E. Acute hemorrhagic erosive gastropathy
1. Definition
   a. Erosive lesions and hemorrhage of the gastric mucosa in the absence of inflammation.
   b. Due to exposure of gastric mucosa to toxic substances or to a reduction in mucosal blood flow.
2. Etiologies
   a. NSAIDs
      i. NSAIDs inhibit cyclooxygenase, thereby decreasing gastric prostaglandin production (necessary for mucosal defense).
   b. Cocaine
      i. Activation of alpha-1 receptors on vascular smooth muscle causes intense vasoconstriction, potentially causing ischemic injury to the stomach and other tissues.
   c. Stress ulcers (severe physiologic stress), mechanisms include:
      i. Severe burns → hypovolemic-induced mucosal ischemia (called "Curling ulcer").
      ii. Head trauma → increased vagal outflow → stimulation of parietal cells to increase production of gastric acid → gastric ulceration (called "Cushing ulcer").
3. Clinical manifestations
   a. Abdominal discomfort/pain.
   b. Nausea, vomiting, and hematemesis (occult or massive bleeding).

F. Ménétrier disease (protein-losing hypertrophic gastropathy)
1. Rare, acquired condition of the stomach associated with giant mucosal folds and hypoalbuminemia, the latter due to a loss of protein-rich gastric secretions.
2. Pathogenesis believed related to the local overproduction of transforming growth factor-alpha, which activates epidermal growth factor signaling and proliferation of mucus-producing cells. The net result is giant gastric rugae and the hypersecretion of a protein-rich mucus (and thus hypoalbuminemia due to protein loss).
3. Clinical manifestations
   a. Epigastric pain, anorexia, nausea, vomiting, and weight loss.
   b. Edema (due to loss of albumin and associated reduction in oncotic pressure).

G. Peptic ulcer disease (PUD)
1. PUD refers to the presence of one (usually) or more ulcers within the stomach and/or duodenum (Fig. 18.8B and C)
2. Two major etiologic factors
   a. *H. pylori*
      i. The most common factor overall (decreasing incidence in developed countries due to improved hygiene).
      ii. Eradication of infection enhances the healing of ulcers and prevents recurrence.
   b. NSAIDs
      i. Via the inhibition of cyclooxygenase, NSAIDs reduce mucosal prostaglandin production (necessary for the maintenance of normal mucosal defense).
         (1) Prostaglandins promote the production of mucous-bicarbonate barrier, microcirculation, and gastric mucosal regeneration.
3. Additional risk factors
   a. Smoking—inhibits ulcer healing and increases recurrence risk.
   b. Alcohol, especially in high concentrations, directly injures the mucosa.
4. Epidemiology
   a. Incidence of peptic ulceration increases with aging.
   b. Duodenal ulcers are more common than gastric ulcers; incidence of bleeding is the same.
5. Pathology
   a. Ulcers are clean, sharply demarcated, and slightly elevated around the edges.
   b. Most gastric ulcers are benign; however, gastric cancers may ulcerate. For this reason, most gastric ulcers are biopsied.
   c. Duodenal ulcers are rarely, if ever, malignant—do not need to be biopsied.
   d. Ulcer base is comprised of necrotic cellular debris, neutrophilic inflammation, granulation tissue, and fibrosis.
   e. Most duodenal ulcers arise within the first portion of the duodenum, whereas gastric ulcers tend to arise on the lesser curvature near the incisura angularis.
6. Clinical manifestations
   a. Epigastric pain (the most common symptom)
      i. Pain usually worse following meals (gastric ulcer).
      ii. Pain developing 2–5 hours after a meal and/or at night between 11:00 p.m. and 2:00 a.m. (peak gastric acid secretion) is characteristic of duodenal ulcers.
7. Complications
   a. Bleeding (hematemesis), the most common complication

i. Gastric ulcers may erode into the left gastric artery (Fig. 18.8E).
ii. Duodenal ulcers erode into the gastroduodenal artery.
b. Perforation (see air under diaphragm on imaging, Fig. 18.8D).
c. Gastric outlet obstruction (due to scarring at the pylorus), the least common complication.
H. Zollinger–Ellison (ZE) syndrome
1. ZE syndrome is characterized by the overproduction of gastric acid due to a gastrin-secreting tumor ("Gastrinoma").
a. Gastrinomas, which are often malignant, most commonly arise within the duodenum. Less commonly, they may be seen in the pancreas and elsewhere.
b. The autonomous secretion of gastrin leads to parietal cell hyperplasia and the release of excess gastric acid.
2. Most are sporadic; however, up to a third are associated with MEN Type I syndrome.

Multiple endocrine neoplasia (MEN) Type I

- Autosomal-dominant mutation in **MEN1**, encodes the tumor-suppressor menin.
- Manifestations can be remembered by the acronym "PPP" (pituitary, pancreas, and parathyroid).
  - Primary hyperparathyroidism (parathyroid adenoma or hyperplasia) is the most common manifestation.
  - Pancreatic neuroendocrine tumors (gastrinoma is most common).
  - Pituitary tumors may be functioning (produce hormones) or nonfunctioning; potential for compressive symptoms (e.g., visual field deficits).
- A personal or family history of parathyroid or pituitary tumors is a clue to the diagnosis of MEN I.

3. Excess gastric acid leads to the development of peptic ulcers; most of which are single and located in the typical locations as discussed above.
a. Other manifestations, which are useful clues to the diagnosis, include the presence of multiple ulcers, ulcers in unusual locations (e.g., distal duodenum and jejunum), ulcers that are resistant to therapy, and/or ulcers in association with diarrhea.
i. Inactivation of pancreatic enzymes in the acidic environment created by the excess acid can cause maldigestion and diarrhea.
4. Clinical findings
a. Epigastric pain (the most common complaint) with weight loss.
b. Heartburn (due to reflux of acidic gastric contents).
c. Single or multiple peptic ulcers.
d. Acid hypersecretion with maldigestion of food (acid interference with pancreatic enzyme activity) and diarrhea.
5. Laboratory findings include:
a. Markedly elevated serum gastrin level >1000 pg/mL (best screen).
b. Secretin stimulation test (provocative test) shows increased serum gastrin.
I. Gastric polyps
1. Definition
a. Small, sessile growths arising from the gastric mucosa.
2. Subtypes
a. Fundic gland polyp
i. Most common subtype in the United States.
ii. Arise in the body and fundus of the stomach.
iii. Often arise sporadically, increased incidence with:
(1) Use of proton pump inhibitors (e.g., omeprazole, lansoprazole, rabeprazole, pantoprazole, and esomeprazole).
(2) Familial adenomatous polyposis (FAP).
b. Hyperplastic polyp
i. Most common gastric polyp in regions of the world where *H. pylori* infection remains prevalent.
ii. Unlike "hyperplastic" colon polyps, hyperplastic gastric polyps are associated with a small risk of malignant transformation.
c. Adenomatous polyp ("gastric adenoma")
i. Adenomatous polyps are dysplastic by definition and therefore associated with a small risk of malignant transformation.
3. Clinical manifestations
a. Gastric polyps are usually asymptomatic and therefore often an incidental finding at endoscopy performed for some other reason.
J. Gastric adenocarcinoma
1. Definition
a. Malignancy of glandular cells of the gastric mucosa.
2. Epidemiology
a. Uncommon in the United States; higher incidence in the Far East (e.g., Japan), Eastern Europe, as well as Central and South America.

3. Risk factors
  a. Intestinal metaplasia of the stomach (usually in association with long-standing H. pylori infection or chronic atrophic gastritis).
  b. Presence of adenomatous gastric polyps.
  c. Ingestion of salt-preserved foods.
  d. Blood group A (reason unknown).
  e. Hereditary diffuse-type gastric cancer
    i. Autosomal dominant; <1% of all gastric cancer.
    ii. Due to mutations in the *CDH1* gene-encoding E-cadherin (see discussion below).
4. Histologic subtypes
  a. Intestinal-type gastric adenocarcinoma
    i. Intestinal metaplasia, a major risk factor.
    ii. Presents as an exophytic, and often ulcerated, mass with infiltrative glands on histologic examination.
  b. Diffuse-type gastric adenocarcinoma
    i. Characterized by the diffuse infiltration of malignant cells (due to loss of the cell adhesion molecule, E-cadherin).
    ii. Stomach may become diffusely thick and rigid ("linitis plastica").
    iii. Tumor cells have "signet ring" appearance due to intracellular mucin vacuole (mucin stains help to identify).
    iv. "Krukenberg tumor" refers to the hematogenous spread of signet ring cells from the stomach (or other sites) to the ovaries (does not represent tumor seeding).
5. Clinical manifestations
  a. Often asymptomatic until late in the disease course.
  b. Weight loss, abdominal pain, anorexia, or early satiety.
  c. Bleeding may occur, potentially resulting in anemia.
  d. Metastasis to the left supraclavicular lymph node (Virchow node) and/or periumbilical region (Sister Mary Joseph nodule).
  e. Paraneoplastic skin lesions
    i. Acanthosis nigricans.
    ii. Sudden appearance of multiple seborrheic keratoses (sign of Leser–Trélat).
6. Diagnosis
  a. Endoscopy with biopsy.
7. Prognosis
  a. Poor in most cases, due to the advanced stage at time of diagnosis.

K. Primary gastric lymphoma
1. The GI tract, particularly the stomach, is the most common site for the development of an extranodal non-Hodgkin lymphoma.
  a. "Extranodal" meaning that the lymphoma did not arise from a lymph node.
2. Most are a "marginal zone" type of non-Hodgkin lymphoma
  a. Low-grade B-cell lymphomas arising from MALT.
  b. Highly associated with long-standing *H. pylori* infection; eradication of the infection may result in cure of the lymphoma.

IV. Intestinal Disorders
A. Bowel obstruction
1. Small bowel is the most common site of obstruction.
2. Diagnosis
  a. Imaging (distention of bowel, air–fluid levels, and absence of air distal to the obstruction).
  b. Free air under the diaphragm (indicative of perforation).
3. Clinical manifestations
  a. Colicky pain (severe pain that alternates with pain-free intervals).
  b. Abdominal distention
    i. Secondary to the accumulation of bowel contents and gas within the bowel lumen.
    ii. As intraluminal pressures increase, patients may develop mucosal ischemia with necrosis, perforation.
    iii. On examination, the abdomen is tympanitic to percussion with high-pitched tinkling sounds on auscultation.
  c. Vomiting
    i. Bilious (bile-stained) if the obstruction is distal to the ampulla of Vater; nonbilious if the obstruction is proximal to the ampulla.
    ii. Prolonged vomiting may lead to hypovolemia, electrolyte imbalance (hypokalemic, hypochloremic metabolic alkalosis).
4. Major etiologies
  a. Serosal adhesions
    i. Fibrous bands between loops of bowel; a complication of peritoneal inflammation (e.g., surgery).

b. Hernia
   i. Defined as a protrusion of tissue through the body wall that normally contains it (e.g., abdominal wall). Globally, the most common cause of intestinal obstruction.
   ii. Protrusion of the bowel through a hernia causes extrinsic compression, potential for obstruction and infarction.
     (1) When bowel or other tissue has entered the defect but cannot be easily returned to its original location, the hernia is said to be "incarcerated."
     (2) Incarcerated hernias are at an increased risk of becoming "strangulated" (i.e., hernia in which the flow of blood, either in or out, is impaired). Strangulated hernias are therefore at an increased risk of infarction.
   iii. Risk factors for the development of a hernia include increased intraabdominal pressure (e.g., heavy lifting) and structural weakness of abdominal wall (e.g., previous surgery).
c. Volvulus
   i. Defined as a twisting of the bowel on its mesenteric attachment.
   ii. Most commonly involves sigmoid colon; however, the small intestine may be affected in some cases.
d. Intussusception
   i. Most common cause of intestinal obstruction in young children.
   ii. Refers to a "telescoping" of an intestinal segment into the immediately distal intestinal segment (due to peristaltic contractions).
     (1) The proximal segment, and its associated mesentery, becomes trapped, causing bowel obstruction and the potential for infarction (compression of vascular supply within the mesentery).
   iii. May or may not have an initiating point that acts as the "leading edge."
     (1) In younger children, the leading edge is often attributed to reactive lymphoid hyperplasia (e.g., following viral infection).
     (2) In older children and adults, the lead point is more likely a mass (e.g., polyp and tumor).

B. GI bleeding
1. Hematochezia
  a. Passage of bright red blood per rectum.
  b. Typically associated with bleeding from the lower GI tract (e.g., colonic diverticular disease, angiodysplasia, hemorrhoids, and anal fissure).
2. Melena
  a. Passage of dark tarry stools; typically signifies an upper GI bleed proximal to the ligament of Treitz (e.g., PUD and hemorrhagic gastropathy).
  b. Due to the conversion of hemoglobin to hematin pigment by gastric acid.

C. Diarrhea
1. Defined clinically as the presence of three or more loose watery stools per day or, objectively, as the passage of >250 g of liquid stool per day.
2. Types of diarrheas
  a. Secretory
    i. Large volume watery stool secondary to abnormal electrolyte transport within the intestinal lumen (e.g., *Vibrio cholerae* toxin, vasoactive intestinal peptide-secreting tumor).
    ii. Does not resolve with fasting.
  b. Osmotic
    i. Due to the ingestion of unabsorbed solutes or nutrients.
    ii. Resolves with fasting.

D. Steatorrhea
1. Excessive loss of fat in the stool (steatorrhea); stools float on the surface of toilet water.
2. Risk of fat-soluble vitamin (A, D, E, and K) deficiencies.
3. Causes of fat malabsorption include:
  a. Exocrine pancreatic insufficiency
    i. Chronic pancreatitis.
    ii. Cystic fibrosis.
  b. Bile salt/acid deficiency
    i. Reduced hepatic synthesis (e.g., cirrhosis).
    ii. Biliary stasis (primary biliary cholangitis or stone in common bile duct).
    iii. Disease of the terminal ileum (e.g., Crohn disease [CD]).
4. Testing for fat malabsorption
  a. Stool 72-hour fecal fat excretion (gold-standard test); excretion of greater than 7 g per day of fat is indicative of malabsorption.
5. Testing for pancreatic insufficiency
  a. Decreased fecal elastase and chymotrypsin levels.
  b. Computed tomography (CT) of the pancreas (often shows dystrophic calcification in chronic pancreatitis).

E. Celiac disease (gluten-sensitive enteropathy)

1. Definition
   a. Chronic autoimmune disorder of the small bowel occurring in genetically susceptible individuals following dietary exposure to gluten (present in wheat, barley, and rye).
2. Epidemiology
   a. Prevalence of ~1 in 200.
   b. More common in those with other autoimmune disorders (e.g., Type 1 diabetes mellitus and autoimmune thyroiditis), Down syndrome, and Turner syndrome.
3. Pathogenesis
   a. Following the ingestion of gluten-containing products, the alcohol-soluble fraction of gluten (gliadin) binds to HLA-DQ2 or HLA-DQ8 on antigen-presenting cells.
      i. Tissue transglutaminase deamidation of gluten peptides enhances binding to HLA-DQ2 and HLA-DQ8 (enhancing their immunogenicity).
      ii. Gliadin is then presented to CD4+ T cells, stimulating the production of pro-inflammatory cytokines (IFN-γ) and activating B-lymphocytes to become plasma cells that secrete antigliadin and antitissue-transglutaminase antibodies.
      iii. The net result is immune-mediated destruction of enterocytes with the eventual destruction of the small intestinal villi (causing villous atrophy; Fig. 18.9).
      iv. As small intestinal villi are destroyed, there is a loss of surface area and malabsorption; the latter causing steatorrhea, weight loss, and vitamin deficiencies.
4. Clinical manifestations
   a. Steatorrhea (fatty stools that float on the surface of toilet water).
   b. Flatulence, weight loss, and in children, a failure to thrive.
   c. Vitamin deficiencies (e.g., anemia due to iron and/or folate deficiency; osteopenia due to vitamin D insufficiency).
   d. Extraintestinal manifestations include dermatitis herpetiformis.
5. Diagnosis
   a. Serologic testing
      i. Antitissue-transglutaminase antibodies (IgA)—the best first test.
      ii. Antiendomysial antibody
      iii. Antigliadin antibodies (lower accuracy, no longer recommended).
   b. Endoscopic biopsy
      i. Villous atrophy, most pronounced within the distal duodenum and proximal jejunum; increased lymphocytic inflammation, and crypt hyperplasia.
      ii. Elimination of gluten from the diet eventually results in normal villous architecture (may be confirmed with biopsy after a period of gluten restriction).
6. Treatment
   a. Life-long dietary avoidance of gluten-containing food.

18.10: Schematic of arteries of the large intestine. The superior mesenteric artery (SMA) supplies most of the small bowel, the ascending and transverse colon up to the left colic flexure (splenic flexure; *interrupted circle*). The inferior mesenteric artery (IMA) supplies the descending and sigmoid colon, proximal rectum (not shown), and upper half of the anal canal (not shown). Note that the colon has the benefit of two blood supplies (SMA and IMA), whereas the small intestine only has one major blood supply (SMA). *(From Moore A, Roy W: Rapid review gross and developmental anatomy, ed 3, Philadelphia, 2010, Mosby Elsevier, p 76, Fig. 3.21.)*

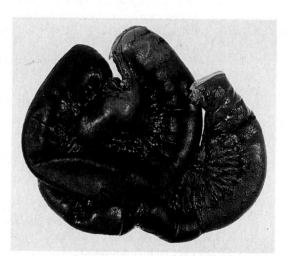

18.11: Small bowel infarction. This segment of small bowel was surgically resected after infarction caused by an embolus from the heart. The infarcted bowel is dilated and nearly black in color. *(From Stevens A, Lowe J, Scott I: Core pathology, ed 3, 2009, Mosby Elsevier, p 267, Fig. 13.18.)*

7. Complications
    a. Increased risk of lymphoma and GI cancer.
F. **Whipple disease**
    1. Rare systemic disease caused by an infection with the Gram-positive bacillus, *Tropheryma whipplei.*
    2. Clinical manifestations
        a. Systemic (arthralgias, weight loss, diarrhea, and abdominal pain).
        b. Neurologic (e.g., ataxia, dementia, and others).
        c. Cardiac (e.g., endocarditis and pericarditis).
    3. Higher prevalence in White males; middle to older age groups.
    4. Biopsies of involved tissue show PAS+ organisms within tissue macrophages (engorged macrophages within small bowel obstruct lymphatics → blocks absorption of nutrients).
    5. Treatment: antibiotics.
G. **Tropical sprue**
    1. Uncommon cause of chronic diarrhea, weight loss, and malabsorption.
    2. Seen in those residing in, or traveling to, a tropical or subtropical region (e.g., Caribbean and Southeast Asia).
    3. Etiology is unknown; however, a bacterial infection is thought most likely.
        a. Theorized that bacterial overgrowth leads to the production of various toxins that damage the small bowel, causing malabsorption of various nutrients (e.g., iron, folate, and vitamin B12).
H. **Vascular disorders of the bowel**
    1. Vascular supply (Fig. 18.10)
        a. Superior mesenteric artery (SMA) supplies all of the small bowel (except for the proximal duodenum) as well as the ascending and transverse colon to the splenic flexure.
        b. SMA and inferior mesenteric artery (IMA) overlap at the splenic flexure (i.e., watershed zone—susceptible to infarction).
        c. The IMA supplies the descending and sigmoid colon, proximal rectum, and the upper half of the anal canal.
    2. Mesenteric ischemia
        a. Defined as a reduction in blood flow to the small intestine.
        b. Acute mesenteric ischemia
            i. Abrupt reduction in small intestinal perfusion, etiologies include:
                (1) Embolic occlusion of the SMA (Fig. 18.11); from the heart (e.g., atrial fibrillation) or aorta (e.g., atheromatous emboli).
                (2) Arterial thrombosis (e.g., atherosclerotic narrowing, vasculitis).
                (3) Generalized reduction of mesenteric blood flow (e.g., cardiogenic shock or use of vasopressors).
                (4) Venous outflow obstruction.
        c. Chronic mesenteric ischemia
            i. Secondary to atherosclerotic narrowing of mesenteric vessels.
            ii. Causes episodic intestinal hypoperfusion (commonly postprandial period).
        d. Clinical and laboratory findings of small bowel infarction include:
            i. Sudden onset of diffuse abdominal pain (pain out of proportion to physical findings), bowel distention, bloody diarrhea, and absence of bowel sounds (ileus).
            ii. Profound neutrophilic leukocytosis, positive stool guaiac.
        e. Diagnosis
            i. CT angiography (gold-standard diagnostic test).
            ii. Plain X-rays may show "thumbprint sign" due to edema in the bowel wall, bowel distention with air–fluid levels.

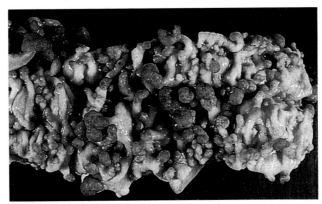

18.12: Familial adenomatous polyposis. Note the numerous adenomatous polyps. *(From Ashar BH, Miller RG, Sisso SD: The Johns Hopkins internal medicine board review, ed 4, 2012, Elsevier, p 441, Fig. 52.2. Taken from Skarin AT, Shaffer K, Wieczorek T, editors: Atlas of diagnostic oncology, ed 3, St. Louis, 2003, Mosby, p 152. In Abeloff MD, Armitage JO, Niederhuber JE, et al: Clinical oncology, ed 3, Philadelphia, 2004, Churchill Livingstone, Fig. 80.7.)*

3. Ischemic colitis
   a. Ischemia-induced inflammation of the large intestine, usually secondary to atherosclerotic vascular disease.
      i. Commonly involves "watershed" zones (e.g., splenic flexure).
   b. Clinical manifestations
      i. Cramping abdominal pain with tenderness, bloody diarrhea (due to mucosal infarction), and weight loss.
   c. Diagnosis
      i. Abdominal CT with contrast (shows segmental edema and thickening of the bowel wall, called "thumbprinting").
      ii. Colonoscopy (gold-standard test in stable patient).
4. Angiodysplasia
   a. Dilated, tortuous mucosal, and submucosal veins, usually of the right colon.
   b. More common in older individuals; pathogenesis is believed related to degenerative changes within the wall of the colon following decades of intermittent venous obstruction.
   c. Presents with hematochezia (dilated superficial veins are prone to rupture).
   d. Diagnosis: colonoscopy and angiography.

I. **Meckel diverticulum**
   1. Congenital diverticulum of the ileum, due to incomplete obliteration of the vitelline duct.
   2. "True" diverticulum (i.e., involves all layers of bowel wall).
   3. Classically described by the "rule of twos"
      a. Two inches in length, located 2 feet proximal to the ileocecal valve, affecting 2% of the population, symptomatic in 2% of patients, usually before the age of 2 years.
   4. May contain heterotopic pancreatic and/or gastric tissue (the latter associated with an increased risk of bleeding due to peptic ulceration).
   5. Clinical manifestations
      a. Usually asymptomatic, may develop bleeding in some patients due to peptic ulceration.
      b. Increased risk of intussusception (diverticulum serves as lead point).
      c. May simulate acute appendicitis if inflamed.
   6. Diagnosis
      a. Meckel scan (99 m technetium pertechnetate has an affinity for gastric mucosa); only identifies diverticula containing heterotopic gastric mucosa (~25% of cases).
      b. Capsule endoscopy.

J. **Small bowel diverticula**
   1. Localized outpouchings of mucosa and submucosa due to herniation through the muscularis propria.
      a. As opposed to a Meckel diverticulum, these are "false" diverticula (consists of mucosa and submucosa only).
      b. Unlike the colon, diverticula are uncommon in the small bowel (increased risk with systemic sclerosis).
   2. Complications include:
      a. Diverticulitis (inflammation of the diverticulum).
      b. Perforation with peritonitis (inflammation of the parietal peritoneum).
      c. Bacterial overgrowth within diverticula (may cause deficiency of bile salts and/or vitamin B12).

K. **Colonic diverticuli**
   1. Definition
      a. Herniations of mucosa and submucosa through areas of weakness in the muscularis propria of the large bowel.
   2. Epidemiology
      a. Common, especially with aging, affecting up to 60% of the population by age 60 years.
   3. Pathogenesis
      a. Elevated intraluminal pressures (e.g., low-fiber diet and straining with defecation) displaces the mucosa and submucosa through areas of weakness along the mesenteric border (where vasa recta enter the muscle wall), most common in the sigmoid colon.
   4. Complications
      a. Inflammation (diverticulitis), perforation (potentially leading to peri-colic abscess), and/or bleeding (usually occult, may be massive).

L. **Inflammatory bowel disease**
   1. Ulcerative colitis (UC)
      a. Chronic relapsing inflammatory disease of undetermined etiology diffusely involving the rectum and extending in a continuous fashion for a variable distance into the colon.
         i. May involve only the rectum ("ulcerative proctitis").
         ii. Does not extend proximal to ileocecal valve (i.e., involves only rectum and colon).
      b. Ulcerations are in continuity and limited to the mucosa.
      c. Any age, bimodal peak (15–30 years and 50–80 years).
      d. Jewish populations at higher risk; smoking associated with lower risk.
      e. Pathology
         i. Inflammation limited to the mucosa, characterized by increased lymphocytes and plasma cells within the lamina propria, crypt branching.
         ii. The presence of neutrophils within crypts (crypt abscess) or within crypt epithelium (acute cryptitis) indicates "active" disease.

    f. Clinical manifestations
- i. Diarrhea (may be bloody), colicky abdominal pain, urgency, tenesmus (feeling of need to have the bowel movement, even when no stool is present).
- ii. Increased risk of colorectal adenocarcinoma (especially with extensive colonic involvement after a period of 8–10 years).
- iii. Extraintestinal manifestations include primary sclerosing cholangitis, arthritis, uveitis, and skin lesions (erythema nodosum and pyoderma gangrenosum).

2. CD
    a. Chronic inflammatory disorder of unknown etiology affecting any region of the GI tract from the mouth to the anus.
- i. Most commonly involves the terminal ileum.

    b. Increased risk in those of Jewish ethnicity and/or cigarette smoking.

    c. Inflammation is discontinuous (areas of inflammation are interspersed between areas of normal mucosa) and transmural (inflammation extends through the entire bowel wall from mucosa to serosa).
- i. Transmural nature of the inflammation increases the risk of developing abscesses, fistulas, and scarring.
- ii. The presence of noncaseating granulomatous inflammation is characteristic (albeit uncommon). Inflammatory infiltrate is otherwise like that seen in UC.

    d. Clinical manifestations
- i. Crampy abdominal pain, diarrhea (with or without gross blood), fatigue, and weight loss.
- ii. Involvement of terminal ileum can be associated with malabsorption (bile salts and vitamin B12).
- iii. Increased risk of oxalate renal stones (enhanced absorption of dietary oxalate → increased urinary excretion [hyperoxaluria]).
- iv. Extraintestinal manifestations similar to those seen with UC.

M. Microscopic colitis
1. Clinical entity characterized by the presence of chronic, nonbloody, watery diarrhea in conjunction with normal endoscopic findings.
2. Two subtypes based on histologic findings.
    a. Lymphocytic colitis is characterized by increased numbers of intraepithelial lymphocytes and surface damage.
    b. Collagenous colitis is characterized by increased intraepithelial lymphocytes in conjunction with an irregular band of subepithelial collagen.
3. More common in women, particularly collagenous colitis.

N. Irritable bowel syndrome
1. Idiopathic condition characterized by recurrent attacks of abdominal pain and altered bowel motility in the absence of structural or other identifiable abnormality.
2. Prevalence of ~10%–15%; a leading cause of work absenteeism.
3. More common in females; often associated with psychosocial stressors, depression, and anxiety.
4. Etiology is unknown; theorized to be hypersensitivity to visceral stimuli, altered fecal microflora.
5. Manifestations
    a. Abdominal pain (sometimes relieved with defecation).
    b. Altered bowel habits (constipation, diarrhea [never nocturnal], or alternating episodes of constipation and diarrhea).
6. Diagnosis based on the presence of characteristic clinical findings in conjunction with a negative workup (i.e., normal C-reactive protein, normal endoscopy, and normal imaging).

O. Necrotizing enterocolitis
1. Ischemic necrosis of bowel seen in infancy.
2. Major risk factor is prematurity.
3. Most common life-threatening emergency of the GI tract in the newborn period.
4. Usually presents in the second to the fourth week of life.
5. Manifestations include:
    a. Temperature instability, metabolic acidosis, hypotension, and disseminated intravascular coagulopathy.
    b. Bloody stools, absent bowel sounds, and/or abdominal tenderness or mass.
6. Radiologic findings
    a. Air within the bowel wall ("intestinal pneumatosis"), ascites, and pneumoperitoneum.

P. Peritonitis
1. Inflammation of the peritoneum, usually secondary to a breach in the abdominal viscera (i.e., perforation).
2. Etiologies include perforated appendix, ruptured ectopic pregnancy, and ruptured ovarian cyst.
3. "Spontaneous bacterial peritonitis"
    a. Peritonitis occurring in those without an evident intraabdominal process; usually seen in those with cirrhosis and ascites.
    b. Severe liver dysfunction is associated with a reduction in serum complement levels and phagocytic function.
    c. Involves the translocation of bacteria from gut lumen into the peritoneum (*Escherichia coli*, the most common agent).
    d. Diagnosis based on the presence of bacteria and neutrophils within ascitic fluid.

Q. Small bowel adenocarcinoma
1. Unlike the colon, adenocarcinoma of the small bowel is uncommon.
2. Increased risk with FAP; see later discussion.

R. Carcinoid (well-differentiated neuroendocrine tumor)
1. Slow-growing tumor of neuroendocrine cells, usually arising within the GI tract (e.g., small intestine, rectum, and appendix).
   a. Most common primary malignancy of the small intestine.
2. Potential for metastatic spread (to the liver), especially from midgut (i.e., jejunum and ileum) tumors.
   a. Those arising in the foregut (e.g., stomach) and/or hindgut (e.g., rectum) are much less likely to metastasize.
3. Carcinoid tumors often produce vasoactive substances (e.g., serotonin and histamine).
   a. Intestinal carcinoids drain, via the portal circulation, into the liver where the various products are metabolized into inactive compounds and excreted in the urine.
      i. Serotonin metabolized to 5-hydroxy-indoleacetic acid (5-HIAA).
4. Because the liver completely metabolizes these substances into inactive metabolites, only those tumors that release serotonin (and other substances) directly into the systemic circulation cause the carcinoid syndrome.
   a. Carcinoid tumors have a characteristic bright yellow gross appearance with "nested" growth pattern on histologic examination.

Carcinoid syndrome

- Constellation of symptoms (e.g., flushing of skin, diarrhea, and bronchospasm) following the release of serotonin and other vasoactive substances from a carcinoid tumor into the systemic circulation.
  - Usually from metastatic carcinoid tumor within the liver.
  - Bronchial carcinoids, although uncommon, may cause the carcinoid syndrome in the absence of hepatic metastasis (serotonin released from these tumors directly enters the systemic circulation).
- Clinical manifestations
  - Flushing of the skin, particularly involving head, neck, and upper torso (due to histamine-induced vasodilation).
  - Diarrhea (due to serotonin-induced increased intestinal secretion and motility).
  - Intermittent wheezing and dyspnea due to bronchospasm.
  - Fibrosis of right-sided heart valves.
  - Niacin deficiency (tryptophan diverted to synthesize serotonin instead of niacin).
- Diagnosis
  - Increase in urinary 5-HIAA.
  - CT or magnetic resonance imaging to detect hepatic metastasis.

S. Intestinal polyps
1. Defined as abnormal tissue growth arising above the mucosal surface; may be sessile (i.e., with flat base) or pedunculated (on a stalk).
2. Hyperplastic polyp
   a. The most common type of colon polyp (adults), usually located within the rectosigmoid colon.
   b. Most are <5 mm in diameter; no risk of malignancy.
   c. Histologically, characterized by a "sawtooth" appearance.
3. Juvenile (retention) polyp
   a. Type of hamartomatous polyp (hamartoma refers to a mass lesion consisting of tissue elements normally found at that site but with disorganized architecture).
   b. Most common in children (thus the name) and the most common type of polyp in children.
   c. Usually located in the rectum; potential for prolapse.
   d. Pathology: smooth surface with enlarged cystic spaces on cross section.
4. Adenomatous polyps
   a. Neoplastic yet benign polypoid tissue growth exhibiting cytologic atypia (dysplasia) of the epithelium.
   b. Premalignant lesions, capable of malignant transformation.
   c. Increasing incidence with aging; males > females.
   d. Histologic subtypes
      i. Tubular adenoma
         (1) Most common type, often pedunculated (on a stalk), analogous to a mushroom.
         (2) Histology reveals mostly tubular (glandular) architecture with cytologic atypia (nuclear hyperchromasia and crowding).
      ii. Tubulovillous adenoma
         (1) Less common; mixture of tubular and villous (finger-like) architecture.
      iii. Villous adenoma
         (1) Least common type.
         (2) Often sessile, comprised of >75% villous architecture.
   e. Risk of malignancy increases with size (>2 cm), number, percent villous architecture, and degree of dysplasia.

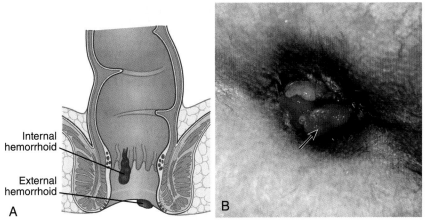

18.13: (A) Schematic showing formation of internal and external hemorrhoids. (B) Prolapsed internal hemorrhoids (*arrow*). *(A, From Kliegman R: Nelson textbook of pediatrics, ed 19, Philadelphia, 2011, Elsevier Saunders, p 1361, Fig. 336.5; B, from Morson BC: Colour atlas of gastrointestinal pathology, London, 1998, Harvey Miller Ltd, pp 275, Fig. 7.16.)*

T. Inherited colon cancer syndromes
1. Familial adenomatous polyposis (FAP)
   a. FAP and its variants are caused by germline mutations in the adenomatous polyposis coli (*APC*) tumor suppressor gene.
   b. FAP, which is inherited in an AD fashion with complete penetrance, is characterized by the development of ≥100 adenomatous polyps throughout the colon, usually developing during the teenage years (Fig. 18.12).
      i. Patients also at increased risk of developing adenomatous polyps within the duodenum and stomach.
   c. Malignant transformation (into colonic adenocarcinoma) by 40 years of age in all patients; reason for prophylactic colectomy by late teens/early twenties.
2. Gardner syndrome
   a. Historical term used to describe a subset of patients with FAP who also exhibit extracolonic manifestations (e.g., osteomas, epidermoid cysts, lipomas, desmoid tumors, and congenital hypertrophy of the retinal pigment epithelium).
3. Turcot syndrome
   a. Historical term describing the occurrence of brain tumors (e.g., medulloblastoma and glioblastoma) in addition to colonic polyposis.
4. Lynch syndrome
   a. Also known as hereditary nonpolyposis colorectal carcinoma.
   b. Most common inherited cause of colon cancer (accounts for ~3% of cases overall).
   c. Autosomal dominant inheritance, due to germline mutation in one of several DNA mismatch repair genes.*MMR*
   d. In addition to colorectal carcinoma, patients are at an increased risk of endometrial (second most common) and other carcinomas.

U. Colorectal carcinoma
1. Definition
   a. Malignancy of colorectal glandular epithelium (i.e., adenocarcinoma).
2. Epidemiology
   a. Globally, colorectal cancer is the third most commonly diagnosed cancer in males and second in females.
   b. Those at average risk in the United States have about a 1 in 25 (4%) chance of developing colorectal carcinoma during their lifetime.
   c. Overall, the incidence increases with age, especially after age 50 years; however, there has been a recent uptick in younger patients.
   d. More common in males, African Americans.
3. Risk factors include:
   a. Increasing age (especially after age 50 years).
   b. Family history (e.g., colon cancer in first degree relative).
   c. Hereditary syndromes (e.g., FAP and Lynch syndrome).
   d. Environmental exposures (e.g., high fat, low-fiber diet, heavy alcohol intake, and obesity).
   e. Inflammatory conditions of colon/rectum (e.g., UC and CD), particularly in those with extensive colonic involvement.
4. Pathogenesis
   a. Carcinogenesis: adenoma → carcinoma sequence.
   b. Involved genes include *APC, KRAS,* and *p53* (in this order).
   c. Mutations involving *APC* are present in most cancers (both sporadic as well as those associated with FAP).

5. Screening beginning at age 45 years (recently lowered from 50 years).
6. Screening options include:
   a. Fecal occult blood test
      i. Guaiac-based test for heme in a stool sample, usually performed annually.
   b. Fecal immunochemical test (FIT)
      i. Antibody test to detect globin in the stool, usually performed annually.
   c. Stool DNA testing
      i. Combination FIT plus an assay to detect common DNA alterations associated with colon cancer; performed every 3 years.
   d. Colonoscopy
      i. Usually considered the best test.
      ii. Can identify and remove polyps prior to malignant transformation; usually performed every 10 years.
7. Clinical manifestations
   a. Change in bowel habits (most common).
   b. Rectal bleeding (melena and hematochezia).
   c. Iron deficiency anemia (secondary to chronic blood loss).
   d. Weight loss.
   e. Abdominal pain/mass.
   f. Intestinal obstruction
      i. More likely in left-sided cancers (diameter of the left colon less than that of the right colon) in which lesions may have annular, "napkin ring" appearance.
   g. Increased incidence of *Streptococcus gallolyticus* (*bovis*) endocarditis.
8. Metastatic spread
   a. Initially to regional mesenteric lymph nodes.
   b. Distant hematogenous metastasis to the liver (most common), lungs, bone, and brain.
9. Prognosis depends upon stage of the disease.
10. Serum carcinoembryonic antigen (CEA) is a tumor marker used to evaluate for recurrence.
    a. Not sensitive or specific, should not be used for screening.

V. Acute appendicitis
1. Definition
   a. Acute inflammation of the vermiform appendix.
2. Epidemiology
   a. Common, lifetime risk of ~7%.
   b. Most common in second to third decade of life.
   c. Males > females.
3. Pathogenesis
   a. Often follows obstruction of the lumen by a fecalith (adults) or lymphoid hyperplasia (children).
   b. Obstruction of appendiceal drainage causes intraluminal and intramural pressures to rise (as pressures rise, perfusion decreases, resulting in ischemic injury).
4. Clinical findings (in sequence)
   a. Abdominal pain (periumbilical initially before localizing to McBurney point in the right lower quadrant).
   b. Anorexia, nausea, and vomiting
      i. Abdominal pain before vomiting—important clue (vomiting before pain suggests bowel obstruction).
   c. Rebound tenderness, pain with the right thigh extension (psoas sign), and pain in the right lower quadrant with palpation of the left lower quadrant (Rovsing sign).
5. Laboratory findings include:
   a. Neutrophilic leukocytosis with left shift, elevated C-reactive protein.
6. Complications
   a. Peri-appendiceal abscess, perforation, peritonitis, and sepsis.
7. Diagnosis
   a. CT scan with intravenous contrast of abdomen and pelvis.
8. Differential diagnosis
   a. Viral gastroenteritis, ruptured ovarian cyst, ruptured ectopic pregnancy, mesenteric lymphadenitis, and Meckel diverticulitis.

W. Appendiceal tumors
1. Neuroendocrine tumors
   a. Well-differentiated neuroendocrine tumor (i.e., carcinoid) is the most common tumor of the appendix.
2. Epithelial tumors (rare)
   a. Adenocarcinoma, low- /high-grade mucinous neoplasms.
   b. Perforation can lead to seeding of peritoneal cavity.
   c. Pseudomyxoma peritonei refers to the presence of copious mucin within the abdominal cavity (most commonly seen in association with mucinous tumors of the appendix).

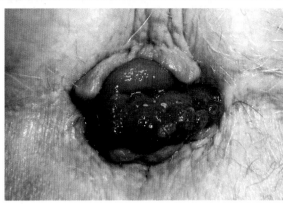

18.14: Rectal prolapse showing hemorrhagic rectal mucosa. *(From Goldman L, Schafer A: Goldman's Cecil medicine, ed 25, 2016, Elsevier Saunders, p 971, Fig. 145.6.)*

V. Anorectal Disorders
A. Hemorrhoids
1. Overview
   a. Hemorrhoids are clusters of vascular tissue (arterioles and venules), smooth muscle, and connective tissue within the anal canal.
   b. Normal anatomic structures; become symptomatic when enlarged, thrombosed, or prolapsed.
   c. Classified as internal or external based on location within the anal canal (Fig. 18.13).
2. External hemorrhoids
   a. Develop from ectoderm, originate below the pectinate line, covered with squamous epithelium.
   b. Drain through the inferior rectal vein into the inferior vena cava.
   c. Innervated by cutaneous nerves (painful when thrombosed).
3. Internal hemorrhoids
   a. Develop from endoderm, originate above the pectinate line, covered by columnar epithelium.
   b. Drain through the superior rectal vein.
   c. Not supplied by somatic sensory nerves (insensitive to pain).
4. Pathophysiology
   a. Impaired venous return from hemorrhoidal tissue leads to engorgement.
      i. Risk factors include advanced age, pregnancy, and straining (e.g., constipation).
      ii. High-fiber diet helps to maintain regular bowel movements, thereby decreasing one's risk of hemorrhoidal complications.
5. Clinical manifestations
   a. Pruritus, prolapse, bleeding, and painful thrombosis (external hemorrhoids).
B. Rectal prolapse (rectal procidentia)
1. Protrusion of the rectal tissue through the anal orifice due to weakening of pelvic floor support.
   a. Partial prolapse includes anal or rectal mucosa only.
   b. Complete prolapse involves all layers of the rectum.
2. Most common in older women, especially those with a history of multiple vaginal deliveries, chronic straining/constipation, and/or prior pelvic surgery.
   a. Cystic fibrosis, a major risk factor in children.
3. Presents with fecal incontinence, mucus-like discharge with bowel movements, incomplete evacuation, rectal bleeding, and/or mass (Fig. 18.14).
C. Pilonidal disease
1. Acquired sinus or cyst within the upper gluteal cleft, due to the traumatic implantation of hair; may become infected to form an abscess.
2. More common in young (15–24 years) adult males.
3. Presents with pain and purulent discharge from a fluctuant mass in the upper gluteal cleft.
D. Anal fissure
1. Painful linear tear in the anal mucosa; usually initiated by the passage of hard stool.
2. Usually located in the midline posteriorly.
   a. Associated findings include skin tag (sentinel pile) at the distal end and hypertrophied anal papilla at the proximal end.
3. Pain and bleeding with defecation.

E. Anal carcinoma
  1. Squamous cell carcinoma (the most common histologic subtype).
  2. Risk factors include:
     a. Active infection with the HPV, especially subtypes 16 and 18.
     b. Smoking.
     c. Receptive anal sex.
     d. Immunosuppression (e.g., HIV and organ transplant recipients).

CHAPTER

19 Hepatobiliary and Pancreatic Disorders

I. Hepatic Microanatomy

A. Hepatic lobule

1. Zone 1 hepatocytes surround the portal tract at the periphery of the lobule. Highest oxygen content (site where blood enters) (Figs. 19.1 and 19.2).
2. Zone 2 hepatocytes are located between zone 1 and zone 3 hepatocytes.
3. Zone 3 hepatocytes are located in the center of the hepatic lobule around the central vein. Lowest oxygen content and thus most susceptible to ischemic injury.

B. Portal tract

1. Located at the periphery of hepatic lobule, contain branches of hepatic artery, portal vein, and bile ductule.

C. Blood flow

1. Blood enters the hepatic lobule at the periphery (portal tract) via branches of hepatic artery and portal vein.
2. Blood then flows along sinusoids before draining into the central vein.
   a. Blood flows by cords of hepatocytes.
   b. Lining the sinusoids are Kupffer cells (macrophages of the liver).
   c. Around the sinusoids, but not visible on light microscopy, are the hepatic stellate cells (function in vitamin A storage).
      i. Activation of stellate cells, in association with hepatocyte inflammation and injury, forms myofibroblasts. Myofibroblasts in turn deposit collagen, explaining the scarring seen in those with severe hepatic injury.
3. Coalescence of blood from central venules drains via the hepatic vein to the inferior vena cava before returning to the heart.

D. Bile flow

1. Bile is actively secreted into bile canaliculi, drains to bile ductule. Coalescence of bile from the various ductules drains via right and left hepatic ducts.

II. Laboratory Evaluation of Liver Cell Injury

A. Bilirubin metabolism in sequence

1. Bilirubin is derived from the breakdown of heme (primarily from senescent red blood cells [RBCs]) (Fig. 19.3A).
2. Senescent RBCs are phagocytosed by macrophages in the spleen, liver, and bone marrow, then catabolized into various components.
   a. Globin chains are broken down into amino acids and recycled.
   b. Heme is oxidized via heme oxygenase, releasing iron (which is recycled), and biliverdin.
   c. Biliverdin converted to bilirubin (by biliverdin reductase).
      i. Heme → biliverdin → bilirubin.
3. At this point, the bilirubin is not water soluble (referred to as "unconjugated bilirubin"—UCB) and must bind to albumin for transport in circulation.
4. Within the liver, the UCB is taken up by hepatocytes and conjugated to glucuronic acid forming conjugated bilirubin (CB).
   a. Uridine-diphosphoglucuronic glucuronosyltransferase (UDPGT) is a family of enzymes, the most physiologically active form of which is UDPGT1A1.

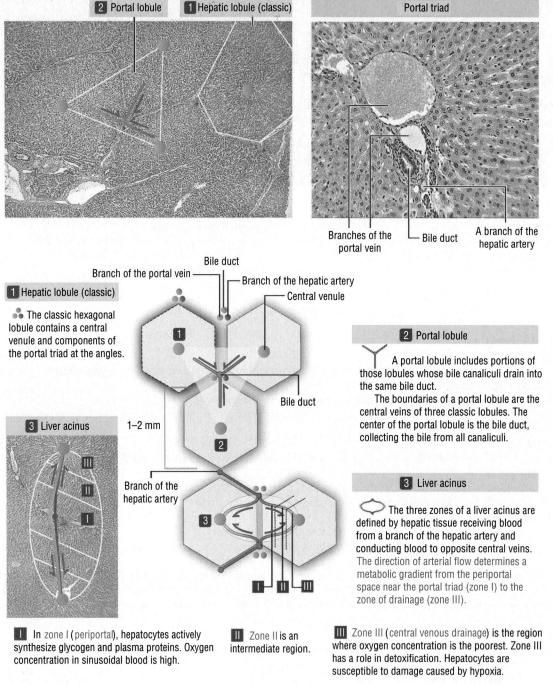

2 Portal lobule   1 Hepatic lobule (classic)

Portal triad

Branches of the
portal vein

Bile duct

A branch of the
hepatic artery

Bile duct

Branch of the portal vein

Branch of the hepatic artery

Central venule

1 Hepatic lobule (classic)

The classic hexagonal lobule contains a central venule and components of the portal triad at the angles.

Bile duct

1–2 mm

Branch of the hepatic artery

2 Portal lobule

A portal lobule includes portions of those lobules whose bile canaliculi drain into the same bile duct.

The boundaries of a portal lobule are the central veins of three classic lobules. The center of the portal lobule is the bile duct, collecting the bile from all canaliculi.

3 Liver acinus

The three zones of a liver acinus are defined by hepatic tissue receiving blood from a branch of the hepatic artery and conducting blood to opposite central veins. The direction of arterial flow determines a metabolic gradient from the periportal space near the portal triad (zone I) to the zone of drainage (zone III).

3 Liver acinus

III
II
I

I In zone I (periportal), hepatocytes actively synthesize glycogen and plasma proteins. Oxygen concentration in sinusoidal blood is high.

II Zone II is an intermediate region.

III Zone III (central venous drainage) is the region where oxygen concentration is the poorest. Zone III has a role in detoxification. Hepatocytes are susceptible to damage caused by hypoxia.

19.1: Hepatic lobule. Hexagonal-shaped hepatic lobule with portal triad at periphery and central vein in the center. *(From Kierszenbaum AL: Histology and cell biology: an introduction to pathology, ed 5, 2020, Fig. 17.12.).*

5. CB, now water soluble, is actively secreted into bile canaliculi (microscopic bile ducts) using the multidrug resistance-associated protein 2.
   a. From the canaliculi, bile drains into hepatic ducts and temporarily stored within the gallbladder.
6. Following the ingestion of a meal, cholecystokinin (CCK), which is released from endocrine cells of the duodenal mucosa, causes the gallbladder to contract → expulsion of bile (containing CB) through the cystic and common bile ducts (CBDs), into the duodenum (ampulla of Vater).

B. **The CB then passes unchanged until it reaches the terminal ileum and colon where bacterial enzymes deconjugate the CB, forming urobilinogen (UBG)**
1. Most (~80%) of the UBG is excreted in the stool (as stercobilin), giving stool its characteristic coloration.
2. Approximately 20% of the UBG is reabsorbed into the portal circulation (enterohepatic circulation) and either re-secreted into the bile or filtered by the kidneys and excreted in the urine.
   a. Normal serum total bilirubin 0.2–1 mg/dL.
   b. In health, most of the bilirubin is unconjugated.
      i. Normal CB <0.2 mg/dL.

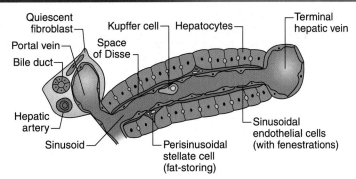

19.2: Normal hepatic microanatomy. Note that blood flows through hepatic sinusoids. *(From Burt AD, Ferrell LD, Portmann BC: MacSween's pathology of the liver, ed 6, St. Louis, 2013, Churchill Livingstone, Elsevier, p 54, Fig. 1.47A.)*

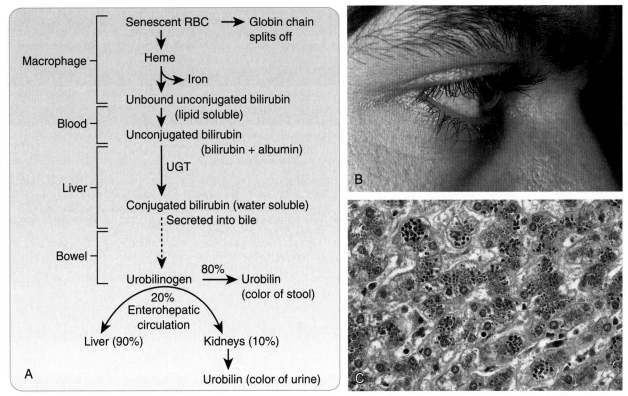

19.3: (A) Bilirubin metabolism. Refer to the text for discussion. (B) Scleral icterus. Note the yellowish discoloration of the sclera. (C) Pigment in lysosomes in Dubin–Johnson syndrome. *RBC*, Red blood cell; *UGT*, uridine glucuronosyltransferase. *(B, From Savin J, Hunter JA, Hepburn NC: Diagnosis in color: skin signs in clinical medicine, London, 1997, Mosby-Wolfe, Fig. 6.28; C, from MacSween R, Burt A, Portmann B, Ishak K, Scheuer P, Anthony P: Pathology of the liver, ed 4, London, 2002, Churchill Livingstone, p 221, Fig. 4.91.)*

3. Excess circulating bilirubin is deposited within the skin and mucous membranes; may be clinically evident as a yellow discoloration known as jaundice.
    a. Jaundice is indicative of hyperbilirubinemia (conjugated, unconjugated, or both); becomes clinically evident when total bilirubin levels exceed ~2.5–3 g/dL.
    b. Bilirubin deposits within sclera ("scleral icterus"—Fig. 19.3B).
C. Laboratory evaluation of jaundice
   1. Total bilirubin:
       a. Further fractionated into "unconjugated" and "conjugated" forms.
           i. UCB sometimes reported as "indirect bilirubin."
           ii. CB sometimes reported as "direct bilirubin."
   2. Bilirubin fractionation can help to narrow the differential diagnosis, depending upon which fraction (conjugated, unconjugated, or both) is elevated:
       a. Unconjugated hyperbilirubinemia (<20% conjugated), causes include
           i. Increased formation (e.g., hemolysis).
           ii. Reduced hepatic uptake.
           iii. Decreased conjugation (e.g., physiologic jaundice of the newborn).

TABLE 19.1 Causes of Jaundice

TYPE OF HYPERBILIRUBINEMIA CB <20% (ALL UCB)	URINE BILIRUBIN	URINE UBG	EXAMPLES OF DISORDERS
Increased production of UCB	Absent	↑	Hemolysis (e.g., hereditary spherocytosis, autoimmune hemolysis)
Decreased conjugation of UCB	Absent	Not useful	• Gilbert syndrome (common, ~5% of population). Second most common cause of jaundice (hepatitis is the most common). Most common hereditary cause of jaundice. Impaired UGT activity (70%–75% decrease in activity). Jaundice occurs with fasting, volume depletion, stress, menses. Serum UCB is rarely >5 mg/dL. All other hepatic laboratory tests are normal. No treatment required. • Crigler–Najjar syndromes: rare, decreased to absent UGT. Type I is autosomal recessive. Characterized by absence of UGT activity; incompatible with life (liver transplantation necessary). Type II is autosomal dominant and is associated with decreased levels of UGT. • Physiologic jaundice of newborn is characterized by jaundice beginning on ~day 3 of life. Caused by the inability of the newborn liver to handle the bilirubin load associated with the normal destruction of fetal RBCs. • Breast milk jaundice: caused by pregnane-3α,20α-diol, which inhibits UGT. No treatment required.
MIXED			
CB 20%–50%	↑	↑	Viral hepatitis: defect in uptake, conjugation of UCB, and secretion of CB
OBSTRUCTIVE			
CB >50%	↑	Absent	• Decreased intrahepatic bile flow (obstructive jaundice) • Drug induced (e.g., oral contraceptive pills) • Primary biliary cholangitis • Dubin–Johnson syndrome: autosomal recessive disorder due to impaired secretion of conjugated bilirubin into intrahepatic bile ducts (mutation involving multidrug resistance protein 2 that is needed for excretion of bilirubin). Black pigment is present in lysosomes of hepatocytes. • Rotor syndrome: Autosomal recessive disorder similar to Dubin–Johnson syndrome but without black pigment. • Decreased extrahepatic bile flow (e.g., gallstone in CBD, carcinoma at head of pancreas causing compression of the CBD).

CB, Conjugated bilirubin; *CBD*, common bile duct; *HDN*, hemolytic disease of newborn; *OCP*, oral contraceptive pill; *UBG*, urobilinogen; *UCB*, unconjugated bilirubin; *UGT*, uridine glucuronosyltransferase.

    b. Mixed hyperbilirubinemia (20%–50% conjugated):
       i. Hepatitis is the most likely etiology (inflamed hepatocytes do not take up, conjugate, or excrete bilirubin normally).
    c. Conjugated hyperbilirubinemia (>50% conjugated):
       i. Biliary tract obstruction likely (e.g., gallstone within CBD, carcinoma at head of pancreas, bile duct stricture).
  3. Causes of jaundice (Table 19.1)
  4. Aminotransferase enzymes:
    a. Elevated with hepatocyte injury:
       i. Alanine aminotransferase (ALT)
         (1) More specific to the liver, present within cytosol of hepatocytes.
         (2) Tends to be higher than aspartate aminotransferase (AST) in viral hepatitis.
       ii. AST
         (1) Not specific to the liver (also present in heart and muscle), present within both the cytosol as well as the mitochondria.
         (2) Disproportionate elevation in alcoholic hepatitis (due to alcohol-induced mitochondrial injury).
    b. Canalicular enzymes:
       i. Alkaline phosphatase (ALP), gamma-glutamyl transferase (GGT)
       ii. Elevated with canalicular injury (e.g., cholestasis).
    c. Prothrombin time (PT) and/or albumin levels:
       i. Useful in the evaluation of hepatic synthetic function.
  D. Summary of laboratory findings in select hepatic disease (Table 19.2)

TABLE 19.2   Summary of Laboratory Findings in Selected Liver Disorders*

DISEASE	% CB	AST	ALT	ALP	GGT	UB	URINE UBG
Normal						Absent	↑
Viral hepatitis	20–50	↑↑↑	↑↑↑↑	↑	↑	↑↑	↑↑
Alcoholic hepatitis	20–50	↑↑	↑	↑	↑↑↑	↑↑	↑↑
Cholestasis	>50	↑	↑↑	↑↑↑	↑↑↑	↑↑↑	Absent
Extravascular hemolysis	<20	↑↑RBCs[†]	N	N	N	Absent	↑↑

*Arrows represent degree of magnitude.
[†]RBCs contain AST.
ALP, Alkaline phosphatase; *ALT*, alanine aminotransferase; *AST*, aspartate aminotransferase; *CB*, conjugated bilirubin; *GGT*, gamma-glutamyl transferase; *UB*, urine bilirubin; *UBG*, urobilinogen.
From Goljan EF, Sloka KI: *Rapid review laboratory testing in clinical medicine*, Philadelphia, 2008, Mosby, p 312, Table 9-20.

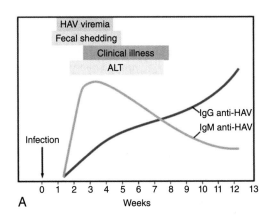
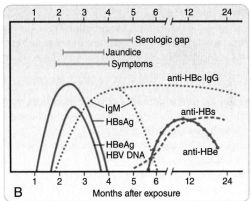

19.4: (A) Clinical course and serologic markers in hepatitis A. (B) Serologic markers in hepatitis B. *ALT*, Alanine aminotransferase; *Anti-HBc*, anti-HBV core antigen; *anti-HBe*, anti-HBV e antigen; *anti-HBs*, anti-HBV surface antibody; *HAV*, hepatitis A virus; *HBeAg*, hepatitis B e antigen; *HBsAg*, hepatitis B surface antigen; *HBV*, hepatitis B virus; *IgG*, immunoglobulin G; *IgM*, immunoglobulin M. *(A, From Mandell GL, Bennett JE, Dolin R:* Principles and practice of infectious diseases, *ed 8, Philadelphia, 2015, Elsevier, Churchill Livingstone, pp 1439–1468. e7, Fig. 119.1A.)*

III. Viral Hepatitis
A. Overview
1. Hepatitis (inflammation of the liver) is most commonly due to an infection by a hepatotropic virus (i.e., hepatitis A, B, C, D, or E).
    a. Other agents (e.g., cytomegalovirus, Epstein–Barr virus, herpes simplex virus, yellow fever) can also infect the liver.
2. Hepatic injury largely secondary to the host immune response against the infecting agent.
B. Clinical manifestations
1. Vary, both between the individuals as well as with the specific virus.
    a. Some patients remain asymptomatic while others develop rapidly progressive hepatic failure.
2. Classically evolve through four phases:
    a. Phase 1: Early asymptomatic stage of infection in which laboratory evidence of hepatitis may be found (elevated AST and ALT).
    b. Phase 2: Prodromal phase characterized by anorexia, nausea, vomiting, malaise, fatigue, aversion to cigarettes.
    c. Phase 3: Obstructive complications (jaundice, dark urine, pale-colored stools), right upper quadrant (RUQ) pain, hepatomegaly.
    d. Phase 4: Symptoms and laboratory abnormalities resolve.
C. Hepatitis A virus (HAV)
1. Transmitted by the fecal–oral route.
2. Incubation ~1 month, usually self-limited.
3. Does not become chronic and fulminant hepatic failure is rare (<1% of cases).
4. Diagnosis:
    a. Anti-HAV IgM: Indicative of acute HAV infection (Fig. 19.4A).
    b. Anti-HAV IgG: Associated with lifelong protective immunity.
        i. Presence of anti-HAV IgG in the absence of anti-HAV IgM is indicative of past infection or vaccination.

TABLE 19.3   Serologic Studies in Hepatitis B Virus

HBsAg	HBeAg HBV DNA	ANTI-HBC IgM	ANTI-HBC IgG	ANTI-HBs	INTERPRETATION
+	–	–	–	–	Earliest phase of acute HBV
+	+	+	–	–	Acute infection
–	–	+	–	–	Window phase, or serologic gap
–	–	–	+	+	Recovered from HBV
–	–	–	–	+	Immunized
+	–	–	+	–	"Healthy" carrier
+	+	–	+	–	Infective carrier

Anti-HBc, Core antibody; *anti-HBs*, surface antibody; *HBeAg*, e antigen; *HBsAg*, surface antigen; *HBV*, hepatitis B virus; +, present; –, absent.

D. **Hepatitis B virus (HBV)**
   1. Transmitted by body fluids (incubation of 1–4 months).
      a. Perinatal transmission common in areas of high prevalence (e.g., Southeast Asia, China).
      b. In the United States, sexual transmission or sharing of needles (IV drug abuse) are common modes of transmission.
   2. Manifestations range from subclinical (most common) to fulminant (rare, <1% of cases).
   3. Potential for development of chronic infection; varies inversely with age at time of infection.
      a. Those infected as newborns have ~90% chance of developing chronic infection while those infected as adults have <5% chance of chronicity.
      b. Important because chronicity increases risk of cirrhosis and hepatocellular carcinoma (HCC).
   4. Acute hepatitis B serology:
      a. Hepatitis B surface antigen (HBsAg)
         i. Appears within 1–10 weeks of exposure (first marker of infection) (Fig. 19.4B).
         ii. Persistence of HBsAg for longer than 6 months implies chronic infection.
      b. Hepatitis B surface antibody (anti-HBs)
         i. Appears after HBsAg.
         ii. Persists for life in most patients (confers long-term immunity).
         iii. "Window period":
            (1) Time period in some patients in which HBsAg has disappeared but anti-HBs still is not detectable.
            (2) During this time, the diagnosis can only be made by the detection of IgM antibodies against hepatitis B core antigen (IgM anti-HBc).
      c. IgM anti-HBc
         i. Confirms acute HBV infection.
         ii. Hepatitis B core antigen (HBcAg) is intracellular and therefore not detectable in serum.
      d. Hepatitis B e antigen (HBeAg) and HBV DNA assays
         i. Both are markers of HBV replication and infectivity.
      e. Summary of hepatitis B serology (Table 19.3).
E. **Hepatitis C virus (HCV)**
   1. Transmitted via body fluids (use of IV drugs is major risk factor).
   2. Most acute infections are asymptomatic; fulminant infection is rare.
   3. High incidence of developing chronic infection (up to 85%).
      a. Important risk factor for the development of cirrhosis
         i. Major indication for liver transplantation in the United States today.
         ii. Potential for progression to HCC.
   4. Laboratory testing:
      a. Both anti-HCV antibody and HCV RNA should be ordered (Fig. 19.5).
      b. If HCV RNA is negative, then acute HCV infection is unlikely.
      c. If HCV RNA is positive and HCV antibody is negative, then an acute HCV infection is likely.
         i. RNA assay detects infection earlier than the serologic test.
      d. If both HCV RNA and HCV antibody are positive, then HCV infection is confirmed (but does not distinguish between acute and chronic infections).
F. **Hepatitis D virus (HDV)**
   1. Transmitted via body fluids.
   2. HDV is dependent upon the presence of HBsAg.
   3. Patients may be infected with both HBV and HDV at the same time (coinfection) or conversely, a patient who was previously infected with HBV may be subsequently infected with HDV (superinfection).

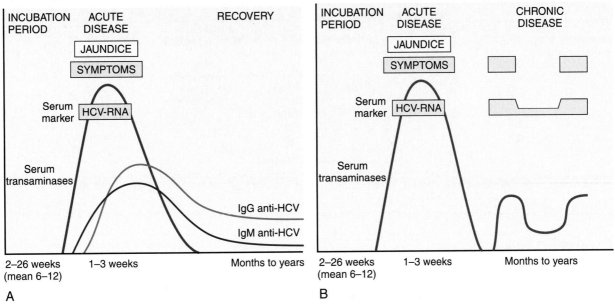

19.5: Sequence of clinical and laboratory findings in HCV. (A) Acute infection. (B) Chronic disease following acute infection. *HCV*, Hepatitis C viruss; *IgG*, immunoglobulin G; *IgM*, immunoglobulin M. *(From Kumar V, Abbas AK, Fausto N [eds]: Robbins Pathologic Basis of Disease, 7th ed. Philadelphia, Elsevier, 2004, p. 895.)*

    a. Coinfection results in acute hepatitis B and acute hepatitis D (indistinguishable from acute hepatitis B; is usually transient and self-limited).

    b. Superinfection may present as a severe acute hepatitis; nearly all will develop chronic HDV infection.

  4. Initial test: total anti-HDV; confirmation with HDV RNA assay.

G. Hepatitis E virus (HEV)

  1. Transmission is fecal–oral.

  2. Fulminant infection uncommon (except in pregnancy in which there is up to 25% mortality).

  3. Chronic infection unlikely except in immunosuppressed patients.

  4. Laboratory testing:

    a. If acute HEV is suspected, then do anti-HEV IgM as the initial test.

    b. If positive, then patient most likely has an acute HEV infection, and the diagnosis is confirmed by detecting HEV RNA in serum.

    c. If the anti-HEV IgM is negative, and there is still a high suspicion for HEV infection, then do HEV RNA assay.

    d. For suspected chronic HEV (uncommon, mostly immunocompromised patients), do HEV RNA assay.

      i. Presence of HEV RNA for longer than 6 months is diagnostic of chronic HEV infection.

    e. Presence of IgG (or total) anti-HEV antibodies is a marker of exposure to HEV (does not distinguish between recent and remote infections).

H. Other laboratory test findings in viral hepatitis

  1. Mixed hyperbilirubinemia (elevated UCB and CB; CB 20%–50%):

    a. UCB is elevated due to impaired hepatic uptake and conjugation.

    b. CB is elevated due to leakage from damaged hepatocytes.

  2. Increased serum aminotransferase enzymes:

    a. ALT > AST:

      i. ALT is the more specific marker of hepatocyte injury.

  3. Increased urine bilirubin:

    a. Leakage of CB from damaged hepatocytes causes elevated conjugated bilirubinemia (filtered by kidneys, excreted in the urine).

    b. Note that UCB is bound to albumin and not filtered (reason that any bilirubin in the urine must be conjugated).

IV. Drug, Toxic, Metabolic, and Autoimmune Hepatitis

A. Reye syndrome

  1. Definition:

    a. Rapidly progressive acute illness characterized by hepatic dysfunction and encephalopathy.

    b. Usually presents after a viral illness (e.g., influenza) treated with aspirin (or other salicylate-containing medication).

  2. Pathogenesis:

    a. Exact etiology unclear, thought to involve mitochondrial injury with disruption of oxidative phosphorylation and fatty acid oxidation.

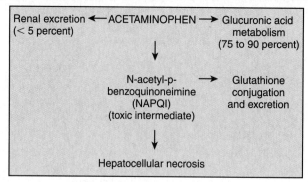

19.6: Acetaminophen metabolism. *(From Bagheri, SC, Clinical review of oral and maxillofacial surgery, ed 2, 2014, Fig. 2.2.)*

3. Laboratory findings:
   a. Markedly elevated aminotransferase enzymes (AST, ALT).
   b. Hyperammonemia.
   c. Hypoglycemia.
4. Pathology:
   a. Fatty infiltration of the liver (microvesicular steatosis).
5. Complications:
   a. Increased intracranial pressure, seizures, and coma.
   b. Mortality ~40%, often due to cerebral herniation.

B. Acetaminophen toxicity
1. Most common cause of acute liver failure in the United States, usually in attempted suicide.
2. Metabolism:
   a. In usual therapeutic doses, majority of the acetaminophen dose (~90%) undergoes conjugation to sulfate and glucuronide conjugates and is excreted in the urine (minor amount excreted unchanged) (Fig. 19.6).
   b. Remainder is metabolized via the hepatic cytochrome P450 mixed-function oxidase into *N*-acetyl-*p*-benzoquinoneimine (NAPQI).
      i. NAPQI is conjugated with glutathione (GSH) to form nontoxic compounds (excreted in the urine).
      ii. In overdose situations, excess NAPQI is formed, thereby depleting GSH stores.
      iii. Remainder of NAPQI (which is toxic) → hepatocellular injury (centrilobular hepatic necrosis).
3. Clinical findings:
   a. Often asymptomatic initially; however, nonspecific manifestations may arise, including nausea, vomiting, anorexia, and malaise.
   b. By days 2–3 following ingestion, patients may develop RUQ pain, renal injury, encephalopathy (sleep abnormalities, confusion, coma); liver failure/death possible.
4. Laboratory findings:
   a. Elevated aminotransferase enzymes (AST and ALT).
   b. Prolonged PT (due to coagulopathy related to hepatic dysfunction).
   c. Elevated serum ammonia (defective urea cycle, contributes to encephalopathy).
   d. Decreased bicarbonate (metabolic acidosis):
      i. Lactic acid accumulation secondary to impaired hepatic clearance, tissue hypoxia.
5. Treatment:
   a. *N*-Acetylcysteine (repletes GSH stores).

C. Hereditary hemochromatosis
1. Definition:
   a. Autosomal recessive (AR) condition characterized by the unrestricted absorption of iron from the small intestine and ultimately, the deposition of excess iron within various tissues of the body.
2. Epidemiology:
   a. Most common genetic disorder in those of Northern European ancestry.
   b. In undiagnosed patients, manifestations begin to appear in males by the fifth decade of life. Females typically present 10–20 years later (i.e., postmenopausal) because menstrual blood losses help to control iron levels.
3. Pathogenesis:
   a. Mutation in the *HFE* gene → unrestricted absorption of iron from the small intestine.
   b. Excess iron accumulates within tissues (e.g., liver, pancreas, heart, pituitary), causing progressive oxidative injury, cellular dysfunction, and fibrosis.
   c. Note that similar consequences may occur in those with iron overload occurring as a result of repeated transfusion of RBCs (iron in RBCs).

4. Clinical manifestations:
   a. Liver disease:
      i. Hepatomegaly, cirrhosis, increased risk of HCC.
   b. Hyperpigmentation:
      i. Mostly a result of increased melanin production that occurs as a result of iron-induced adrenal injury (primary adrenal insufficiency). Loss of cortisol causes pituitary to release more pro-opiomelanocortin (POMC), a precursor for adrenocorticotropic hormone (ACTH) and melanocyte-stimulating hormone (MSH). ↑ MSH causes hyperpigmentation.
   c. Diabetes mellitus:
      i. Iron-induced destruction of β-islet cells in pancreas.
   d. Cardiac effects:
      i. Conduction defects, restrictive cardiomyopathy, dilated cardiomyopathy (later finding)
   e. Pituitary gland dysfunction:
      i. Hypogonadotropic hypogonadism
         (1) Reduced follicle-stimulating hormone and luteinizing hormone from pituitary.
      ii. Secondary hypothyroidism
         (1) Reduced pituitary release of thyroid-stimulating hormone.
5. Laboratory findings:
   a. Increased serum iron, transferrin saturation, and serum ferritin.
      i. Transferrin saturation is the best screening test; values >45% suggest hemochromatosis.
   b. Decreased total iron binding capacity (TIBC)
      i. TIBC is a measure of transferrin.
      ii. Varies inversely with ferritin levels (↑ ferritin, ↓ TIBC).
6. Screening test:
   a. Iron studies (serum iron, TIBC, transferrin saturation, and serum ferritin).
      i. Transferrin–iron saturation >45% should prompt further evaluation.
7. Diagnosis:
   a. *HFE* gene testing (also used to screen relatives for hemochromatosis).
   b. Liver biopsy in some cases.

D. Wilson disease (hepatolenticular degeneration)
   1. Definition:
      a. AR disorder of impaired hepatic copper excretion.
   2. Pathogenesis:
      a. Inherited mutation in *ATP7B* gene (encodes for the copper transport protein, ATP7B), impairs biliary excretion of copper.
      b. Accumulation of copper → oxidative injury (e.g., liver, brain).
   3. Clinical manifestations (usually presents in the first two decades of life).
      a. Liver disease can range from acute liver failure to chronic liver disease/cirrhosis.
      b. Kayser–Fleischer ring is due to deposits of copper in Descemet membrane in the cornea; nonspecific, but highly suggestive of the diagnosis.
      c. Neurologic manifestations may include
         i. Parkinson disease-like manifestations with tremor ("wing-beating" tremor).
         ii. Psychiatric manifestations (e.g., depression, irritability, personality changes).
   4. Diagnosis:
      a. Low serum ceruloplasmin.
      b. Low serum copper (due to reduced serum ceruloplasmin).
      c. Increased 24-hour urinary copper excretion (reflects non-ceruloplasmin-bound copper concentration in plasma).
      d. Elevated hepatic copper concentration.
      e. Molecular testing for *ATP7B* mutation.
   5. Treatment:
      a. Copper chelation (e.g., trientine, penicillamine).
E. Alpha-1-antitrypsin (AAT) deficiency (Pi*ZZ)
   1. Definition:
      a. Autosomal codominant inherited condition in which there is a deficiency of the protease inhibitor, AAT.
      b. AAT, which is synthesized in the liver, inhibits various proteases (e.g., trypsin, chymotrypsin, elastase) released from neutrophils.
         i. Normal allele "M" while the most common variant is "Z."
         ii. Each allele is inherited in a codominant fashion.
         iii. AAT is described in terms of "PI" (for protease inhibitor) followed by the alleles that are present (thus "PI*MM" refers to homozygosity for the normal gene), while PI*ZZ indicates homozygosity for the Z allele.
   2. Epidemiology:
      a. Most commonly identified in Whites of Northern European descent.

3. Pathogenesis:
   a. Deficiency of functioning AAT results in unregulated protease activity within the airways that, over time, causes progressive loss of elastic tissue and the development of panacinar emphysema.
   b. PI*ZZ (and some other mutant alleles) leads to the production of structurally abnormal AAT that is "trapped" within hepatocytes (causing hepatocellular injury).
      i. Periodic acid–Schiff-stained liver biopsies show retained mutant AAT protein (appear as red globules within the cytoplasm of hepatocytes).
4. Clinical manifestations:
   a. Panacinar emphysema (usually developing by age 45, especially in smokers).
   b. Progressive liver disease → cirrhosis (potential for development of HCC).

F. **Autoimmune hepatitis**
   1. Definition:
      a. Chronic inflammatory disease of the liver associated with the presence of autoantibodies and elevated immunoglobulin levels.
      b. Diagnosis of exclusion (must exclude other causes of hepatitis first).
   2. Epidemiology:
      a. More common in women; often young to middle age.
      b. More common in those with other autoimmune disorders (e.g., autoimmune thyroiditis, celiac disease, rheumatoid arthritis).
   3. Pathogenesis:
      a. Unclear, likely involves a combination of genetic susceptibility in association with an unknown environmental trigger (e.g., virus, medication).
   4. Laboratory findings:
      a. Elevated aminotransferase enzymes (ALT and AST)
      b. Presence of autoantibodies:
         i. Antinuclear antibodies—most common, but nonspecific.
         ii. Antismooth muscle antibodies and anti-liver–kidney microsomal-1 antibodies are less common but more specific for autoimmune hepatitis.
      c. Elevated total serum gamma-globulin.
   5. May progress to chronic liver disease and cirrhosis.

V. **Circulatory Disorders of the Liver**
   A. **Review of hepatic blood flow**
      1. Dual blood supply to the liver via the hepatic artery and the portal vein.
      2. Tributaries of these vessels enter at the periphery of hepatic lobules (within portal tracts).
      3. Blood flows within hepatic sinusoids before draining into the central vein (at the center of the lobule).
      4. Blood drains from the liver via the hepatic vein.
   B. **Disruption of blood flow may occur at several sites**
      1. Prehepatic (before the liver):
         a. Obstruction of either the hepatic artery or portal vein (from a thrombus, embolus, tumor, or extrinsic compression) can cause localized infarct (widespread infarction is unlikely given the dual blood supply).
      2. Intrahepatic (within the liver):
         a. Cirrhosis is the most common cause of impaired blood flow through the liver.
      3. Posthepatic (after the liver):
         a. Hepatic vein thrombosis results in hepatic congestion, pain, and ascites (Budd-Chiari syndrome).
         b. Etiologies include inherited or acquired thrombophilia (e.g., antiphospholipid antibody syndrome), myeloproliferative neoplasms (e.g., polycythemia vera), invasion of hepatic vein by HCC.
         c. High mortality.
   C. **Passive hepatic congestion/centrilobular necrosis**
      1. Etiologies:
         a. Right-sided heart failure → hepatic congestion and necrosis of zone III hepatocytes ("centrilobular necrosis"):
            i. Liver becomes enlarged with mottled red coloration ("nutmeg" liver).
            ii. Congestion of central venules and sinusoids is prominent.
         b. Left-sided heart failure → hypoperfusion of the liver:
            i. Zone III hepatocytes are most susceptible to ischemic injury (receive the least oxygen as they are further downstream of blood entering at the portal tract).
      2. Clinical manifestations:
         a. Painful hepatomegaly with or without jaundice.
      3. Laboratory findings:
         a. Elevated serum aminotransferase enzymes (due to necrosis of hepatocytes).

VI. **Alcoholic Liver Disease**
   A. **Overview**
      1. Excessive ingestion of alcohol is a major cause of liver disease with a wide range of manifestations.

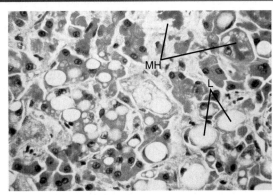

19.7: Alcoholic hepatitis. Hepatocytes contain lipid (L) droplets (triglyceride), and eosinophilic MH. *MH*, Mallory hyaline. *(From Damjanov I: Pathology for the health professions, ed 4, Philadelphia, 2012, Saunders Elsevier, p 277, Fig. 11.13.)*

B. **Pathologic effects on liver**
1. Fatty change (steatosis):
    a. Definition:
        i.   Accumulation of fat vacuoles within hepatocytes; most common effect of alcohol.
    b. Pathogenesis:
        i.   Alcohol dehydrogenase is the major enzyme system for metabolism of alcohol (requires nicotinamide adenine dinucleotide [NAD]), produces acetaldehyde and reduced NAD (NADH).
        ii. The decreased NAD+/NADH redox ratio impairs glycolysis and gluconeogenesis (contributing to hypoglycemia), impairs oxidation of fatty acids (contributing to steatosis), and increases the production of acetyl-CoA (increased fatty acid synthesis, contributing to steatosis).
    c. Pathology:
        i.   Accumulation of large fat vacuoles within cytoplasm of hepatocytes.
    d. Clinical findings:
        i.   Usually asymptomatic, hepatic enlargement/tenderness possible.
    e. Laboratory findings:
        i.   Mildly increased serum bilirubin and ALP.
2. Alcoholic steatohepatitis:
    a. Definition:
        i.   Inflammatory disease of the liver characterized by steatosis, neutrophilic inflammation, and hepatocellular injury.
    b. Pathogenesis:
        i.   Acetaldehyde, the major metabolite of alcohol, has both direct and indirect toxic effects (e.g., oxidative injury).
    c. Pathology:
        i.   Steatosis (fatty change), neutrophilic inflammation, cytoplasmic Mallory-Denk bodies (represent damaged cytokeratin intermediate filaments), and perivenular fibrosis (Fig. 19.7).
    d. Clinical manifestations:
        i.   Fever, painful hepatomegaly, ascites, hepatic encephalopathy; risk of progression to cirrhosis.
    e. Laboratory findings:
        i.   Neutrophilic leukocytosis.
        ii.   Disproportionate elevation of AST over ALT (>2:1).
            (1) AST is present within mitochondria as well as cytosol. Alcohol is a mitochondrial toxin, reason for disproportionate increase of AST relative to ALT.
        iii. Increased GGT.
3. Cirrhosis
    a. Represents end-stage fibrosis of the liver with regenerative nodule formation.
    b. Risk of HCC.

VII. **Liver Tumors and Tumor-like Disorders**
A. Definition:
1. Nonalcoholic fatty liver disease (NAFLD) refers to hepatocellular injury occurring as a result of excessive fat deposits within the liver in those who do not consume alcohol or have another explanation (e.g., medication) for fat accumulation within the liver.
B. **Epidemiology:**
1. Common cause of chronic liver disease in the United States, usually in association with the metabolic syndrome (e.g., obesity, insulin resistance, hyperlipidemia).

C. **Pathogenesis:**
  1. Exact mechanism is unclear; however, insulin resistance appears to be the major factor.
     a. Increased hepatic uptake of free fatty acids.
     b. Increased synthesis of pro-inflammatory cytokines (e.g., tumor necrosis factor-α [TNF-α]), the latter potentially leading to the development of nonalcoholic steatohepatitis (NASH). NASH is characterized by hepatic steatosis in conjunction with inflammation and hepatocyte injury (with associated elevated aminotransferase enzyme levels).
D. **Complications:**
  1. Progression to cirrhosis (analogous to alcoholic liver disease) and concomitant increased risk of developing HCC.

VIII. **Cholestatic Liver Disease**
  A. Definition:
    1. Cholestasis refers to a reduction in the flow of bile; may be secondary to either impaired hepatic secretion of bile and/or obstruction of biliary drainage (either intra- or extrahepatic).
    2. Net result is the accumulation of bilirubin (causing jaundice) and the potential for secondary hepatocellular injury.
  B. **Etiologies:**
    1. Causes of intrahepatic cholestasis include
      a. Drugs:
        i.   Oral contraceptives, anabolic steroids, and others.
      b. Primary biliary cholangitis:
        i.   Previously known as primary biliary cirrhosis.
        ii. Characterized by immune-mediated destruction of intrahepatic bile ductules with granulomatous inflammation.
        iii. Coexisting autoimmune disorder (e.g., Sjögren syndrome, rheumatoid arthritis, systemic sclerosis) often present.
        iv. Pathogenesis is a combination of genetic susceptibility in conjunction with an unknown environmental insult that modifies mitochondrial proteins.
          (1) E2 component of mitochondrial pyruvate dehydrogenase complex (PDC-E2) is autoantigen.
        v.   Subsequent CD8+ T-cell mediated attack on intralobular biliary ductules.
        vi. Primarily a disorder of women (>90% of cases), usually presenting in middle age (40–50 years).
        vii. Clinical findings:
          (1) Often asymptomatic; fatigue and pruritus are common early manifestations.
            (a) Mechanism of pruritus unclear, severity does not correlate with serum bilirubin; some evidence suggests an association with increased levels of endogenous opioids.
          (2) RUQ pain, hepatosplenomegaly.
          (3) Jaundice (late finding once majority of intralobular ducts have been destroyed).
          (4) Potential for cirrhosis, HCC.
        viii. Laboratory findings:
          (1) Antimitochondrial antibodies (nearly always present, key diagnostic finding).
          (2) Increase in serum IgM (characteristic finding).
          (3) Increased serum ALP and GGT.
        ix. Liver transplantation improves survival.
      c. Intrahepatic cholestasis of pregnancy:
        i.   Reversible type cholestasis occurring in genetically predisposed women, usually late in pregnancy.
        ii. Characterized by intense pruritus, with or without jaundice.
        iii. Not well understood, likely associated with increased sensitivity to cholestatic effects of estrogen.
    2. Causes of extrahepatic cholestasis include
      a. CBD obstruction:
        i.   Gallstone within CBD (most common cause).
        ii. Carcinoma at the head of the pancreas.
        iii. CBD stricture.
      b. Biliary atresia:
        i.   Heterogeneous condition in which extrahepatic biliary ducts undergo progressive obliteration (causing loss of patency, impaired biliary drainage) during the first few months of life.
        ii. Presents with jaundice, acholic (light-colored) stools, dark urine, and hepatomegaly with or without splenomegaly.
        iii. Hepatic biopsy shows proliferation of bile ductules and the accumulation of bile.
        iv. Common indication for liver transplantation in children.
      c. Primary sclerosing cholangitis (PSC)
        i.   Definition:
          (1) Chronic progressive cholestatic disorder characterized by periductal fibrosis ("onion skinning") and chronic inflammation of both intra- and extrahepatic bile ducts.
        ii. Epidemiology:
          (1) Male dominant disease (65% of cases), usually presenting between 30 and 40 years of age.

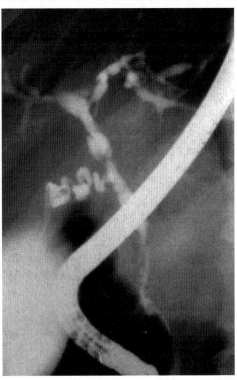

19.8: Primary sclerosing cholangitis. Extrahepatic and large intrahepatic bile ducts show alternating areas of beading and strictures. *(From Iacobuzio-Donahue CA, Montgomery E, Goldblum JR: Gastrointestinal and liver pathology, ed 2, Philadelphia, 2012, Saunders Elsevier, p 617, Fig. 19.20.)*

      (2) Many (>80%) have underlying inflammatory bowel disease (ulcerative colitis > Crohn disease).
   iii. Pathogenesis:
      (1) Cause unknown; likely immunologically mediated disorder (i.e., autoimmune).
      (2) Likely involves genetic predisposition in conjunction with unknown environmental trigger.
   iv. Clinical manifestations:
      (1) Fatigue, pruritus, RUQ pain, jaundice, hepatosplenomegaly.
   v. Laboratory findings:
      (1) Elevated total and CB.
      (2) Bilirubinuria.
      (3) Absent urine UBG, light-colored stools (bilirubin does not enter the bowel for conversion to UBG).
      (4) Increased serum ALP, GGT.
   vi. Complications:
      (1) Cirrhosis.
      (2) Cholangiocarcinoma (cancer of the bile ducts).
   vii. Diagnosis:
      (1) Contrast cholangiography (e.g., endoscopic retrograde cholangiopancreatography—ERCP) shows narrowing and dilation of bile ducts ("beading") (Fig. 19.8).
3. Pathologic findings in cholestasis:
  a. Hepatic enlargement with green discoloration.
  b. Bile ducts distended with bile, bile lakes, and bile infarcts.
4. Clinical manifestations of cholestasis:
  a. Jaundice (deposition of bilirubin in skin and mucous membranes).
  b. Pruritus.
  c. Fat malabsorption (lack of adequate bile salts).
  d. Pale "clay colored" stools (failure of CB to enter the gut prevents formation of stercobilin, the pigment responsible for normal stool coloration).
5. Laboratory findings of cholestasis include
  a. Increased total bilirubin (>50% conjugated).
  b. Increased urine bilirubin (secondary to leakage of CB into circulation and filtration by kidney).
  c. Absence of urine UBG.
    i. Formation of UBG requires bile to be present within the gut (conversion of CB into UBG by gut bacteria).
  d. Increased ALP and GGT (released from injured bile ducts).

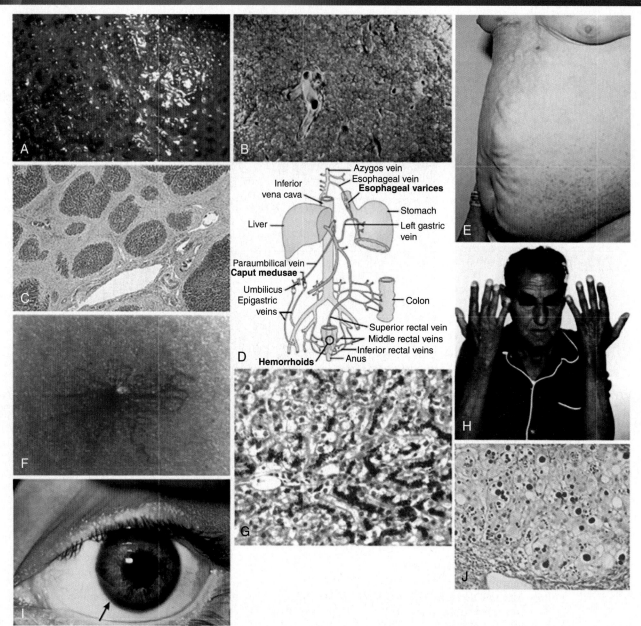

19.9: (A) Surface of a cirrhotic liver. (B) Cut section of a liver with alcoholic cirrhosis, showing regenerative nodules surrounded by collagen. (C) Trichrome-stained section of a liver with alcoholic cirrhosis. Note the regenerative nodules (*red*) and the fibrotic tissue (*blue*). (D) Portal vein anatomy and anastomoses. Note that the portal vein derives from the splenic vein and the superior mesenteric veins. Portacaval anastomoses occur when there is reversed blood flow in portal hypertension. These lead to the development of esophageal varices (via anastomoses of the left gastric vein [portal] and the azygous vein [systemic]), caput medusae (via anastomoses of the paraumbilical vein [portal] with the superficial veins of the anterior abdominal wall [systemic]), and hemorrhoids (via anastomoses of the superior rectal vein [portal] and inferior rectal [systemic] veins). (E) Patient with alcoholic cirrhosis showing ascites (abdominal distention), caput medusae (dilated superficial abdominal wall veins), and bilateral gynecomastia. (F) Spider angioma (telangiectasia) showing a single central arteriole and numerous radiating capillaries. (G) Liver biopsy stained with Prussian blue in a patient with hereditary hemochromatosis. The hepatocytes are filled with blue iron granules. This is an early stage before parenchymal damage and fibrosis develop. (H) Hemochromatosis in a male patient showing the characteristic bronze appearance of the skin. The hyperpigmentation results from the combination of iron deposited in skin plus an increase in melanin synthesis. (I) Kayser–Fleischer ring (*arrow*). This shows deposition of a copper-colored pigment in the Descemet membrane in the cornea. (J) Alpha-1-antitrypsin (AAT) deficiency. The globules of AAT accumulating in hepatocytes are periodic acid–Schiff positive. *(A, C, and J, From MacSween R, Burt A, Portmann B, Ishak K, Scheuer P, Anthony P: Pathology of the liver, ed 4, London, 2002, Churchill Livingstone, pp 596, 280, 176, respectively, Figs. 13.13, 6.9, 4.21, respectively; B, from Damjanov I, Linder J: Pathology: a color atlas, St. Louis, 2000, Mosby, p 154, Fig. 8.42; D, from Moore A, Roy W: Rapid review gross and developmental anatomy, ed 3, Philadelphia, 2010, Mosby Elsevier, p 95, Fig. 3.40; E, from Swartz M: Textbook of physical diagnosis history and examination, ed 5, Philadelphia, 2006, Saunders Elsevier, p 497, Fig. 17.14; F, from Gitlin M, Strauss R: Atlas of clinical hepatology, Philadelphia, 1995, Saunders, pp 3, 22, Figs. 1-4 and 2-9, respectively; G, from Kumar V, Fausto N, Abbas A: Robbins and Cotran pathologic basis of disease, ed 7, Philadelphia, 2004, Saunders, p 910, Fig. 18.28; H, from Gitlin N, Straauss R: Atlas of clinical hepatology, Philadelphia, 1995, Saunders, p22, Fig. 2.9; I, from Perkin GD: Mosby's color atlas and text of neurology, St. Louis, 2002, Mosby, p 151, Fig. 8.15.)*

IX. **Hepatic Cirrhosis**
  A. Definition:
    1. End-stage liver disease characterized by progressive hepatic fibrosis (Fig. 19.9).
    2. Altered hepatic architecture with diffuse fibrosis and "regenerative" nodules.
    3. Impaired blood flow through the liver → elevated pressures within the portal vein (i.e., portal hypertension).
  B. Etiologies:
    1. Hepatitis C, alcohol abuse, and NAFLD:
      a. Major factors (together, account for ~80% of cirrhosis in the United States).
    2. Secondary biliary cirrhosis:
      a. Refers to the development of cirrhosis as a complication of chronic biliary obstruction.
      b. An example is cystic fibrosis in which the viscous bile causes cholestasis, hepatocellular damage, and eventually cirrhosis.
  C. Complications:
    1. Impaired synthetic and metabolic function of liver:
      a. Bleeding complications due to decreased coagulation factor synthesis.
      b. Thrombotic complications due to decreased synthesis of natural anticoagulant proteins (e.g., antithrombin, protein C, protein S).
      c. Edema due to decreased hepatic synthesis of albumin (loss of intravascular oncotic pressure).
      d. Hepatic encephalopathy (related to elevated levels of ammonia):
        i. Ammonia, a product of protein metabolism, is normally metabolized to urea by the hepatic urea cycle (impaired in severe hepatic disease).
        ii. Most important precipitating factor is increased protein absorption (e.g., high protein diet, absorption of blood in the gastrointestinal tract).
        iii. Manifestations include altered mental status, somnolence, disordered sleep, asterixis (flapping tremor), coma, and death.
    2. Portal hypertension:
      a. Portal vein is formed by the convergence of the superior mesenteric and splenic veins.
      b. Increased pressure within the portal vein ("portal hypertension") occurs due to increased resistance to blood flow through the cirrhotic liver (altered hepatic architecture in cirrhosis due to fibrosis and regenerative nodule formation).
        i. Portal hypertension can also occur in those with thrombosis of the portal or hepatic vein, tumor invasion of either vessel.
      c. Complications of portal hypertension include
        i. Congestive splenomegaly:
          (1) Secondary to increased hydrostatic pressure within the splenic vein.
          (2) May be associated with various cytopenias (e.g., thrombocytopenia) due to sequestration of blood cells within the enlarged spleen.
        ii. Esophageal varices:
          (1) Bleeding esophageal varices is the single most life-threatening complication of portal hypertension.
        iii. Hemorrhoids.
        iv. Periumbilical venous collaterals (caput medusae).
        v. Ascites:
          (1) Excess peritoneal fluid, usually a transudate.
          (2) Due to elevated hydrostatic pressure within the portal vein in conjunction with a reduction in oncotic pressure (decreased albumin synthesis in damaged liver).
          (3) On exam, ascites is associated with abdominal distention, fluid wave, shifting dullness to percussion.
          (4) Risk of developing spontaneous bacterial peritonitis.
    3. Hepatorenal syndrome:
      a. Renal dysfunction secondary to advanced liver disease.
      b. High mortality; potentially reversible with correction of the hepatic dysfunction.
    4. Hyperestrogenism
      a. Impaired hepatic metabolism of estrogen and adrenal androgens (e.g., androstenedione).
        i. Adrenal androgens are converted into estrogen by aromatase (an enzyme present in adipose tissue and other sites).
      b. Clinical manifestations:
        i. Gynecomastia, palmar erythema, spider telangiectasia (dilation of capillaries causing a spider-like appearance).
X. **Liver Tumors and Tumor-Like Disorders**
  A. **Focal nodular hyperplasia**
    1. Benign liver lesion characterized by the proliferation of hepatocytes in response to a vascular abnormality (e.g., vascular malformation).
    2. Predominantly middle-aged females, second most common benign liver lesion (hemangioma is most common).

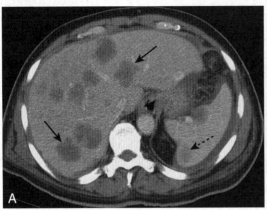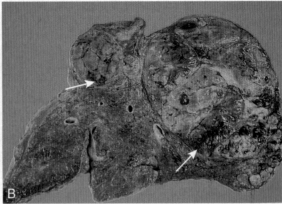

19.10: (A) Computed tomography image showing metastases to the liver and spleen. Metastases usually appear as multiple, low-attenuation masses (*solid black arrows*). There are also low-attenuation lesions in the spleen (*dotted black arrow*). The patient had a primary adenocarcinoma of the colon. (B) Hepatocellular carcinoma, gross image showing hemorrhagic tumor masses within liver. (*A, From Herring W: Learning radiology recognizing the basics, ed 2, Philadelphia, 2012, Elsevier Saunders, p 187, Fig. 18.31; B, from Damjanov I, Linder J: A color atlas, St. Louis, 2000, Mosby, p 161, Fig. 8.70.*)

    3. Gross: Well-circumscribed nodule with central depressed stellate scar.
    4. Diagnosis: Imaging studies of the liver (e.g., computed tomography [CT], magnetic resonance imaging [MRI]).
    5. Treatment only necessary if symptomatic (pain).
B. Cysts/abscesses
    1. Simple cyst:
       a. Benign cyst of liver occurring in ~1% of the adult population, somewhat more common in females.
       b. Usually asymptomatic, may cause abdominal pain.
    2. Echinococcal (hydatid) cyst:
       a. Uncommon in the United States; seen in sheep herders (acquired from sheepdogs); caused by larval form of *Echinococcus granulosus.*
       b. Often asymptomatic, may cause compressive symptoms or rupture (the latter potentially causing anaphylaxis).
C. Benign tumors of the liver
    1. Hepatic hemangioma:
       a. Benign tumor of endothelial cells (most common benign hepatic tumor).
       b. Often described as a "cavernous" hemangioma due to the large dilated "cave-like" vascular spaces seen on histologic examination.
       c. Typically, an incidental finding (most are asymptomatic).
       d. Small risk of hemorrhage (either spontaneous or following needle biopsy).
    2. Hepatocellular adenoma:
       a. Uncommon benign liver tumor associated with the use of exogenous steroids (oral contraceptives, anabolic steroids); may regress upon discontinuation.
       b. More common in women than in men.
       c. Complications include hemorrhage; small risk of malignant transformation (into HCC).
D. Malignant tumors of the liver

Risk factors for the development of gallstones

- Obesity (increased biliary secretion of cholesterol).
- Female sex/estrogen exposure (e.g., oral contraceptives, pregnancy, hormone replacement therapy); estrogen raises cholesterol levels in the bile and slows gallbladder motility.
- Increasing age (>40 years).
- Ethnicity (Native Americans, Mexican Americans).
- Rapid weight loss (biliary stasis in absence of food intake).
- Disease of terminal ileum (e.g., Crohn disease) impairs reabsorption of bile acids.
- Chronic hemolysis (e.g., hereditary spherocytosis).
  - Stones are dark black in color, comprising calcium bilirubinate.
- Infection of CBD; bacterial (e.g., *Escherichia coli*); parasitic (e.g., *Clonorchis sinensis*).
  - More common in Asia; stones are brown in color, comprising calcium salts, cholesterol, and bilirubin.

The most common hepatic malignancy is metastatic tumor from elsewhere. Primary sites include colorectal carcinoma (most common), lung, and breast cancer. May appear as single or multiple lesions (Fig. 19.10A).

1. HCC:
   a. Definition:
      i. Primary tumor of hepatocytes.
   b. Epidemiology:
      i. Most common primary malignancy of the liver in adults.
      ii. Third most common cancer worldwide (due to the high prevalence of chronic hepatitis B and C).
      iii. Increasing incidence in the United States, largely due to chronic hepatitis C.
      iv. More common in males than females.
      v. Peaks around fifth to sixth decades of life.
   c. Etiologies include
      i. Cirrhosis (e.g., chronic hepatitis B/C, alcohol, NAFLD).
      ii. Aflatoxins (from *Aspergillus* mold in grains and peanuts).
   d. Pathology:
      i. HCC may present as single or multiple hepatic masses, usually (~90%) in association with preexisting cirrhosis (Fig. 19.10B).
      ii. May invade the portal and/or hepatic vein with associated manifestations (e.g., portal hypertension).
      iii. Microscopically characterized by malignant cells containing bile.
   e. Clinical manifestations:
      i. Abdominal pain/mass, weight loss.
      ii. Paraneoplastic syndromes (hypoglycemia, erythrocytosis, hypercalcemia), see below.
      iii. Fever (due to tumor necrosis).
      iv. Obstructive jaundice possible (due to invasion of bile ducts).
      v. Lung is the most common site for metastasis.
   f. Laboratory findings:
      i. Increased serum α-fetoprotein (AFP).
      ii. Production of ectopic hormones:
         (1) Erythropoietin causing erythrocytosis.
         (2) Insulin-like factor producing hypoglycemia.
         (3) Parathyroid hormone-related peptide producing hypercalcemia.
   g. Diagnosis
      i. Imaging studies (CT scan, ultrasound) are used to localize the lesion.
      ii. Angiography shows pooling and increased vascularity of the tumor.
      iii. Biopsy for histologic confirmation.
   h. Prognosis:
      i. Poor, if unresectable most patients die within months.
2. Fibrolamellar carcinoma:
   a. **Definition**:
      i. Rare malignant tumor of the liver.
      ii. Historically considered a variant of HCC; however, the tumor cells have been found to exhibit markers of both hepatocytes as well as biliary epithelium (and unlike conventional HCC, does not secrete AFP).
   b. Epidemiology:
      i. No known risk factors and no sex predisposition.
      ii. Usually arises in childhood to young adulthood (5–35 years).
   c. Treatment:
      i. Resection (~60% 5-year survival).
3. Angiosarcoma:
   a. Rare malignant neoplasm of endothelial cells.
   b. Risk factors include exposure to vinyl chloride, arsenic, and thorium dioxide.
XI. **Gallbladder and Biliary Tract Disease**
   A. **Choledochal cyst**
      1. Congenital bile duct anomaly characterized by cystic dilatation of the biliary tract (extrahepatic, intrahepatic, or both).
      2. Clinical manifestations:
         a. Jaundice, RUQ pain and/or mass.
      3. Complications:
         a. Increased risk of cholangitis, pancreatitis, and cholangiocarcinoma (cancer of bile ducts).
      4. Diagnosis: Abdominal ultrasound, cholangiography.
   B. **Caroli disease/syndrome**
      1. Congenital conditions characterized by focally dilated regions of large intrahepatic ducts.
         a. Caroli syndrome, which is more common, is characterized by dilated bile ducts plus congenital hepatic fibrosis.
         b. Caroli disease is characterized by ductal dilatation alone.
      2. Complications:
         a. Biliary lithiasis (stone formation within biliary tree).

    b. Cholangitis (inflammation/infection of biliary tree).

    c. Cholangiocarcinoma (see below).

C. Cholangiocarcinoma

1. Malignancy of the bile duct epithelium (may be intrahepatic or extrahepatic).

2. Second most common primary hepatic malignancy (behind HCC).

    a. Relatively rare in the United States, more common in Asia (e.g., Thailand) in association with liver fluke infestation.

3. Major risk factor is chronic inflammation of biliary tract:

    a. PSC—most common cause of cholangiocarcinoma in the United States.

    b. *Clonorchis sinensis* (Chinese liver fluke; particularly in northern Thailand).

    c. Choledochal cyst, Caroli disease/syndrome.

4. May arise at any location (intra- or extrahepatic):

    a. Intrahepatic (20%–25% of cases).

    b. Confluence of the right and left hepatic bile ducts (i.e., liver hilum; ~60% of cases; called "Klatskin" tumor).

    c. Distal CBD (20% of cases).

5. Clinical manifestations:

    a. Upper abdominal pain, weight loss, obstructive jaundice, hepatomegaly.

6. Diagnosis:

    a. Ultrasound, cholangiography, CT, MRI.

7. Prognosis:

    a. Poor, most cases are unresectable.

D. Gallstones (cholelithiasis)

1. Overview:

    a. Gallbladder concentrates and stores bile between meals.

    b. Following a meal, CCK is released by endocrine cells in the proximal small intestine.

    c. CCK stimulates gallbladder contraction, resulting in the expulsion of bile through the cystic duct and CBD into the duodenum through the ampulla of Vater.

    d. Saturation of bile with cholesterol, with or without stasis, leads to the development of gallstones (calculi).

2. Cholesterol stones:

    a. Most common type in Western countries (~80%).

    b. Comprised of crystalline cholesterol monohydrate (develop following the supersaturation of bile with cholesterol).

3. Pigment stones:

    a. Infection of bile duct, chronic hemolysis.

4. Clinical manifestations:

    a. Most stones remain asymptomatic.

    b. Biliary colic (steady constant pain in right upper abdomen with radiation to right scapula).

       i. Often follows meals, persists for few hours.

       ii. May be accompanied by nausea, bloating, flatulence.

    c. Acute cholecystitis:

       i. Definition:

         (1) Syndrome of RUQ pain, fever, and neutrophilic leukocytosis in conjunction with inflammation of the gallbladder; usually secondary to obstruction of the cystic duct by a gallstone.

       ii. Clinical manifestations:

         (1) RUQ/epigastric pain arising ~1 hour after the ingestion of a meal (especially fatty meals). Pain is typically severe, steady, and prolonged for several hours; may radiate to the right scapula.

         (2) Fever, nausea, vomiting.

         (3) Positive Murphy sign (pain on deep palpation of the RUQ as the inflamed gallbladder comes into contact with the examiner's hand during inspiration).

       iii. Laboratory findings:

         (1) Absolute neutrophilic leukocytosis with left shift (increased band neutrophils).

         (2) Other findings (e.g., elevated AST/ALT, lipase/amylase, ALP, GGT, and bilirubin) are possible if the stone obstructs the CBD.

5. Diagnosis of gallstones

    a. Abdominal ultrasound (preferred initial test).

       i. Used to identify presence of stones and to evaluate for edema and thickening of the gallbladder wall.

       ii. Ultrasound is less effective in the identification of CBD stones (cholangiography better choice).

    b. Cholescintigraphy (hepatic iminodiacetic acid scan)

       i. Used if ultrasound is not diagnostic.

       ii. Involves the injection of a radioactive tracer that is taken up selectively by hepatocytes and excreted into bile.

       iii. If cystic duct is patent, the tracer will enter the gallbladder; also useful for demonstrating patency of the CBD and ampulla.

6. Complications of cholecystitis:
   a. Cholecystoenteric fistula (connection between an inflamed gallbladder and the bowel; usually the duodenum).
   b. Gallstone ileus (bowel obstruction following the passage of a gallstone through a cholecystoenteric fistula into the bowel).
   c. Gangrenous cholecystitis (ischemic necrosis of gallbladder).
   d. Emphysematous cholecystitis (secondary infection of the gallbladder by gas-forming organisms).
   e. Chronic cholecystitis (chronic inflammation of the gallbladder, usually associated with the presence of gallstones).

E. **Gallbladder cancer**
   1. Definition:
      a. An adenocarcinoma (tumor of glandular epithelial cells) arising from the gallbladder mucosa.
   2. Epidemiology:
      a. More common in women, usually older.
   3. Risk factors:
      a. Gallstone (nearly always present).
      b. "Porcelain gallbladder" (calcification of the gallbladder wall, seen in those with chronic gallstone-induced mucosal injury).
      c. Chronic *Salmonella* infection of gallbladder.
   4. Often found incidentally at time of cholecystectomy, poor prognosis.

XII. **Pancreatic Disorders**
A. **Congenital abnormalities of the pancreas**
   1. Pancreatic divisum:
      a. Most common congenital malformation of pancreas.
      b. Though most are asymptomatic, there is an increased risk of recurrent pancreatitis secondary to impaired pancreatic drainage.
   2. Annular pancreas:
      a. Congenital anomaly characterized by a ring of pancreatic tissue around the duodenum.
      b. Due to incomplete rotation of the ventral pancreatic bud.
      c. Often asymptomatic, may obstruct duodenum.
   3. Pancreatic heterotopia:
      a. Presence of pancreatic tissue in aberrant locations (e.g., stomach, duodenum, jejunum, Meckel diverticulum).
      b. An incidental finding in a surgical specimen or at autopsy.

B. **Acute pancreatitis**
   1. Definition:
      a. Episode of pancreatic inflammation and parenchymal injury resulting in abdominal pain, nausea, and vomiting.
   2. Pathogenesis:
      a. Variety of triggers (discussed below), all of which essentially cause premature activation of pancreatic digestive enzymes and thus "autodigestion" of pancreatic tissue.
      b. Recovery may or may not be complete, depending upon degree of tissue injury.
   3. Etiologies:
      a. Gallstones:
         i. Obstruction of the CBD at the level of the ampulla of Vater → increased pressure within pancreatic ducts → damages pancreatic acini (the cells of the exocrine pancreas) → release and activation of digestive enzymes → pancreatic parenchymal injury (edema, hemorrhage).
         ii. Most common cause of acute pancreatitis.
      b. Alcohol:
         i. Mechanism of alcoholic pancreatitis is unclear.
         ii. May be secondary to increased synthesis of digestive enzymes by pancreatic acinar cells.
         iii. Second most common cause of acute pancreatitis.
      c. Genetic factors (e.g., *PRSS1*, *SPINK1*, *CFTR* gene mutations).
         i. *PRSS1* gene mutations result in an abnormal form of trypsinogen that resists inactivation.
         ii. *SPINK1* gene mutations impair function of a trypsin inhibitor.
         iii. *CFTR* mutations (cause of cystic fibrosis) impair ion channels, causing thickened pancreatic secretions, partial obstruction of pancreatic duct.
      d. Metabolic disorders (e.g., hypertriglyceridemia, hypercalcemia).
      e. Infections (e.g., mumps, coxsackievirus).
      f. Trauma (e.g., ERCP).
   4. Clinical manifestations:
      a. Persistent epigastric or periumbilical pain with radiation into the back (pancreas is retroperitoneal).
      b. Nausea, vomiting, dehydration.
      c. Retroperitoneal bleeding in some cases (Grey-Turner sign: flank ecchymosis; Cullen sign: periumbilical ecchymosis).

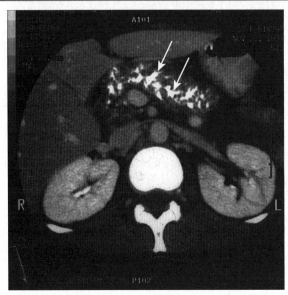

19.11: Computed tomography image showing diffuse dystrophic calcification of the pancreas in a patient with chronic pancreatitis (*white arrows*). (*From Goldman L, Schafer A:* Goldman's Cecil medicine, *ed 25, Philadelphia, 2016, Elsevier Saunders, p 964, Fig. 144.2.*)

    5. Complications:
      a. Hypovolemic shock:
        i. Due to leakage of fluid and blood.
      b. Disseminated intravascular coagulation:
        i. Due to activation of prothrombin by trypsin.
      c. Hypocalcemia:
        i. Due to binding of calcium to fatty acids released in areas of enzymatic fat necrosis. May result in tetany (muscle spasms associated with a decrease in serum ionized calcium).
      d. Pancreatic pseudocyst:
        i. Nonepithelialized peripancreatic fluid collection.
        ii. Presents with persistence of pain, nausea, weight loss, and elevated pancreatic enzyme levels several weeks after the episode of acute pancreatitis.
        iii. May require surgical drainage (fluid characteristically has high levels of amylase).
      e. Acute respiratory distress syndrome:
        i. Due to inactivation of surfactant by circulating pancreatic enzymes.
      f. Chronic pancreatitis:
        i. Secondary to repeated attacks of acute pancreatitis and parenchymal fibrosis.
    6. Diagnosis of acute pancreatitis:
      a. Increase in serum amylase and/or lipase to three times normal (lipase is more specific).
      b. Imaging (e.g., CT of abdomen) showing pancreatic edema and necrosis.
C. Chronic pancreatitis
    1. Definition:
      a. Syndrome of chronic abdominal pain and pancreatic insufficiency due to the fibrous replacement of damaged pancreatic parenchyma. Usually arises following repeated episodes of acute pancreatitis.
    2. Manifestations:
      a. Chronic severe abdominal pain with radiation into the back.
      b. Malabsorption (due to loss of exocrine pancreatic enzymes).
      c. Type 1 diabetes mellitus (due to loss of β-islet cells).
    3. Laboratory and radiographic findings include
      a. Variable levels of amylase and lipase (may be normal).
      b. Increased fecal fat (loss of exocrine pancreatic function).
      c. Decreased fecal elastase and chymotrypsin.
      d. CT of abdomen (pancreatic atrophy with multiple parenchymal and intraductal calcifications are characteristic findings of chronic pancreatitis; see Fig. 19.11).
D. Pancreatic adenocarcinoma
    1. Definition:
      a. Malignancy of pancreatic ductal epithelial cells.

2. Epidemiology:
   a. Tenth leading cause of cancer in the United States but the fourth leading cause of cancer-related death (i.e., high mortality rate).
   b. Most arise in older adults (mean age ~70 years).
   c. Most common pancreatic malignancy (>90%).
3. Risk factors
   a. Cigarette smoking (major environmental risk factor), chronic pancreatitis, diabetes mellitus.
   b. Inherited genetic mutations, including:
      i. *PRSS1*: Familial pancreatitis (40% lifetime risk pancreatic cancer).
      ii. *STK11*: Peutz-Jeghers syndrome (>100-fold increased risk).
      iii. *CDKN2A*: Familial atypical mole and multiple melanoma syndrome (40-fold increased risk).
4. Pathogenesis:
   a. Mutations in the *KRAS* oncogene results in unregulated cell proliferation (present in >90% of tumors).
   b. Mutations in tumor suppressor genes (*TP53*, *CDKN2A*) are also commonly found.
5. Clinical manifestations:
   a. Nausea, vague abdominal pain, weight loss.
      i. Those arising within the head of pancreas (~75% of cases) may cause jaundice, pale-colored stools, and palpable gallbladder (Courvoisier sign) secondary to the obstruction of biliary drainage at the ampulla/distal CBD.
   b. Superficial migratory thrombophlebitis (Trousseau syndrome).
   c. Periumbilical metastasis (Sister Mary Joseph nodule); nonspecific, also occurs in stomach cancer.
6. Laboratory findings:
   a. Increase serum CA19.9 (gold standard tumor marker).
   b. If tumor obstructs biliary flow through the ampulla, then total bilirubin, ALP, and aminotransferase enzymes will all be elevated.
7. Imaging:
   a. Abdominal CT scan useful for identification of the mass and for guidance of needle biopsy in order to confirm the diagnosis.
8. Prognosis:
   a. Poor (80% are unresectable); overall 5-year survival of 5%.

I. Renal Anatomy

A. Blood supply

1. The renal artery, a branch of the aorta, delivers oxygenated blood to the kidneys.
2. Branches of the renal artery are as follows (Fig. 20.1):
   a. Renal artery → segmental arteries → lobar arteries → interlobar arteries → arcuate arteries → interlobular arteries → afferent arterioles → glomerulus.
3. Afferent arteries deliver blood to the glomerulus.
   a. Blood flow through afferent arteries is controlled by prostaglandins E_2 and I_2.
      i. Released from the kidney, these prostaglandins cause vasodilation of afferent arteriole and thus an increase in renal blood flow and glomerular filtration.
      ii. Nonsteroidal antiinflammatory drugs (NSAIDs) inhibit this effect (by inhibiting cyclooxygenase, they block prostaglandin synthesis). This is of particular concern when there is a decrease in actual (hypovolemia) or effective blood volume (e.g., heart failure), potentially contributing to renal injury.
4. Glomerular capillaries (glomerulus)
   a. Site of blood filtration (see below).
5. Efferent arterioles
   a. Efferent arterioles drain glomeruli, eventually form vasa recta.
   b. Flow through efferent arterioles is controlled by angiotensin II (AT II) (causes vasoconstriction).
6. Glomerulus (Fig. 20.2)
   a. Network of capillaries, site of blood filtration.
   b. Three layers (Fig. 20.3)
      i. Glomerular capillary endothelium (fenestrated).
      ii. Glomerular basement membrane (GBM)
         (1) Composed of Type IV collagen with a net negative charge (acts as a size and charge barrier).
         (2) Normally impermeable to negatively charged or large proteins (e.g., albumin).
      iii. Visceral epithelial cells
         (1) Contain foot-like processes known as podocytes (filtration slits between podocytes).
7. Mesangium
   a. Supportive cells of mesenchymal origin.
   b. Lie between glomerular capillaries; various functions (contractile, phagocytic, and secretory).
8. Parietal epithelial cells (lining cells of Bowman capsule).

II. Renal Function

A. Excretes harmful waste products (e.g., urea, creatinine [Cr], and uric acid).
B. Maintains acid–base homeostasis.
C. Reabsorps essential substances (e.g., sodium, glucose, and amino acids).
D. Regulates water balance via changes in urine concentration.
E. Regulates total body sodium levels.
F. Regulates blood pressure/volume via release of renin.

1. Activation of the renin–angiotensin–aldosterone system
   a. Renin (released from the juxtaglomerular apparatus in the kidney) cleaves angiotensinogen into angiotensin I (AT I).
   b. AT I is converted into AT II by angiotensin-converting enzyme (ACE).

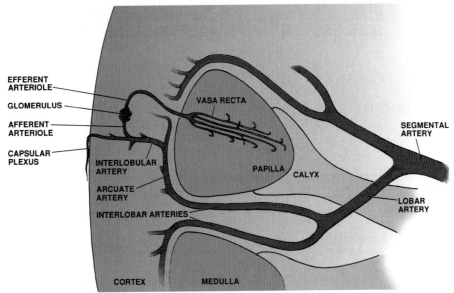

20.1: Intrarenal arterial anatomy. *(From Campbell-Walsh-Wein urology, ed 12, Copyright © 2021 by Elsevier, Inc, eFig. 84.17.)*

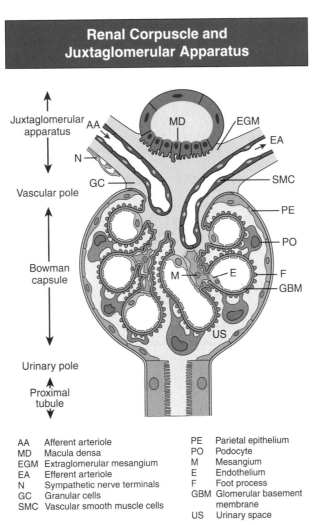

AA	Afferent arteriole
MD	Macula densa
EGM	Extraglomerular mesangium
EA	Efferent arteriole
N	Sympathetic nerve terminals
GC	Granular cells
SMC	Vascular smooth muscle cells

PE	Parietal epithelium
PO	Podocyte
M	Mesangium
E	Endothelium
F	Foot process
GBM	Glomerular basement membrane
US	Urinary space

20.2: Structure of glomerulus. *(From Kriz W, Kaissling B: Structural organization of the mammalian kidney. In Seldin DW, Giebisch G, editors: The kidney, ed 3, Philadelphia, 2000, Lippincott Williams & Wilkens, pp 587–654.)*

Peripheral Portion of a Glomerular Lobule

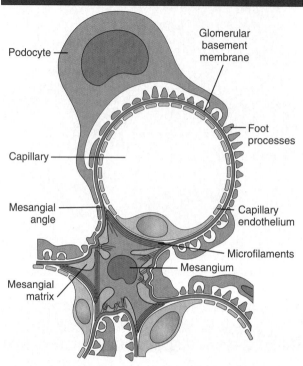

20.3: Layers of glomerular membrane. *(From Comprehensive clinical nephrology, ed 6, © 2019, Elsevier Inc, Fig. 1.6.)*

    c. AG II has two effects:
      i. Direct vasoconstriction of peripheral vascular resistance arterioles.
      ii. Stimulation of aldosterone release from the zona glomerulosa of the adrenal cortex (enhances reabsorption of sodium from the distal convoluted tubule, thereby increasing blood volume).

G. Erythropoietin (EPO) production
  1. Renal hypoxia stimulates fibroblasts within the renal cortex to release EPO.
  2. EPO stimulates the proliferation and differentiation of erythrocyte precursors in the bone marrow (thereby increasing red cell mass).

H. Maintenance of calcium homeostasis (Fig. 20.4)
  1. 7-Dehydrocholesterol (skin) hydroxylated to 25-hydroxycholecalciferol (liver) and subsequently to 1,25-dihydroxy-cholecalciferol (calcitriol) by 1α-hydroxylase (kidney).
    a. Calcitriol is the active form of vitamin D.
    b. The final step of vitamin D biosynthesis (i.e., 1α-hydroxylase) is under the control of parathyroid hormone (PTH).
  2. By increasing the absorption of calcium from the gut, and enhancing the reabsorption of calcium from the kidneys, calcitriol maintains serum calcium and promotes bone mineralization.

III. Renal Laboratory Interpretation
  A. Urinalysis
    1. Gold-standard test is the initial workup of the renal disease.
    2. Hematuria
      a. Blood in the urine (gross or microscopic); may arise from the disease of the upper or lower urinary tract.
      b. Upper urinary tract (i.e., kidneys and ureter) etiologies include:
        i. Nephrolithiasis (renal stone; most common).
        ii. Glomerular disease
          (1) Clue is the presence of dysmorphic red blood cells (RBCs) and/or RBC casts in the urinary sediment.
        iii. Pyelonephritis (infection of the kidney).
        iv. Neoplasms (e.g., renal cell carcinoma [RCC] and urothelial carcinoma).
        v. Renal papillary necrosis (e.g., sickle cell disease, diabetes mellitus, and analgesic abuse).
      c. Lower urinary tract (bladder, urethra, and prostate) etiologies include:
        i. Urinary tract infection (most common).
        ii. Urothelial carcinoma.
        iii. Prostatic hyperplasia and prostate cancer.

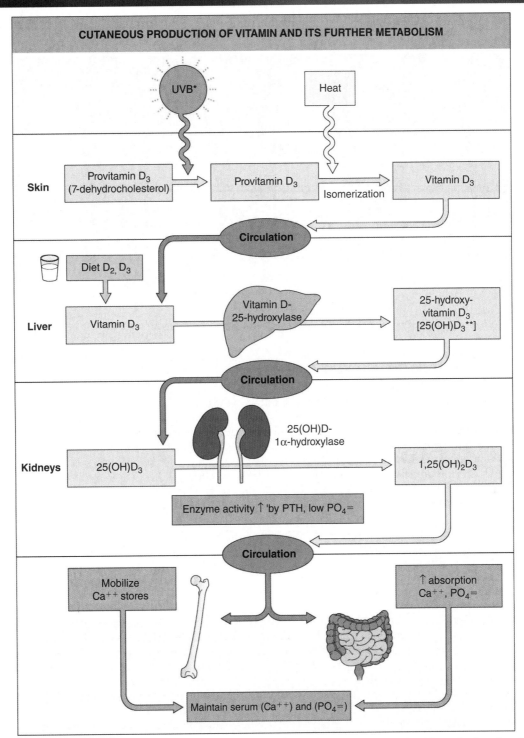

CUTANEOUS PRODUCTION OF VITAMIN AND ITS FURTHER METABOLISM

20.4: Vitamin D synthesis. Exposure to ultraviolet radiation converts 7-dehydrocholesterol within the skin to the inactive vitamin D3. After binding to carrier proteins, vitamin D is transported to the liver, where it is enzymatically hydroxylated to 25-hydroxyvitamin D [25(OH)D], the major circulating form of vitamin D. 25(OH)D is then converted into its active form, 1,25-dihydroxyvitmain D [1,25(OH)2D], within the kidney by the enzyme 1α-hydroxylase. 1,25(OH)2D decreases its own synthesis via feedback inhibition and decreases the synthesis and secretion of parathyroid hormone by the parathyroid glands. 1,25(OH)2D also enhances intestinal calcium absorption in the small intestine and acts to maintain calcium and phosphorus levels. *Most effective wavelength = 300 ± 5 nm. **Measurement of this form most commonly done to assess vitamin D status. *(From Dermatology, ed 4, © 2018, Elsevier Limited, Fig. 51.11.)*

3. Proteinuria
   a. Definition
      i. Urinary protein excretion of more than 150 mg/24 hours.
      ii. In health, only minimal (<30 mg/24 hours) protein is lost in the urine; mostly Tamm–Horsfall protein, a glycoprotein synthesized by the thick ascending limb of the loop of Henle.

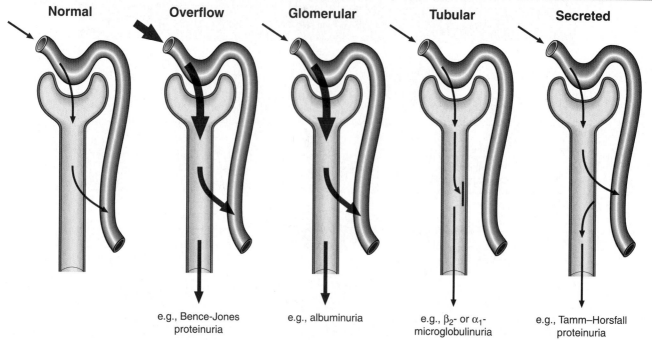

Normal	Overflow	Glomerular	Tubular	Secreted
	e.g., Bence-Jones proteinuria	e.g., albuminuria	e.g., β₂- or α₁- microglobulinuria	e.g., Tamm–Horsfall proteinuria

20.5: Mechanisms of proteinuria. See text for discussion. *(From Gaw A, Murphy MJ, Srivastava R, Cowan RA, O'Reilly Denis St J: Clinical biochemistry: an illustrated colour text, ed 5, St. Louis, 2013, Churchill Livingstone Elsevier, p 34, Fig. 17.1.)*

       iii. Large proteins (e.g., albumin) are not normally found in the urine.
    b. Etiologies (Fig. 20.5)
       i. Overflow (number of filtered proteins exceed tubular reabsorption capacity).
       ii. Damage to the glomerular filtration barrier.
       iii. Impaired tubular reabsorption of filtered proteins.
       iv. Loss of white blood cells in the urine (e.g., urinary tract infection).
    c. Persistent proteinuria usually indicates renal disease.
       i. Tests to identify protein in the urine
          (1) Dipsticks
             (a) Specific for albumin, only sensitive down to a level of ~20 mg/dL (i.e., albuminuria of <20 mg/dL will be missed by this method).
          (2) Sulfosalicylic acid
             (a) Detects all proteins, including albumin and globulins (i.e., more sensitive).
    d. Twenty-four-hour urine collection used to quantitate protein excretion.

B. Blood urea nitrogen (BUN)
    1. Urea, an end product of protein catabolism, is produced primarily in the liver (urea cycle).
    2. Rate of production is not constant, an elevated BUN level may be seen following the ingestion of large quantities of dietary protein or in association with increased resorption of tissue protein (e.g., absorption of blood from the gastrointestinal tract).
    3. Reference range 10–20 mg/dL (adult).
    4. Urea is filtered at the glomerulus and also partially reabsorbed in the proximal tubule; the amount reabsorbed is dependent on renal blood flow.
       a. As renal blood flow slows (e.g., as would be seen in a patient with volume depletion or heart failure), more urea is reabsorbed.
    5. BUN levels depend on the following:
       a. Glomerular filtration rate (GFR) (↑ GFR, ↓ BUN; ↓ GFR, ↑ BUN).
       b. Protein content in the diet (↑ dietary protein, ↑ BUN).
       c. Reabsorption in the proximal tubule.
       d. Functional status of the urea cycle in the liver (liver disease → decreased urea synthesis [↓ BUN]).

C. Serum Cr
    1. Cr is formed at a relatively constant rate in muscle; serum levels are proportional to muscle mass.
    2. Cr is filtered at the glomerulus but not appreciably reabsorbed or secreted by the renal tubules.
    3. With stable muscle mass, serum Cr levels correlate with renal function (GFR).
    4. Normal serum Cr concentration is 0.6–1.2 mg/dL.
    5. Creatinine clearance (CCr) is widely used to estimate GFR.
       a. Important to consider CCr when dosing nephrotoxic drugs (e.g., aminoglycosides) to prevent renal toxicity.

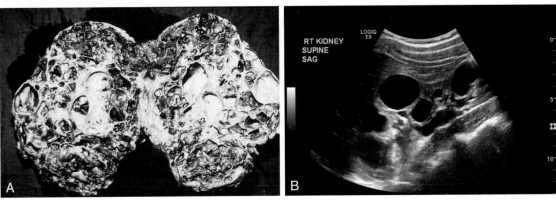

20.6: Autosomal dominant polycystic kidney disease. (A) Gross specimen. (B) Ultrasonography. *(From Zitelli and Davis' atlas of pediatric physical diagnosis, ed 7, Copyright © 2018 by Elsevier, Fig. 14.32.)*

   b. Calculation of CCr
     i. CrCl (mL/min) = [UCr (mg/dL)/SCr (mg/dL)] × [urine volume (mL)/collection time (minutes)].
  D. **Fractional excretion of sodium (FENa)**
     1. Measure of the percent of filtered sodium that is excreted in the urine.
     2. Can be used to differentiate between types of acute kidney injury (AKI) (see later discussion).
IV. **Congenital Diseases of the Kidneys**
  A. **Horseshoe kidney**
     1. Most common congenital abnormality (~1 in 1000 newborns); more common in males.
     2. Increased incidence in Turner syndrome; trisomies 13, 18, and 21.
     3. Most (~90%) are fused at the inferior pole; renal ascent halted by the root of the inferior mesenteric artery.
     4. Usually asymptomatic; increased risk of infection, stone formation, and hydronephrosis.
  B. **Renal agenesis**
     1. Defined as congenital absence of renal parenchymal tissue.
     2. More common in males, due to disrupted metanephric development at an early stage.
     3. Variety of associations, including genetic mutations (e.g., *RET*) and environmental exposures.
     4. Unilateral renal agenesis is usually asymptomatic.
        a. Risk of renal insufficiency later in life secondary to hyperfiltration.
     5. Bilateral renal agenesis is incompatible with life.
        a. The absence of kidneys leads to a lack of amniotic fluid (anhydramnios) with pulmonary hypoplasia, characteristic facies (e.g., flattened nose and ears), and positional limb deformities (constellation of findings known as Potter sequence).
  C. **Autosomal dominant polycystic kidney disease (ADPKD)**
     1. Definition
        a. Inherited disorder (autosomal dominant [AD]) characterized by the development of multiple renal cysts (Fig. 20.6).
     2. Epidemiology
        a. Most common inherited kidney disease (~1:1000).
     3. Pathogenesis
        a. Mutations in *PKD1* (~80% of cases), encodes for a protein (polycystin 1) involved in cell–cell adherence and ciliary function.
        b. Mutations in *PKD2* (~15% of cases), encodes for a protein (polycystin 2) involved in calcium ion signaling.
     4. Clinical manifestations
        a. Usually asymptomatic for approximately the first three decades of life.
        b. Over time, progressive cyst formation leads to bilateral renal enlargement, hematuria, and worsening renal impairment.
        c. Hypertension (due to the upregulation of the renin–angiotensin–aldosterone system) is common.
        d. Increased incidence of hepatic cysts, intracranial aneurysms, and mitral valve prolapse.
V. **Glomerular Diseases**
  A. **Overview**
     1. Disorders of the glomeruli have a wide spectrum of disease manifestations, ranging from asymptomatic to rapidly progressive disease with renal failure.
        a. Glomerular disease typically presents as either a "nephritic" or "nephrotic" syndrome (see later discussion and Table 20.1).
     2. A common underlying theme of glomerular disease is the presence of inflammation within the glomerulus (glomerulonephritis—detailed below) with diagnosis often dependent upon renal biopsy.

TABLE 20.1 **Characteristics of Nephritic and Nephrotic Syndromes**

	NEPHROTIC	NEPHRITIC
Onset	Insidious	Abrupt
Edema	++++	++
Blood pressure	Normal	Elevated
Proteinuria	++++	++
Hematuria	±	+++
Red cell casts	Absent	Present
Serum albumin	Low	Normal to slightly reduced

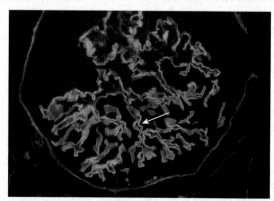

20.7: Direct immunofluorescence showing linear immunofluorescent staining in patient with antiglomerular basement membrane disease. *(From Fogo AB, Kashgarian M: Diagnostic atlas of renal pathology, ed 2, St. Louis, 2012, Elsevier, p 256, Fig. 1.324.)*

   3. In addition to routine microscopic examination, biopsies of the kidney are routinely evaluated by special techniques to further delineate the underlying pathology.
     a. Immunofluorescence (IF)
       i. Site and pattern of staining, using specific fluorochrome "tagged" antibodies.
       ii. Example: linear deposits of IgG in anti-GBM disease (Fig. 20.7).
     b. Electron microscopy (EM)
       i. Used to detect submicroscopic defects in the glomerulus (e.g., fusion of podocytes, presence and site of immune complex deposits).
       ii. Immune complex deposits between the endothelial cell and the GBM are classified as "subendothelial," whereas those between the GBM and podocytes are "subepithelial."
       iii. "Intramembranous" deposits represent immune complexes within the GBM.
       iv. "Mesangial" deposits represent immune complexes within the mesangium.
B. Pathogenesis
   1. Deposition of immune complexes (Type III hypersensitivity reaction [HSR]).
     a. Most are formed in situ (circulating antibodies bind to intrinsic renal antigens or to extrinsic antigens that have been "planted" within the glomerulus). Less commonly, immune complexes form elsewhere and secondarily deposit within the glomeruli.
       i. Immune complexes appear "granular" on IF (antibodies bound to specific antigens).
   2. Immune complex formation triggers an inflammatory reaction that causes localized injury.
     a. Involves the activation of complement, leukocyte recruitment, and cytokine release.
C. Nephritic syndrome
   1. Glomerular disease in which the major findings include hematuria, hypertension, and edema (often periorbital).
   2. Urine characteristically contains RBC casts and has a "smoky" or "cola-colored" appearance.
   3. Proteinuria may be present as well, usually in small amounts.
   4. Reduction in GFR results in oliguria (decreased urinary output), edema (due to fluid retention), and azotemia (elevated BUN and serum Cr).
D. Nephrotic syndrome
   1. Glomerular disease characterized by sufficient structural damage that proteins leak across the glomerular filtration barrier (which in health, normally excludes most proteins) and defined by the presence of heavy proteinuria (>3.5 g/day), hypoalbuminemia, peripheral edema, and hypercholesterolemia.

2. Increased risk of thromboses (due to the loss of anticoagulant proteins in the urine) and infection (due to the loss of immunoglobulins and complement in the urine).
3. Hyperlipidemia (hypercholesterolemia and hypertriglyceridemia) due to the increased production and decreased catabolism.
    a. Urine contains "Maltese crosses" and "oval fat bodies."

E. **Inflammatory diseases of the glomeruli (glomerulonephritides)**
1. Acute postinfectious glomerulonephritis (APIGN).
    a. Any age, most common in children; causes the nephritic syndrome.
       i. Most common cause of nephritic syndrome in children.
    b. Most common underlying infection is group A streptococcus (GAS).
    c. Arises 1–3 weeks after a throat or skin infection by certain "nephritogenic" strains of GAS.
       i. Streptococcal antigens (primarily streptococcal pyogenic exotoxin B) deposit within glomeruli.
       ii. Antibodies bind to the streptococcal antigen, initially in a subendothelial location, triggering an injurious inflammatory reaction.
       iii. Subsequently, via an unknown mechanism, the immune complexes dissociate, migrate to a subepithelial location, and reform.
    d. Diagnostic clues
       i. History of recent streptococcal infection, elevated antistreptococcal antibody titers, and low serum complement (C3).
       ii. Granular immune deposits within glomeruli on IF.
       iii. Discrete, electron-dense subepithelial deposits on EM.
    e. Clinical presentation
       i. APIGN typically presents in children (usually 2–14 years old, with a 2:1 male predominance) with periorbital edema, hypertension, and hematuria (smoky-colored urine).
    f. Prognosis in children is favorable, most (~95%) recover renal function, less favorable prognosis in adults.
2. IgA nephropathy (Berger disease)
    a. Characterized by mesangial deposits of IgA and subsequent glomerular injury resulting in hematuria with or without mild proteinuria.
       i. Rarely may present with nephrotic range proteinuria.
    b. Etiology unknown, likely autoimmune as it is often preceded by a respiratory tract infection.
    c. May arise at any age, but peak incidence is in the second and third decades of life with 2:1 male predominance.
    d. Most common form of glomerulonephritis in most developed countries (and the most common form of glomerulonephritis to cause renal failure, often requiring renal transplantation).
3. Rapidly progressive glomerulonephritis (RPGN)
    a. Usually presents as nephritic syndrome.

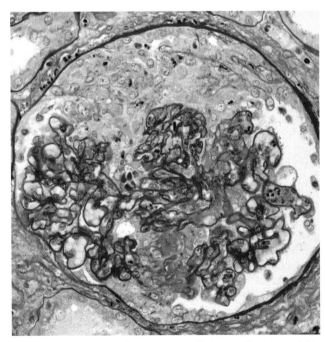

20.8: Crescentic glomerulonephritis. Crescent (*top of image*) represents cellular proliferation within Bowman space. (*From Brenner and Rector's the kidney, ed 11, Copyright © 2020 by Elsevier, Fig. 31.34.*)

b. Not a specific disease but rather a clinical syndrome characterized by a progressive loss of kidney function over a short period of time (days to a few months) in conjunction with the presence of "crescents" within Bowman space (Fig. 20.8).

c. Crescents are formed by a proliferation of glomerular epithelial cells along with an influx of monocytes and macrophages into Bowman space (thought to represent a nonspecific response to severe glomerular injury).

d. Also known as "crescentic glomerulonephritis" because of the histologic findings, RPGN may be a complication of various conditions, often further classified by immunologic findings.

   i. Linear deposits of IgG (and often C3) within the GBM

     (1) Known as antiglomerular basement membrane (anti-GBM) disease; represents a rare small vessel vasculitis affecting glomerular capillaries, pulmonary capillaries, or both.

     (2) Antibodies are directed against the noncollagen-1 domain of the alpha-3 chain of Type IV collagen (see Chapter 17 for the discussion of pulmonary involvement).

     (3) Untreated cases progress rapidly to end-stage renal disease.

   ii. Immune complex glomerulonephritis

     (1) For example, IgA nephropathy and APIGN.

   iii. Pauci-immune

     (1) Refers to the lack of detectable anti-GBM antibodies or immune complexes.

     (2) Etiologies include systemic vasculitides (e.g., granulomatosis with polyangiitis and microscopic polyangiitis).

4. Minimal change disease

a. Presents as a nephrotic syndrome (the most common cause of nephrotic syndrome in children).

b. Characterized by a good response to steroids.

c. Idiopathic in most cases (sometimes seen in association with Hodgkin lymphoma).

d. Normal by light microscopy and no immune deposits on IF; diagnosis dependent on EM (shows effacement of foot processes).

5. Focal segmental glomerulosclerosis (FSGS)

a. FSGS refers to a histologic pattern of glomerular injury in which there is sclerosis (scarring) of some, but not all, glomeruli (i.e., focal) with only a portion of each glomeruli affected (i.e., segmental).

b. Common cause of nephrotic syndrome in adults (~35% of all cases), particularly in Blacks.

   i. Although it may be a cause of nephrotic syndrome in children, it is much less common than minimal change disease.

c. Some cases are idiopathic, whereas others occur in a variety of settings (e.g., human immunodeficiency virus, heroin, sickle cell disease).

6. Membranous nephropathy

a. Second major cause of nephrotic syndrome in adults, especially Whites.

b. Characterized by diffuse thickening of the glomerular capillary wall due to subepithelial deposits of immunoglobulins.

c. Primary membranous nephropathy is an autoimmune disease caused by antibodies against the M-type phospholipase A2 receptor.

d. Secondary causes of membranous nephropathy include drugs, systemic lupus, and infection (e.g., hepatitis B).

7. Membranoproliferative glomerulonephritis

a. Unique in that it may present as either nephritic or nephrotic pattern.

b. Not a specific disease entity but rather a pattern of glomerular injury characterized histologically by hypercellularity and thickening of the GBM.

F. Hereditary glomerular diseases

1. Hereditary nephritis (Alport syndrome)

a. Inherited (mostly X-linked) disorder characterized by impaired synthesis of alpha-3, alpha-4, and alpha-5 chains of Type IV collagen.

   i. Normally found in the GBM, the cochlea, and the eye.

b. Manifestations include:

   i. Hematuria, proteinuria, and progressive renal failure.

   ii. Sensorineural hearing loss.

   iii. Cataracts, anterior lenticonus.

2. Thin basement membrane disease ("benign familial hematuria")

a. Common (affects ~1% of the population).

b. Due to mutations in the genes that encode for α-3 or α-4 chains of Type IV collagen.

c. The net result is thinning of the GBM with asymptomatic hematuria.

d. Long-term prognosis is good in most patients.

G. Systemic diseases affecting the glomerulus

1. Diabetes mellitus (DM)

a. Diabetic nephropathy is a clinical syndrome characterized by proteinuria, progressive decline in GFR, and hypertension.

b. Diabetes is a major cause of chronic kidney disease (CKD) and is the single most common cause of the end-stage renal disease.
  i. Renal failure is the second most common cause of death in those with DM, second only to myocardial infarction.
c. May be a complication of either Type 1 or Type 2 DM.
d. Pathogenesis is complex, mechanisms of injury include:
  i. Nonenzymatic glycosylation of proteins to form advanced glycation end products that subsequently bind to receptor for advanced glycation end products (RAGE) causing a variety of effects:
    (1) Generation of reactive oxygen species.
    (2) Increased procoagulant activity.
    (3) Proliferation of vascular smooth muscle cells and increased synthesis of extracellular matrix.
    (4) Increased release of various growth factors such as vascular endothelial growth factor (VEGF) and transforming growth factor-β (TGF-β).
  ii. Activation of protein kinase C
    (1) Signaling pathway, leads to the increased production of VEGF, TGF-β, and plasminogen activator inhibitor-1
  iii. Oxidative stress/polyol pathway
    (1) Glucose $\rightarrow$ sorbitol (aldose reductase).
    (2) Reaction uses NADPH which is necessary to maintain glutathione in a reduced state. Lack of reduced glutathione increases susceptibility to oxidative stress.
e. Pathology (Fig. 20.9)
  i. Thickening of GBM.
  ii. Mesangial sclerosis.
  iii. Nodular glomerulosclerosis (Kimmelstiel–Wilson lesion).
  iv. Vascular disease (atherosclerosis and hyaline arteriolosclerosis).
f. Clinical manifestations
  i. Albuminuria (>300 mg/day).
  ii. Progressive kidney disease (declining GFR and increasing serum Cr).
  iii. Hypertension.
2. Amyloidosis
  a. Amyloid refers to extracellular deposits of fibrillar proteins.
  b. Not a single protein; over 30 different proteins have been identified as components of amyloid in various clinical settings.
    i. Consistent among these proteins is a β-pleated sheet configuration.
      (1) Explains the insoluble nature of these proteins as well as the staining characteristics apparent on microscopic examination.
  c. Common causes of renal amyloidosis include:
    i. Amyloid light chain protein
      (1) Comprised of immunoglobulin light chains secreted from monoclonal plasma cells (e.g., multiple myeloma [MM]).
    ii. Amyloid-associated (AA) protein
      (1) AA is created by the proteolysis of serum amyloid A, an acute phase reactant elevated in those with chronic inflammatory states.
  d. Amyloid deposits primarily within vessels (including glomeruli), ultimately narrowing/obliterating their lumen.
    i. Renal manifestations include proteinuria and renal insufficiency.
  e. Diagnosed with the use of a Congo red stain
    i. Highlights tissue deposits of amyloid (appear apple-green under polarized light microscopy).

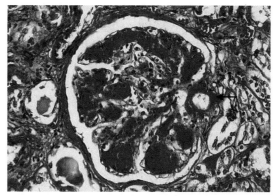

20.9: Nodular glomerulosclerosis of diabetes (Kimmelstiel–Wilson lesion). Note the hyaline arteriolosclerosis involving one of the arterioles (*arrow*). (*From Damjanov I: Pathology for the health professions, ed 4, Philadelphia, 2012, Saunders Elsevier, p 313, Fig. 13.11.*)

   3. Systemic lupus erythematosus (SLE)
      a. Renal involvement is seen in up to 50% of those with SLE.
      b. Glomerular deposits of DNA/anti-dsDNA immune complexes (Type III HSR).
      c. Causes renal insufficiency with elevated Cr, proteinuria, hematuria, and hypertension.

VI. **Disorders of the Tubules and Interstitium**
   A. **Acute kidney injury (AKI)**
      1. Definition
         a. Previously known as acute renal failure, AKI represents an acute deterioration in renal function occurring over hours to days and is characterized by a reduced GFR and azotemia (elevated BUN and serum Cr levels).
      2. Clinical manifestations
         a. Reduced urine output (oliguria) to absent urine output (anuria).
         b. Edema, weight gain (volume overload).
         c. Confusion, altered mental status.
      3. Classification of AKI based on cause
         a. Prerenal
            i. Renal dysfunction secondary to decreased renal perfusion (e.g., hypovolemia, heart failure, sepsis).
               (1) No renal parenchymal injury present.
         b. Postrenal
            i. Azotemia developing as a result of obstructed urinary flow (e.g., prostatic hyperplasia/cancer or retroperitoneal fibrosis).
         c. Renal (intrinsic renal disease)
            i. Definition
               (1) An acute reduction in renal function secondary to renal injury.
               (2) Etiologies include:
                  (a) Disorders of the renal vasculature (e.g., renal artery stenosis or thrombosis, emboli, vasculitis, and severe hypertension).
                  (b) Acute glomerulonephritis (e.g., RPGN or hemolytic uremic syndrome).
                  (c) Acute tubular injury (ATI) (see later discussion).
         d. Differentiation between types of AKI
            i. Prerenal
               (1) BUN-to-serum Cr ratio of >20:1.
               (2) FENa < 1%.
            ii. Renal
               (1) BUN-to-serum ratio is ≤15.
               (2) FENa varies (>3% in acute tubular necrosis [ATN]).
            iii. Postrenal
               (1) BUN-to-serum Cr and FENa vary.

   B. **Acute tubular injury (ATI)**
      1. Abrupt rapid decline in renal function secondary to renal tubular injury.
      2. ATI is the most common cause of acute renal injury; when accompanied by necrosis of tubular epithelium, the term "acute tubular necrosis (ATN)" is used.
      3. Two major mechanisms (ischemic, nephrotoxic)
         a. Ischemic ATI
            i. Injury to renal tubular cells secondary to reduced perfusion.
            ii. Etiologies include impaired cardiac function (e.g., myocardial infarction), widespread loss of peripheral vascular tone (e.g., septic shock), or severe hypovolemia (e.g., vomiting, diarrhea, sweating, and poor oral intake).
            iii. Renal tubular epithelial cells, particularly the proximal convoluted tubule and ascending limb of the loop of Henle, are prone to ischemic injury.
         b. Nephrotoxic ATI
            i. A variety of agents are toxic to renal tubule cells, including:
               (1) Medications (e.g., cisplatin, gentamicin, amphotericin B, and NSAIDs).
               (2) Radiocontrast agents.
               (3) Myoglobin (e.g., rhabdomyolysis and crush injuries).
               (4) Hemoglobin (e.g., intravascular hemolysis).
               (5) Free immunoglobulin light chains (e.g., myeloma).
      4. Findings in ATI
         a. With a severe injury, sloughing of necrotic tubular epithelial cells forms casts.
         b. Urine microscopy shows "muddy brown" granular epithelial cell casts and sloughed tubular epithelial cells (Fig. 20.10).
         c. Casts and sloughed epithelial cells obstruct tubules.
         d. Decreased GFR, urine output; increased FENa.

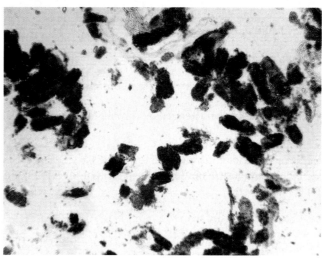

20.10: Muddy brown, granular casts, a finding consistent with a diagnosis of acute tubular necrosis. *(From Ferri's clinical advisor, 2022, Copyright © 2022 by Elsevier, Inc, Fig. E.1.)*

C. **Tubulointerstitial nephritis**
   1. Inflammatory process involving renal interstitium and tubules.
   2. May eventually lead to scarring of the interstitium and tubular atrophy.
   3. Acute interstitial nephritis is classically characterized by fever, rash, and eosinophilia.
      a. Presence of eosinophils in urine is a clue to diagnosis.
   4. Etiologies include:
      a. Drugs (e.g., beta-lactam antibiotics, NSAIDs, allopurinol, and others).
      b. Infections (e.g., *Legionella*, *Leptospira*, and cytomegalovirus).
      c. Systemic disease (e.g., SLE, sarcoidosis, and Sjögren syndrome).
D. **Acute pyelonephritis**
   1. Definition
      a. Inflammation of the renal parenchyma, usually secondary to a bacterial infection (most commonly *Escherichia coli*).
   2. Epidemiology
      a. Overall, more common in females (especially those of childbearing age).
      b. With increasing age, males are increasingly affected (obstruction of urinary flow in relation to prostatic hyperplasia).
   3. Risk factors
      a. Urinary tract obstruction
         i. Prevents the flushing effect of urination and allows for the pooling of urine. Etiologies include renal stones and prostatic hyperplasia.
      b. Sexual intercourse
         i. Promotes colonization of female urethra by enteric organisms (e.g., *E. coli*).
      c. Diabetes mellitus
         i. Glycosuria (glucose in the urine is a good growth media for bacteria).
         ii. Urinary stasis (secondary to autonomic neuropathy).
         iii. Impaired leukocyte function.
      d. Vesicoureteral reflux (VUR)
         i. During micturition, contraction of the bladder normally compresses the intravesical portions of the ureters (which traverse the bladder wall at an angle). An anatomic abnormality that impairs this effect allows for the retrograde flow of the urine into the ureter during micturition (i.e., VUR).
   4. Pathogenesis
      a. Ascending infection
         i. Most urinary tract infections, whether involving the bladder (cystitis) or kidney (pyelonephritis), are due to an ascending infection by enteric bacteria (most commonly *E. coli*).
      b. Hematogenous dissemination
         i. Uncommon, risk factors include intravenous drug use or infective endocarditis; especially consider when urine culture reveals *Staphylococcus aureus*.
   5. Clinical manifestations
      a. Fever, chills, flank pain, and costovertebral angle (CVA) tenderness.
      b. Manifestations of cystitis (e.g., frequency, dysuria, and suprapubic tenderness) often present as well.

    6. Laboratory findings
       a. White blood cell casts (key finding)
       b. Pyuria (pus in urine)
       c. Bacteriuria (usually *E. coli*, a Gram-negative rod)
       d. Hematuria
    7. Those with an underlying disorder of the urinary tract (e.g., obstruction), are at increased risk of complications, such as sepsis or chronic pyelonephritis.
       a. Chronic pyelonephritis is a disorder characterized by chronic tubulointerstitial inflammation and scarring of renal calyces and pelvis.

E. Renal papillary necrosis
    1. Renal papillae represent the apical end of the medullary pyramids.
    2. Ischemic necrosis of the renal medullary pyramids and papillae can cause sloughing of necrotic cellular debris and the potential for obstruction.
    3. Risk factors
       a. DM, sickle cell disease, and analgesic abuse.
    4. Manifestations
       a. Hematuria, proteinuria, and flank pain.

F. Urate nephropathy
    1. Defined as a renal injury occurring secondary to the deposition of uric acid crystals within the renal tubules and interstitium.
    2. The major risk factor is tumor lysis syndrome (TLS).
       a. TLS is a constellation of metabolic effects secondary to the acute breakdown of tumor cells.
       b. As tumor cells are broken down, there is a massive release of potentially injurious intracellular contents; resulting in hyperphosphatemia, hyperkalemia, and hyperuricemia.
          i. Hyperuricemia is due to the release of purines, which are metabolized to uric acid by hepatic xanthine oxidase.
       c. Uric acid is not very soluble at the low pH of the renal tubules (urate crystals obstruct distal tubules and collecting ducts).
       d. Prevention includes the use of medications (e.g., allopurinol and febuxostat) that inhibit xanthine oxidase along with good hydration.

G. Lead nephropathy
    1. Acute lead exposure can cause proximal tubule dysfunction (Fanconi syndrome).
    2. Chronic low-grade exposure, usually in an occupational setting, can cause CKD with hyperuricemia (lead impairs the renal excretion of uric acid).
    3. Histologic findings include tubular atrophy and interstitial fibrosis.

H. Multiple myeloma (MM)
    1. Impairs renal function via multiple mechanisms:
       a. Direct tubular injury
          i. Bence-Jones proteins (light chains) are directly toxic to the proximal tubule epithelium.
          ii. Binding of free light chains to Tamm–Horsfall protein leads to the formation of casts that obstruct tubular lumina.
       b. Calcification of renal tubules (nephrocalcinosis)
          i. Hypercalcemia is a common complication of myeloma (related to osteolytic bone lesions). Excess calcium is excreted through the urine (hypercalciuria), potentially leading to calcification of tubules.
       c. Amyloidosis
          i. Free light chains may deposit as amyloid (insoluble proteins with β-pleated sheet configuration) causing glomerular injury with proteinuria.

VII. Chronic Kidney Disease
  A. Definition
    1. Historically known as chronic renal failure (CRF), CKD refers to a chronic (>3 months) reduction of renal function in association with renal injury (or a GFR < 60 mL/min/1.73 m^2).
  B. Epidemiology
    1. Common disorder affecting 15% of the adult population in the United States; the ninth leading cause of death.
  C. Etiologic factors
    1. DM and hypertension (the most common factors).
    2. Urinary tract obstruction (e.g., recurrent renal stones and prostatic hyperplasia).
    3. Vascular diseases (e.g., renal artery stenosis and vasculitis).
    4. Autoimmune disorders (e.g., SLE).
    5. Drugs/toxins (e.g., heroin, gold, penicillamine, and heavy metals).
    6. ADPKD.
    7. Hereditary nephritis (Alport syndrome).

D. **Five stages**
1. Stage description GFR (mL/min/1.73 m^2)
   a. Kidney damage with normal or ↑GFR → ≥90.
   b. Kidney damage with mild or ↓GFR → 60–89.
   c. Moderate ↓GFR → 30–59.
   d. Severe ↓GFR → 15–29.
   e. Kidney failure → <15 (or on dialysis).
E. **Manifestations of CKD (uremia) include:**
1. Impaired salt and water excretion
   a. If severe, may lead to hypertension and edema.
2. Normochromic, normocytic anemia
   a. Due to impaired renal secretion of EPO.
   b. Causes fatigue and reduced exercise tolerance.
3. Electrolyte abnormalities
   a. Hyperkalemia and hyperphosphatemia (decreased urinary excretion).
   b. Hypocalcemia (mostly secondary to vitamin D deficiency)
      i. Recall that the renal enzyme 1α hydroxylase is required for the final hydroxylation step in the activation of vitamin D (calcitriol).
4. Secondary hyperparathyroidism
   a. Chronic hypocalcemia-induced release of PTH leads to excessive bone resorption (osteitis fibrosa cystica).
5. Metabolic acidosis, a variety of mechanisms
   a. Impaired renal acid excretion of hydrogen ions (Type 1 renal tubular acidosis [RTA]).
   b. Decreased reabsorption of filtered bicarbonate (Type 2 RTA).
6. Neuropathy.
7. Immune dysfunction (increased risk of infections).
8. Increased risk cardiovascular disease (e.g., myocardial infarction, pericarditis, and peripheral arterial disease).

VIII. **Vascular Diseases of the Kidney**
A. **Nephrosclerosis (narrowing of renal arterioles, small arteries)**
1. Hyaline arteriolosclerosis
   a. Thickening and "hyalinization" of arteriolar walls due to extravasation of plasma proteins.
   b. Causes narrowing of lumina and ischemic injury; potential for glomerular and tubulointerstitial scarring.
   c. Kidneys become atrophic with fine granularity of cortex (due to subcapsular scarring).
   d. Major risk factors include long-standing hypertension and DM.
2. Hyperplastic arteriolosclerosis
   a. Complication of severe hypertension.
   b. Concentric proliferation of smooth muscle cells ("onion skin" appearance) within the walls of arterioles (Fig. 20.11) and luminal narrowing.
B. **Renal infarction**
1. Infarction of renal parenchyma, relatively common due to the lack of collateral blood flow.
2. Usually secondary to emboli, sources include:
   a. Heart
      i. Most common source of emboli.
      ii. Risk factors include atrial fibrillation and poor contractility (e.g., following myocardial infarction).

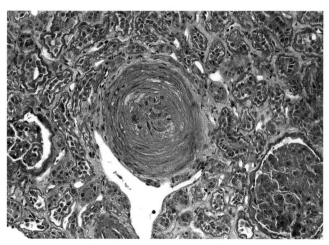

20.11: Hyperplastic arteriolosclerosis, a finding associated with severe hypertension. *(From Rosai and Ackerman's surgical pathology, ed 11, Copyright © 2018 by Elsevier Inc, Fig. 23.90.)*

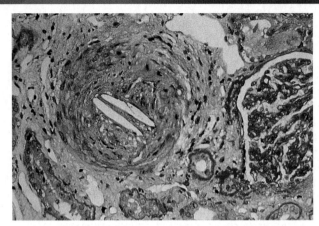

20.12: Cholesterol emboli (*elongated clefts*) in kidney biopsy specimen. *(From Dr. Robert G. Horn: Laboratory for kidney pathology, Inc., Nashville TN.)*

    b. Atherosclerotic plaque ("atheroemboli")
      i. Typically older patients with diffuse atherosclerotic vascular disease, particularly following surgical manipulation of the aorta.
      ii. Pathology reveals cholesterol emboli within small renal arteries (Fig. 20.12).
  3. Pathologic findings
    a. Wedge-shaped pale infarction of renal cortex (base against cortical surface with apex pointing toward renal medulla).
  4. Clinical and laboratory findings
    a. Sudden onset of severe flank pain and hematuria.
    b. Transient elevation serum Cr.
    c. Elevated lactate dehydrogenase (a marker of tissue necrosis).

Sickle cell nephropathy

- In both sickle cell anemia and sickle cell trait, the physiologic characteristics of the renal medulla (e.g., relative hypoxia, acidosis, and hyperosmolarity) make it a prime site for sickling of erythrocytes.
- Resulting ischemic injury and microinfarcts can lead to hematuria (typically asymptomatic) and hyposthenuria (excretion of urine of low specific gravity due to an inability to concentrate the urine).

IX. **Obstructive Disorders of the Kidney**
  A. Hydronephrosis
    1. Definition
      a. Distention of the renal calyces and pelvis secondary to obstruction of urine flow distal to the renal pelvis.
    2. Etiologies
      a. Anatomic abnormalities (e.g., urethral valves, stenosis at the ureterovesical or ureteropelvic junction) are most common in children.
      b. In adults, ureteral stones are most common; however, with aging one must consider extrinsic compression of ureter (e.g., prostatic hyperplasia/carcinoma, retroperitoneal fibrosis, or cervical cancer).
    3. Gross findings
      a. Dilated renal pelvis (Fig. 20.13) as well as compression atrophy from increased intraluminal pressure.
  B. Renal stones (urolithiasis)
    1. Definition
      a. Formation of small mineral concretions within the urinary tract, usually the kidney.
    2. Epidemiology
      a. Common; affects up to 1 in 5 men (or 1 in 10 women) during their lifetime.
      b. Highest incidence is in the southeastern United States (reason unclear).
    3. Risk factors
      a. Elevated urinary calcium excretion (hypercalciuria), possible mechanisms include:
        i. Increased intestinal calcium absorption ("absorptive hypercalciuria").
        ii. Increased bone resorption ("resorptive hypercalciuria").
        iii. Defective renal calcium reabsorption ("renal hypercalciuria").

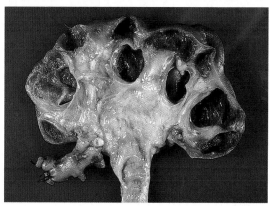

20.13: Hydronephrosis. Note the dilated renal calyces. *(From King TS: Elsevier's integrated pathology, St. Louis, 2007, Mosby Elsevier, p 297, Fig. 12.5.)*

    b. Low urine volume
       i. Stones are more likely to form in highly concentrated urine.
    c. Reduced urinary citrate
       i. Citrate binds to calcium in the tubular lumen thereby reducing the amount of free calcium available to form stones.
    d. Urine pH alterations
       i. Alkaline urine pH promotes the formation of calcium phosphate and struvite (magnesium ammonium phosphate) stones.
       ii. Acidic urine pH favors crystallization of uric acid and thus the formation of urate stones.
    e. Dietary factors
       i. Reduced fluid intake
         (1) Highly concentrated urine predisposes to stone formation.
       ii. Increased consumption of animal protein (and lower intake of fruits and vegetables)
         (1) Increases urine acidity (increases risk of developing urate stones).
       iii. High-dose vitamin C
         (1) Metabolism of vitamin C generates oxalate (increasing risk of forming oxalate stones).
    f. Elevated serum oxalate
       i. Disease of the terminal ileum (e.g., Crohn disease) can lead to increased absorption of dietary oxalate.
    g. Tumor lysis syndrome (TLS)
       i. Rapid breakdown of tumor cells with the release of massive quantities of intracellular contents (e.g., purines metabolized to uric acid).
       ii. Hyperuricemia leads to increased urinary excretion of uric acid and thus an increased risk of urate stones.
    h. Primary hyperparathyroidism
       i. ↑ PTH → ↑ serum calcium → ↑ urinary calcium excretion (thereby increasing one's risk of forming calcium stones).
    i. Urinary infection by urease-producing organisms (e.g., *Proteus* and *Klebsiella*).
       i. Urease converts urea into ammonia → alkaline urine → precipitation of magnesium ammonium phosphate salts → struvite stone formation.
  4. Stone types
    a. Calcium stones (the most common type of stone).
       i. Most are comprised of calcium oxalate, either alone or in combination with calcium phosphate.
       ii. Risk factors include hypercalciuria (most common), hyperoxaluria (malabsorption), and decreased urine citrate (e.g., RTA and diarrhea).
    b. Magnesium ammonium phosphate (struvite) stone
       i. Second most common type.
       ii. May grow rapidly over weeks to months to fill the intrarenal calyces; branched shape ("staghorn calculus").
       iii. Occurs when there is an upper urinary tract infection by urease-producing organisms (e.g., *Proteus* and *Klebsiella*) that alkalinize the urine (a clue is the smell of ammonia).
       iv. Large size of stones often requires surgical removal.
    c. Uric acid stones
       i. Major risk factors include low urinary pH and volume, elevated serum uric acid levels (high dietary protein, TLS).

d. Cystine stones
    i. Least common (1% of cases); major risk factor is cystinuria, an autosomal disorder characterized by impaired renal reabsorption of cystine, resulting in elevated urinary cystine levels.
  5. Clinical manifestations
    a. Sudden onset of severe flank pain radiating into the ipsilateral groin.
    b. Hematuria (common)
    c. Presence of crystals in urine.
    d. Hypercalcemia (if present, rule out primary hyperparathyroidism).
  6. Diagnosis
    a. Noncontrast computed tomography (CT).
  7. Treatment
    a. Urine should be strained to collect the stone for analysis (treatment is tailored to the type of stone).
    b. Hydration is a key to stone prevention.
X. **Tumors of the Kidney and Renal Pelvis**
  A. **Angiomyolipoma**
    1. Uncommon benign neoplasm derived from perivascular epithelial cells.
    2. Comprised of blood vessels, smooth muscle, and adipose tissue.
    3. Increased incidence in association with tuberous sclerosis.
    4. Treatment is surgical excision.
  B. **Oncocytoma**
    1. Benign epithelial tumor of the kidney arising from intercalated cells of the collecting ducts.
    2. Characteristic mahogany brown color with central stellate scar.
    3. Tumor cells are eosinophilic and finely granular (due to mitochondria).
    4. Treatment is surgical excision.
  C. **Renal cell carcinoma (RCC)**
    1. Overview
      a. RCC is the most common primary renal malignancy (~85%).
      b. More common in males, older patients (sixth to eighth decade).
    2. Histologic subtypes
      a. Clear cell carcinoma, the most common subtype, arises from proximal convoluted tubules; associated with deletions of chromosome 3p (region containing the *VHL* tumor suppressor gene).
      b. Papillary carcinoma is the second most common histologic subtype; arises from the distal convoluted tubules.
    3. Risk factors
      a. Smoking (major factor).
      b. Obesity.
      c. Acquired and inherited cystic diseases of the kidney (e.g., ADPKD).
      d. Von Hippel–Lindau disease (VHL)
        i. Autosomal dominant disorder associated with the development of cerebellar and retinal hemangioblastomas, pheochromocytoma, and RCC.
    4. Pathologic findings
      a. Bright yellow, focally cystic cut surface with areas of hemorrhage.
      b. Clear cells contain lipid and glycogen (Fig. 20.14).
      c. Tendency for renal vein invasion (portends poor prognosis); may extend into the inferior vena cava and right side of heart.
      d. Unlike most carcinomas, RCC spreads hematogenously to the lungs, bones, brain, liver, and other sites.

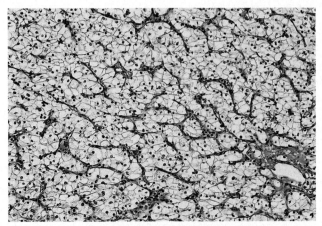

20.14: Renal cell carcinoma. Note the clear cells. *(From Diagnostic histopathology of tumors, ed 5, Copyright © 2021 by Elsevier, Fig. 12A.13.)*

5. Clinical findings
   a. RCC may remain clinically silent for long periods, often an incidental finding on imaging.
   b. Classic triad of hematuria, abdominal mass, and flank pain.
   c. Left-sided varicocele can be a clue (extension of tumor into the left renal vein impedes drainage of left spermatic vein).
6. Laboratory findings
   a. Normocytic anemia (anemia of chronic disease).
      i. Some may develop polycythemia (↑ RBC mass); due to ectopic EPO released by the tumor (paraneoplastic effect).
   b. Hypercalcemia
      i. Due to lytic bone metastasis and/or the release of PTH-related peptide from the tumor (paraneoplastic effect).
7. Diagnosis is with imaging (ultrasound, abdominal CT, and magnetic resonance imaging).
8. Treatment is surgical excision.
9. Prognosis depends on stage
   a. Stage I and II tumors (i.e., those limited to the kidney) have good prognosis.
   b. Stage III (extension into perinephric fat or renal vein) and stage IV tumors (metastatic disease) have much less favorable prognosis.

D. Urothelial carcinoma of the renal pelvis
1. Malignant tumor arising from the urothelial cells lining the renal pelvis.
2. Second most common primary tumor of the kidney (accounting for 5%–10% of cases).
3. Presence of a second urothelial carcinoma elsewhere in the urinary system (e.g., bladder) is common—so-called "field effect."

E. Wilms tumor (nephroblastoma)
1. Malignant tumor of the kidney derived from the metanephric blastema (i.e., embryologic precursor cells to nephrons and the collecting ducts).
2. Most common primary renal malignancy in childhood (~5% of childhood cancers) with nearly all cases occurring before the age of 10.
3. Higher risk in African Americans.
4. Most are sporadic; however, some occur as a component of a genetic condition.
   a. WAGR syndrome (chromosomal deletion of the *WT1* gene)
      i. **W**ilms tumor, **a**niridia (absent iris), **g**enitourinary abnormalities, mental **r**etardation (intellectual disability).
   b. Denys–Drash syndrome (point mutation *WT1*)
      i. Wilms tumor, progressive renal disease, male pseudohermaphroditism.
   c. Beckwith–Wiedemann syndrome (mutation *WT2*)
      i. Wilms tumor, macrosomia, macroglossia, omphalocele, prominent eyes, ear creases, large kidneys, pancreatic hyperplasia, and hemihypertrophy.
5. Pathology
   a. Necrotic, gray-tan tumor with areas of hemorrhage and necrosis.
   b. Microscopically appears as sheets of primitive "small blue cells" (blastemal component) along with primitive-appearing tubules.
6. Clinical manifestations
   a. Palpable abdominal mass (may be bilateral in some cases).
   b. May have hematuria, hypertension.
   c. Risk of pulmonary metastasis.
7. Prognosis is good with approximately 80%–90% survival.

I. Disorders of the Ureters

A. Megaureter
1. Defined as an abnormally large, dilated ureter.
2. Possible etiologies include vesicoureteral reflux (VUR) and ureteral obstruction (usually at the junction with the bladder).

B. Ureteral stones
1. Kidney stones (nephrolith), especially those larger than 4 mm in diameter, may lodge within the ureter causing pain, hematuria, and the potential for obstruction.

C. Retroperitoneal fibrosis
1. Rare condition characterized by inflammation and fibrosis of the infrarenal aorta, iliac arteries, and surrounding structures (e.g., ureters, inferior vena cava).
2. Most cases (~70%) are idiopathic and may be immune-mediated (some have coexisting autoimmune disease).
3. Secondary causes include:
   a. Methysergide and other ergot alkaloids.
   b. Therapeutic radiation exposure.
4. Complications
   a. Hydronephrosis (potential for acute kidney injury).
   b. Varicocele (obstruction of spermatic vein).
   c. Deep venous thrombosis and lower extremity edema (due to impaired venous drainage from legs).

D. Ureteral cancers
1. Urothelial carcinoma is the most common primary malignancy of the ureter (discussed under Urinary Bladder).

II. Disorders of the Urinary Bladder

A. Congenital abnormalities of the urinary bladder
1. Vesicoureteral reflux (VUR)
   a. During micturition, the ureter is normally compressed as it traverses the bladder wall (i.e., at the ureterovesical junction).
   b. Failure of this antireflux mechanism causes reflux of urine from the bladder into the ureter ("VUR").
   c. Any bacteria present within the bladder may be carried up the ureters into the kidney (causing pyelonephritis).
2. Exstrophy of the bladder
   a. Congenital anomaly of anterior abdominal wall and bladder in which the bladder has been "turned inside out" (i.e., the mucosa is exposed) and open to the body surface (Fig. 21.1).
   b. Increased risk of glandular metaplasia of the bladder and the potential for malignant transformation (adenocarcinoma).

B. Acute cystitis
1. Defined as acute inflammation of the urinary bladder, usually secondary to an infectious process.
2. Risk factors for the development of cystitis include:
   a. Female sex
      i. Shorter distance from the anus to the urethra, and shorter urethra, allows for easier access of pathogens into the urinary bladder (ascending infection).
   b. Presence of indwelling urinary catheters.
   c. Sexual intercourse ("Honeymoon cystitis")

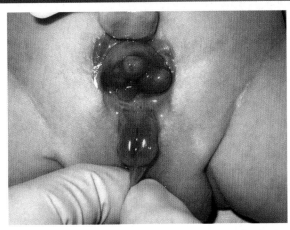

21.1: Exstrophy of the bladder. *(From Nelson textbook of pediatrics, Copyright © 2020 Elsevier Inc., Fig. 556.1.)*

      i. Voiding after intercourse reduces the risk of infection by flushing out any bacteria that may have entered the urethra.
   d. Urinary stasis (e.g., neurogenic bladder or bladder outlet obstruction).
  3. Microbial pathogens
   a. *Escherichia coli* (the most common pathogen) and other Enterobacteriaceae (e.g., *Klebsiella* and *Proteus*).
   b. *Staphylococcus saprophyticus*
     i. Particularly in young, sexually active women
  4. Clinical manifestations
   a. Pain/burning on urination (dysuria).
   b. Increased urinary urgency or frequency.
   c. Suprapubic pain.
   d. Hematuria (gross or microscopic).
  5. Laboratory findings
   a. Presence of leukocytes within a midstream urine specimen.
     i. Note that white cell *casts* indicate the inflammation of the renal tubules and is therefore not seen with acute uncomplicated cystitis.
   b. Dipstick testing
     i. Leukocyte esterase positivity (indicates the presence of neutrophils).
     ii. Nitrite positivity indicates the presence of bacteria that produce nitrate reductase, an enzyme that reduces nitrate to nitrite (e.g., *E. coli*, *Klebsiella*, and *Enterobacter*).

C. Schistosomiasis
  1. Infection acquired via contact with water contaminated with cercariae, the infectious form of the parasite.
  2. Contact of skin with contaminated water allows the cercariae to penetrate the skin and gain access to circulation; ultimately, growing into adults within the liver.
  3. Adult worms, in the case of *Schistosoma haematobium*, migrate to the venous plexus of the bladder and deposit their eggs.
   a. *S. haematobium* is present in Africa and the Middle East.
   b. Eggs identified by the presence of a large terminal spine (Fig. 21.2).
  4. The immune response against the eggs causes bladder ulceration, chronic granulomatous inflammation, and the potential for developing bladder cancer, especially squamous cell carcinoma.

D. Bladder pain syndrome (interstitial cystitis)
  1. Chronic bladder pain with urinary frequency and urgency in the absence of infection or other identifiable cause.
  2. Characteristic findings include reddened areas of the bladder mucosa and chronic ulcers ("Hunner ulcer").
  3. If performed, bladder biopsies characteristically reveal increased numbers of mast cells.

E. Hemorrhagic cystitis
  1. Noninfectious form of cystitis characterized by gross hematuria.
  2. Usually seen following the use of various chemotherapeutic agents (e.g., ifosfamide or cyclophosphamide).

F. Asymptomatic bacteriuria
  1. Defined as the presence of bacteria in an appropriately collected urine specimen from an individual without symptoms of urinary tract infection.
  2. Usually of no clinical consequence; antibiotics are not required, except in pregnancy.
   a. Pregnant women should be treated to reduce the risk of pyelonephritis and/or pregnancy complications (e.g., preterm birth).

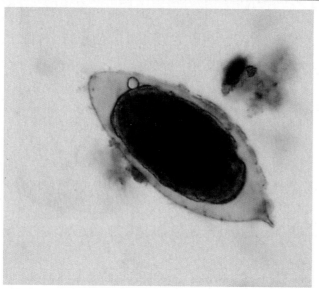

21.2: *Schistosoma haematobium* egg. Note the terminal spine. *(From Medical microbiology, ed 9, © 2021, Elsevier Inc., Fig. 75.13.)*

G. Bladder cancer
1. Urothelial carcinoma
    a. Most common histologic type of bladder cancer.
    b. Arises from the lining epithelium of the bladder (i.e., urothelium).
    c. Historically known as "transitional cell" carcinoma; these tumors may also arise, albeit less commonly, within the renal pelvis, ureter, and/or urethra.
    d. Most commonly seen in older adults (most over 65 years) with the highest incidence in White males.
    e. Risk factors include a variety of environmental exposures:
        i. Cigarette smoking (major factor).
        ii. Occupational exposure (e.g., paint, rubber, and leather industries) to chemical carcinogens.
        iii. Cyclophosphamide
            (1) A metabolite (acrolein) is believed responsible for the increased incidence of hemorrhagic cystitis and bladder cancer in those treated with cyclophosphamide.
    f. Pathologic findings
        i. Varies with histologic grade of the tumor.
        ii. Low-grade tumors are more likely to exhibit a papillary architecture and are often noninvasive.
        iii. High-grade tumors are less likely to exhibit papillary architecture and are usually invasive.
    g. Clinical manifestations
        i. Gross or microscopic hematuria (most common sign).
        ii. Irritative voiding symptoms (e.g., dysuria and increased frequency).
        iii. Pain (indicative of locally advanced or metastatic disease).
    h. Diagnosis
        i. Cystoscopy with biopsy.
        ii. Intravenous pyelogram is especially useful for the evaluation of the upper urinary tract (e.g., ureter and renal pelvis).
2. Squamous cell carcinoma
    a. Uncommon (<5%) in the United States; associated with long-standing bladder inflammation (e.g., *S. haematobium*).
    b. Chronic bladder inflammation/irritation → squamous metaplasia → dysplasia → squamous cell carcinoma.
3. Adenocarcinoma
    a. Uncommon (<1%); characterized by the formation of infiltrative glands.
    b. Most arise from urachal remnants or exstrophy of the urinary bladder.
4. Embryonal rhabdomyosarcoma (sarcoma botryoides)
    a. Malignant tumor of rhabdomyoblasts, the embryonic derivative of skeletal muscle tissue.
    b. Uncommon, primarily during childhood (boys > girls).
        i. In girls, embryonal rhabdomyosarcoma is more likely to arise within the vagina.
    c. Presents as "grape-like" mass protruding from the urethral orifice (or the vagina in girls).
5. Secondary tumor involvement
    a. Cervical cancer and prostate cancer may secondarily involve the bladder by direct extension.
    b. Encasement of the urethra and/or ureters may cause urinary obstruction resulting in hydronephrosis, postrenal azotemia, renal failure, and death.

III. Urethral Diseases
A. Urethritis
1. Inflammation of the urethra, typically in association with sexually transmitted infections (most common in young, sexually active males).
2. Etiologies include *Neisseria gonorrhoeae* and *Chlamydia trachomatis*.
3. Clinical manifestations
   a. Dysuria (painful urination)—major symptom.
   b. Urethral discharge.

B. Posterior urethral valve
1. Congenital membranous mucosal fold within the lumen of the posterior urethra.
2. Most common cause of the urinary tract obstruction in the newborn male.
3. Prenatal diagnosis (by ultrasound) may reveal oligohydramnios (decreased amniotic fluid), bilateral hydronephrosis, dilated bladder, and dilated posterior urethra.
4. Postnatally, may present with respiratory distress due to lung hypoplasia (amniotic fluid needed for lung development), difficulty voiding, urinary tract infections, VUR, and chronic kidney disease.
5. Diagnosis: voiding cystourethrogram.

C. Urethral cancer
1. Uncommon, most are secondary to chronic irritation associated with urethral stricture in men and urethral diverticula in women.
   a. Some cases seen in association with human papilloma virus (HPV 16).
2. Histologic subtype
   a. In men, most are urothelial carcinoma.
   b. In women, most are squamous cell carcinoma.
3. Clinical manifestations
   a. Hematuria, dysuria.
4. Lymphatic drainage
   a. Distal one-third of urethra → superficial or deep inguinal nodes.
   b. Proximal two-thirds of urethra → pelvic lymph nodes.

IV. Disorders of the Penis
A. Hypospadias
1. Congenital anomaly of the male urethra characterized by an abnormal ventral placement of the urethral opening proximal to its usual location at the tip of the penis.
2. Relatively common (~1 in 300); risk factors include preterm birth and intrauterine growth restriction.
3. In some cases, genetic mutations involving androgenic stimulation (production, receptors) have been implicated (androgens necessary for the development of external male genitalia).
4. Some have an associated ventral penile curvature.

B. Epispadias
1. Abnormal opening of the urethral meatus on the dorsal surface of the penis.
2. Rare, often seen in association with exstrophy of the bladder.

C. Phimosis
1. Defined as an inability to retract the foreskin over the glans penis.
   a. Interferes with cleansing of the glans and increases the risk of balanitis (inflammation of the glans penis).
2. If a phimotic foreskin is forcibly retracted over the glans, paraphimosis may occur.
   a. Paraphimosis is retracted foreskin that cannot be returned to the normal position; constriction of foreskin around the distal penile shaft may have a "tourniquet" effect (causing ischemia of the distal penis).

D. Balanoposthitis
1. Inflammation of the glans penis and foreskin (prepuce) in an uncircumcised male.
   a. Balanitis is inflammation of the glans penis.
   b. Posthitis is inflammation of the foreskin.
2. Increased risk of balanoposthitis in those with phimosis due to inability to properly cleanse.
   a. Smegma, an oily sebaceous secretion, accumulates under the foreskin.
3. Inflammatory scarring may produce acquired phimosis.

E. Peyronie disease
1. Acquired, localized fibrotic disorder of the tunica albuginea resulting in lateral curvature of the erect penis.
2. Estimated to affect 5% of men, increasing incidence with age.
3. May cause pain on erection, painful intercourse.

F. Priapism
1. Persistent and painful erection; commonly seen in sickle cell disease.

G. Squamous cell carcinoma in situ (Erythroplasia of Queyrat)
1. Commonly associated with chronic irritation and inflammation of the glans.
2. Typical patient is middle-aged to older and uncircumcised (poor hygiene, chronic infection).

3. Presents with redness, crusting, and scaling, ulceration possible.
4. May evolve into invasive squamous cell carcinoma.

H. Squamous cell carcinoma
1. Most common malignancy of the penis.
2. Risk factors include:
   a. Lack of circumcision (major factor)
      i. Due to retained smegma, poor hygiene.
   b. Squamous cell carcinoma in situ (previous discussion).
   c. HPV.
   d. Tobacco exposure.
3. Most common sites include the glans and/or mucosal surface of the prepuce.

V. Disorders of the Testis, Scrotal Sac, and Epididymis
A. Cryptorchidism
1. Failure of testicles to descend to their normal location in the scrotum by 4 months of age.
2. Normal testicular descent occurs in two phases.
   a. Transabdominal phase
      i. The first phase, occurring between 8 and 15 weeks' gestation.
      ii. Descent to the pelvic brim in the lower abdomen; controlled by insulin-like hormone 3 from the Leydig cells.
   b. Inguinoscrotal phase
      i. The second phase, occurring between 25 and 35 weeks.
      ii. Descent of testes through the inguinal canal into the scrotal sac.
      iii. Mediated by the androgen-induced release of calcitonin gene–related peptide from the genitofemoral nerve.
3. Failure of either of these phases results in cryptorchidism.
   a. Testis is usually located within the inguinal canal but may remain within the abdomen (Fig. 21.3).
4. Epidemiology
   a. Most common genitourinary disorder of boys (present in up to 5% of full-term and ~30% of preterm male infants).
5. Clinical presentation
   a. Lack of testis within the scrotum, usually unilateral.
   b. May have palpable mass within the inguinal canal.
   c. Many spontaneously descend within the first several months of life.
6. Complications (if uncorrected)
   a. Infertility
      i. Due to scarring of seminiferous tubules, loss of spermatogenesis, and testicular atrophy; similar changes may occur in the normally descended contralateral testis.
   b. Increased risk of testicular cancer
      i. Normally descended testicle also at increased risk.
   c. Increased risk of torsion (see later).
7. Orchitis
   a. Defined as inflammation of one or both testes.
   b. Presents with testicular pain and swelling.
   c. Etiologies include mumps virus (usually children) and sexually transmitted infections (e.g., *N. gonorrhoeae* and *C. trachomatis*).

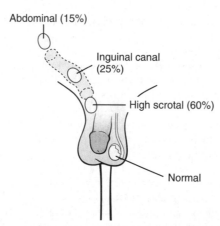

21.3: In cryptorchidism, the testis is not in the scrotum but may be found in the inguinal canal or the abdominal cavity. (*From Ivan Damjanov, MD, PhD: Pathology for the health professions, ed 4, Philadelphia, 2012, Saunders Elsevier, p 325, Fig. 14.3.*)

8. Epididymitis
   a. Inflammation of the epididymis (e.g., etiologies include infection and trauma).
      i. Acute epididymitis is the most common cause of scrotal pain in adults.
   b. Pathogens
      i. Common pathogens in younger (<35 years) sexually active patients include *N. gonorrhoeae* and *C. trachomatis*.
      ii. In older men (>35 years), *E. coli* and *Pseudomonas aeruginosa* are more likely (often secondary to urinary obstruction related to prostatic hyperplasia).
      iii. *Mycobacterium tuberculosis* may involve the epididymis (before spreading to the seminal vesicles, prostate, and testicles).
   c. Clinical findings
      i. Unilateral scrotal pain with radiation into the spermatic cord or flank.
      ii. Scrotal swelling and epididymal tenderness.
      iii. Urethral discharge (with sexually transmitted infections).
      iv. Manual elevation of the affected hemiscrotum will decrease the pain (positive Prehn sign).
      v. Positive cremasteric reflex (testis pulls up when the ipsilateral thigh is stroked).
9. Testicular torsion
   a. Twisting (torsion) of the spermatic cord/testis; due to inadequate fixation of the testis to the tunica vaginalis.
   b. Torsion reduces arterial inflow and impairs venous outflow (i.e., causes ischemia).
   c. Can arise at any age (commonly neonates and post pubertal).
      i. May occur spontaneously or after an inciting event (e.g., trauma or vigorous physical activity).
   d. Clinical manifestations
      i. Acute onset of severe testicular pain, tenderness, and swelling.
      ii. Absence of ipsilateral cremasteric reflex.
      iii. Classic finding of asymmetrically high-riding testis with its long axis oriented horizontally instead of vertically.
   e. Urologic emergency; requires manual and/or surgical reduction.
10. Varicocele
    a. Definition
       i. Collection of dilated and tortuous veins of pampiniform plexus of the spermatic cord within the scrotum (Fig. 21.4).
    b. Pathogenesis
       i. Impaired drainage of spermatic vein.
       ii. More common on the left (left spermatic vein enters the renal vein at a 90-degree angle; thereby increasing resistance to blood flow).
          (1) Obstruction of the left renal vein (e.g., renal cell carcinoma) can present with left-sided varicocele.

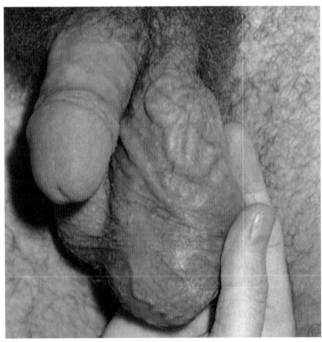

21.4: Varicocele in the left scrotal sac. Note the "bag of worms" appearance. *(From Swartz MH: Textbook of physical diagnosis, ed 5, Philadelphia, 2006, Saunders Elsevier, p 545, Fig. 18.27.)*

  iii. Conversely, right-sided varicoceles are less common (less resistance to drainage of right spermatic vein which inserts directly into the inferior vena cava).

 c. Clinical manifestations

  i. Often asymptomatic, may have heaviness or dull ache in scrotum with prolonged standing; relieved by lying down.

  ii. Visible "bag of worms" appearance that resolves once a patient is supine or increases with Valsalva maneuver.

 d. Complications

  i. Infertility (believed related to elevated scrotal temperatures that occur with the increase in vascularity).

11. Hydrocele

 a. Collection of serous fluid between the two layers of the tunica vaginalis causing scrotal mass.

 b. Most common cause of scrotal enlargement in boys.

 c. Pathogenesis

  i. Failure of the tunica vaginalis to close, fluid accumulation between layers of the tunica vaginalis.

  ii. Invariably associated with an indirect inguinal hernia.

 d. Diagnosis

  i. Transillumination or ultrasound (distinguishes fluid versus testicular mass).

12. Other fluid accumulations

 a. Hematocele (contains blood).

 b. Spermatocele (contains sperm)

  i. Common in adolescents; located in the upper pole of the epididymis.

13. Testicular tumors

 a. Epidemiology

  i. One percent of male cancers in the United States.

  ii. Most common type of carcinoma in males between the ages of 15 and 35 years.

  iii. More common in Whites.

 b. Risk factors

  i. Cryptorchid testis

   (1) Particularly those that remain intraabdominal.

   (2) Contralateral normally descended testis also at somewhat increased risk.

   (3) Surgical correction of the undescended testis (orchiopexy) reduces, but does not eliminate, risk.

  ii. Personal or family history of testicular cancer.

  iii. Human immunodeficiency virus infection (increased risk of seminoma).

  iv. Androgen insensitivity syndrome.

  v. Peutz–Jeghers syndrome (increased risk Sertoli cell tumor).

 c. Types of testicular tumors

  i. Germ cell tumors (GCT)

   (1) Represent 95% of all testicular tumors.

   (2) Classified as seminoma or nonseminomatous GCTs.

    (a) Seminoma

     a. Most common type of GCT.

    (b) Nonseminomatous GCTs include

     a. Yolk sac tumor

     b. Teratoma

     c. Embryonal carcinoma

     d. Choriocarcinoma

   (3) GCTs are often comprised of an admixture of tumor subtypes (e.g., seminoma + embryonal carcinoma; teratoma + embryonal carcinoma).

   (4) Although most arise within the testis, GCTs can also arise in other locations (e.g., pineal gland or mediastinum).

  ii. Primary malignant lymphoma of the testis

   (1) Older men.

 d. Clinical manifestations of testicular cancer

  i. Unilateral, painless testicular mass.

  ii. Tumor markers

   (1) α-Fetoprotein (AFP): elevated with yolk sac tumor (nonspecific).

   (2) β-Human chorionic gonadotropin (hCG): markedly elevated with choriocarcinoma; elevated to a lesser degree in some with seminoma.

    (a) Note that hCG has a similar structure to TSH (↑ hCG can therefore stimulate the thyroid gland to produce thyroid hormone).

  iii. Most commonly metastasizes to ipsilateral retroperitoneal lymph nodes.

  iv. Distant metastatic sites include lungs (producing dyspnea, cough, or hemoptysis) as well as liver, bone, and brain.

(1) Choriocarcinoma is notorious for early, hematogenous metastasis.
  e. Diagnosis
    i. Physical examination and ultrasound.
  f. Staging workup
    i. Computed tomography scan of the abdomen and pelvis.
    ii. Chest X-ray.
    iii. Tumor markers (AFP and hCG).

VI. Disease of the Prostate
A. Overview
  1. Prostate is comprised of glands and fibromuscular stroma.
  2. Growth dependent upon testicular androgens, castration leads to atrophy.

B. Acute bacterial prostatitis
  1. Acute onset of urogenital symptoms accompanied by bacterial infection of the prostate gland.
    a. Involvement of prostate ascertained by the presence of inflammatory cells in, or bacterial growth from, prostatic secretions.
  2. Etiologic organisms include:
    a. *E. coli* (most common); *Proteus, Klebsiella, Enterobacter, Pseudomonas*.
    b. *N. gonorrhoeae* and *C. trachomatis* (young, sexually active patients).
  3. Transmission of infection
    a. Intraprostatic reflux of contaminated urine from the urethra or urinary bladder.
    b. Hematogenous seeding from distant infection (less common).
  4. Clinical manifestations
    a. Fever, chills, malaise, dysuria, and pelvic or perineal pain.
    b. Urinary symptoms (e.g., frequency and urgency).
    c. Edema and tenderness on prostate examination.
  5. Complications
    a. Spread of infection in the blood (bacteremia) or elsewhere (e.g., epididymitis), chronic prostatitis, and prostatic abscess.

C. Chronic bacterial prostatitis
  1. Chronic urogenital symptoms in conjunction with bacterial infection of the prostate.
  2. Etiologies include *E. coli* (most common), *Proteus, Klebsiella*, and *Pseudomonas* spp.
  3. Clinical manifestations
    a. May be asymptomatic; some exhibit symptoms of recurrent urinary tract infection (e.g., frequency, dysuria, and urgency).

D. Benign prostatic hyperplasia (BPH)
  1. BPH is a pathologic diagnosis characterized by hyperplasia of the glandular and stromal elements of the prostate.
    a. Hyperplasia (increased cell number), not hypertrophy (which refers to an increase in cell size).
    b. BPH begins in the transition/periurethral zone of the prostate.
    c. As the name suggests, BPH is a benign process (no increased risk of prostate cancer).
  2. Epidemiology
    a. Age-dependent change that eventually affects the majority of men.
    b. Usually begins around age 40 years, increasing in prevalence with age.
  3. Pathogenesis
    a. Circulating testosterone is metabolized locally by 5α-reductase to dihydrotestosterone, a potent androgen that stimulates growth of prostatic tissue.
  4. Gross and microscopic findings
    a. Hyperplasia of glandular and stromal tissue forms nodules within the periurethral zone, eventually compressing the prostatic urethra (causing manifestations of bladder outlet obstruction).
  5. Clinical manifestations
    a. Signs of bladder outlet obstruction (most common)
      i.   Difficulty initiating and/or maintaining urine stream (i.e., straining to urinate).
      ii. Incomplete emptying of the urinary bladder.
      iii. Nocturia (nighttime urination).
      iv. Increased urinary frequency and/or urgency.
      v.   Hematuria (usually microscopic).
      vi. Normal to slight elevation prostate-specific antigen (PSA).
  6. Complications, due to obstruction of prostatic urethra, include:
    a. Bilateral hydronephrosis.
    b. Bladder diverticula (secondary to increased intravesical pressure required to initiate and maintain the urine stream).
    c. Hypertrophy and hyperplasia of the bladder muscle.
    d. Recurrent urinary tract infections.
    e. Risk of renal insufficiency (postrenal azotemia).

E. **Prostate cancer**
   1. Definition
      a. Malignancy of prostatic glandular epithelium (adenocarcinoma).
      b. Usually begins in the peripheral zone of the prostate.
   2. Epidemiology
      a. Most common noncutaneous malignancy in men.
      b. In the United States, prostate cancer is second only to lung cancer as a cause of cancer-related death.
      c. More common in African Americans.
      d. Rare before age 40 years, increasing prevalence with age.
   3. Risk factors
      a. Increasing age (primary factor).
      b. Family history, African American ethnicity, and obesity.
   4. Pathology
      a. Adenocarcinomas usually begin within the peripheral zone of the prostate and therefore may be palpable on digital rectal examination (DRE).
      b. Tumor grading (Gleason) based on the degree of differentiation.
         i. Low Gleason score = well-differentiated tumor, likely exhibits slow tumor growth.
         ii. High Gleason score = poorly differentiated tumor, likely to exhibit more aggressive growth.
   5. Clinical manifestations
      a. Early-stage disease is usually asymptomatic.
      b. Obstructive urinary symptoms (e.g., hesitancy, and decreased urinary stream) may ultimately occur with growth of the tumor around the prostatic urethra or bladder neck.
      c. Metastasis to regional pelvic lymph nodes (may lead to lower extremity edema and/or perineal discomfort).
      d. Distant metastasis (most commonly to bone)
         i. Prostate cancer spreads via the Batson venous plexus.
         ii. Bone metastasis may be painful, risk of pathologic fracture, and spinal cord compression.
         iii. Elevation of serum alkaline phosphatase (malignant cells release cytokines that stimulate osteoblasts to form bone).
         iv. Imaging reveals increased bone density (osteoblastic metastasis).
   6. Screening
      a. Screening for prostate cancer is controversial; usually involves the use of serum PSA.
      b. US Preventive Services Task Force currently recommends that men aged 55–69 years be counseled about the use of PSA for screening with the decision being individualized (i.e., no set guidelines for the population as a whole).
         i. Note that a normal serum PSA (0–4 ng/mL) does not exclude the possibility of prostate cancer (patient with cancer may have normal PSA).
         ii. In addition, an elevated PSA is not specific for cancer (may also be seen with BPH, prostatitis).
      c. DRE is generally not recommended unless a patient presents with urinary or rectal symptoms. If performed, the DRE may identify tumors within the posterior and lateral regions of the prostate (stony hard and asymmetrical nodule).
   7. Diagnosis
      a. Ultrasound-guided transrectal needle core biopsy.
   8. Spread of prostate cancer
      a. Perineural invasion.
      b. Lymphatic spread to regional lymph nodes (internal iliac nodes).
      c. Hematogenous spread
         i. Bone is the most common extranodal site of metastasis, especially lumbar spine, proximal femur, and pelvis.

VII. **Male Reproduction**
   A. **Follicle-stimulating hormone (FSH)**
      1. Stimulates spermatogenesis by seminiferous tubules of testes (Fig. 21.5).
   B. **Luteinizing hormone (LH)**
      1. LH stimulates testosterone synthesis by the Leydig cells of the testes.
   C. **Testosterone**
      1. Maintains male secondary sex characteristics and increases libido (sexual desire).
      2. Enhances spermatogenesis in the seminiferous tubules.
      3. Decreased levels associated with a loss of muscle mass, decreased libido, testicular atrophy, and infertility.
   D. **Sex hormone–binding globulin (SHBG)**
      1. Produced by the liver, SHBG is the binding protein for testosterone (as well as estrogen).
      2. Estrogen promotes the synthesis of SHBG.
      3. Androgens, insulin, obesity, and hypothyroidism all suppress the synthesis of SHBG.
      4. SHBG has a higher binding affinity for testosterone than estrogen.
         a. Increased serum SHBG → decreased free serum testosterone.
         b. Decreased SHBG → increased free serum testosterone.

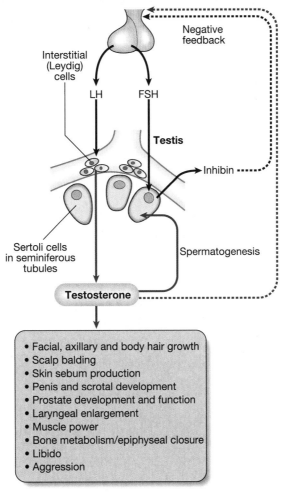

21.5: Male reproductive physiology. See text for discussion. *FSH,* Follicle-stimulating hormone; *LH,* luteinizing hormone. *(From Walker BR, Colledge NR, Ralston SH, Penman ID: Davidson's principles and practice of medicine, ed 22, St. Louis, 2014, Churchill Livingstone Elsevier, p 756, Fig. 20.12.)*

E. Male hypogonadism
1. Clinical syndrome related to a reduction in sperm and/or testosterone production (i.e., testicular failure).
2. Primary hypogonadism (hypergonadotropic hypogonadism)
   a. Abnormality of the testes with decreased serum testosterone and/or sperm count. The loss of negative feedback of testosterone on the hypothalamus and pituitary causes gonadotropins to be elevated.
      i. Decreased testosterone, increased gonadotropin-releasing hormone (GnRH), LH, and FSH.
   b. Causes include:
      i. Klinefelter syndrome
         (1) Defined by the presence of an extra X chromosome in the male (usually 47,XXY).
         (2) Small testes, infertility, and varying degrees of androgen deficiency despite elevated gonadotropin concentrations.
      ii. Cryptorchidism
         (1) If unilateral, sperm count may be low and serum FSH concentration will be slightly elevated.
         (2) If bilateral, sperm count is usually markedly decreased (serum testosterone may also be reduced).
      iii. Mumps orchitis
         (1) More likely to cause testicular damage/impairment when infection occurs as an adult.
      iv. Radiation/chemotherapeutic agents
         (1) Damages seminiferous tubules, less likely to decrease testosterone production.
      v. Genetic mutations involving LH and FSH receptors.
      vi. Ketoconazole (antifungal agent) inhibits testosterone synthesis.
3. Secondary hypogonadism (hypogonadotropic hypogonadism)
   a. Reduction in testicular function secondary to a lack of gonadotropins.
      i. Serum testosterone, LH, and FSH are all decreased.

    b. Due to hypothalamic or pituitary dysfunction, causes include:

        i. Suppression of gonadotropins (e.g., GnRH analogs, hyperprolactinemia, and anabolic steroids).

        ii. Damage to hypothalamus (e.g., sarcoidosis) and/or pituitary (e.g., head trauma, hemochromatosis).

        iii. Kallmann syndrome

           (1) Inherited deficiency of GnRH plus anosmia (lack of ability to smell).

    4. Manifestations of hypogonadism

      a. Depends upon the age at presentation.

        i. Hypogonadism developing prior to the completion of puberty results in small genitalia (testes and penis), decreased muscle mass, and failure of the voice to deepen.

        ii. Hypogonadism developing in adulthood causes decreased libido and depressed mood.

F. Male infertility

  1. Defined as an inability to cause pregnancy in a fertile woman for a least 1 year.

  2. Etiologies include:

    a. Defective spermatogenesis (the most common cause)

      i. Most are idiopathic, other etiologies include Klinefelter syndrome (47,XXY), cryptorchidism.

    b. Pituitary and/or hypothalamic dysfunction (i.e., hypogonadotropic; hypogonadism with decreased LH, FSH, and testosterone)

      i. Infiltrative disorders (e.g., sarcoidosis, tuberculosis, and fungal infection).

      ii. Hyperprolactinemia.

      iii. Head trauma (damage to hypothalamus and/or pituitary).

      iv. Iron overload (damages endocrine organs, e.g., pituitary).

      v. Congenital GnRH deficiency (Kallmann syndrome).

    c. Abnormal sperm transport

      i. Abnormality of vas deferens (e.g., vasectomy).

      ii. Congenital absence of the vas deferens (e.g., cystic fibrosis).

    d. Idiopathic

      i. Semen analysis is normal, no other apparent cause of infertility.

  3. Laboratory tests for infertility

    a. Semen analysis (gold-standard test for infertility).

      i. Normal sperm count of 20–150 million sperm/mL.

      ii. Sperm motility.

    b. Serum gonadotropins, testosterone

VIII. Erectile Dysfunction (ED)

  A. Definition: Persistent inability to obtain or maintain a penile erection adequate for coitus.

  B. Causes

    1. Psychogenic

      a. Most common cause in younger men; usually secondary to stress, depression, relationship conflicts, and/or performance anxiety.

        i. The presence of normally occurring erections during sleep ("nocturnal penile tumescence") is a clue. All other causes of ED are associated with a loss of nocturnal penile tumescence.

    2. Vascular insufficiency

      a. Most common cause of ED in men >50 years of age.

      b. Usually secondary to aortoiliac atherosclerosis with associated reduction in penile blood flow.

      c. May be accompanied by claudication (cramping pain when walking), diminished femoral pulse.

    3. Neurologic disease

      a. Parasympathetic nervous system (S2–S4) necessary for erection.

        i. Sympathetic nervous system necessary for ejaculation.

      b. Various neurologic conditions (e.g., spinal cord injury, nerve damage secondary to prostatectomy, multisystem atrophy, etc.) may cause ED.

    4. Hormonal

      a. Hypogonadism

        i. Decreased testosterone → decreased libido.

      b. Hyperprolactinemia

        i. Etiologies include pituitary adenoma and medications.

        ii. Prolactin suppresses the release of GnRH → decreased LH, FSH → decreased testosterone.

      c. Thyroid disease

        i. Hyperthyroidism: excess thyroid hormone stimulates production of SHBG, thereby lowering testosterone bioavailability.

        ii. Primary hypothyroidism → increased release of thyrotropin-releasing hormone → stimulates production of prolactin.

Female Reproductive Disorders and Breast Disorders

I. **Genital Infections**
   A. **Overview of genital infections (Figs. 22.1–22.4).**
II. **Disorders of the Vulva**
   A. **Overview**
      1. The vulva (external female genitalia) consists of the labia majora, labia minora, clitoris, vestibule, Bartholin's glands, and vaginal opening.
      2. Primary lymphatic drainage is to the superficial inguinal lymph nodes.
      3. Bartholin glands produce lubricating mucus and drain via ducts into the vestibule at approximately the 4-o'clock and 8-o'clock positions.
   B. **Bartholin gland cyst**
      1. Vulvar mass of lower vestibular region caused by the obstruction of Bartholin duct.
      2. Usually less than 3 cm in diameter, Bartholin cysts are often asymptomatic; however, some develop vulvar pain and dyspareunia (painful intercourse).
   C. **Bartholin gland abscess**
      1. Infectious complication of Bartholin gland cyst (e.g., *Staphylococcus* and *Escherichia coli*).
      2. Characterized by the presence of the tender fluctuant mass of lower vestibule with edema and erythema; may have purulent discharge.
   D. **Vulvar lichen sclerosus**
      1. Chronic inflammatory disorder of the vulva and perineum characterized by thinning of the epidermis and hyalinization of the dermal collagen.
      2. Most common in prepubertal girls and postmenopausal women.
      3. Etiology unknown; increased risk in those with autoimmune disorders.
      4. Manifests as a white parchment paper-like lesion around introitus and perianal region ("keyhole" distribution), pruritus, and dyspareunia.
      5. Confers a small increased risk of squamous cell carcinoma (SCC).
   E. **Low-grade squamous intraepithelial lesion of the vulva (vulvar LSIL)**
      1. Formerly known as vulvar intraepithelial neoplasia 1.
      2. Associated with low-risk human papillomavirus (HPV) subtypes (6 and 11); self-limited, not considered premalignant.
   F. **High-grade squamous intraepithelial lesion of the vulva (vulvar HSIL)**
      1. Associated with high-risk HPV subtypes (e.g., 16 and 18) that integrate into the host genome.
         a. The E6 and E7 genes of high-risk HPV types encode oncoproteins that interfere with the activity of cellular tumor suppressor proteins. E6 protein increases turnover of p53 while E7 proteins act by associating with members of the retinoblastoma (*Rb*) family.
         b. Allows for unregulated cell growth and the potential for malignant transformation (SCC).

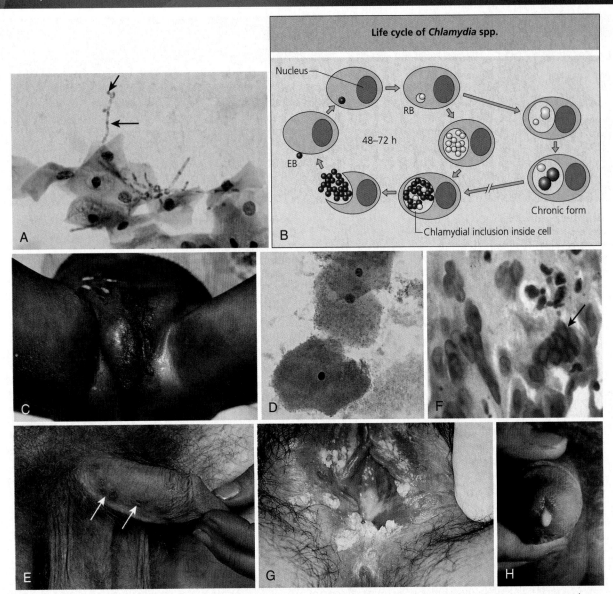

22.1: Genital infections. (A) *Candida* spp. The bottom arrow shows elongated yeasts (pseudohyphae); the top arrow shows yeasts. (B) *Chlamydia trachomatis* life cycle. (C) *Lymphogranuloma venereum* (*C. trachomatis* subspecies). The patient has unilateral vulvar lymph-edema and inguinal ulcerations (*four white areas*). (D) *Gardnerella vaginalis.* Superficial squamous cells (SCs) are covered by granular material representing bacterial organisms attached to (not invading) the surface. (E) Genital herpes. Arrows show ulcerated, red lesions on the shaft of the penis. (F) Genital herpes. Biopsy showing a multinucleated SC with smudged, "ground-glass" nuclei with intranuclear inclusions (*arrow*). (G) Human papillomavirus. Numerous keratotic papillary processes are present on the surface of the labia (condylo-mata acuminata). (H) *Neisseria gonorrhoeae* urethritis. (*A and F, From Atkinson BF: Atlas of diagnostic cytopathology, Philadelphia, 1992, Saunders, pp 76, 78, 80, respectively, Figs. 2.49B, 2.55, and 2.63, respectively; B, from Cohen J, Opal SM, Powderly WG: Infectious diseases, ed 3, St. Louis, 2010, Mosby Elsevier, p 1817, Fig. 177.1; C, from Cohen J, Powderly W: Infectious diseases, ed 2, St. Louis, 2004, Mosby; D and G, from Ivan Damjanov, MD, PhD, Linder J: Pathology: a color atlas, St. Louis, 2000, Mosby, pp 261, 260, respectively, Figs. 13.10B, 13.8, respectively; E, from Bouloux P-M: Self-assessment picture tests: medicine, Vol 1, London, 1996, Mosby-Wolfe, p 17, Fig. 33; H, from Marx J: Rosen's emergency medicine concepts and clinical practice, ed 7, Philadelphia, 2010, Mosby Elsevier, p 1291, Fig. 96.10; I, from Greer I, Cameron IT, Kitchener HC, Prentice A: Mosby's color atlas and text of obstetrics and gynecology, St. Louis, 2000, Mosby, p 274, Fig. 10-50; J and L, from Swartz MH: Textbook of physical diagnosis, ed 5, Philadelphia, 2006, Saunders Elsevier, p 537, 553, respectively, Fig. 18.13, 18.39, respectively; K, from Lookingbill D, Marks J: Principles of dermatology, ed 3, Philadelphia, 2000, Saunders, p 124, Fig. 10.17; M, from Kumar V, Fausto N, Abbas A: Robbins and Cotran pathologic basis of disease, ed 7, Philadelphia, 2004, Saunders, p 1064, Fig. 22.4.*)

    2. Histology reveals atypical pleomorphic cells and increased mitotic activity extending from the base into the upper layers of the vulvar epithelium.

G. Differentiated vulvar intraepithelial neoplasia

    1. Describes lesions not associated with HPV but rather with vulvar dermatoses (e.g., lichen sclerosus).

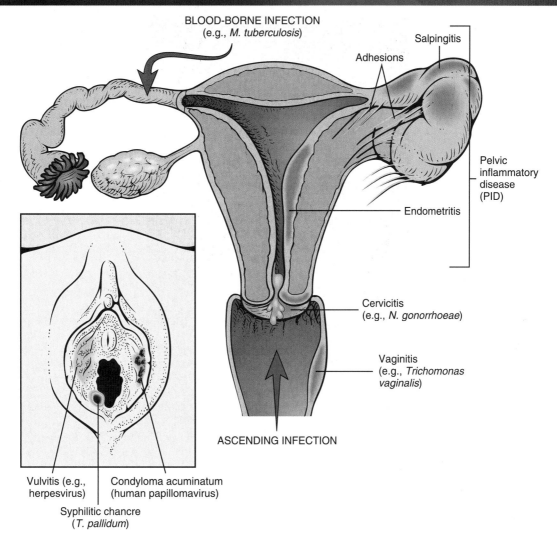

BLOOD-BORNE INFECTION
(e.g., *M. tuberculosis*)

Salpingitis

Adhesions

Pelvic
inflammatory
disease
(PID)

Endometritis

Cervicitis
(e.g., *N. gonorrhoeae*)

Vaginitis
(e.g., *Trichomonas
vaginalis*)

ASCENDING INFECTION

Vulvitis (e.g.,
herpesvirus)

Condyloma acuminatum
(human papillomavirus)

Syphilitic chancre
(*T. pallidum*)

22.2: Overview of the pathology and pathogenesis of infections involving the female genital organs. Ascending infections are usually caused by sexual contact, pregnancy, or instrumentation. *(From Damjanov I: Pathology for the health professions, ed 4, Philadelphia, 2012, Saunders Elsevier, p 344, Fig. 15.4.)*

H. SCC of the vulva
1. Most common type of vulvar malignancy (~85% of cases).
2. Predominantly postmenopausal (mean 68 years).
3. Risk factors
   a. Infection by high-risk HPV serotype; primarily HPV 16.
   b. Smoking cigarettes.
   c. Immunodeficiency (e.g., acquired immunodeficiency syndrome).
   d. Lichen sclerosus.
4. Manifestations
   a. Vulvar mass, pruritus, pain, bleeding, and malodorous discharge.
5. Metastatic spread
   a. Depends on a specific location, primarily to inguinal nodes.

I. Melanoma
1. Second most common primary malignancy of the vulva (~5%).
2. Predominantly seen in White postmenopausal women (mean 61 years).
3. Treatment is surgical resection, high-risk recurrence, and metastatic spread.

J. Extramammary Paget disease
1. Intraepithelial adenocarcinoma of the vulva.
2. Uncommon; <1% of vulvar malignancies.
3. Clinical manifestations

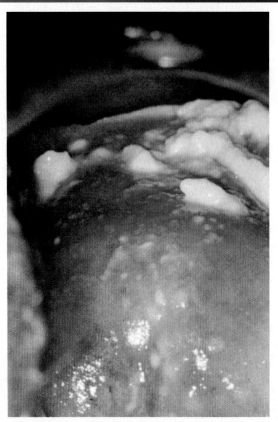

22.3: Vulvovaginal candidiasis. A curd-like discharge is commonly present in candidiasis. *(Courtesy of Bingham JS, Pocket Picture Guide Series: Sexually transmitted diseases, London, 1984, Gower Medical Publishing Ltd.)*

    a. Pruritus (the most common symptom).
    b. Eczematous, well-demarcated lesion on a red background.
  4. Malignant cells (called Paget cells) contain mucin, spread along the epithelium (Fig. 22.5).
    a. Mucin stains (e.g., periodic acid-Schiff) can be useful diagnostically to identify the Paget cells.

III. **Disorders of the Vagina**
  A. **Imperforate hymen**
    1. The hymen, a fibrous membrane overlying the vaginal opening, normally undergoes degeneration during fetal life.
    2. If the usual degenerative process does not occur (i.e., imperforate hymen), then vaginal obstruction occurs.
    3. May present during the newborn period with bulging of the hymenal membrane as mucus collects behind the obstruction.
    4. Note that vaginal mucus is produced in response to stimulation by maternal estradiol. As estrogen levels decline following delivery, mucus is resorbed. For this reason, the diagnosis may not be made during the newborn period.
      a. Many cases go undiagnosed until puberty when the patient presents with primary amenorrhea (menstrual blood collects behind the imperforate hymen).
  B. **Mayer–Rokitansky–Küster–Hauser syndrome**
    1. Müllerian ducts form the upper vagina, cervix, uterine corpus, and fallopian tubes.
    2. Prevalence of ~1 in 5000 females; characterized by complete Müllerian agenesis (i.e., patients do not develop any of the aforementioned Müllerian structures).
    3. Patients have a short vagina that ends in a blind pouch.
    4. Often presents with primary amenorrhea.
    5. Ovaries are present and function (not of Müllerian origin; therefore patients develop secondary sex characteristics [breasts, pubic hair, and axillary hair]).
  C. **Gartner duct cyst of the vagina**
    1. Cyst within the lateral vaginal wall (mesonephric remnant).
    2. Usually asymptomatic, may cause dyspareunia.
  D. **Embryonal rhabdomyosarcoma (sarcoma botryoides)**
    1. Malignant tumor of rhabdomyoblasts.
    2. Most common malignancy of the vagina in girls less than 5 years of age.
    3. Presents with bleeding and/or as a "grape-like" mass arising from the vagina with protrusion through the vaginal os (Fig. 22.6A).

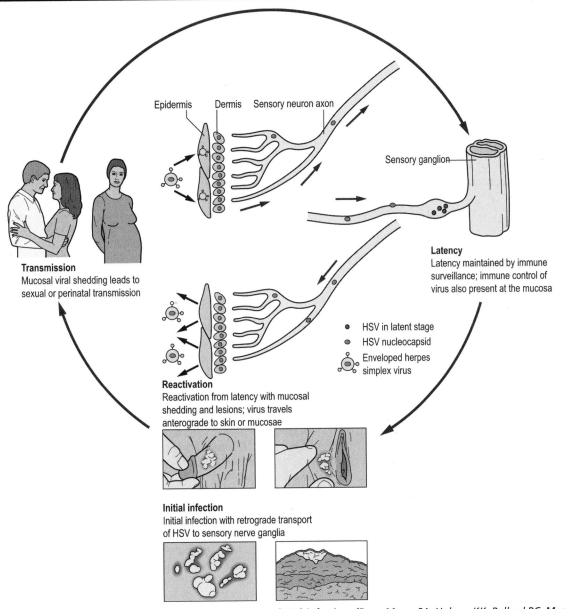

Epidermis   Dermis   Sensory neuron axon

Sensory ganglion

Latency
Latency maintained by immune
surveillance; immune control of
virus also present at the mucosa

- HSV in latent stage
- HSV nucleocapsid
- Enveloped herpes
  simplex virus

Transmission
Mucosal viral shedding leads to
sexual or perinatal transmission

Reactivation
Reactivation from latency with mucosal
shedding and lesions; virus travels
anterograde to skin or mucosae

Initial infection
Initial infection with retrograde transport
of HSV to sensory nerve ganglia

22.4: Pathogenesis and transmission of genital herpes simplex virus (HSV) infection. *(From Morse SA, Holmes KK, Ballard RC, Moreland AA: Atlas of sexually transmitted diseases and AIDS, ed 4, Philadelphia, 2010, Saunders Elsevier, p 171, Fig. 10.5.)*

E. **Clear cell adenocarcinoma of the vagina (Fig. 22.6B)**
  1. Rare adenocarcinoma of the upper vagina and/or cervix arising from an area of adenosis.
     a. Adenosis refers to the presence of columnar (glandular) epithelium, rather than the usual squamous epithelium within the vagina Fig. 22.6B.
  2. Historically seen in young adult women exposed to diethylstilbestrol (DES) during prenatal life.
     a. A synthetic estrogen used in the past to prevent pregnancy complications, DES was discontinued in the 1970s due to its teratogenic and carcinogenic properties.
F. **SCC of the vagina**
  1. Tumor of squamous epithelial cells.
  2. Although SCC is the most common primary vaginal malignancy, it is rare. Most vaginal malignancies represent a tumor arising elsewhere (e.g., SCC of cervix).
  3. Lymphatic drainage (from the upper vagina) is to pelvic and paraaortic lymph nodes.
  4. Lymphatic drainage (from the distal vagina) is to inguinal and femoral lymph nodes.
IV. **Disorders of the Uterine Cervix**
  A. **Overview**
    1. Uterine cervix is comprised of the ectocervix and endocervix.
       a. Ectocervix is lined by nonkeratinized stratified squamous epithelium.
       b. Endocervix is lined by mucus-secreting columnar (glandular) epithelium.

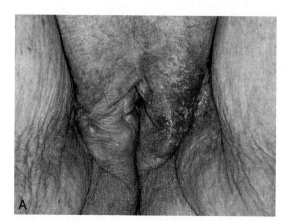

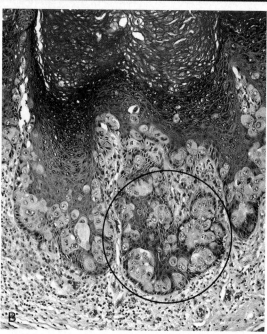

22.5: (A) Paget disease of the vulva. The patient's left vulva is erythematous and superficially ulcerated from scratching. (B) Pale, malignant mucin-filled columnar cells infiltrating the epidermis. *(A, From Crum CP, Nucci MR, Lee KR, Boyd TK, Granter SR, Haefner HK, Peters WA: Diagnostic gynecologic and obstetric pathology, ed 2, Philadelphia, 2011, Saunders Elsevier, pp 136, 137, Figs. 7-2, 3A, respectively.)*

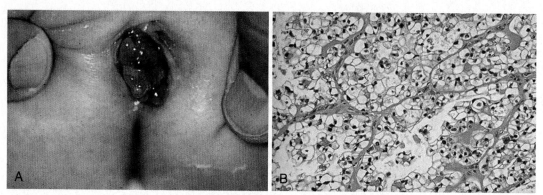

22.6: (A) Embryonal rhabdomyosarcoma of the vagina. Note the bloody, necrotic mass protruding out of the vagina. (B) Clear cell carcinoma of the vagina. Note the clear, vacuolated cells with ill-defined glandular spaces. *(A, From Ivan Damjanov, MD, PhD, Linder J: Pathology: a color atlas, St. Louis, 2000, Mosby, p 266, Fig. 13.29; B, from Klatt E: Robbins and Cotran atlas of pathology, Philadelphia, 2006, Saunders, p 295, Fig. 13.12.)*

2. During the reproductive years, the mucus-secreting glandular epithelium of the endocervix is partially replaced by stratified squamous epithelium (called "squamous metaplasia").
   a. Columnar epithelium → stratified squamous epithelium.
3. This process, although benign, results in an epithelium that is susceptible to infection by HPV.
   a. Explains the importance of sampling this region ("transformation zone") during a cervical Papanicolaou (Pap) smear.
4. Obstruction of endocervical drainage by metaplastic squamous cells can result in the formation of benign mucus-filled cysts ("Nabothian cyst").

B. Cervicitis
1. Cervicitis is defined as inflammation of the uterine cervix; primarily involves the columnar epithelium of the endocervix.
   a. Cervix and vagina are normally resistant to infection because of the acidic pH (4.0–4.5); due to the presence of *Lactobacilli* within vaginal flora.
2. Despite the acidic pH, infections can occur, usually as a result of sexual transmission (e.g., *Chlamydia trachomatis, Neisseria gonorrhoeae,* and *Trichomonas vaginalis*).
3. Clinical manifestations
   a. Vaginal discharge (most common)

i. Note that the most common cause of vaginal discharge in the United States is bacterial vaginosis (BV). For unknown reasons, the vaginal microbiome in some women may shift away from the usual lactobacilli, causing the vaginal pH to rise. BV, which technically is not an infection since it represents an overgrowth of *Gardnerella vaginalis*, is characterized by a malodorous watery vaginal discharge and "fishy" odor (particularly after coitus). Clues to the diagnosis include a positive "whiff test" (fishy smell following the addition of potassium hydroxide to a sample of the vaginal discharge), as well as the presence of "clue cells" on the microscopic examination (squamous epithelial cells covered by bacteria).

b. Vaginal bleeding, often postcoital.

c. Dyspareunia (painful intercourse).

d. On examination, the cervix is erythematous and friable (i.e., bleeds easily when touched with swab).

   i. May see punctate hemorrhages in cases of *T. vaginalis* cervicitis ("strawberry cervix").

4. Diagnosis

  a. Purulent cervical discharge.

  b. Nucleic acid amplification testing (NAAT)

    i. Used to detect *C. trachomatis* and *N. gonorrhoeae*.

  c. Microscopic examination ("Wet mount")

    i. Prominent neutrophilic inflammation.

    ii. *T. vaginalis* are pear-shaped and exhibit jerky movement (due to flagella).

    iii. *C. trachomatis* is likely if lymphoid follicles are identified (either on cervical cytology [Pap smear] or biopsy specimen).

5. Complications

  a. Pelvic inflammatory disease (PID)—see later.

  b. Neonatal infection (conjunctivitis and pneumonia)

    i. Due to contact with infected secretions during delivery.

    ii. Conjunctivitis (ophthalmia neonatorum)

      (1) *N. gonorrhoeae* (presents the first week of life).

      (2) *C. trachomatis* (longer incubation period—presents during the second week of life).

C. Hormonal changes by Pap smear

1. Superficial squamous cells indicate estrogen stimulation.

  a. Presence of 100% superficial squamous cells indicates predominant estrogen effect (e.g., taking estrogen without progesterone, exposure to estrogen-secreting tumor—e.g., granulosa cell tumor of the ovary).

2. Intermediate squamous cells indicate progesterone stimulation.

  a. Pregnant women should have 100% intermediate squamous cells (progesterone is the primary hormone of pregnancy).

3. Parabasal cells indicate the lack of hormonal stimulation.

  a. Presence of only parabasal cells suggests that the patient is postmenopausal.

4. In health, normal nonpregnant women have ~70% superficial squamous cells and 30% intermediate squamous cells.

D. Endocervical polyp

1. Nonneoplastic polypoid mass of endocervical tissue.

2. Most commonly seen in women between 30 and 50 years of age.

3. Usually an incidental finding, may cause postcoital bleeding or vaginal discharge.

4. Etiology unknown; chronic inflammation and/or hormonal factors may be contributory.

E. Cervical intraepithelial neoplasia (CIN)

1. Premalignant condition of cervix caused by HPV.

  a. Low-risk HPV types (HPV 6 and 11) do not integrate into the host genome but may cause genital warts (condyloma acuminata) and cause low-grade dysplasia (CIN 1).

  b. High-risk HPV types (e.g., 16 and 18) integrate into the host genome; viral oncoproteins E6 and E7 interfere with host tumor suppressor proteins p53 and Rb, respectively, resulting in unregulated cell growth.

2. Classification

  a. CIN 1

    i. Low-grade lesion characterized by atypia involving the lower third of the epithelium.

    ii. Koilocytes represent the viral cytopathic effect of HPV-infected squamous cells; identified by a wrinkled nucleus with surrounding clear zone (Fig. 22.7B).

  b. CIN 2

    i. High-grade lesion with cellular atypia involving the lower two-thirds of the epithelium.

  c. CIN 3

    i. High-grade lesion with cellular atypia involving more than the lower two-thirds of the epithelium; may be full thickness ("carcinoma in situ").

3. Progression of dysplasia is not inevitable.

  a. Most cases of CIN 1 will regress.

  b. CIN 2 and CIN 3 are more likely to progress; potential for malignant transformation over a period of several years (SCC).

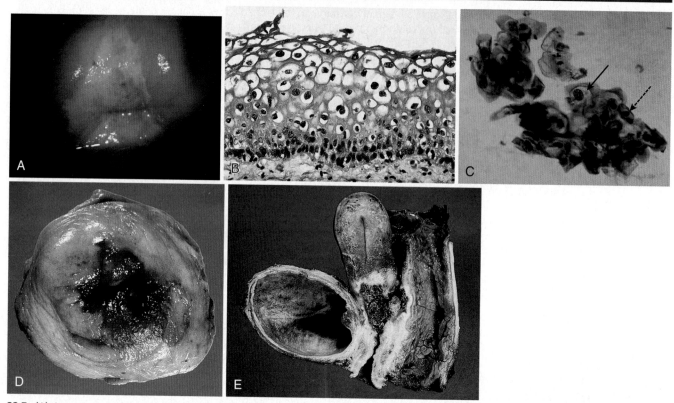

22.7: (A) Appearance of the cervix after application of 3%–5% acetic acid. Note the well-defined, opaque acetowhite area, with regular margins, involving a large part of the visible squamocolumnar junction. (B) Koilocytosis caused by human papillomavirus (HPV). The squamous cells have wrinkled pyknotic nuclei surrounded by a clear halo. (C) Papanicolaou stain of the exfoliated cervicovaginal squamous epithelial cells, showing the perinuclear cytoplasmic vacuolization termed koilocytosis (vacuolated cytoplasm; *solid arrow*) and nuclear pyknosis (*interrupted arrow*) characteristic of HPV infection. (D) Squamous cell carcinoma (SCC) of the cervix. Note the bleeding and ulceration in the cervical os. (E) SCC of cervix with extension down into the vagina, wall of the urinary bladder (on left), and wall of the rectum (on the right). *(A, From Cohen J, Opal SM, Powderly WG: Infectious diseases, ed 3, St. Louis, 2010, Mosby Elsevier, p 653, Fig. 59.2; B, from Rosai J, Ackerman LV: Surgical pathology, ed 9, St. Louis, 2004, Mosby, p 1530, Fig. 19.74; C, from Murray PR, Rosenthal KS, Pfaller MA: Medical microbiology, ed 6, Philadelphia, 2009, Mosby Elsevier, p 504, Fig. 51.7; D and E, courtesy of Dr. Hector Rodriguez-Martinez, Mexico City, Mexico.)*

     c. Average age for the development of cervical cancer (~50 years) is 8–10 years later than the peak incidence of high-grade CIN.
  4. Risk factors
     a. Infection by a high-risk serotype of HPV (e.g., 16 and 18).
     b. Cigarette smoking (synergistic effect with HPV).
     c. Persistent infection is more likely in immunosuppressed (e.g., human immunodeficiency virus [HIV]).
     d. Higher risk of infection in those with the early onset of sexual activity (<18 years of age), multiple sexual partners (>6), and/or engaging in sex with high-risk partners (e.g., those with a history of multiple sexual partners).
  5. Clinical findings
     a. CIN is not usually visible to the naked eye.
     b. Colposcopy, the direct visualization of the cervix following the application of a 3% acetic acid, is used to identify dysplastic mucosa (dysplasia is characteristically white with vascular changes).

F. Cervical cancer
  1. Malignancy of uterine cervix; highly associated with infection by HPV (especially types 16 and 18).
  2. May be in situ (i.e., full thickness atypia) or invasive.
     a. Tumor is said to be "invasive" once it has penetrated the basement membrane into underlying stroma.
  3. Histologic types
     a. SCC
       i. Most common type: refers to a malignancy of squamous epithelial cells. Typically arises within the transformation zone.
     b. Adenocarcinoma
       i. Second most common type; arises from endocervical glandular epithelial cells.
  4. Epidemiology
     a. Cervical cancer is the third most common type of gynecologic cancer (after endometrium and ovary) in the United States.

   i. Incidence is higher in countries with a limited access to health care (lack of screening Pap smears).
   b. In the United States, cervical cancer is more common in Hispanic and African Americans with a mean age at diagnosis of 50 years.
   5. Clinical manifestations
   a. Abnormal vaginal bleeding (most common), usually postcoital.
   b. Malodorous discharge.
   c. Tumor may grow into the bladder and/or ureters causing urinary tract obstruction (renal failure is a common cause of death).
V. **Reproductive Physiology and Selected Hormone Disorders**
   A. **Sequence to menarche**
   1. Breast budding (thelarche) → growth spurt → pubic hair → menarche.
   2. Menarche: beginning of menses, averages ~12 years.
   B. **Synthesis of sex hormones in theca cells of the ovary (Fig. 22.8).**
   C. **Hormonal changes during the menstrual cycle involve the ovary and endometrium (Fig. 22.9).**
   1. Ovarian cycle
   a. Follicular phase
   i. Development of a dominant follicle.
   ii. Increasing estrogen (E) levels 24–36 hours before ovulation stimulate the release of luteinizing hormone (LH) from the anterior pituitary (called the "LH surge").
   (1) E surge → LH surge → ovulation.
   b. Ovulation
   i. Release of the ovum from the ovary.
   ii. Recognized clinically by an increase in body temperature (progesterone effect) and Mittelschmerz (pelvic discomfort due to local peritoneal irritation).
   c. Luteal phase
   i. Secretion of progesterone from the corpus luteum.
   2. Endometrial cycle
   a. Menses
   i. The first day of menses is the first day of the menstrual cycle.
   ii. In the absence of implantation, decreasing levels of serum estradiol and progesterone cause sloughing of the superficial endometrium (stratum functionalis) with bleeding (i.e., menses).
   iii. The stratum basalis (basal layer of endometrium) does not shed; allows for endometrial regeneration following menses.

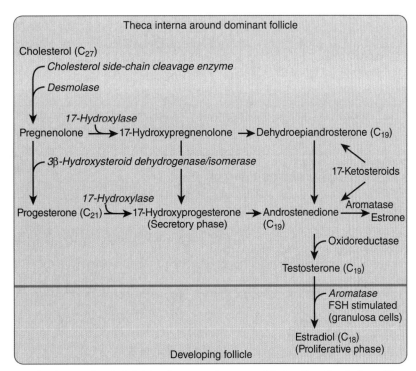

22.8: Synthesis of sex hormones in the ovaries. Luteinizing hormone is responsible for the stimulation of hormone synthesis in the theca interna surrounding the developing follicle. Follicle-stimulating hormone increases the synthesis of aromatase in granulosa cells. Aromatase converts testosterone to estradiol. *(Modified from Goljan EF: Star series: pathology, Philadelphia, 1998, Saunders, Fig. 18.1.)*

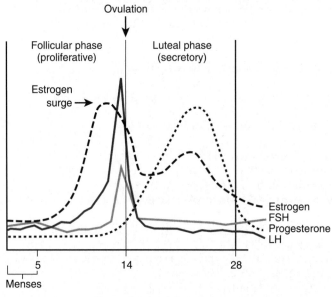

22.9: Menstrual cycle. Estrogen is most important in the proliferative phase and progesterone in the secretory phase of the cycle. Estrogen surge causes the luteinizing hormone (LH) surge, which initiates ovulation. Note the positive feedback of estrogen on LH is greater than follicle-stimulating hormone (FSH). *(From Brown TA: Rapid review physiology, Philadelphia, 2007, Mosby, p 99, Fig. 3.15.)*

  iv. Maternal estrogens cause growth of the fetal endometrium. The rapid decline of maternal hormones following delivery causes sloughing, resulting in the vaginal bleeding seen in some newborns.
 b. Proliferative phase
  i. Estrogen-induced growth (proliferation) of endometrial tissue.
  ii. Most variable phase of the menstrual cycle.
 c. Secretory phase
  i. Least variable phase of the menstrual cycle.
  ii. Primary hormone is progesterone (produced by the corpus luteum).
  iii. Prepares endometrium for possible implantation.
  iv. Glands become tortuous, begin to produce secretions.

> An endometrial biopsy on day 21 of the cycle can be useful in a fertility workup. The presence of secretory-type endometrium (e.g., subnuclear vacuoles) confirms that ovulation has occurred (Fig. 22.10).

D. Menopause
 1. Menopause is defined as a permanent cessation of menses.
  a. Determined retrospectively by the absence of menses (amenorrhea) for 12 months in the absence of a pathologic etiology.
 2. Average age of menopause is 51.3 years.
 3. Menopause before 40 years of age is called premature ovarian failure.
 4. Clinical manifestations
  a. Amenorrhea (>12 months).
  b. Hot flashes
   i. Episodic sudden sensation of heat, especially involving the upper chest and face, lasting 2–4 minutes; may be accompanied by sweating and feeling of anxiety.
   ii. Due to alterations in the hypothalamic thermoregulatory center associated with the withdrawal of estrogen.
  c. Vaginal dryness/irritation
   i. Low estrogen levels cause thinning of vaginal mucosa (vaginal atrophy) and reduced secretions (causing vaginal dryness and dyspareunia).
 5. Long-term effects of estrogen deficiency
  a. Osteoporosis (increased fracture risk).
  b. Cardiovascular effects (increased total and low-density lipoprotein cholesterol).
 6. Laboratory findings in menopause
  a. Decreased estrogen and progesterone levels.
  b. Increase in serum follicle-stimulating hormone (FSH) and serum LH.
   i. Elevated serum FSH is the best marker of menopause.

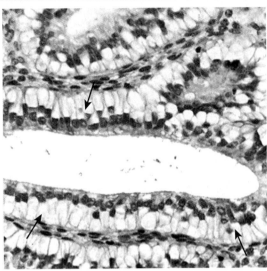

22.10: Subnuclear vacuoles (*arrows*) containing mucin push the nuclei of the endometrial cells toward the apex of the cell. Eventually, the mucin passes the nucleus and enters the lumen, marking the beginning of the secretory phase. *(From Kumar V, Fausto N, Abbas A: Robbins and Cotran pathologic basis of disease, ed 7, Philadelphia, 2004, Saunders, p 1081, Fig. 21.5B.)*

E. Hirsutism and virilization in females

1. Hirsutism refers to excessive terminal hair growth (course, dark hair) in androgen-sensitive regions (e.g., upper lip, chin, and upper abdomen).
2. Virilization refers to hirsutism plus other manifestations, such as clitoral enlargement and acne (see later).
   a. Both are secondary to elevated levels of androgens.
3. Sites of androgen production in the female include the ovary, adrenal glands, and peripheral tissues.
   a. Ovaries secrete 25% of circulating testosterone (dependent upon LH from the anterior pituitary).
   b. Adrenals secrete 25% of circulating testosterone (dependent upon adrenocorticotropic hormone from the anterior pituitary).
      i. Dehydroepiandrosterone-sulfate (DHEA-S) is an androgen entirely produced by the adrenal glands (can be used as a marker of adrenal androgen production).
   c. Peripheral tissues (adipose and skin)
      i. Weak androgens (androstenedione and DHEA) are converted to testosterone (accounting for 50% of testosterone in females).
      ii. Enzyme 5 alpha-reductase converts testosterone to dihydrotestosterone (DHT)—the most potent androgen.
4. Testosterone is largely bound, primarily to sex hormone-binding globulin (SHBG); changes in SHBG concentration will affect testosterone bioavailability.
   a. Elevated levels of SHBG (e.g., estrogen, pregnancy, and hyperthyroidism) cause more testosterone to be bound (decreasing testosterone effect).
   b. Decreased levels of SHBG (e.g., androgens, hypothyroidism, hyperinsulinemia, and obesity) cause more testosterone to be free (increasing testosterone effect).
5. Androgen excess (virilization) is characterized by hirsutism, acne, male pattern baldness, menstrual abnormalities (oligomenorrhea or amenorrhea), clitoromegaly, and deepening voice.
   a. Causes of hirsutism
      i. Polycystic ovary syndrome (PCOS)
         (1) Most common cause: ~75% of cases (see later).
      ii. Idiopathic hirsutism
         (1) Normal serum androgen concentrations, no menstrual irregularity.
      iii. Congenital adrenal hyperplasia
         (1) Most commonly due to 21-hydroxylase (P450c21) deficiency; causes an increase in adrenal androgens (e.g., androstenedione).
      iv. Androgen-secreting tumors of the ovary (e.g., Sertoli–Leydig cell tumor).
      v. Adrenal adenoma or carcinoma
         (1) May produce androgens as well as cortisol (may present with manifestations of Cushing syndrome).
      vi. Obesity and hypothyroidism
         (1) Both decrease SHBG thereby increasing testosterone bioavailability (more testosterone available to bind androgen receptors).

6. PCOS
   a. PCOS is a condition characterized by any two of the following:
      i. Decreased to absent ovulation.
      ii. Elevated serum androgens.
      iii. Polycystic ovaries on ultrasound.
   b. Etiology
      i. Altered gonadotropin-releasing hormone (GnRH) release causes a disproportionate increase in LH compared to FSH (LH > FSH).
      ii. LH stimulates ovaries to increase the production of androgens.
      iii. FSH regulates aromatase enzyme in ovarian granulosa cells. Those with PCOS have less FSH and therefore decreased aromatization of androgens into estrogen.
         (1) Increased intrafollicular androgen levels cause follicular atresia and the formation of subcortical cysts.
      iv. Elevated insulin (hyperinsulinism) is a common contributing factor.
         (1) Insulin not only enhances the ovarian production of androgens but also decreases the hepatic synthesis of SHBG. As levels of SHBG decline, more testosterone is unbound (i.e., free to bind to androgen receptors).
   c. Clinical manifestations
      i. Menstrual irregularities (oligomenorrhea or amenorrhea), hirsutism, and acne (usually beginning during puberty).
      ii. Patients commonly are obese with impaired glucose intolerance.
   d. Laboratory findings
      i. LH/FSH ratio > 3.
      ii. Increased "free" serum testosterone.

F. Heavy menstrual bleeding (formerly menorrhagia)
   1. Excessively heavy menstrual bleeding (>80 mL total); discussed further under abnormal uterine bleeding (AUB).

G. Premenstrual syndrome
   1. Definition
      a. Physical and/or behavioral symptoms that occur repetitively near the end of the menstrual cycle, resolving around the time of menses.
   2. Manifestations
      a. Abdominal bloating, breast tenderness, headaches, irritability, depression, and mood swings.
   3. Pathogenesis
      a. Etiology is unknown; likely involves interaction between changing hormone levels and central neurotransmission (e.g., serotonin).
   4. Diagnosis
      a. Clinical (i.e., the presence of the aforementioned clinical findings).
      b. No specific laboratory tests are required.

H. Dysmenorrhea
   1. Definition
      a. Painful menstruation (recurrent, crampy within the lower abdomen/pelvis).
   2. Primary versus secondary dysmenorrhea
      a. Primary dysmenorrhea
         i. Describes dysmenorrhea occurring in the absence of an underlying disease process that could explain the symptoms.
         ii. Usually occurs in adolescents and young women.
         iii. Prostaglandins (PGE_2 and $PGF_{2\alpha}$) from the endometrium stimulate uterine contractions. Uterine contractions cause intrauterine pressure to rise. Once intrauterine pressure exceeds arterial pressure, then uterine ischemia occurs, resulting in the accumulation of anaerobic metabolites that stimulate type C pain fibers.
      b. Secondary dysmenorrhea
         i. Similar clinical manifestations but due to an underlying pathologic condition (e.g., endometriosis, adenomyosis, or uterine leiomyoma).

I. Abnormal uterine bleeding (AUB)
   1. Definition
      a. Abnormalities in the menstrual cycle occurring outside of pregnancy. Includes variations in
         i. Frequency (normal menses occurs every 24–38 days).
         ii. Duration (normal menses lasts ≤8 days).
         iii. Volume (normal menstrual blood loss of <80 mL total).
   2. Etiologies (PALM-COEIN is a useful acronym)
         P: Polyp
         A: Adenomyosis
         L: Leiomyoma
         M: Malignancy and hyperplasia
         C: Coagulopathy

O: Ovulatory dysfunction: in the absence of ovulation, no corpus luteum forms and thus patients do not develop sufficient progestin to prevent endometrial breakdown (thereby causing irregular and heavy bleeding).

E: Endometrial disorders

I: Iatrogenic

N: Not otherwise classified

J. **Amenorrhea**

1. Definition

a. The absence of menses in a woman of reproductive age.

2. Primary amenorrhea

a. Absence of menses by 15 years of age in the presence of normal growth and secondary sexual characteristics (e.g., breast development and pubic hair) or by 13 years in the absence of secondary sexual characteristics.

b. Etiologies include

i. Turner syndrome.

ii. Müllerian agenesis (absence of vagina/uterus).

iii. "Constitutional delay" (family history of delayed menarche).

iv. Polycystic ovarian syndrome.

v. Weight loss/anorexia nervosa.

vi. Kallman syndrome (isolated GnRH deficiency plus anosmia).

vii. Imperforate hymen.

c. Workup of primary amenorrhea

i. Initial laboratories include β-human chorionic gonadotropin (hCG), prolactin, thyroid-stimulating hormone (TSH), LH, and FSH (Fig. 22.11).

3. Secondary amenorrhea

a. The absence of menses for >3 months in a patient who has had normal previous menstrual cycles (or >6 months in a patient with previously irregular menstrual cycles).

b. Etiologies

i. Pregnancy

(1) Most common cause; order pregnancy test (β-hCG).

ii. Thyroid disorders

(1) Order TSH.

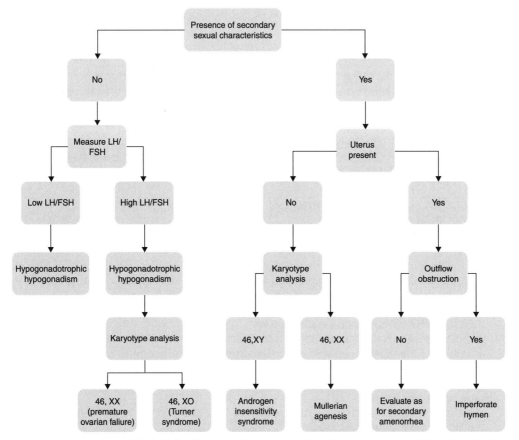

22.11: Workup of primary amenorrhea. *FSH,* Follicle-stimulating hormone; *LH,* luteinizing hormone; *TSH,* thyroid-stimulating hormone. *(From Klein DA, Poth MA: Amenorrhea: an approach to diagnosis and management, Am Fam Physician 87:781–788, 2013.)*

      iii. Hyperprolactinemia
        (1) Prolactin suppresses hypothalamic GnRH secretion.
        (2) ↑ Prolactin, ↓ GnRH, ↓ FSH/LH, ↓ estradiol.
        (3) Causes include drugs (e.g., antipsychotics) and prolactin-secreting pituitary tumor (order magnetic resonance imaging [MRI] of head).
      iv. Hypothalamic dysfunction
        (1) Decreased GnRH release → decreased LH/FSH.
        (2) Causes include anorexia nervosa, excessive exercise, and stress.
      v. Androgen excess (e.g., hirsutism and virilization)
        (1) Order androgen levels (e.g., free testosterone).
        (2) Perform ultrasound of ovaries (probable polycystic ovarian syndrome).
      vi. Ovarian disorder
        (1) Hypergonadotropic hypogonadism (↑ FSH, ↑ LH, and low estradiol).
        (2) Causes include premature ovarian failure (e.g., Turner syndrome, autoimmune destruction ovaries, and chemo/radiation).
      vii. End-organ (target organ) defect
        (1) Any defect that prevents the normal egress of blood (e.g., imperforate hymen) would cause primary amenorrhea.
        (2) History of uterine instrumentation (in conjunction with normal laboratory testing) suggests Asherman syndrome (intrauterine adhesions secondary to trauma; usually following repeated endometrial curettage).
   c. Workup of secondary amenorrhea
      i. Initial laboratories include β-hCG, prolactin, TSH, LH, and FSH (Fig. 22.12).

VI. Uterine Disorders

A. Uterine prolapse
1. Descent of the uterus into the vagina; due to the relaxation of support structures.
2. Usually asymptomatic; may have a feeling of pressure or vaginal "bulge."
3. Symptoms commonly worsen with standing, heavy lifting, or straining.
4. In some cases, the uterus prolapses through the vaginal introitus (called uterine procidentia).
5. Predisposing conditions include multiparity (stretching and tearing of tissues during childbirth) and increased intra-abdominal pressure (e.g., obesity and straining).

B. Endometritis
1. Infection of the endometrium; usually pregnancy-related (follows childbirth or abortion).
2. Acute endometritis
   a. Acute inflammation of the endometrium, most commonly secondary to bacterial infection following childbirth (vaginal or cesarean).
      i. More likely following prolonged labor and/or prolonged rupture of membranes.
      ii. Manifestations include fever, abdominal pain, uterine tenderness, and purulent vaginal discharge.

Chronic endometritis

- Chronic inflammation of the endometrium (plasma cells are the key microscopic finding).
- Etiologies include retained placental tissue, use of an intrauterine device; the latter is classically associated with *Actinomyces israelii* (see yellow granular material called "sulfur granules").

C. Adenomyosis
1. Defined as the presence of endometrial tissue (glands and stroma) within the myometrium.
2. Common, usually in mid to late 40s.
3. May cause enlargement of the uterus (Fig. 22.13A), AUB, and/or dysmenorrhea.

D. Endometriosis
1. Defined as the presence of endometrial tissue (glands and stroma) outside the confines of the uterus.
2. Common condition affecting ~10% of reproductive-aged women. Peak prevalence in those 25–30 years of age.
3. Pathogenesis is unclear, favored theories include:
   a. Retrograde menstruation theory
      i. Believed to be the most common mechanism.
      ii. Refers to the retrograde flow of endometrial tissue through the fallopian tubes followed by the implantation of viable endometrial cells in various locations throughout the peritoneum.
   b. Vascular or lymphatic spread theory
      i. Explains the presence of endometrial implants in areas outside the abdomen and pelvis.
   c. Coelomic metaplasia theory
      i. Believed that some endometriosis may be derived from pluripotent stem cells within the peritoneum that transform into endometrial tissue.

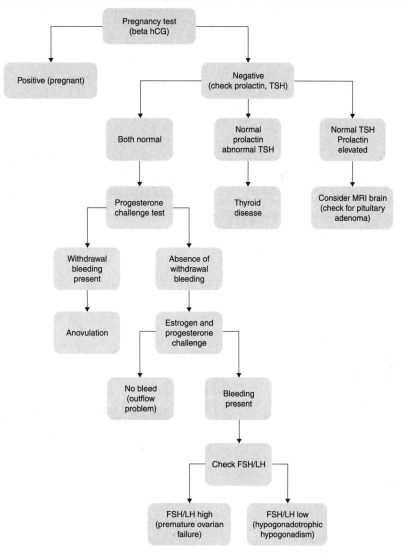

22.12: Workup of secondary amenorrhea. *DHEA-S*, Dehydroepiandrosterone-sulfate; *FSH*, follicle-stimulating hormone; *LH*, luteinizing hormone; *MRI*, magnetic resonance imaging; *TSH*, thyroid-stimulating hormone. *(From Klein DA, Poth MA: Amenorrhea: an approach to diagnosis and management. Am Fam Physician 87:781–788, 2013.)*

4. Common sites of endometriosis
   a. Ovaries (the most common site)
   b. Uterine ligaments
   c. Cul-de-sac (pouch of Douglas)
      i. Region anterior to the rectum and posterior to the uterus.
      ii. Most dependent portion of the female pelvis (may be palpated on digital rectal examination).
      iii. Common site for blood (e.g., following ruptured tubal pregnancy), malignant cells (e.g., seeding by ovarian cancer), endometriosis, and pus (e.g., PID).
   d. Fallopian tubes
   e. Intestines
5. Clinical manifestations
   a. Pain
      i. May be chronic or occur only during menses (dysmenorrhea).
      ii. Painful intercourse (dyspareunia).
      iii. Painful bowel movements (due to stretching of endometrial implants on the rectal serosa).
   b. Increased risk for ectopic pregnancy
      i. Due to scarring of fallopian tubes by endometrial implants.
   c. Increased risk of infertility
      i. Due to distortion of tubal and ovarian architecture (e.g., implants of endometriosis on ovaries causing blood-filled cysts).

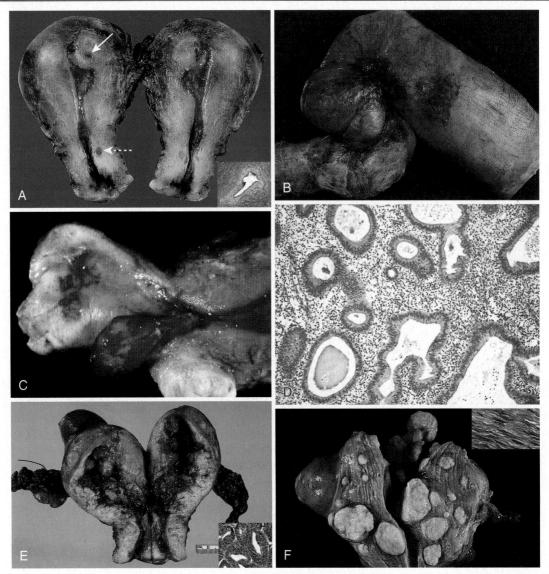

22.13: (A) Adenomyosis. The solid arrow shows an area of hemorrhage surrounded by irregularly thickened endometrial stroma. The interrupted arrow shows a Nabothian cyst in the endocervical canal. The microscopic section shows an endometrial gland and stroma in the myometrium. (B) Endometriosis implants on a loop of intestine. Note that the serosal surface has multiple areas of hemorrhage with a "powder burn" appearance. (C) Endometrial polyp. (D) Simple hyperplasia of endometrial glands showing cystic dilation and focal areas of glandular outpouching. (E) Endometrial carcinoma showing necrotic tumor filling the uterine cavity and extending through the uterine wall and into the endocervical canal. Snippet in right lower quadrant is a well-differentiated adenocarcinoma with crowding of the glands and hyperchromatic nuclei. (F) Leiomyomas. In sagittal section, multiple well-circumscribed, gray-white nodules (leiomyomas) are dispersed throughout the myometrium. Submucosal leiomyomas are a common cause of uterine bleeding. Snippet in the right upper corner shows elongated spindle-shaped smooth muscle cells. *(A and E, From Rosai J, Ackerman LV: Surgical pathology, ed 9, St. Louis, 2004, Mosby, pp 1578, 1586, respectively, Figs. 19.123, 19.136B, respectively. Snippet in corner of (A and E) from Rosai J, Ackerman LV: Surgical pathology, ed 10, St. Louis, 2011, Mosby, p 1485, Fig. 19.124, 137A, respectively; B and F, from Ivan Damjanov, MD, PhD, Linder J: Pathology: a color atlas, St. Louis, 2000, Mosby, pp 126, 277, respectively, Figs. 7.77, 13.49.)*

    6. Diagnosis
       a. Laparoscopy (implants have a "powder burn" appearance, see Fig. 22.13B).
E. Endometrial polyp
    1. Defined as an overgrowth of benign endometrial tissue.
    2. Appears as a polypoid mass arising from the surface of the endometrium, may range up to a few centimeter in diameter (Fig. 22.13C).
    3. Often asymptomatic, may cause AUB or protrude through the cervical os into the vagina.
    4. Diagnosis: vaginal ultrasound and hysteroscopy.
F. Endometrial hyperplasia
    1. Definition
       a. Overgrowth of endometrial glands (of variable size and shape) resulting in an increased gland-to-stroma ratio.

2. Classification system (World Health Organization)
   a. Hyperplasia without atypia.
      i. Overgrowth of endometrial tissue with normal appearing glandular epithelial cells.
   b. Atypical hyperplasia
      i. Overgrowth of endometrial tissue with glands that exhibit cytologic and nuclear atypia, increased mitotic activity.
      ii. Increased risk of malignant transformation.
3. Pathogenesis
   a. Continuous exposure of the endometrium to unopposed estrogen (without progestin).
4. Risk factors
   a. Obesity
      i. Aromatase enzyme in adipose tissue converts androgens into estrogens (androstenedione to estrone; testosterone to estradiol).
   b. Ovulatory dysfunction
      i. Without ovulation, there is no corpus luteum and therefore insufficient progesterone (causing a lack of endometrial breakdown).
   c. Unopposed exogenous estrogen therapy.
   d. Lynch syndrome (hereditary nonpolyposis colorectal cancer).
5. Clinical manifestations
   a. AUB, typically in a perimenopausal or postmenopausal patient.
6. Diagnosis
   a. Endometrial biopsy (Fig. 22.13D).

G. **Endometrial carcinoma**
1. Definition
   a. Malignancy of the endometrium; most commonly arising from the glandular epithelium (i.e., adenocarcinoma).
2. Epidemiology
   a. Most common gynecologic cancer in the United States (ovarian cancer is the second most common).
   b. Second most common gynecologic malignancy leading to death (behind ovarian).
   c. Median age at presentation: 60 years.
3. Pathogenesis
   a. Prolonged estrogen stimulation (same as for endometrial hyperplasia).
4. Cancer characteristics
   a. Endometrial carcinoma invades into the myometrium and the cervix (Fig. 22.13E).
   b. Metastasis to regional lymph nodes and elsewhere (e.g., lungs).
5. Clinical manifestations
   a. Vaginal bleeding (often postmenopausal).
6. Diagnosis
   a. Endometrial biopsy.

H. **Uterine leiomyoma (fibroids)**
1. Definition
   a. Benign tumor of smooth muscle.
2. Epidemiology
   a. Most common pelvic tumor in women.
   b. Blacks > Whites.
3. Pathogenesis
   a. Leiomyomas are derived from a progenitor myocyte, sensitive to estrogen and progesterone stimulation (progesterone is believed to be the most important factor).
      i. Estrogen functions to upregulate and maintain progesterone receptors (PRs).
   b. Common for a leiomyoma to outgrow its blood supply resulting in degenerative changes (e.g., calcification and hemorrhage).
4. Clinical manifestations
   a. May be single or multiple (Fig. 22.13F).
   b. May arise throughout the myometrium (i.e., submucosal, intramural, and/or subserosal).
   c. Submucosal leiomyomas may ulcerate and bleed, possibly interfere with implantation.
   d. Larger leiomyomata may cause compressive manifestations.
      i. Increased urinary frequency, urgency, and incontinence (compression of bladder).
      ii. Constipation (compression of rectum).
   e. No risk of malignant transformation (i.e., do not transform into leiomyosarcoma).
5. Diagnosis
   a. Ultrasound.

I. **Uterine leiomyosarcoma**
1. Definition
   a. Malignant tumor of smooth muscle.
      i. Recall that sarcomas are malignancies of mesenchymal tissue (derived from the mesoderm).
      ii. Arise de nova (not from leiomyoma).

2. Epidemiology
   a. Uncommon
3. Pathology
   a. Increased cellularity, mitoses (often abnormal), and necrosis.
      i.   Key findings that differentiate them from leiomyoma.
   b. Frequently contain inactivating mutations in tumor protein p53 (*TP53*) and retinoblastoma gene (*RB1*).*RB1*
   c. Aggressive; poor prognosis.
4. Clinical manifestations
   a. AUB, abdominal pain, and distention.

J. Carcinosarcoma
1. Carcinosarcomas are tumors comprised of both malignant glandular tissue (i.e., adenocarcinoma) and malignant stromal tissue (i.e., sarcoma).
2. Rare, primarily postmenopausal. Strong association with previous irradiation; poor prognosis.

VII. Fallopian Tube Disorders
A. Hydatid cysts of Morgagni
1. Benign cystic Müllerian remnants most often located near the fimbriated end of the fallopian tube.
2. Typically, an incidental finding on pathologic specimens.
B. Pelvic inflammatory disease (PID)
1. Definition
   a. Acute infection of the upper genital tract (i.e., uterus, fallopian tubes, and ovaries) and surrounding peritoneum causing inflammation of affected structures (e.g., endometritis, salpingitis, oophoritis, and peritonitis).
   b. Usually begins during or immediately following menstruation.
2. Pathogenesis
   a. Typically begins as a sexually transmitted infection followed by ascension of the organism from the vagina/cervix into the upper genital tract.
   b. Unclear why some infections ascend into the upper genital tract (possibly related to heavy bacterial load, decreased viscosity of cervical mucus, and impaired host immune response).
3. Risk factors
   a. Sexual activity
      i.   Nearly all cases begin as a sexually transmitted infection.
      ii.   Those with multiple sexual partners and/or high-risk sexual partners (i.e., a partner with known sexually transmitted infection) are at an increased risk.
      iii. Most common in those 15–25 years of age.
4. Etiologic agents
   a. PID is usually polymicrobial; common agents include *N. gonorrhoeae* and *C. trachomatis*.
5. Pathology
   a. During acute infection, the fallopian tubes fill with pus. Then, following the resolution of the infection, the pus is resorbed leaving behind clear fluid and distention of the fallopian tube ("hydrosalpinx").
   b. Perihepatitis (inflammation of the liver capsule, commonly known as the Fitz–Hugh Curtis syndrome); presents with the right upper quadrant pain/tenderness.
   c. Tubo-ovarian abscess (inflammatory mass involving the fallopian tube and ovary).

Clinical manifestations of pelvic inflammatory disease

- Lower abdominal pain with vaginal discharge (usually purulent).
- Cervical motion and adnexal tenderness on pelvic examination.
- Advanced cases may exhibit rebound tenderness, fever, and diminished bowel sounds.
- Increased risk of ectopic pregnancy and infertility due to scarring of the fallopian tube.

6. Diagnosis is based on clinical findings, including:
   a. Examination (cervical motion and adnexal tenderness, purulent vaginal discharge).
   b. Increased white cells in vaginal discharge.
   c. Documentation of cervical infection (e.g., *N. gonorrhoeae* and *C. trachomatis*) by NAAT.
C. Ectopic pregnancy
1. Definition
   a. Implantation of the fertilized ovum outside the endometrial lining of the uterus; the most common site is within the fallopian tube.
2. Pathogenesis
   a. Scarring of a tube (e.g., previous episode of PID, endometriosis or previous tubal ligation).
3. Clinical manifestations
   a. First-trimester vaginal bleeding and/or abdominal pain.

4. Diagnosis
  a. Confirm pregnancy (serum hCG).
     i. Serum, not urine (more sensitive; hCG can be detected in the serum as early as 21 days after the first day of the last menstrual period).
  b. Transvaginal ultrasound.
5. Complications of ectopic pregnancy
  a. Rupture of the fallopian tube with intra-abdominal hemorrhage
     i. Risk of hypovolemic shock (the most common cause of maternal death in early pregnancy).
  b. Hematosalpinx
     i. Blood in the fallopian tube; if present, most likely due to ectopic pregnancy.

VIII. **Ovarian Disorders**
  A. **Overview**
    1. Patient's age and menstrual status are important considerations when evaluating adnexal structures (e.g., ovaries and fallopian tubes).
    2. If a patient is having regular menstrual cycles, then any adnexal abnormality is likely benign (e.g., follicular cyst).
    3. In general, malignancy is more likely as the patient ages.
  B. **Follicular cyst**
    1. Nonneoplastic benign fluid accumulation within a follicle.
    2. Most regress spontaneously, however, rupture may cause sterile peritonitis with pain.
  C. **Corpus luteum cyst**
    1. Hemorrhage into corpus luteum following ovulation (benign and nonneoplastic).
    2. Most common ovarian mass in pregnancy.
    3. Most regress spontaneously.
  D. **Oophoritis**
    1. Definition: inflammation of one or both ovaries.
    2. Etiologies include mumps infection and PID.
  E. **Ovarian torsion**
    1. Definition
      a. Rotation of the adnexa on its fibrovascular pedicle with compromise of blood flow, potentially causing infarction of the tube and/or ovary.
    2. Epidemiology
      a. Torsion in an infant or child is usually associated with an otherwise normal ovary.
      b. In adults, torsion is more likely to be secondary to an underlying ovarian cyst or tumor.
    3. Clinical presentation
      a. Acute abdominal pain (may mimic acute appendicitis).
      b. Nausea and vomiting.
      c. Palpable pelvic mass.
    4. Pathology
      a. Enlarged, dark red with bloody fluid seen on sectioning of the gross specimen.
      b. Necrosis and hemorrhage on histologic examination.
  F. **Ovarian tumors**
    1. Overview
      a. Ovarian neoplasms may originate from the surface (Müllerian) epithelium, germ cells, or sex cord-stromal cells (Fig. 22.14).
      b. Most (~80%) ovarian tumors are benign, especially in younger patients (<45 years of age).
      c. Risk of malignancy increases with age; most ovarian malignancies occur in women >45 years of age.

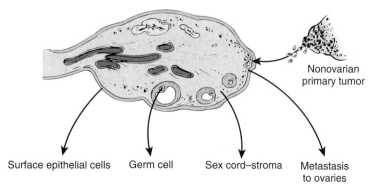

22.14: Schematic showing the derivation of primary ovarian tumors. *(From Kumar V, Abbas AK, Fausto N, Mitchell RN: Robbins basic pathology, ed 8, Philadelphia, 2007, Saunders Elsevier, p 729, Fig. 19.16.)*

2. Risk factors
   a. Inherited genetic predisposition
      i. *BRCA1* and *BRCA2* gene mutations interfere with DNA repair mechanisms. Risk of ovarian cancer is particularly high with a *BRCA1* mutation (~40%–50%).
   b. Nulliparity, early menarche, and late menopause
      i. Each associated with longer periods of repetitive ovulation and therefore repeated episodes in which there is disruption of the ovarian surface (increased risk of developing ovarian carcinoma arising from the surface epithelium).
      ii. Conversely, long periods of anovulation (e.g., use of oral contraceptives or breastfeeding) decreases one's risk.
3. Surface-derived (epithelial) ovarian tumors
   a. Comprise 70% of ovarian neoplasms (most now believed to originate within fallopian tube fimbria); usually arise in mid to late adulthood.
      i. Serous tumors (benign, borderline, and malignant).
      ii. Mucinous tumors (benign, borderline, and malignant).
   b. Detachment of cells from an epithelial ovarian carcinoma may "seed" the peritoneal cavity (peritoneal carcinomatosis).
4. Germ cell tumors
   a. Comprise ~15% of ovarian tumors; usually arise in the late teens to early 20s.
   b. Derive from primitive germ cells of the embryonic gonad.
   c. Mature teratoma (benign)—the most common germ cell tumor.
   d. Dysgerminoma is the most common malignant germ cell tumor (analogous to seminoma in the male).
5. Sex cord-stromal tumors (SCST)
   a. Comprise ~10% of all ovarian tumors, most are benign.
   b. Develop from the sex cord (e.g., Sertoli cell tumor and granulosa cell tumor), stromal cells (e.g., fibroma, thecoma, and Leydig cell tumor), or both (e.g., Sertoli–Leydig cell tumor).
   c. Fibroma is the most common benign SCST.
      i. Meig's syndrome refers to the presence of an ovarian fibroma, ascites, and/or pleural effusion. Removal of the tumor results in the resolution of the ascites and pleural effusion.
   d. Granulosa cell tumor is the most common potentially malignant SCST.
   e. Some produce hormones (e.g., estrogen from granulosa cell tumors and androgen from Sertoli–Leydig tumors).
   f. Sex cord tumor with annular tubules is a rare SCST, commonly associated with Peutz–Jeghers syndrome.
6. Metastasis to the ovaries
   a. Primary sites include uterus, fallopian tubes, contralateral ovary, breast, and gastrointestinal tract (e.g., colon and stomach).
      i. Krukenberg tumor (signet ring cell tumor metastatic to the ovary) usually arises in the stomach (diffuse gastric carcinoma) or the breast.
7. Clinical manifestations
   a. Abdominal enlargement (the most common sign), commonly due to ascites.
   b. Induration of the rectal pouch (palpated on the digital rectal examination).
   c. Palpable ovarian mass in a postmenopausal woman (ovaries not normally palpable in postmenopausal women due to atrophy).
   d. Malignant pleural effusion (pleural cavity is a common site for ovarian cancer metastasis, may cause shortness of breath).
   e. Signs of excess estrogen (granulosa cell tumor secretes estrogen).
      i. Vaginal bleeding (secondary to estrogen-induced endometrial hyperplasia or cancer).
      ii. Hundred percent superficial squamous cells in a cervical Pap smear.
   f. Signs of androgen excess (e.g., hirsutism, virilization) from Sertoli–Leydig cell tumors.
8. Tumor markers
   a. Cancer antigen (CA) 125 is often elevated in those with a nonmucinous epithelial ovarian carcinoma (e.g., serous carcinoma).
      i. Most useful for monitoring women following treatment.
      ii. Low sensitivity and specificity preclude its use as a screening test of ovarian cancer.

IX. **Gestational Disorders**
   A. **Placental anatomy**
      1. Fetal surface
         a. Meconium-staining of the placenta is often a sign of fetal distress.
            i. Meconium is a sterile, thick, black-green, material from the fetal intestine (consists of desquamated cells, mucin, amniotic fluid (AF), and intestinal secretions).
         b. Meconium aspiration syndrome
            i. Rare complication in which the newborn aspirates meconium into the airways during his/her initial breaths.
            ii. Obstructs airway and causes a chemical pneumonitis (inflammation of lungs).

2. Maternal surface
   a. Chorionic villi are lined by trophoblastic tissue.
   b. Outer layer of chorionic villi composed of syncytiotrophoblast.
      i. Syncytiotrophoblasts synthesize hCG and human placental lactogen (hPL).
      ii. Amount of hPL directly correlates with the placental mass and has antiinsulin activity (similar to human growth hormone).
      iii. Inside layer of the chorionic villi is composed of cytotrophoblast.
      iv. Vessels within chorionic villi coalesce to form the umbilical vein (containing oxygenated fetal blood).
   c. Umbilical cord
      i. Contains one umbilical vein and two umbilical arteries.
      ii. Unlike most veins, the umbilical vein contains highly oxygenated blood.
      iii. Single umbilical artery is sometimes associated with congenital anomalies.

B. Placental infections
1. Most are ascending bacterial infections from the vagina.
   a. Group B streptococcus (*Streptococcus agalactiae*) is a common pathogen in the vagina.
   b. Complications include premature rupture of membranes.
2. Chorioamnionitis
   a. Definition
      i. Infection of the fetal membranes (amnion and chorion).
      ii. Associated with an increased risk of neonatal sepsis and meningitis.
3. Transmission of infection from mother to fetus (vertical transmission).
   a. Occurs during intrauterine life (prenatal) or as the baby passes through the birth canal (perinatal).
   b. Pathogens include cytomegalovirus, toxoplasmosis, HIV, rubella, syphilis, and others.

C. Placenta previa
1. Definition
   a. Implantation of the placenta over the internal cervical os (opening of the cervix).
2. Risk factors
      i. Previous cesarean section.
      ii. Previous placenta previa (recurs in 4%–8% of subsequent pregnancies).
      iii. Multiple gestations.
3. Clinical findings
   a. Painless vaginal bleeding, beginning in the second trimester.
      i. Can be life-threatening to the mother.
      ii. May necessitate preterm delivery with associated neonatal complications.
   b. Precludes vaginal delivery (i.e., must deliver infant by cesarean section).
4. Diagnosis
   a. Transabdominal ultrasound (identifies placental location over the cervical os).
   b. Digital vaginal examination is contraindicated due to the risk of vaginal hemorrhage.

D. Placental abruption (abruptio placentae)
1. Definition
   a. Partial or complete detachment of the placenta prior to delivery of the fetus.
2. Pathogenesis
   a. Ruptured maternal vessels in the decidua basalis → accumulation of blood between the placenta and uterine wall (i.e., retroplacental) → placenta separates from the uterus.
3. Clinical findings
   a. Abrupt onset of vaginal bleeding, abdominal and/or back pain, and uterine tenderness.
      i. Maternal bleeding may be life-threatening.
      ii. Disseminated intravascular coagulation (DIC) is a potential complication.
   b. Fetal distress
      i. Evidenced by nonreassuring fetal heart rate pattern.
      ii. Lack of oxygen delivery to the fetus increases the risk of intrauterine fetal demise.
      iii. Requires delivery of the infant (if preterm, associated with risk of respiratory distress syndrome).
4. Risk factors for abruption
   a. Previous abruption (a major factor)
   b. Maternal hypertension
   c. Smoking
   d. Cocaine use
   e. Abdominal trauma
5. Diagnosis
   a. Ultrasound (to identify the retroplacental hematoma).

E. **Placenta accrete spectrum (accreta, increta, and percreta)**
  1. Defined as an abnormal trophoblast invasion into the myometrium.
     a. Placenta accreta refers to the attachment of placental villi to the myometrium (rather than decidua).
     b. Placenta increta refers to the penetration of the villi into the myometrium.
     c. Placenta percreta refers to the penetration of chorionic villi through the myometrium to the uterine serosa.
  2. Potential for life-threatening hemorrhage after delivery.
     a. Due to failure of the placental tissue to separate from the myometrium; may necessitate hysterectomy.
  3. Major risk factor is placenta previa in a patient with a previous cesarean section.

F. **Velamentous cord insertion**
  1. Defined as insertion of the umbilical vessels into the placental membranes away from the placental surface.
     a. Lack of the protective substance of the cord (called "Wharton Jelly") around the vessels makes them susceptible to rupture or compression.
  2. Diagnosed by ultrasound.
  3. May require cesarean delivery to prevent a tear or compression of the vessels during vaginal delivery.

G. **Marginal cord insertion (battledore placenta)**
  1. The umbilical cord normally inserts at or near the center of the placenta.
  2. Insertion of the cord at the margin of the placenta is associated with a small increased risk of adverse outcome (less risk than with velamentous cord insertion).

H. **Succenturiate placenta**
  1. Defined as a placenta in which one or more lobes are separate from the main placental disk.
  2. Extra lobe functions normally; however, there is a potential for hemorrhage or postpartum infection if the extra lobe is retained within the uterus (i.e., it is important to confirm completeness of placental delivery).

I. **Placentomegaly**
  1. Defined as an abnormally large placenta (weight >90% percentile).
  2. Commonly seen in infants of diabetic mothers (due to associated fetal hyperinsulinemia).

J. **Twin placentation (Fig. 22.15)**
  1. Monozygotic ("identical") twins are due to fertilization of a single ovum by a single sperm with subsequent division of the zygote.
     a. Timing of egg division determines placentation.
  2. Monozygotic twins may have two separate placentas (dichorionic/diamniotic) or one placenta (usually monochorionic/diamniotic but rarely monochorionic/monoamniotic).
     a. Fetal-to-fetal transfusion can occur in either type.
  3. Monochorionic diamniotic placenta
     a. Twins share placenta (i.e., blood supply) but have separate amniotic sacs.
  4. Monochorionic monoamniotic placenta
     a. Placentation in which there is a single placenta and a single amniotic sac.
        i. Associated with risk of cord entanglement.
        ii. Type seen in conjoined twins.
  5. Dizygotic ("fraternal") twins is due to fertilization of two oocytes by two sperm.
     a. Results in dichorionic/diamniotic placentation (two separate placentas).
     b. Placentas can be fused (40%) or separate (60%).

K. **Preeclampsia and eclampsia (toxemia of pregnancy)**
  1. Preeclampsia is the new onset of hypertension and proteinuria or the new onset of hypertension and significant end-organ dysfunction (e.g., altered mental status, headache, and visual changes) near the end of pregnancy.

		Identical	Fraternal
A	Monochorionic monoamniotic	X	
B	Monochorionic diamniotic	X	
C	Dichorionic diamniotic (fused)	X	X
D	Dichorionic diamniotic (separate)	X	X

22.15: Twin placentas. See text for description. (*Redrawn from Goljan EF: Star series: pathology, Philadelphia, 1998, Saunders, Fig. 18.2.*)

    2. Risk factors for preeclampsia
       a. Nulliparity.
       b. History of preeclampsia in the previous pregnancy.
       c. Obesity.
       d. Advanced maternal age (>35 years).
       e. Multiple gestations.
    3. Pathogenesis of preeclampsia
       a. Shallow placentation and failure of spiral artery remodeling with inadequate uteroplacental blood flow → oxidative stress and inadequate oxygenation of the placenta.
       b. In response, the placenta releases various injurious factors into the maternal circulation causing widespread endothelial injury and dysfunction.
       c. The net result is hypertension, proteinuria, etc.
    4. Clinical manifestations of preeclampsia
       a. Hypertension ($\geq 140/\geq 90$ mm Hg).
       b. Proteinuria (>300 mg/day)
         i. Note that urinary protein excretion is normally higher in pregnancy compared to healthy nonpregnant individuals in whom the upper limit of daily protein excretion is 150 mg.
       c. Any of the following indicates more severe disease:
         i. Persistent and/or severe headache, altered mental status, visual abnormalities (e.g., blurred vision and photophobia), and upper abdominal pain.
    5. Complications
       a. Maternal complications include cerebral hemorrhage, stroke, hepatic rupture, renal failure, pulmonary edema, seizure, and placental abruption.
       b. Eclampsia (new onset, generalized, tonic-clonic seizures in a patient with preeclampsia).
       c. Increased risk of fetal death.
    6. Treatment
       a. Delivery of the baby.

L. HELLP syndrome
    1. HELLP is an acronym (hemolysis, elevated liver enzymes, and a low platelet count).
    2. Thought to represent a severe form of preeclampsia (pathogenesis is similar).
       a. Compared to the usual presentation of preeclampsia, however, there is a more pronounced activation of coagulation and hepatic inflammation (reason unknown).
    3. Clinical presentation
       a. Abdominal pain (most common), nausea, vomiting, and malaise.
    4. Maternal complications include:
       a. Acute renal failure, DIC, bleeding, hepatic hemorrhage, and/or rupture.
    5. Laboratory findings
       a. Thrombocytopenia.
       b. Schistocytes, elevated bilirubin, decreased haptoglobin (findings of intravascular hemolysis).
       c. Elevated aminotransferase enzymes (indicative of hepatic inflammation).
         i. ↑ Aspartate aminotransferase.
         ii. ↑ Alanine aminotransferase.

M. Gestational trophoblastic disease (GTD)
    1. Group of related conditions characterized by abnormal proliferation of trophoblastic cells (cells that form the placenta).
    2. Hydatidiform mole (i.e., molar pregnancy)
       a. Most common form of GTD.
       b. Described as complete, partial, or invasive based on the karyotype, gross, and histologic appearance.
       c. Complete mole
         i. Diploid karyotype
           (1) 46, XX (90%) due to the fertilization of an "empty" ovum lacking maternal chromosomes by a haploid sperm that then duplicates.
           (2) 46, XY (10%) due to the fertilization of an "empty" ovum by two sperm.
         ii. Absence of fetal tissue; all villi are edematous and exhibit hyperplasia of the trophoblasts.
         iii. Manifestations include:
           (1) Vaginal bleeding and pelvic pain/pressure.
           (2) Excessive uterine enlargement for gestational age.
           (3) hCG levels higher than expected for gestational age.
           (4) Hyperemesis gravidarum (excessive vomiting).
         iv. Ultrasound shows "snowstorm pattern."

d. Partial mole
  i. Triploid karyotype (69XXX, 69XXY, or 69XYY); usually due to fertilization of the ovum by two sperm.
  ii. Mixture of normal and abnormal villi (some of the villi are edematous with trophoblastic hyperplasia); the presence of fetal tissue.
  iii. Usually presents as a spontaneous abortion (i.e., vaginal bleeding and the absence of fetal heart tones).
e. Invasive mole
  i. Hydatidiform mole with abnormally enlarged and hydropic villi invading into the myometrium.

N. **Gestational trophoblastic neoplasia (GTN)**
1. Group of malignant neoplasms of trophoblastic tissue.
2. May arise in either a molar (hydatidiform mole) or a nonmolar pregnancy.
3. Invasive mole that does not resolve spontaneously is also considered a type of GTN.
4. Choriocarcinoma
  a. Highly malignant and aggressive tumor of malignant trophoblasts.
  b. Risk of invasion into myometrium and vascular spaces.
  c. Widespread hematogenous metastasis to the lungs (most common), vagina, central nervous system, and liver.

X. **Amniotic Fluid**
A. **Overview**
1. Liquid that surrounds the fetus during gestation.
2. Produced by the fetus (fetal urine and lung secretions) and removed by fetal swallowing.
3. Variety of physiologic functions necessary for normal growth and development of the fetus.
  a. Protection of the fetus from trauma and infection.
  b. Prevents cord compression.
  c. Provides space and growth factors for fetal lung maturation.
B. **Polyhydramnios**
1. Refers to an excessive amount of AF in the amniotic sac.
2. Pathogenesis is primarily one of two mechanisms:
  a. Decreased fetal swallowing (e.g., anencephaly; esophageal or duodenal atresia).
  b. Increased fetal urine production (e.g., maternal diabetes → fetal hyperglycemia → polyuria).
3. May be associated with preterm birth and fetal anomalies (as noted above).
C. **Oligohydramnios**
1. Refers to an AF volume that is less than expected for gestational age.
2. Pathogenesis
  a. Decreased fetal urine formation (e.g., uteroplacental insufficiency or renal anomalies).
  b. Fluid loss (preterm rupture of membranes).
3. Complications include:
  a. Compression of umbilical cord with subsequent reduction in fetal perfusion.
  b. Severe oligohydramnios can cause compression of the fetus, resulting in limb and facial deformities, pulmonary hypoplasia (Potter sequence).

XI. **Prenatal Screening (Quadruple Test)**
A. **Used for the prenatal diagnosis of a disease.**
B. **Usually performed in the early second trimester.**
C. **Maternal serum concentrations of the following are measured (α-fetoprotein, unconjugated estriol, total or free beta subunit of hCG, and inhibin A).**
D. **Interpretation (Table 22.1).**

XII. **Breast Disorders**
A. **Lymph nodes**
1. Outer quadrant of the breast (the site of most breast tissue and thus most common location of breast cancer) drains to the axillary lymph nodes.
2. Cancers from the inner quadrants drain to the internal mammary nodes.
B. **Nipple discharge**
1. Galactorrhea
  a. Nipple discharge unrelated to pregnancy or breastfeeding.
  b. Usually secondary to elevated prolactin.

TABLE 22.1 Interpretation of Prenatal Screening

DIAGNOSIS	AFP	hCG	Estriol	Inhibin A
Trisomy 18	↓	↓	↓	Normal
Trisomy 21	↓	↑	↓	↑
Neural tube defect	↑	Normal	Normal	Normal

AFP, α-Fetoprotein; *hCG*, human chorionic gonadotropin.

    c. Causes of hyperprolactinemia include:
       i.   Prolactin-secreting pituitary adenoma (prolactinoma).
      ii.   Drugs (e.g., antipsychotics)
          (1) Recall that dopamine from the hypothalamus suppresses the release of prolactin from the pituitary. Blockage of the dopamine receptor by medications will therefore increase prolactin release.
     iii.   Renal failure → decreased clearance of prolactin.
  2. Bloody nipple discharge
    a. Concerning for ductal cancer (especially in women older than 40 years).
    b. Intraductal papilloma (benign) most likely in younger women.
  3. Purulent nipple discharge
    a. Indicative of mastitis (e.g., *Staphylococcus aureus*).

C. Nonproliferative benign breast lesions
  1. Fibrocystic change
    a. Very common (affects ~50% of women) condition of premenopausal women in which there is a variable amount of stromal fibrosis and cystic change within the breast.
    b. Cysts are due to dilated lobules, may vary in size during the menstrual cycle, and often contain hemorrhagic fluid ("blue-dome cysts").
    c. Clinically recognizable as a diffuse nodularity ("lumpy bumpy"); no well-defined mass and breast pain (that also may vary during the menstrual cycle).
    d. No increased risk of breast cancer.
  2. Fat necrosis
    a. Necrosis of adipose tissue, secondary to trauma or surgery.
    b. May form a palpable mass (thus raising concern for malignancy).
    c. Histology reveals necrotic fat, lipid-laden macrophages, and foreign body giant cells.
    d. No increased risk of cancer.

D. Proliferative breast changes
  1. Usual ductal hyperplasia
    a. Usually, an incidental finding in a biopsy obtained for some other reason.
    b. Characterized by an increased number of cytologically benign cells within the ductal space.
    c. No treatment necessary, small increased risk of cancer.
  2. Atypical ductal hyperplasia
    a. Microcalcification on mammography is a common finding.
    b. Characterized by proliferation of atypical-appearing ductal epithelial cells.
    c. Associated with an increased risk of breast cancer.
    d. Requires excisional breast biopsy to exclude malignancy.

XIII. Breast Tumors

Fibroadenoma

- Most common benign tumor in the breast (usually arise between 15 and 35 years).
- Etiology is unknown; hormonal relationship is likely because they often increase in size during pregnancy or with estrogen therapy and typically regress after menopause.
- Presents as a well-defined, mobile mass (or a solid mass on ultrasound).
- Tumor of stromal cells; leads to the compression of surrounding ducts.
- Diagnosis is by needle biopsy (either fine needle aspiration [FNA] or core biopsy).

A. Phyllodes tumor
  1. Most commonly diagnosed between 40 and 50 years.
  2. Rare neoplasm with variable biologic behavior (benign, borderline, and malignant).
    a. Although usually benign, certain histologic features (e.g., increased cellularity, increased mitotic activity) indicate increased risk of aggressive behavior (recurrence and/or metastasis).
  3. Pathology
    a. Round to oval, multinodular mass, may be several centimeter in diameter.
    b. Histology reveals papillary projections of epithelial-lined stroma extending into cleft-like spaces ("leaf-like" architecture).
  4. Treatment is complete surgical excision.

B. Intraductal papilloma
  1. Benign tumor arising within lactiferous ducts or sinuses.
  2. Most common cause of a bloody nipple discharge in women <40 years.
  3. No increased risk of cancer.

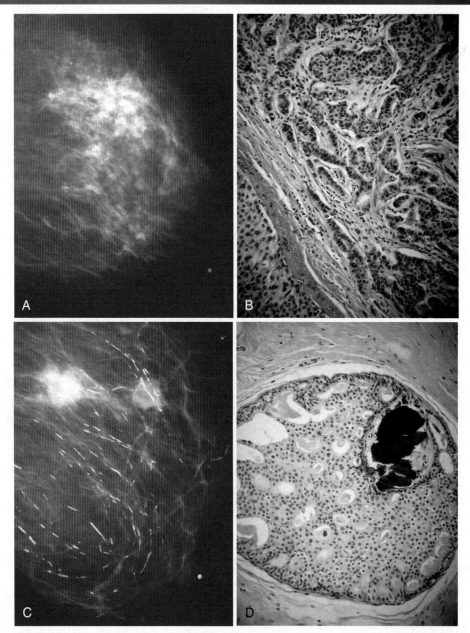

22.16: Invasive (A and B) and noninvasive ductal carcinomas (C and D). (A) Mammogram. Carcinoma has poorly defined edges that have begun to extend into surrounding tissue. Fibrous, or scar-like, tissue may form as a reaction to the invading cancer cells. (B) Histology of sample from the patient in (A) shows a random configuration of cells extending through the periductal connective tissue. (C) Mammogram. Noninvasive ductal carcinoma (also known as intraductal carcinoma or ductal carcinoma in situ) contains breast duct cells that have malignant characteristics but have not invaded the surrounding tissue. (D) Histology of sample from the patient in (C) shows proliferating malignant ductal cells limited to existing ductal units without invasion through the basement membrane. The blue material is dystrophic calcification, which shows up in mammograms. *(Courtesy of Dr. Juan Lee, Mercer University School of Medicine, Georgia, and Dr. Emil Goergi, Dodge County Hospital, Georgia.)*

C. **Invasive breast carcinoma (Figs. 22.16 and 22.17)**
1. Epidemiology
   a. Most common noncutaneous malignancy of women (~one in eight chance of developing breast cancer during lifetime).
   b. Rarely occurs in men (≤1% of cases).
   c. Second most common cancer leading to death in women (lung cancer #1).
   d. Risk increases with age, and the most common breast mass in women over 50 years of age.
2. Risk factors
   a. Increasing age.
   b. Female sex (100 times more frequent in females).
   c. History of breast cancer in a first-degree relative (e.g., mother or sister).

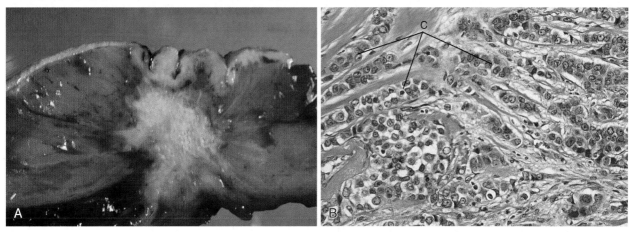

22.17: Breast carcinoma. (A) On gross inspection, the tumor appears to be grayish white as a result of the abundance of connective tissue between the tumor cells. Such desmoplastic tumors are firm and gritty on sectioning and allows the tumor to be palpable, depending on its size. Note irregular extension of the tumor into tissue. (B) Histologic appearance of an infiltrating duct carcinoma of the breast. Note the groups and strands of cancer cells (C) surrounded by abundant pink-staining collagenous connective tissue. *(From Damjanov I: Pathology for the health professions, ed 4, Philadelphia, 2012, Saunders Elsevier, p 372, Fig. 16.7.)*

     d. Presence of *BRCA1* or *BRCA2* gene mutation (up to 70% lifetime risk of breast cancer).
     e. Prolonged elevated levels of estrogen
        i. Early menarche, late menopause, and nulliparity.
        ii. Postmenopausal obesity (aromatase enzyme in adipose tissue converts androgens to estrogens).
        iii. Postmenopausal hormone replacement therapy.
     f. Personal history of breast cancer (either in situ or invasive).
     g. Smoking.
     h. Therapeutic radiation to the chest at the early age.
3. Clinical manifestations
     a. Breast mass (usually painless)
        i. Most commonly located within the upper outer quadrant (location of a majority of breast tissue).
     b. Skin or nipple retraction.
     c. Painless axillary adenopathy.
     d. Hepatomegaly and/or bone pain may herald the presence of metastatic disease.
4. Screening
     a. Mammography (used for screening and diagnosis).
        i. Used to detect nonpalpable mass.
        ii. The first imaging study performed following the discovery of a breast mass.
        iii. Screening recommendations vary, often beginning around 40–50 years.
        iv. Findings suspicious for malignancy include the presence of microcalcifications and/or a spiculated mass.
           (1) Microcalcifications often indicative of atypical ductal hyperplasia or ductal carcinoma in situ (DCIS).
     b. MRI screening reserved for high-risk patients (e.g., those harboring *BRCA* gene mutation).
     c. Suspicious lesions are biopsied.
        i. FNA can detect the presence of malignant cells but does not distinguish between in situ and invasive tumors.
        ii. Core needle biopsy (or excisional biopsy) can differentiate in situ from invasive.
     d. Breast carcinoma initially spreads via the lymphatics to regional lymph nodes.
        i. Cancers in outer quadrants spread to the axillary nodes.
        ii. Cancers of inner quadrants spread to the internal mammary nodes.
     e. Over time, tumor cells gain access to the vasculature and spread hematogenously.
        i. Common sites of metastatic disease include the lungs, bone, liver, and brain (sometimes many years after initial diagnosis/treatment).
5. Important diagnostic evaluations
     a. Sentinel lymph node biopsy
        i. The sentinel lymph node is the first lymph node(s) that the cancer drains into (i.e., the first site of lymph node metastasis).
        ii. Commonly biopsied as a method of evaluating for the presence of nodal metastasis.
           (1) If no tumor is identified within the sentinel lymph node, then the remaining nodes are likely negative as well (i.e., no reason to resect remaining nodes).
           (2) If, however, the sentinel lymph node contains metastatic tumor, then the remaining nodes may contain metastatic disease as well and must be surgically resected.

    b. Estrogen receptor (ER) and PR assays
- i. Hormone receptor assays (ER/PR); more likely to be positive in postmenopausal women.
- ii. ER and/or PR positive breast cancers have an overall better prognosis (antiestrogen agents often useful adjunct).

    c. Human epidermal growth factor receptor 2 (HER2)
- i. *HER2* oncogene encodes for a glycoprotein receptor with intracellular tyrosine kinase activity.
- ii. Amplification or overexpression of *HER2* is seen in ~15% of invasive breast cancer.
- iii. Historically associated with a worse prognosis; however, the use of anti-HER2 therapy (e.g., trastuzumab) has resulted in improved outcomes.

6. Surgical procedures in breast cancer
   - a. Modified radical mastectomy includes the nipple–areolar complex, all the breast tissue, and an axillary lymph node dissection.
   - b. Lumpectomy involves complete removal of the mass with a surrounding rim of benign tissue.

XIV. Disorders of the Male Breast

A. Gynecomastia
1. Benign glandular enlargement of the male breast.
2. Trimodal age distribution: infancy, puberty, and old age.
3. Presents as a rubbery firm subareolar mass.
4. Pathogenesis is related to an imbalance between estrogens and androgens (increased estrogen/decreased androgen).
5. Etiologies include:
   - a. Transplacental transfer of maternal estrogens.
   - b. Obesity (aromatase enzyme in adipose tissues converts androgens into estrogens).
     - i. Testosterone → estradiol; androstenedione → estrone.
   - c. Cirrhosis
     - i. Caused by increased adrenal production of androstenedione and subsequent aromatization of androstenedione to estrone.
   - d. Spironolactone
     - i. Increased aromatization of testosterone to estradiol, decreased testicular production of testosterone, displacement of androgens from SHBG, and direct androgen receptor blockade.
   - e. Hypogonadism
     - i. Decreased androgen production (e.g., aging).

B. Breast cancer
1. Breast cancer in men is rare ($\leq$1% of all cases of breast cancer).
2. Risk factors
   - a. Family history of breast cancer in the first-degree relative.
   - b. Genetic mutations
     - i. *BRCA2* is an especially important cause of male breast cancer.
   - c. Klinefelter syndrome
     - i. Inheritance of an extra X chromosome (47, XXY).
     - ii. ↓ Serum total and free testosterone.
     - iii. ↑ FSH and LH.
     - iv. ↑ SHBG concentrations.
3. Stage for stage, breast cancer in men has the same prognosis as in women.

I. Overview of Endocrine Disease
A. Negative feedback loops
1. Common in biologic systems; play an important role in the maintenance of homeostasis.
2. Characterized by an inverse relationship between the concentration of a hormone and its stimulatory agent.
3. Examples:
   a. Parathyroid hormone (PTH) and ionized calcium concentration
      i. Increased ionized calcium → decreases PTH release.
      ii. Decreased ionized calcium → increases PTH release.
   b. Adrenocorticotropic hormone (ACTH) and serum cortisol
      i. Increased serum cortisol → decreases ACTH release.
      ii. Decreased serum cortisol → increases ACTH release.
B. Positive feedback loops
1. Uncommon in biologic systems, a positive feedback loop is characterized by changes in the same direction as the initial change (serves to amplify the effect).
2. An example is breastfeeding.
   a. Prolactin promotes the production of breast milk.
   b. Stimulation of the breast by the suckling infant further enhances the release of prolactin to promote breast milk production.
C. Causes of endocrine hypofunction
1. Autoimmune destruction of endocrine organ
   a. Most common cause of endocrine hypofunction; for example:
      i. Addison disease (autoimmune destruction of the adrenal cortex).
      ii. Hashimoto thyroiditis (autoimmune destruction of the thyroid).
      iii. Type I diabetes mellitus (DM) (autoimmune destruction of pancreatic β-islet cells).
2. Infarction of endocrine organ
   a. Sheehan syndrome (postpartum pituitary necrosis)
      i. During pregnancy, the pituitary enlarges due to hypertrophy and hyperplasia of lactotrophs (prolactin-secreting cells).
      ii. Severe bleeding during delivery can cause hypovolemia-induced ischemic necrosis of the pituitary.
      iii. Manifestations are those of decreased tropic hormones:
         (1) Failure to lactate (↓ prolactin).
         (2) Failure to resume menses, infertility, vaginal atrophy, and dyspareunia (↓ gonadotropins).
         (3) Secondary hypothyroidism (↓ thyroid-stimulating hormone [TSH]).
         (4) Secondary adrenal insufficiency (↓ ACTH).
3. Hypothalamic and/or pituitary dysfunction
   a. Variety of etiologies, including:
      i. Infection (e.g., *Mycobacterium tuberculosis* and fungal infection).
      ii. Trauma (e.g., surgery).
      iii. Neoplasms (e.g., metastatic carcinoma).
      iv. Infiltrative processes (e.g., sarcoidosis and Langerhans cell histiocytosis).

D. **Causes of endocrine hyperfunction**
1. Benign tumors (the most common cause)
   a. Cushing syndrome (hypercortisolism) is a classic example.
      i. Elevated serum cortisol due to the autonomous secretion by an adrenal cortical adenoma or an ACTH-producing pituitary adenoma ("Cushing disease").
2. Malignant tumors
   a. Adrenal cortical carcinoma (rare cause of Cushing syndrome).
   b. Paraneoplastic effect
      i. Small-cell carcinoma of the lung (and others) sometimes produces various tropic hormones, including:
         (1) Antidiuretic hormone (ADH) → "Syndrome of inappropriate ADH."
         (2) ACTH → "Cushing syndrome."
3. Hyperplasia
   a. Parathyroid gland hyperplasia → hypercalcemia.
   b. Adrenal cortical hyperplasia → hypercortisolism.
4. Acute inflammation
   a. Acute inflammation of the thyroid (acute thyroiditis) results in the release of a stored hormone (causing hyperthyroidism).

II. **Hypothalamus**
A. **Hypothalamic-pituitary axis (Fig. 23.1).**
B. **Hypothalamic dysfunction can arise from any number of conditions, including:**
1. Primary intracranial tumors (e.g., craniopharyngioma)
   a. Craniopharyngioma, a rare tumor arising from remnants of Rathke pouch, commonly presents in childhood (5–15 years) or older adulthood (>50 years). Manifestations include visual changes, headache, and hypothalamic dysfunction (e.g., diabetes insipidus). Pathology reveals both solid and cystic components with focal calcification; cysts contain turbid fluid with cholesterol (Fig. 23.1). The treatment is surgical resection.
   b. Metastatic tumors (e.g., breast cancer).
   c. Head trauma.
   d. Inflammatory disorders (e.g., sarcoidosis and *M. tuberculosis*).
C. **Manifestations of hypothalamic dysfunction**
1. Secondary hypopituitarism (deficiency of tropic factors).
   a. Decreased gonadotropin-releasing hormone (GnRH) → decreased follicle-stimulating hormone (FSH) and luteinizing hormone (LH) from the anterior pituitary.

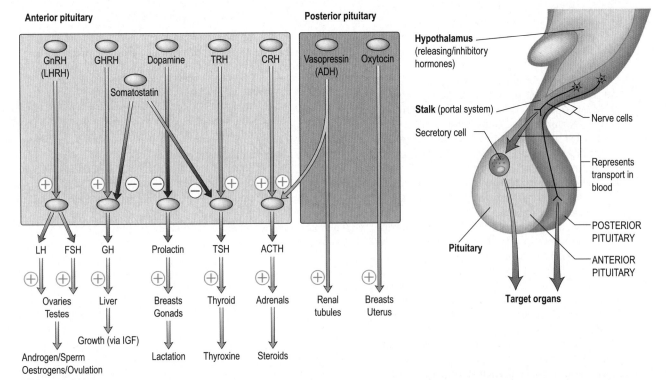

23.1: Hypothalamic releasing hormones and the pituitary tropic hormones. *ADH*, Antidiuretic hormone; *CRH*, corticotropin-releasing hormone; *FSH*, follicle-stimulating hormone; *GH*, growth hormone; *GHRH*, growth hormone-releasing hormone; *GnRH*, gonadotropin-releasing hormone; *IGF*, insulin-like growth factor; *LH*, luteinizing hormone; *TRH*, thyrotropin-releasing hormone. (*From Kumar and Clark's clinical medicine, ed 10, © 2021, Elsevier, Fig. 21.7.*)

       i. Kallman syndrome refers to a deficiency of GnRH plus anosmia (lack of smell).

   b. Decreased corticotropin-releasing hormone (CRH) → decreased ACTH from the anterior pituitary.

   c. Decreased ADH → central diabetes insipidus.

   d. Decreased dopamine → hyperprolactinemia

       i. Recall that dopamine (from hypothalamus) suppresses the release of prolactin from the anterior pituitary. For this reason, a decrease in dopamine from the hypothalamus is associated with hyperprolactinemia and associated manifestations (e.g., galactorrhea).

   e. Decreased growth hormone-releasing hormone → decreased release of growth hormone (GH).

III. Pineal Gland

A. Overview of the pineal gland

1. Located in the midline of the brain near the third ventricle.
2. Calcifies with age (useful marker in imaging).
3. Innervation is sympathetic (from the superior cervical ganglia).
4. Receives and conveys information regarding the light-dark cycle.
5. Produces melatonin from the amino acid tryptophan.
6. Nocturnal release of melatonin into the cerebrospinal fluid (CSF) and bloodstream helps to regulate sleep and circadian rhythms.

B. Tumors of the pineal gland

1. Tumors of the pineal gland are rare; most are germ-cell tumors.
2. Neurologic manifestations may arise secondary to direct invasion, compression, and/or obstruction of CSF flow (obstructive hydrocephalus).
   a. Hydrocephalus often presents with headache and lethargy.
   b. Paralysis of upward conjugate gaze (Parinaud syndrome).

IV. Pituitary Gland

A. Hypopituitarism

1. Deficiency of one or more pituitary hormones.
2. Etiologies include:
   a. Nonfunctioning pituitary adenoma (the most common cause in adults).
   b. Iatrogenic (e.g., surgery or radiation effect on pituitary).
   c. Hereditary hemochromatosis (excess iron damages the pituitary).
   d. Autoimmune destruction (lymphocytic hypophysitis).
   e. Infarction (Sheehan syndrome and sickle cell anemia).
   f. Pituitary apoplexy
      i. Sudden hemorrhage into the pituitary gland.
      ii. Acute onset of headache, diplopia, and hypopituitarism (potential for cardiovascular collapse and sudden death).
   g. "Empty sella syndrome"
      i. Refers to an imaging finding of CSF within the sella turcica.
      ii. Due to a defect in the diaphragma sella that allows CSF pressure to enlarge the sella.
      iii. Pituitary function usually remains normal.
   h. Hypothalamic dysfunction (see the previous discussion).
      i. Traumatic brain injury, radiation, and tumor
         (1) Craniopharyngioma (hypothalamic tumor derived from remnant of Rathke pouch) is the most common cause of hypopituitarism in children.

B. Posterior pituitary

1. Stores and releases ADH and oxytocin, both of which are produced by the supraoptic and paraventricular nuclei of the hypothalamus.
2. ADH controls water balance by increasing the reabsorption of free water from the collecting ducts.
   a. Central diabetes insipidus (the absence of ADH) is characterized by the loss of free water in the urine (urine is dilute, serum is concentrated).
3. Oxytocin has two physiologic effects.
   a. Enhances uterine contractions during labor.
   b. Stimulates the ejection of milk during breastfeeding.
      i. Suckling infant enhances the release of oxytocin, causing contraction of myoepithelial cells and the expulsion of milk into the breast ducts.

C. Hyperpituitarism

1. Definition
   a. Excessive secretion of pituitary hormone, usually from a functioning pituitary adenoma.
2. Types of pituitary adenomas
   a. Prolactinoma
      i. Benign prolactin-secreting tumor of the anterior pituitary gland.
      ii. Most common tumor of the pituitary.

     iii. Prolactin enhances the production of milk but inhibits the release of GnRH.

     iv. Clinical and laboratory findings

        (1) Galactorrhea

           (a) Milk production in the absence of pregnancy (prolactin effect).

        (2) Hypogonadotropic hypogonadism

           (a) Decreased GnRH, LH, and FSH.

           (b) Decreased estrogen causes amenorrhea, infertility, vaginal dryness, and decreased bone mineralization.

           (c) Decreased testosterone causes erectile dysfunction and decreased libido.

        (3) Larger tumors (macroadenoma) can present with headache, deficits of other pituitary hormones, and/or visual field defects (bitemporal hemianopia).

  b. GH adenoma

     i. Benign GH-secreting pituitary tumor.

     ii. Second most common functioning pituitary adenoma.

     iii. Effects of GH, many of which are mediated by insulin-like growth factor 1 (IGF-1) include:

        (1) Increased amino acid uptake and protein synthesis (causing the growth of bone and muscle).

        (2) Increased lipolysis (releases free fatty acids).

        (3) Hyperglycemia (decreased glucose uptake and increased gluconeogenesis). Note that GH has a negative feedback with glucose (↑ glucose inhibits the release of GH; ↓ glucose stimulates the release of GH).

     iv. Clinical and laboratory findings

        (1) Gigantism (in children)

           (a) Prior to the closure of the growth plates, excess GH increases linear bone growth (tall stature).

        (2) Acromegaly (in adults)

           (a) After the closure of growth plates, excess GH causes lateral bone growth.

           (b) Manifestations include enlargement of jaw, hands, and feet (may have increased glove and shoe size), coarsening of facial features with increased spacing between teeth (Fig. 23.2), prominence of forehead (frontal bossing), and increased hat size.

           (c) Cardiovascular manifestations include hypertension and cardiomyopathy (a common cause of death).

           (d) Headache and visual field defects (compressive effects of tumor).

           (e) Serum GH and IGF-1 are both increased, the latter being more sensitive.

           (f) Elevated serum glucose secondary to the diabetogenic effect of GH.

     v. Diagnosis

        (1) First measure the serum IGF-1 level.

        (2) If elevated, then measure GH levels during an oral glucose tolerance test (those with acromegaly will not exhibit the expected suppression of GH following the ingestion of glucose).

        (3) Magnetic resonance imaging (MRI) is used to further evaluate the lesion.

  c. Other pituitary adenomas

     i. ACTH-secreting pituitary adenoma (7% of adenomas).

        (1) Causes "Cushing disease."

     ii. TSH-, LH-, or FSH-secreting pituitary adenomas are all uncommon, each accounting for 1% of tumors.

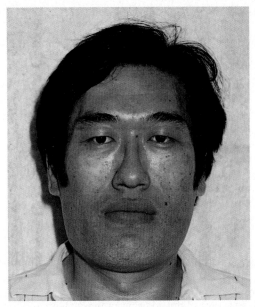

23.2: Acromegaly: facial characteristics. *(From Swartz MH: Textbook of physical diagnosis: history and examination, ed 7, Philadelphia, 2014, Saunders Elsevier, p 37, Fig. 1.2.)*

V. Thyroid Gland
  A. Overview
    1. Thyroid gland produces and secretes thyroid hormones: thyroxine (T4) and triiodothyronine (T3).
      a. T4 is the primary hormone released; however, T3 exhibits most physiologic activity.
        i. Majority of T3 is derived from T4 (an outer ring deiodinase converts T4 to T3).
    2. Both bound and unbound thyroid hormones
      a. Unbound "free" thyroid hormone exhibits physiologic activity.
      b. Remainder bound, largely to thyroid-binding globulin (TBG).
    3. Changes in TBG levels will therefore affect *total* hormone levels, but not the active "free" thyroid hormone.
      a. Estrogens stimulate the synthesis of TBG.
      b. Androgens and hepatic failure decrease the synthesis of TBG.
        i. TBG levels lower in nephrotic syndrome as well (lost in the urine).
    4. Total thyroid hormone level comprised of bound and unbound fractions.
  B. Functions of thyroid hormone
      a. Controls the basal metabolic rate (BMR), growth and maturation of tissues (e.g., brain), as well as the turnover of hormones and vitamins.
      b. Controls the synthesis of low-density lipoprotein (LDL) and β-adrenergic receptors.
  C. Thyroid function tests
    1. Total T4
      a. Represents T4 bound to TBG plus free (unbound) T4 (FT4).
      b. As noted above, changes in TBG will alter the total serum T4 but not the phsiologically active free form.
        i. Changes in TBG also have no effect on TSH. This is because feedback on the hypothalamic-pituitary axis is with free thyroid hormone (FT4).
      c. Using estrogen as an example:
        i. Estrogen increases the hepatic synthesis of TBG.
        ii. As TBG levels rise, the total T4 increases (increased bound T4).
          (1) ↑ TBG → ↑ total serum T4
          (2) Free T4 remains within normal limits (i.e., patient is euthyroid).
        iii. Conversely, a reduction in TBG (e.g., nephrotic syndrome or liver failure) results in fewer binding sites available (decreased total T4).
          (1) ↓ TBG → ↓ total serum T4.
          (2) Free T4 remains within normal limits (patient is euthyroid).
      d. Clinical situations
        i. Graves disease (increased synthesis of thyroid hormones)
          (1) FT4/FT3 increased, TBG normal, and total T3/T4 increased.
        ii. Thyroiditis (release of free T4 from colloid)
          (1) FT4/FT3 increased, TBG normal, and total T3/T4 increased.
        iii. Hypothyroidism
          (1) FT4/FT3 decreased, TBG normal, and total T3/T4 decreased.
        iv. Use of anabolic steroids
          (1) FT4/FT3 normal, TBG decreased, and total T3/T4 decreased.
        v. Nephrotic syndrome
          (1) FT4/FT3 normal, TBG decreased, and total T3/T4 decreased.
        vi. Use of exogenous estrogens or pregnancy
          (1) FT4/FT3 normal, TBG increased, and total T3/T4 increased.
    2. TSH
      a. Excellent screening test to evaluate thyroid function.
      b. Examples of serum TSH alterations
        i. Primary hypothyroidism
          (1) Decreased FT4/FT3 (decreased thyroid production) → increased serum TSH (due to the loss of the negative feedback by FT4/FT3).
        ii. Thyrotoxicosis (e.g., Graves disease)
          (1) Increased FT4/FT3 (due to autoimmune stimulation of thyrotropin receptor and thus increased thyroid hormone production) → decreased serum TSH (due to the negative feedback with FT3/FT4).
        iii. Hypopituitarism (secondary hypothyroidism)
          (1) Decreased TSH → decreased synthesis of FT4/FT3.
        iv. Hypothalamic dysfunction (tertiary hypothyroidism)
          (1) Decreased thyrotropin-releasing hormone (TRH) → decreased synthesis and release of TSH from the anterior pituitary → decreased synthesis of FT4/FT3.
    3. Radioactive iodine uptake (^{123}I)
      a. Used to evaluate the synthetic activity of the thyroid gland.
        i. Iodide [I] is used to synthesize thyroid hormone.

  b. Increased uptake is indicative of a hyperactive thyroid.
    i. Example: Graves disease.
  c. Decreased uptake is indicative of a hypoactive thyroid.
    i. Example: a patient taking exogenous thyroid hormone.
  d. Used to evaluate the functional status of thyroid nodules (see later).
    i. Decreased ^{123}I uptake ("cold" nodule).
      (1) Adenoma (e.g., follicular adenoma) and thyroid cancer.
    ii. Increased ^{123}I uptake ("hot" nodule)
      (1) Multinodular goiter.
4. Serum thyroglobulin (Tg)
  a. Thyroid-specific glycoprotein, useful in the follow-up of thyroid carcinoma.
    i. Being thyroid-specific, serum Tg concentrations should be very low/undetectable following thyroid resection.

D. Hypothyroidism
  1. Definition
    a. Deficiency of thyroid hormone.
  2. Classification
    a. Primary hypothyroidism
      i. Most common type of hypothyroidism, refers to dysfunction of the thyroid gland.
    b. Secondary hypothyroidism
      i. Hypothyroidism secondary to an inadequate release of TSH from the pituitary.
    c. Tertiary hypothyroidism
      i. Hypothyroidism occurring as a result of inadequate TRH from the hypothalamus.
  3. Epidemiology
    a. Incidence of hypothyroidism increases with age, more common in females.
  4. Etiologies
    a. Chronic autoimmune (Hashimoto) thyroiditis (Fig. 23.3).
      i. Most common cause in iodine-sufficient areas of the world (see later discussion).
    b. Iodine deficiency
      i. Most common cause worldwide.
    c. Medications
      i. Lithium inhibits thyroidal iodine uptake, iodotyrosine coupling, and secretion of thyroid hormone.
      ii. Amiodarone metabolism releases iodine into the circulation and interferes with the conversion of T4 to T3.
    d. Radiation to the neck (e.g., treatment of cancer).
    e. Infiltrative disorders of the thyroid (e.g., Reidel thyroiditis and hemochromatosis).
  5. Clinical manifestations
    a. Slowing of mental activity (e.g., depressed mood and cognitive changes).
    b. Slowing of physical activity (fatigue, weakness, and lethargy).
    c. Slowing of metabolic activity (decreased BMR)
      i. Weight gain, cold intolerance, decreased perspiration, constipation, menstrual disturbances, and impaired fertility.
    d. Cutaneous changes (e.g., dry skin and hair loss)

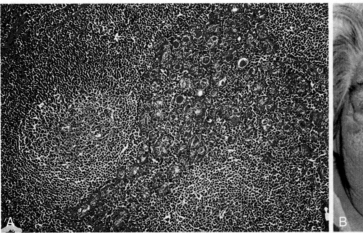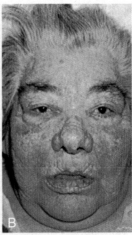

23.3: (A) Microscopic section of Hashimoto thyroiditis. Note the prominent secondary lymphoid follicle and heavy infiltrate of lymphocytes throughout the gland with destruction of the thyroid follicles. (B) Primary hypothyroidism in a patient with Hashimoto thyroiditis. Note the facial puffiness. *(A, From Rosai J, Ackerman LV: Surgical pathology, ed 9, St. Louis, 2004, Mosby, p 522, Fig. 9.10; B, from Forbes C, Jackson W: Color atlas and text of clinical medicine, ed 2, London, 2002, Mosby, p 325, Fig. 7.72.)*

  e. Myxedema coma

   i. Rare, life-threatening manifestation of severe hypothyroidism.

   ii. Characterized by hypotension, bradycardia, altered mental status, and hypothermia.

   iii. Usually seen in a known hypothyroid patient with superimposed acute event (e.g., infection, myocardial infarction, or surgery) that causes acute worsening of thyroid function.

   iv. Medical emergency with high mortality.

  f. Congenital hypothyroidism

   i. Refers to the existence of hypothyroidism in the fetus/newborn.

   ii. Thyroid hormone is required for neurologic development; therefore manifestations are those of impaired mental and motor development.

   iii. Etiologies include:

    (1) Thyroid dysgenesis

     (a) Abnormal embryologic formation of the thyroid gland.

     (b) Most cases are sporadic, some are associated with inherited mutations that affect thyroid development (e.g., *PAX8* and *TTF2*).

    (2) Dyshormonogenesis

     (a) Defective thyroid hormone synthesis (e.g., enzymatic defects, TSH receptor gene mutations, and defective TSH production).

    (3) Iodine deficiency

     (a) Major cause worldwide.

   iv. Clinical manifestations

    (1) Delayed mental and motor development, poor growth, feeding difficulties, macroglossia (enlarged tongue), hoarse cry, umbilical hernia, and facial puffiness.

 6. Laboratory findings in hypothyroidism

  a. Decreased serum T3/T4 and increased serum TSH.

  b. Antithyroid antibodies (Hashimoto thyroiditis)

   i. Antithyroid peroxidase and antithyroglobulin antibodies.

  c. Elevated total and LDL cholesterol

   i. Thyroid hormone required for the synthesis of LDL receptors (lack of thyroid hormone impairs LDL clearance).

E. Hyperthyroidism

 1. Definition

  a. Excessive levels of thyroid hormone in circulation.

 2. Etiologies

  a. Graves disease

   i. Definition

    (1) Hypermetabolic state characterized by the production of IgG autoantibodies that directly stimulate TSH receptors (i.e., thyroid-stimulating immunoglobulins).

    (2) Binding of the antibody to receptor mimics action of TSH (stimulates the release of thyroid hormone).

   ii. Epidemiology

    (1) Most common cause of hyperthyroidism.

    (2) Female > male; usual onset between 20 and 40 years of age.

    (3) Patients at increased risk of other autoimmune disorders (e.g., systemic lupus erythematosus, Type I DM, Addison disease, and pernicious anemia).

   iii. Clinical manifestations

    (1) Weight loss, tachycardia, increased perspiration, lid lag, stare, and atrial fibrillation.

    (2) Diffuse enlargement of the thyroid gland.

    (3) Other manifestations unique to Graves

     (a) Ophthalmopathy

     Inflammation of the extraocular muscles and orbital fat.

     Causes proptosis (exophthalmos) and periorbital edema (Fig. 23.4).

     (b) Pretibial myxedema

     Bilateral, thickening and induration of the skin, usually in a pretibial location, due to the dermal accumulation of glycosaminoglycans and lymphocytic inflammation.

   iv. Pathology

    (1) Diffuse hypertrophy and hyperplasia of thyroid follicular epithelial cells with papillary infoldings of the glands.

    (2) Lymphoid infiltrates, primarily T cells, throughout the glands.

  b. Toxic multinodular goiter

   i. Enlarged nodular thyroid with autonomous production of thyroid hormone.

   ii. Second most common cause of hyperthyroidism (after Graves disease).

   iii. Caused by activating mutations in TSH receptor genes (thyroid hormone synthesis and release are autonomous).

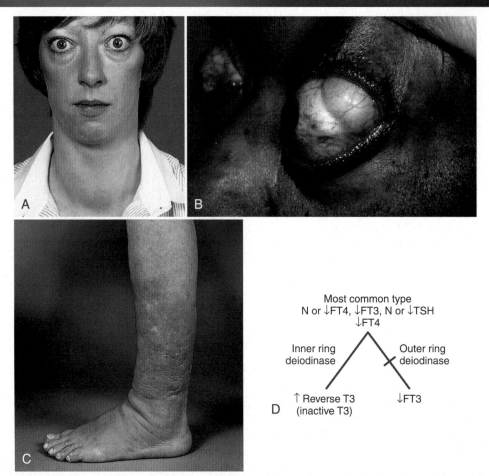

23.4: (A) Graves disease. The patient has exophthalmos and a diffuse enlargement of the thyroid gland (goiter). (B) Severe exophthalmos in Graves disease. (C) Pretibial myxedema in Graves disease. Note the thickened area of erythema involving the pretibial area. (D) Schematic of euthyroid sick syndrome (ESS). In ESS, the outer ring deiodinase is blocked, and the inner ring deiodinase converts T4 to reverse T3, which is inactive. *(A, From Forbes C, Jackson W: Color atlas and text of clinical medicine, ed 2, London, 2002, Mosby, 2002, p 323, Fig. 7.61; B from Swartz MH: Textbook of physical diagnosis, ed 5, Philadelphia, 2006, Saunders Elsevier, p 232, Fig. 10.35; C, courtesy of R.A. Marsden, MD, St. George's Hospital, London; D, courtesy of Edward Goljan, MD.)*

      iv. Radioactive iodine uptake reveals "hot" nodules (indicative of increased 123I uptake).
      v. As opposed to Graves, there is no exophthalmos or pretibial myxedema.
  3. Clinical manifestations
    a. Warm, moist skin with thin, fine hair.
    b. Sweating, heat intolerance, and weight loss (increased metabolic rate).
    c. Tachycardia, systolic hypertension, risk of atrial fibrillation.
    d. Bone loss (thyroid hormone stimulates bone resorption).
    e. Neuropsychiatric manifestations (e.g., psychosis, agitation, anxiety, insomnia, and emotional lability).
F. Laboratory findings of excess thyroid hormone
  1. Increased serum T3/T4 and decreased serum TSH.
  2. Increased 123I uptake
    a. Graves disease: uptake diffusely increased.
    b. Toxic multinodular goiter: uptake limited to overactive nodules.
  3. Decreased 123I uptake
    a. Thyroiditis (inflamed thyroid glands).
    b. Excess exogenous thyroid hormone (suppresses TSH, thyroid is therefore not stimulated to take up the 123I).
  4. Hypocholesterolemia (low serum total and high-density lipoprotein [HDL] cholesterol).
  5. Hypercalcemia (increased bone resorption).
G. Thyroid (thyrotoxic) storm
  1. Rare, life-threatening condition characterized by severe thyrotoxicosis.
  2. Usually arises in an individual with unrecognized or inadequately treated thyrotoxicosis with a superimposed physiologic stressor (e.g., surgery, infection, or myocardial infarction).
  3. Manifestations include tachycardia, hyperpyrexia (marked temperature elevation), psychosis, agitation, weakness, and muscle wasting.

H. Euthyroid sick syndrome (nonthyroidal illness syndrome)
1. Phenomenon in which a patient without preexisting thyroid disease develops abnormal thyroid function tests in conjunction with a nonthyroidal illness.
2. Most common finding is a low serum T3.
3. Pathogenesis
   a. Most T3 is derived from the peripheral conversion of T4 via an outer ring deiodinase.
   b. In nonthyroidal illness, the outer ring deiodinase is blocked, while an inner ring deiodinase is activated (Fig. 23.4D).
   c. Blockage of the outer ring deiodinase decreases the conversion of T4 to T3 and reduces the metabolism of reverse T3 (rT3).
   d. Induction of the inner ring deiodinase enhances the conversion of T4 to rT3 and the metabolism of T3.
   e. The net effect is low T3 and elevated reverse T3.
4. No treatment is required (other than the underlying illness).
5. Laboratory findings return to normal following resolution of the underlying illness.

I. Goiter
1. Enlarged thyroid gland; may be diffuse or nodular.
   a. Thyroid hormone production may be increased, decreased, or normal.
   b. Etiologies include Hashimoto thyroiditis and iodide deficiency, the latter being the most common cause worldwide.
2. Clinical manifestations
   a. Most are asymptomatic (slow growth over decades).
   b. Some, such as Hashimoto thyroiditis or iodide deficiency, present with manifestations of hypothyroidism.
   c. Compressive effect of the enlarged thyroid may be seen.
      i. Exertional dyspnea due to compression of the trachea.
      ii. Dysphagia due to compression of the esophagus.
      iii. Hoarseness due to compression of recurrent laryngeal nerve.
      iv. Horner syndrome due to compression of the cervical sympathetic chain.

J. Thyroiditis
1. Inflammation of the thyroid gland, several etiologies.
2. Acute suppurative thyroiditis
   a. Bacterial infection of the thyroid gland.
   b. Usually secondary to hematogenous seeding of the thyroid.
   c. May be euthyroid or have a transient period of hyperthyroidism due to the release of preformed hormone from the inflamed gland.
   d. Manifests with neck tenderness, pain, fever, chills, and leukocytosis with left shift.
   e. Complete recovery is typical with a return of thyroid function to normal.
3. Subacute (granulomatous, de Quervain) thyroiditis
   a. Self-limited inflammatory disorder of the thyroid gland, thought likely due to a viral infection as most patients give a history of recent upper respiratory infection prior to the onset of thyroiditis.
      i. Usually presents in young to middle-aged adults; more common in females.
   b. Clinical manifestations
      i. Thyroid enlargement and pain (the most common cause of a painful thyroid).
      ii. Initial period of hyperthyroidism secondary to the release of the stored hormone (↑ T4 and T3, ↓ TSH, and ↓ iodine uptake).
      iii. Resolution of the inflammation over several weeks is followed by recovery of normal gland function.
      iv. Sequence of findings is as follows:
         (1) Hyperthyroid → euthyroid → hypothyroid → euthyroid (i.e., normal thyroid function is restored).
4. Chronic autoimmune (Hashimoto) thyroiditis
   a. Autoimmune-mediated destruction of the thyroid gland resulting in the development of hypothyroidism.
      i. Most common cause of primary hypothyroidism in iodine-sufficient areas of the world.
      ii. Usual onset between 30 and 50 years; more common in females.
      iii. Genetic susceptibility (e.g., HLA-DR3, Down syndrome).
   b. Pathology
      i. Diffuse lymphocytic infiltration of the thyroid, lymphoid follicles, and destruction of thyroid follicles.
      ii. Gland destruction is largely mediated by T cells (Type IV hypersensitivity reaction) and associated cytokine release.
         (1) Autoantibodies against one or more thyroid antigens (e.g., Tg, thyroid peroxidase) are identified but are thought to be a secondary phenomenon elicited by thyroid damage.
      iii. As the gland is destroyed, previously synthesized (stored) thyroid hormone is released; potentially causing an initial transient period of thyrotoxicosis (called "hashitoxicosis").
         (1) Over time, as the stored hormone is depleted, patients develop hypothyroidism.
         (2) Sequence: hyperthyroid → euthyroid → hypothyroid.
   c. Clinical manifestations are those of hypothyroidism:
      i. Cold intolerance, fatigue, lethargy, anorexia, weakness, constipation, and weight gain.
      ii. Bradycardia, dry cool skin, alopecia, dull facial expression, hoarseness, and delayed deep tendon reflexes.

    d. Diagnosis
      i. Elevated TSH (loss of negative feedback with thyroid hormone), low free T4.
      ii. Once a patient is confirmed to be hypothyroid, then antithyroid antibody tests are ordered.
        (1) Antithyroid peroxidase (preferred), if negative then order antithyroglobulin.
  5. Fibrous (Riedel) thyroiditis
    a. Rare, chronic inflammatory disease of the thyroid characterized by fibrosis of the thyroid and adjacent neck structures (key feature).
    b. Complications include airway obstruction, hoarseness, and dysphagia.
K. Thyroid nodules/tumors
  1. Overview
    a. Estimated that up to 6% of adult women and 2% of adult men will have a palpable solitary thyroid nodule during their lifetime.
    b. Most thyroid nodules are benign (e.g., cysts or follicular adenoma), only a small fraction are malignant.
      i. Radiation exposure of the thyroid during childhood is a risk factor for the development of a thyroid neoplasm.
    c. Clues that suggest malignancy in a thyroid nodule include:
      i. Rapid growth
      ii. Fixation to surrounding tissues
      iii. Ipsilateral cervical lymphadenopathy
    d. Cell of origin differs.
      i. Papillary carcinoma, follicular carcinoma, and anaplastic carcinoma all derive from follicular epithelial cells.
      ii. Medullary carcinoma is derived from parafollicular (C cells).
  2. Papillary carcinoma of the thyroid
    a. Most common primary thyroid malignancy (85% of cases).
      i. More common in women than men (3:1).
      ii. Usually young- to middle-aged adults (30–50 years).
    b. Pathology
      i. Malignant tumor of follicular epithelial cells, often with papillary architecture (thus the name).
      ii. Important diagnostic clues include crowded, overlapping cells with nuclear grooves, pseudoinclusions (i.e., clear space in nucleus ["Orphan Annie nuclei"]), and psammoma bodies.
      iii. Initially spreads via lymphatics to cervical lymph nodes.
      iv. Distant metastasis (advanced stage disease) to lungs, bone, brain, and adrenals.
  3. Diagnosis
    a. Fine needle aspiration (FNA).
  4. Prognosis
    a. Psammoma bodies represent concentric calcifications of necrotic tumor cells (Fig. 23.5). In addition to papillary carcinoma of the thyroid, they are also commonly found in papillary serous carcinomas of the ovary and endometrium (see Chapter 22) as well as meningioma (see Chapter 26).
    b. Good, >90% 5-year survival.
  5. Follicular carcinoma
    a. Second most common primary thyroid malignancy (~9%); also arises from follicular cells.
    b. More common in females; usually 40–60 years.
    c. Gross and microscopic findings
      i. The presence of capsular and/or vascular invasion differentiates these tumors from a follicular adenoma.
      ii. More likely to spread via the hematogenous route (to lungs and bones) rather than the lymphatics.
      iii. Five-year survival rate is ~80%.

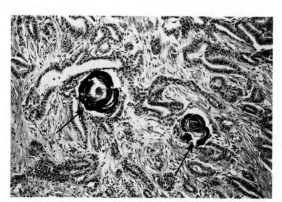

23.5: Papillary carcinoma of thyroid showing branching papillae and areas of concentric calcification (arrows) representing "psammoma bodies." *(From Rosai J, Ackerman LV: Surgical pathology, ed 9, St. Louis, 2004, Mosby, p 534, Fig. 9.37A.)*

6. Anaplastic carcinoma of the thyroid
   a. Uncommon type of thyroid malignancy (<1% of all thyroid cancer) occurring in older adulthood (>65 years).
   b. Undifferentiated tumor of follicular cells; rapidly aggressive and uniformly fatal.
7. Medullary carcinoma
   a. Uncommon, represents ~5% of all thyroid cancers.
   b. Unlike other cancers, medullary carcinoma is a malignancy of parafollicular cells.
      i. C-cell hyperplasia is a precursor lesion for medullary carcinoma.
      ii. Recall that parafollicular cells synthesize and release calcitonin (calcitonin lowers blood calcium levels).
      iii. Calcitonin is used as a tumor marker for medullary thyroid carcinoma; can be converted into amyloid (histologic clue to the diagnosis of medullary carcinoma).
   c. Pathogenesis
      i. Activating point mutations in the *RET* proto-oncogene.
      ii. Familial in 20%; autosomal dominant multiple endocrine neoplasia (MEN) syndromes (Types IIa and IIb) (Fig. 23.6).
         (1) MEN IIa syndrome (medullary carcinoma, primary hyperparathyroidism, and pheochromocytoma).
         (2) MEN IIb syndrome (medullary carcinoma, mucosal neuromas of the lips and tongue, pheochromocytoma, and Marfanoid body habitus).
   d. Diagnosis
      i. FNA and elevated serum calcitonin.
8. Primary B-cell malignant lymphoma
   a. Uncommon type of thyroid malignancy (<1% of cases) typically arising as a complication of Hashimoto thyroiditis.

VI. Parathyroid Gland Disorders
A. Overview
1. Four parathyroid glands, each located immediately posterior to the superior and inferior poles of each thyroid lobe.
   a. Superior parathyroids derived from the endoderm of the fourth pharyngeal pouches.
   b. Inferior parathyroids, as well as the thymus, are derived from the endoderm of the third pharyngeal pouches.
2. Function in calcium regulation (Fig. 23.7)
   a. Parathyroid cells contain a "calcium-sensing receptor" that detects changes in extracellular calcium.
   b. Secretes PTH in response to hypocalcemia.
      i. Feedback with ionized, unbound calcium ions.
   c. PTH raises serum calcium levels via several mechanisms.
      i. Enhances renal reabsorption of calcium.
      ii. Stimulates vitamin D synthesis via the activation of 1α-hydroxylase enzyme in the kidney.
         (1) Vitamin D (calcitriol) increases the absorption of dietary calcium.
      iii. Induces osteoclast-mediated bone resorption.
B. Serum calcium
1. Total serum calcium is comprised of both bound and unbound (ionized) forms.
2. Calcium binds primarily to negative charges on albumin; levels vary with albumin concentration and pH.

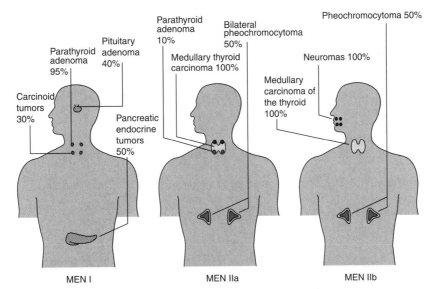

23.6: Multiple endocrine neoplasia (MEN) syndromes (autosomal dominant). In MEN Ia, the most common pituitary tumor is a prolactinoma. Pancreatic tumors can secrete gastrin, insulin, vasointestinal peptide, glucagon, or somatostatin. *(From Gaw A, Murphy MJ, Srivastava R, Cowan RA, O'Reilly Denis St J: Clinical biochemistry: an illustrated colour text, ed 5, Churchill 2013, Livingstone Elsevier, p 142, Fig. 71.1.)*

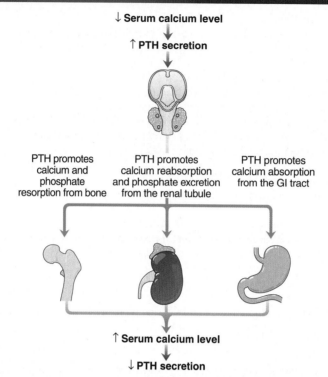

↓ Serum calcium level

↑ PTH secretion

PTH promotes calcium and phosphate resorption from bone

PTH promotes calcium reabsorption and phosphate excretion from the renal tubule

PTH promotes calcium absorption from the GI tract

↑ Serum calcium level

↓ PTH secretion

23.7: Parathyroid hormone (PTH) increases serum calcium level through its effects on bone, renal tubules, and intestine. *GI*, Gastrointestinal. *(From Copstead LE, Banasik JL: Pathophysiology, ed 5, Philadelphia, 2013, Elsevier Saunders, p 812, Fig. 40.12.)*

   a. Hypoalbuminemia causes a decrease in total serum calcium as there is less albumin available to bind with calcium.
   b. With hypoalbuminemia, ionized calcium and PTH remain within normal limits and thus there are no manifestations of hypocalcemia.
      i. Levels of ionized calcium, the metabolically active form, are normal.
   c. To correct total serum calcium for hypoalbuminemia:
      i. Corrected total serum calcium = [0.8 × (normal albumin − patient's albumin)] + measured serum calcium level.
        (1) Normal albumin is 4 g/dL.
      ii. Example: a patient with the measured serum calcium of 7.5 g/dL and albumin of 3 g/dL has a corrected calcium of 8.3 g/dL [0.8 (4 − 3) + 7.5].
  3. Alkalosis
   a. At a normal pH of 7.4, ~40% of the acidic groups on albumin are free to bind to the positively charged calcium ions (Ca^{2+}).
      i. Alkalosis increases the number of negative charges available to bind ionized calcium. As pH rises, more binding sites become available for binding with calcium (Fig. 23.8).
      ii. As more calcium binds with albumin, ionized calcium levels decline and patients may develop clinical manifestations of hypocalcemia (e.g., perioral numbness and tingling).
      iii. In response to the reduced ionized calcium, PTH is released (restoring ionized calcium to normal).
C. Hypoparathyroidism
  1. Definition
   a. Deficiency in the secretion or action of PTH.
   b. Characterized by decreased serum levels of PTH and calcium; elevated serum phosphate.
  2. Etiologies
   a. Loss of parathyroid tissue as a complication of neck surgery (the most common cause).
   b. Autoimmune destruction of parathyroids (the second most common cause).
   c. Agenesis of the parathyroid glands (e.g., DiGeorge syndrome).
   d. Hypomagnesemia
      i. Magnesium is required for PTH activation and secretion.
      ii. Causes of hypomagnesemia include the use of diuretics, alcohol, nephrotoxic medications (e.g., aminoglycosides), and/or stool losses (e.g., diarrhea).
  3. Manifestations of acute hypocalcemia include:
   a. Tetany (neuromuscular irritability)
      i. Usually begins with paresthesia of the fingers, toes, and around the mouth (perioral).
      ii. Muscle stiffness, spasms, and seizures are possible.

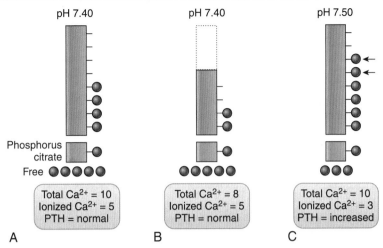

pH 7.40   pH 7.40   pH 7.50

Phosphorus
citrate
Free

Total Ca²⁺ = 10
Ionized Ca²⁺ = 5
PTH = normal

Total Ca²⁺ = 8
Ionized Ca²⁺ = 5
PTH = normal

Total Ca²⁺ = 10
Ionized Ca²⁺ = 3
PTH = increased

A   B   C

23.8: Total serum calcium in a normal individual with a normal pH (A), an individual with hypoalbuminemia and normal pH (B), and an individual with respiratory alkalosis and alkaline pH (C). Refer to the text for discussion. *PTH*, Parathyroid hormone.

b. Trousseau sign
   i. Induced carpal spasm with adduction of thumb into palm and wrist flexion (follows inflation of a sphygmomanometer on the upper arm for 3 minutes).
c. Chvostek sign
   i. Twitching of the circumoral facial muscles in response to tapping over the facial nerve just anterior to the ear.
d. Laboratory findings in hypoparathyroidism
   i. Hypocalcemia, hyperphosphatemia, and decreased serum PTH.

D. Primary hyperparathyroidism
1. Refers to excessive release of PTH from parathyroid glands.
2. Most common cause of hypercalcemia in an outpatient setting.
3. Etiologies include:
  a. Parathyroid adenoma (~80% of cases)
    i. Histology: sheets of chief cells with no intervening adipose.
  b. Parathyroid hyperplasia (~20% of cases)
    i. Increased number of parathyroid cells involving all glands.
  c. Parathyroid carcinoma (rare)
4. Association with MEN I and IIa.
5. Effects of excessive PTH/elevated calcium
  a. Skeletal abnormalities (osteitis fibrosa cystica)
    i. PTH increases osteoclast-mediated bone resorption (decreased bone mineral density) and increases fracture risk.
  b. Renal abnormalities
    i. Nephrolithiasis (calcium stones), nephrocalcinosis (calcification of tubules); potential for chronic kidney disease.
    ii. Nephrogenic diabetes insipidus (due to ADH refractoriness).
  c. Gastrointestinal findings
    i. Constipation (decreased smooth muscle tone).
    ii. Peptic ulcer disease (calcium stimulates gastrin release, increasing production of gastric acid).
    iii. Acute pancreatitis (calcium activates trypsinogen within pancreatic parenchyma).
  d. Central nervous system findings
    i. Anxiety, depression, cognitive dysfunction, psychosis, and coma.
  e. Useful mnemonic: "Bones, stones, abdominal moans, and psychic groans."
  f. Electrocardiogram shows shortening of the QT interval.
6. Laboratory findings in primary hyperparathyroidism
  a. Increased serum PTH (intact serum PTH assay is the best initial screening test).
  b. Increased serum calcium (hypercalcemia) and decreased serum phosphate (hypophosphatemia).
  c. Primary hyperparathyroidism is the most common cause of hypercalcemia in an outpatient setting.
  d. Malignancy is the most common cause of hypercalcemia in the hospital setting.
  e. Together, account for ~90% of all cases of hypercalcemia.
  f. Serum PTH can usually differentiate.
  g. PTH is increased in primary hyperparathyroidism.
  h. PTH is often decreased in hypercalcemia of malignancy (PTH-related peptide may be increased).
  i. Parathyroid adenoma localized using a technetium-99m-sestamibi radionuclide scan.

E. **Secondary hyperparathyroidism**
  1. Hyperparathyroidism developing as a result of chronic hypocalcemia.
      a. Usually due to chronic kidney disease ($\downarrow$ synthesis vitamin D).
      b. Chronic hypocalcemia → increased PTH secretion (i.e., secondary hyperparathyroidism).
      c. In secondary hyperparathyroidism, all four parathyroid glands become hyperplastic to compensate for chronic hypocalcemia.
  2. Although PTH levels are increased, patients continue to exhibit hypocalcemia.
      a. Potential for the development of tertiary hyperparathyroidism (glands become autonomous regardless of the calcium level).

F. **Hypophosphatemia**
  1. Causes
      a. Decreased intestinal absorption
          i. Use of phosphate-binding medications.
          ii. Chronic diarrhea.
          iii. Inadequate dietary intake.
      b. Redistribution of phosphate from extracellular space into cells
          i. Acute respiratory alkalosis
              (1) Rise in intracellular pH stimulates glycolysis.
      c. Increased urinary excretion
          i. Diuretics.
          ii. Hyperparathyroidism (PTH enhances renal excretion of phosphate).
          iii. Impaired proximal tubule reabsorption.
  2. Clinical manifestations
      a. Decreased adenosine triphosphate synthesis
          i. Decreased myocardial contractility, weakness, hemolysis, and encephalopathy.
      b. Decreased levels of 2,3-bisphosphoglycerate
          i. Reduces the release of oxygen from red blood cells to the tissues.

G. **Hyperphosphatemia**
  1. Etiologies
      a. Decreased renal excretion.
          i. Acute or chronic kidney disease is the most common cause.
      b. Acidosis
          i. Causes a transcellular shift of phosphate out of cells.
      c. Acute cellular catabolism
          i. Rhabdomyolysis, intravascular hemolysis, and tumor lysis syndrome.
      d. Increased phosphate absorption
          i. Vitamin D toxicity and bisphosphonates
  2. Clinical manifestations
      a. Although often asymptomatic, patients may develop manifestations of hypocalcemia due to phosphate binding with calcium and/or renal failure (due to deposits of calcium phosphate within renal tubules).

VII. **Adrenal Gland**
  A. **Overview**
      1. Comprised of an outer cortex (a site of steroid hormone synthesis) and an inner medulla (a site of catecholamine synthesis).
      2. Steroid hormones of the adrenal cortex are synthesized using cholesterol as the precursor molecule (Fig. 23.9).
          a. Adrenal cortical hormones
              i. Zona glomerulosa produces mineralocorticoids (aldosterone and deoxycorticosterone).
              ii. Zona fasciculata produces glucocorticoids (cortisol and corticosterone).
              iii. Zona reticularis produces adrenal androgens (dehydroepiandrosterone [DHEA], DHEA-sulfate, and androstenedione).
      3. Adrenal medullary hormones
          a. Tyrosine (an amino acid) is the initial precursor molecule for the synthesis of catecholamines.
              i. Cells of the adrenal medulla are of neural crest origin.
              ii. Produce catecholamines (epinephrine [EPI], norepinephrine [NOR], and dopamine).
              iii. Metabolites of EPI and NOR include metanephrine and normetanephrine, both of which are further metabolized to vanillylmandelic acid (VMA).
              iv. Dopamine metabolized to homovanillic acid (HVA).
  B. **Primary adrenal insufficiency**
      1. Acute or chronic disorder characterized by reduced glucocorticoid release by the adrenal gland.
          a. May or may not be accompanied by reduced mineralocorticoids and/or adrenal androgens.
      2. Etiologies include:
          a. Abrupt withdrawal of corticosteroids
              i. Most common acute cause; due to exogenous hormone suppression of ACTH release by the pituitary.

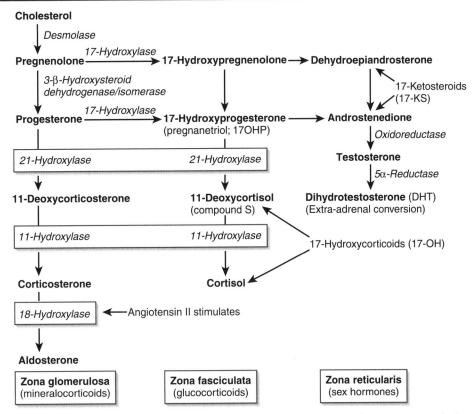

23.9: Adrenocortical hormone synthesis. The zona glomerulosa produces mineralocorticoids (e.g., aldosterone), the zona fasciculata produces glucocorticoids (e.g., cortisol), and the zona reticularis produces sex hormones (e.g., testosterone). The 17-hydroxycorticoids (17-OH) are 11-deoxycortisol and cortisol. The 17-ketosteroids (17-KSs; weak androgens) are dehydroepiandrosterone and androstenedione. Testosterone is converted to dihydrotestosterone (DHT) by 5α-reductase in extra-adrenal tissue. *17-OHP*, 17-Hydroxyprogesterone.

   b. Autoimmune destruction (Addison disease)
      i. Most common cause of chronic adrenal insufficiency.
   c. Infectious adrenalitis (e.g., tuberculosis and fungal).
   d. Adrenal hemorrhage
      i. Trauma (e.g., motor vehicle accident).
      ii. Anticoagulation.
      iii. Hemorrhagic infarction (Waterhouse–Friderichsen syndrome) is often secondary to meningococcal sepsis.
3. Clinical manifestations
   a. Acute deficiency (adrenal crisis)
      i. Cardiovascular collapse with shock, abdominal pain/tenderness, and reduced consciousness.
   b. Chronic deficiency
      i. Fatigue, weight loss, anorexia, nausea, and vomiting.
      ii. Postural hypotension (dizziness upon standing).
      iii. Hyperpigmentation (particularly skin creases, mucosal membranes, and breast areola).
        (1) Chronic elevation of ACTH (secondary to ↓ cortisol) stimulates melanocytes and causes increased pigmentation (Fig. 23.10).
      iv. Psychiatric symptoms (e.g., cognitive changes, depression, and psychosis).
4. Diagnosis
   a. Low morning serum cortisol is suggestive, but must be confirmed with subnormal response to corticotropin (ACTH) stimulation.
   b. Additional workup is dependent upon specific patient characteristics (e.g., autoantibodies against 21-hydroxylase to evaluate for autoimmune adrenalitis; imaging to evaluate for hemorrhage, infection, or infiltrative processes of adrenals).
5. Laboratory findings
   a. Elevated blood urea nitrogen (BUN) and creatinine
      i. Loss of mineralocorticoid effect results in hypovolemia (causing prerenal azotemia).
   b. Hyponatremia, hyperkalemia
      i. Due to lack of mineralocorticoids.
   c. Fasting hypoglycemia
      i. Lack of glucocorticoids → decreased gluconeogenesis.

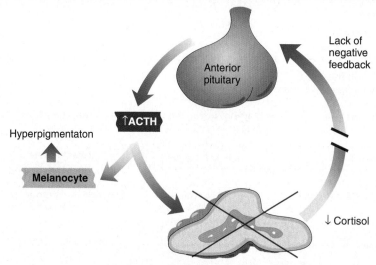

23.10: Primary adrenocortical insufficiency (decreased cortisol production) leads to hypersecretion of adrenocorticotropic hormone (ACTH) due to the lack of negative feedback. ACTH binds to receptors on melanocytes and stimulates pigment development in the skin. Even though ACTH levels are high, the adrenal gland is unable to produce adequate levels of cortisol. *(From Copstead LE, Banasik JL: Pathophysiology, ed 5, Philadelphia, 2013, Elsevier Saunders, p 807, Fig. 40.7.)*

C. Congenital adrenal hyperplasia
1. Autosomal recessive (AR) condition due to a deficiency of one or more enzymes of cortisol synthesis.
2. Failure to synthesize cortisol with associated loss of negative feedback on the pituitary.
   a. Stimulates the release of ACTH and, subsequently, the growth of adrenal cortical cells (i.e., adrenal cortical hyperplasia).
3. Proximal to the enzyme block, precursors are diverted to the formation of androgens (may cause female infants to have ambiguous genitalia).
   a. If genitalia are ambiguous, first determine genetic sex.
4. Pathogenesis
   a. 21-Hydroxylase enzyme deficiency
      i. Mutation of *CYP21A2* gene.
      ii. Most common cause congenital adrenal hyperplasia (90%–95% of cases).
      iii. Clinical manifestations vary depending upon the degree of enzyme deficiency.
         (1) The most severe "salt-wasting" form is associated with a complete absence of enzyme activity (causing hypotension).
         (2) Conversely, a low but detectable level of enzyme activity results in a less severe "simple-virilizing" form (some mineralocorticoids are formed).
         (3) Enzymes proximal to the block (e.g., 17-hydroxyprogesterone [17-OHP]) are increased.
   b. 11-Hydroxylase (11-OHase) deficiency
      i. Second most common enzyme deficiency.
      ii. The deficiency of 11-hydroxylase impairs synthesis of cortisol (distal to the block).
      iii. The loss of cortisol feedback on the pituitary leads to increased ACTH release and hyperplasia of the adrenal gland.
      iv. As with 21-hydroxylase deficiency, hormones proximal to the block (e.g., 17-OHP and androgens) are increased.
      v. Elevated androgens may cause genitalia of the female to appear ambiguous (as before, must determine genetic sex).
      vi. In milder deficiency states, clinical effects of elevated androgens may not appear until later in childhood.
      vii. Increased levels of the weak mineralocorticoid, 11-deoxycorticosterone (proximal to the enzyme block) cause salt retention and hypertension.
5. Screening for congenital adrenal hyperplasia
   a. Serum 17-OHP
      i. Because it is proximal to the enzyme block in both 21- and 11-OHase deficiency states, levels will be increased.
      ii. Screening performed routinely in newborns.

D. Adrenal hyperfunction (hypercortisolism, Cushing syndrome)
1. Definition
   a. Refers to the clinical manifestations associated with elevated serum cortisol levels.

2. Etiologies
   a. Iatrogenic
      i. Exogenous glucocorticoid administration (common cause).
      ii. Laboratory findings: increased serum cortisol; decreased ACTH.
   b. ACTH-producing pituitary adenoma ("Cushing disease").
      i. Laboratory findings: increased serum cortisol; increased ACTH.
   c. Adrenal neoplasm
      i. Autonomous release of cortisol by an adrenal neoplasm (usually adrenal cortical adenoma).
      ii. Laboratory findings: increased serum cortisol; decreased ACTH.
   d. Ectopic ACTH
      i. Ectopic secretion of ACTH by tumor (small-cell carcinoma of the lung is most common).
      ii. Laboratory findings: increased serum cortisol; increased ACTH.
3. Clinical manifestations
   a. Glucose intolerance (cortisol stimulates gluconeogenesis).
   b. Obesity (increased fat storage; most pronounced centrally).
      i. Facial rounding ("moon facies").
      ii. Shoulder ("buffalo hump").
      iii. Abdomen.
   c. Skin atrophy, easy bruising, and dermal stria (catabolic effects of glucocorticoids).
   d. Hyperpigmentation
      i. Not due to cortisol but rather the stimulation of melanin synthesis by melanocyte-stimulating hormone (MSH).
      ii. ACTH and MSH are released together as a prohormone (pro-opiomelanocortin [POMC]).
      iii. Stimulation of ACTH release → increased release of MSH (explaining the hyperpigmentation).
   e. Proximal muscle wasting and weakness (catabolic effects of glucocorticoids).
   f. Psychosis, paranoia, and depression.
4. Screening for Cushing syndrome, either:
   a. Twenty-four-hour urine-free cortisol (if elevated, supports a diagnosis of Cushing syndrome).
   b. Low-dose dexamethasone (cortisol analog) suppression test
      i. A low dose of dexamethasone will not suppress cortisol in a patient with Cushing syndrome of any cause.
   c. Once the diagnosis of Cushing syndrome is made, then one must distinguish between the various causes.
      i. Use high dose dexamethasone suppression test, along with a measurement of ACTH.
      ii. If ACTH is undetectable/decreased and cortisol does not suppress, then a patient has an adrenal cause of Cushing syndrome (e.g., adenoma or carcinoma).
      iii. If ACTH is increased and cortisol does not suppress, then a patient ectopic ACTH production.
      iv. If ACTH is increased and partial suppression of cortisol occurs, then a patient has an ACTH-producing pituitary adenoma (called "Cushing disease").
5. Nelson syndrome
   a. Refers to complications associated with enlargement of the pituitary (and ACTH release) following bilateral adrenalectomy.
      i. Following bilateral adrenalectomy, serum cortisol levels decline, thereby removing the suppressive effect of cortisol on the hypothalamus.
      ii. Loss of negative feedback by cortisol causes the hypothalamus to increase the production of CRH.
      iii. CRH stimulates the pituitary to release ACTH, causing diffuse hyperpigmentation (via stimulation of melanocytes) and pituitary enlargement.
         (1) The latter may lead to compression of surrounding structures (e.g., optic chiasm causing bitemporal hemianopia), headache.

E. Hyperaldosteronism
1. Primary aldosteronism
   a. Refers to the autonomous secretion of excess aldosterone from an adrenal cortical process.
      i. Bilateral idiopathic adrenal hyperplasia (most common).
      ii. Unilateral adrenal adenoma (second most common).
      iii. Adrenal carcinoma (rare).
   b. Excessive aldosterone enhances the renal reabsorption of sodium (causing hypernatremia) in exchange with potassium (causing hypokalemia).
   c. Clinical manifestations
      i. Hypertension (excess sodium reabsorption).
      ii. Hypokalemia.
   d. Diagnosis
      i. Increased plasma aldosterone concentration in conjunction with a decreased plasma renin activity.
         (1) As plasma volume increases (aldosterone effect), so does renal blood flow (suppressing renin release).
2. Secondary aldosteronism
   a. Elevated aldosterone secondary to a reduction in effective blood volume (reduced renal blood flow).

b. Decreased renal blood flow stimulates the release of renin and thus activation of renin–angiotensin–aldosterone system.

c. Both plasma aldosterone and plasma renin are increased.

F. **Adrenal medulla**

1. Overview

a. Cells of the adrenal medulla are of neural crest origin; also known as chromaffin cells (because they stain with chromium salts).

b. Similar cells outside the adrenal medulla form "paraganglia."

i. Example is the organ of Zuckerkandl, located near the aorta between the renal arteries and the aortic bifurcation.

2. Pheochromocytoma

a. Definition

i. Catecholamine-secreting tumor arising from the chromaffin cells of the adrenal medulla or sympathetic ganglia.

(1) The latter are known as "extra-adrenal pheochromocytomas" or "catecholamine-secreting paragangliomas."

ii. Most pheochromocytomas (90%) are located within the adrenal medulla, are unilateral, and benign.

b. Epidemiology

i. Rare tumors; most common in the fourth to fifth decades.

ii. Incidence equal between males and females.

iii. Most are sporadic; however, up to 25% are familial and associated with genetic disorders, including:

(1) MEN Type II

(2) Von Hippel–Lindau disease

(3) Neurofibromatosis Type 1

c. Clinical manifestations

i. Hypertension (paroxysmal or sustained)

ii. Headache (often paroxysmal, severe, "pounding").

iii. Palpitations

iv. Hyperhidrosis (increased sweating)

v. Note that these manifestations are often paroxysmal in association with the episodic release of catecholamines by the tumor (patients often asymptomatic between the episodes).

d. Diagnosis

i. Plasma free and urinary metanephrines (e.g., metanephrine and normetanephrine).

ii. Imaging (computed tomography or MRI) of abdomen and pelvis.

3. Neuroblastoma

a. Definition

i. Tumors of primordial neural crest cells arising within the adrenal or extra-adrenal paraganglia.

b. Epidemiology

i. Nearly always arises in children, median age at diagnosis is ~17 months.

ii. Third most common malignancy in children (behind leukemia and brain tumors).

c. Pathology

i. Can develop anywhere within the sympathetic nervous system, primarily within the adrenal gland; remainder arise from paraspinal sympathetic ganglia.

ii. Composed of malignant neuroblasts.

iii. Prognosis highly dependent upon age at presentation (those beyond the newborn stage but <18 months have more favorable prognosis).

d. Clinical manifestations

i. Varies with stage of disease, localized disease may present as an asymptomatic mass or abdominal pain.

ii. Manifestations of metastatic disease are common.

(1) Bone pain and anemia (secondary to bone metastasis).

(2) Hepatomegaly (metastasis to liver)

(3) Proptosis (metastasis to orbit)

(4) Subcutaneous nodules

(5) Compression of spinal cord

e. Diagnosis

i. Increased urinary catecholamine metabolites (HVA and VMA).

ii. Tissue biopsy for confirmation (small round blue cells with Homer-Wright rosettes representing neuroblasts localized around a central space).

iii. Electron microscopy shows cytoplasmic neurosecretory granules.

VIII. **Endocrine Disorders of the Pancreas**

A. **Insulinoma**

1. Tumor of pancreatic β-islet cells.

a. Beta-islet cells are the site of insulin formation (cleavage of proinsulin into insulin and C-peptide).
b. Both serum insulin and C-peptide are increased in those with an insulinoma.
    i.   Conversely, those with excess exogenous insulin have elevation of serum insulin alone.
2. Manifestations
    a. Hypoglycemia and associated symptoms (e.g., sweating, palpitations, weakness, confusion, and loss of consciousness).
3. Diagnosis
    a. Overnight fasting blood glucose in conjunction with plasma insulin and C-peptide levels.

B. Diabetes mellitus (DM)
1. Definition
    a. Chronic metabolic syndrome characterized by elevated levels of blood glucose (hyperglycemia) in association with insufficient levels and/or function of insulin.
    b. Broadly classified into Type I DM and Type II DM.
2. Epidemiology
    a. Type I usually presents in childhood, especially around puberty.
    b. Type II usually presents during adulthood (affects ~10% of the population in the United States), increased incidence with age.
    c. Increased incidence in Blacks, Hispanics, and Native Americans.
    d. More common in obese individuals.
    e. Leading cause of blindness, peripheral neuropathy, chronic kidney disease, and peripheral vascular disease.
3. Classification
    a. Types I and II DM
        i.   Type I DM
            (1) Hyperglycemia in Type I DM is secondary to an absolute deficiency of insulin resulting from autoimmune destruction of β-islet cells.
            (2) HLA-DR3/4 association; the presence of autoantibodies against insulin and glutamic acid decarboxylase (GAD).
            (3) Histology shows lymphocytic inflammation around islets ("insulitis").
            (4) Often presents during childhood, especially teens.
            (5) Manifestations include polyuria, polydipsia, and weight loss.
            (6) May present with diabetic ketoacidosis (DKA), see later discussion.
            (7) Chronic complications include cardiovascular disease, neuropathy, nephropathy, and retinopathy.
        ii.   Type II DM
            (1) Characterized by relative insulin deficiency in conjunction with insulin resistance and increased gluconeogenesis.
            (2) Highly associated with obesity and is typically a disease of adults; however, the obesity epidemic in children has been accompanied by increased incidence of Type II DM.
            (3) Hyperglycemia-induced osmotic diuresis can result in severe volume loss (hyperglycemic hyperosmolar state, see later discussion).
            (4) Chronic complications include cardiovascular disease, nephropathy, neuropathy, and retinopathy.
    b. Secondary causes of DM
        i.   Pancreatic disease (e.g., cystic fibrosis, chronic pancreatitis, and hemochromatosis).
        ii.   Drugs (e.g., glucocorticoids, pentamidine, and thiazides).
        iii.   Endocrine disease (e.g., pheochromocytoma, glucagonoma, and Cushing syndrome).
        iv.   Maturity onset diabetes of the young—MODY
            (1) MODY refers to a monogenic form of diabetes presenting in adolescence to young adulthood.
            (2) Accounts for up to 5% of all cases of diabetes.
            (3) Not associated with autoantibodies but rather inherited genetic mutations that impair glucose sensing and insulin secretion.
                (a) Most common mutation is in the hepatocyte nuclear factor-1-alpha (*HNF1A*) gene.
        v.   Metabolic syndrome
            (1) Insulin resistance syndrome characterized by hyperglycemia, dyslipidemia, abdominal obesity, and hypertension.
            (2) Affects ~25% of adults in the United States.
            (3) Diagnostic criteria (any three of the five are sufficient for the diagnosis).
                (a) Abdominal obesity (waist circumference $\geq$ 40 inches in males or 35 inches in females).
                (b) Hypertriglyceridemia ($\geq$150 mg/dL).
                (c) HDL cholesterol <40 mg/dL in males or <50 mg/dL in females.
                (d) Elevated blood pressure ($\geq$130/85 mm Hg).
                (e) Elevated fasting plasma glucose $\geq$100 mg/dL.

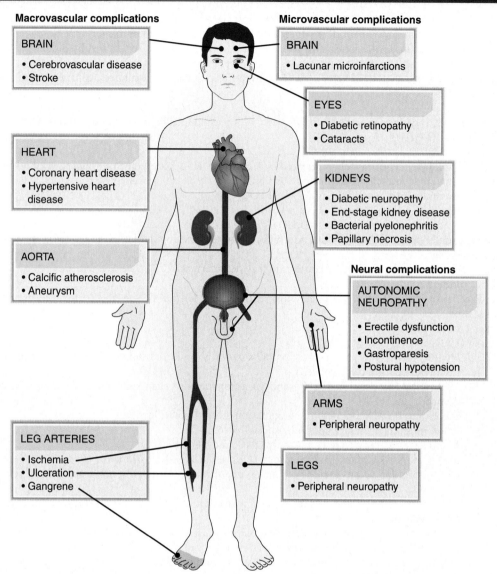

Macrovascular complications

BRAIN
- Cerebrovascular disease
- Stroke

HEART
- Coronary heart disease
- Hypertensive heart disease

AORTA
- Calcific atherosclerosis
- Aneurysm

LEG ARTERIES
- Ischemia
- Ulceration
- Gangrene

Microvascular complications

BRAIN
- Lacunar microinfarctions

EYES
- Diabetic retinopathy
- Cataracts

KIDNEYS
- Diabetic neuropathy
- End-stage kidney disease
- Bacterial pyelonephritis
- Papillary necrosis

Neural complications

AUTONOMIC NEUROPATHY
- Erectile dysfunction
- Incontinence
- Gastroparesis
- Postural hypotension

ARMS
- Peripheral neuropathy

LEGS
- Peripheral neuropathy

23.11: Clinically important complications of diabetes mellitus. Clinical findings may result from pathologic changes in large blood vessels (macrovascular complications), small blood vessels (microvascular complications), and nerves (neural complications). *(From Damjanov I,: Pathophysiology, Philadelphia, 2009, Saunders Elsevier, p 358, Fig. 10.12.)*

4. Complications (Fig. 23.11)
   a. Long-term effects of diabetes are largely related to chronic hyperglycemia-induced vascular injury.
   b. Macrovascular disease
      i. Hyperglycemia is pro-atherogenic; leads to the development of atherosclerotic plaques within medium to large arteries (e.g., ischemic heart disease, strokes, and peripheral arterial disease).
   c. Microvascular disease
      i. Hyperglycemia contributes to endothelial dysfunction of capillaries and arterioles; has both direct and indirect effects (e.g., oxidative stress, cellular swelling, and nonenzymatic glycosylation).
      ii. Damage to retinal vessels causes retinal hypoxia, triggering neovascularization (new blood vessel formation). The newly formed vessels are prone to rupture, explaining retinal hemorrhages and visual changes.
   d. Neuropathy (affects peripheral and autonomic nervous systems).
      i. Distal symmetrical polyneuropathy (pain, paresthesia, and numbness; typically, in a "stocking and glove" distribution).
      ii. Loss of sensation results in gait instability, skin ulceration, and infection.
   e. Nephropathy
      i. Increased synthesis of Type IV collagen in the basement membranes and mesangium of the renal glomeruli.
      ii. Alterations in glomerular basement membrane lead to the development of proteinuria (loss of albumin in the urine is the first clinical sign of nephropathy).

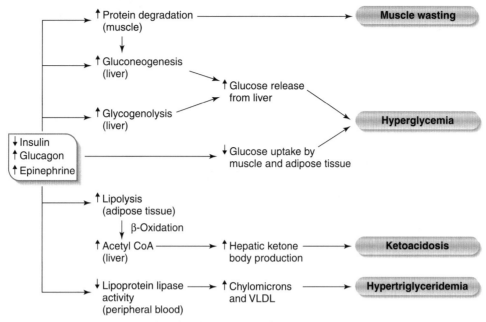

23.12: Metabolic changes in diabetic ketoacidosis (DKA). Refer to the text for discussion. *VLDL*, Very-low-density lipoprotein. *(From Pelley J, Goljan FF: Rapid review: biochemistry, Philadelphia, 2004, Mosby, p 176, Fig. 9.5.)*

    f. Iatrogenic hypoglycemia
       i. Risk of irreversible brain damage; due to excessive insulin and/or other medications.
      ii. Manifestations include sweating, tachycardia, palpitations, and tremulousness. Potential for focal neurologic deficits, mental confusion, and coma.
    g. DKA
       i. Life-threatening complication of poorly controlled Type I DM.
      ii. Precipitated by medical illness and/or omission of insulin.
      iii. Characterized by hyperglycemia-induced osmotic diuresis, severe volume depletion, and metabolic acidosis.
      iv. Pathophysiology of DKA
         (1) Insulin reduces blood glucose by two major mechanisms:
            (a) Enhanced peripheral glucose uptake.
            (b) Inhibition of glycogenolysis and gluconeogenesis.
         (2) Lack of insulin, as occurs when a patient with Type I DM omits insulin dose, results in severe hyperglycemia.
         (3) The hyperglycemia causes an osmotic diuresis with volume depletion (Fig. 23.12).
         (4) Concurrent elevated levels of counter-regulatory hormones (e.g., glucagon, EPI, cortisol, and GH) enhance hormone sensitive lipase activity, causing the release of free fatty acids and glycerol.
         (5) Hepatic beta-oxidation of fatty acids into acetyl-CoA leads to the formation of ketone bodies.
            (a) Acetoacetic acid, beta-hydroxybutyric acid, and acetone (the first two being ketoacids, partially explaining the acidosis).
      v. Laboratory findings in DKA
         (1) Hyperglycemia (blood glucose usually 250–800 mg/dL).
         (2) Pseudohyponatremia (osmotic movement of fluid into the vasculature causes dilutional effect).
         (3) Increased anion gap metabolic acidosis
            (a) Due to accumulation of ketoacids and lactic acid (the latter due to decreased tissue perfusion associated with hypovolemia).
         (4) Hyperkalemia
            (a) Buffering of excess acid (i.e., K^+ moves out of cells as H^+ moves into cells).
            (b) Note however that the osmotic diuresis is associated with urinary loss of potassium. Once the acidosis has been corrected, and K^+ moves back into cells, the patients develop hypokalemia.
            (c) Treatment of DKA requires insulin, fluid replacement, and replenishment of potassium stores.
         (5) Elevated BUN and creatinine
            (a) Reduced blood volume (osmotic diuresis) → reduced renal blood flow (i.e., prerenal azotemia).
    h. Hyperosmolar hyperglycemic state (HHS)
       i. Complication of Type II DM
         (1) In Type II DM, there is enough insulin to prevent ketoacidosis but not enough to prevent hyperglycemia.
         (2) Hyperglycemia-induced osmotic diuresis causes volume depletion (and elevated serum osmolarity).

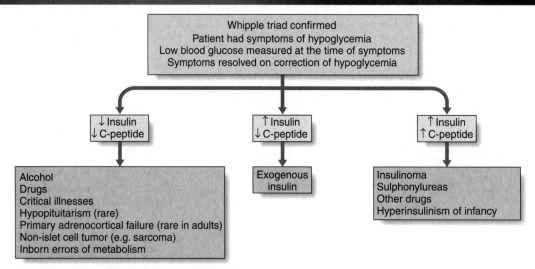

23.13: Differential diagnosis of spontaneous hypoglycemia. Measurement of insulin and C-peptide concentrations during an episode is helpful in determining the underlying cause. *(From Walker BR, Colledge NR, Ralston SH, Penman ID: Davidson's principles and practice of medicine, ed 22, 2014, Churchill Livingstone Elsevier, p 783, Fig. 20.24.)*

5. Criteria for the diagnosis of DM
   a. Fasting plasma glucose level of ≥126 mg/dL.
   b. Two-hour oral glucose tolerance test result of ≥ 200 mg/dL.
   c. Hemoglobin A1C level of ≥6.5%.
   d. Random plasma glucose of ≥200 mg/dL in the presence of the classic signs and symptoms of hyperglycemia (e.g., polyuria, polydipsia, polyphagia, weakness, and weight loss).
6. Gestational DM
   a. Defined as the development of glucose intolerance during pregnancy.
   b. Although it usually resolves following delivery, patients are at increased risk developing diabetes in the future.
   c. Newborns of diabetic mothers are at an increased risk of:
      i. Macrosomia (enlarged fetal size)—due to elevated levels of fetal insulin necessary to handle the excess load of glucose from the mother. Insulin increases fat and muscle mass.
      ii. Respiratory distress syndrome.
         (1) Insulin inhibits fetal production of surfactant.
      iii. Neonatal hypoglycemia
         (1) When mother's blood glucose is elevated, the baby responds by increasing insulin production.
         (2) After delivery, when maternal glucose is no longer present, yet the child still has elevated levels of insulin, the infant may develop severe hypoglycemia (with concomitant risk of neurologic injury).
   d. Screening for GDM occurs between 24th and 28th weeks of gestation.

C. **Hypoglycemia**
   1. Technically defined as blood glucose <70 mg/dL (normal fasting glucose is 70–100 mg/dL); however, not everyone will develop manifestations at a specific glucose value.
   2. To confirm that patient's symptoms are due to hypoglycemia, the "Whipple triad" is used (Fig. 23.13).
      a. A patient must meet all three criteria to be considered to have manifestations associated with hypoglycemia.
      b. Whipple triad includes:
         i. Signs and symptoms compatible with hypoglycemia.
         ii. Low blood glucose level.
         iii. Resolution of clinical manifestations once the blood glucose has returned to normal.
      c. Etiologies of hypoglycemia include:
         (1) Iatrogenic (excess exogenous insulin or oral hypoglycemic agents).
         (2) Insulinoma (endogenous production of insulin by tumor).

IX. **Autoimmune Polyglandular Syndromes**
   A. **Type I polyglandular syndrome**
      1. Rare AR disease caused by loss-of-function mutations in the autoimmune regulator gene (*AIRE*).
      2. Patients develop autoreactive T cells and autoantibodies against multiple tissues.
      3. Typically presents during childhood with the following (in order of presentation):
         a. Mucocutaneous candidiasis
         b. Primary hypoparathyroidism
         c. Primary adrenal insufficiency

B. Type II polyglandular syndrome
1. More common than Type I polyglandular syndrome; typically presents in middle-aged females.
2. Endocrinologic abnormalities include Type I DM and thyroid dysfunction (either autoimmune hypothyroidism or Graves disease).
3. Additional endocrinologic abnormalities may occur as well (e.g., adrenocortical insufficiency, pernicious anemia, and celiac disease).

I. Bone Disorders

A. Osteogenesis imperfecta (brittle bone disease)

1. Autosomal dominant disorder of Type I collagen synthesis (usually due to a mutation in *COL1A1* or *COL1A2* gene). Recall that type I collagen is an important component of bones, tendons, ligaments, as well as the skin and sclerae.
2. Manifestations include:
   a. Extreme skeletal fragility ("brittle bones")
      i. Fractures occur with minimal or no trauma.
      ii. Milder forms may present with premature osteoporosis.
   b. Blue sclera (the lack of collagen makes underlying choroid visible).
   c. Hearing loss (due to abnormalities of middle ear bones).
   d. Small misshapen teeth.

B. Achondroplasia

1. Autosomal dominant disorder characterized by gain-of-function mutations in the fibroblast growth factor receptor 3 (*FGFR3*) gene.
   a. Most (80%) cases are secondary to new mutations; homozygous inheritance is lethal.
2. Impaired endochondral bone growth → short stature.
   a. Particularly affects the long bones of proximal extremities (short arms and legs) and head (causing enlarged head with the bulging forehead).
3. No effect on longevity, cognition, or fertility.

C. Osteopetrosis (marble bone disease)

1. Rare disorder of increased bone density secondary to impaired osteoclast function (impaired acidification of osteoclast resorption pits).
2. Bone is dense but brittle and easily fractured.
3. Some may develop pancytopenia secondary to replacement of the bone marrow by dense bone.
   a. Complications are related to the various cytopenias (e.g., fatigue from anemia, infection due to neutropenia, and bleeding due to thrombocytopenia).
4. Cranial nerve deficits (e.g., visual and hearing loss) secondary to narrowing of neural foramina by dense bone.

D. Osteomyelitis

1. Overview
   a. Infection of bone, usually bacterial.
   b. *Staphylococcus aureus* is the most common etiologic agent.
   c. Increased risk of *Salmonella* osteomyelitis in those with sickle cell disease; related to the loss of splenic function.
2. Acute osteomyelitis
   a. Infection of bone evolving over several days with characteristic clinical manifestations of inflammation (pain, warmth, erythema, and swelling).
      i. Fever, malaise, and other systemic manifestations may be present as well.
      ii. Osteomyelitis in children usually affects long bones (e.g., tibia and femur); typically, secondary to hematogenous dissemination. Patients may present with irritability, limp, and failure to use the limb.
   b. Routes of infection include:
      i. Extension from contiguous site
         (1) Extension of an infection from a foot ulcer into underlying bone (common in diabetics).
      ii. Hematogenous dissemination
         (1) Bacteremia (bacteria in the bloodstream) commonly seeds the metaphysis.

(2) In young children, infection may extend into the epiphysis and potentially the adjacent joint space (risk of joint deformity).

(3) *Mycobacterium tuberculosis* commonly involves bone, particularly the vertebral column (called "Pott disease").

(4) Use of intravenous (IV) drugs is an additional important risk factor for the development of bacteremia and osteomyelitis.

    iii. Direct implantation

      (1) Following penetrating injury (e.g., trauma).

3. Chronic osteomyelitis

  a. Chronic infection of the bone (months to years); occurs when the treatment of acute osteomyelitis fails to clear the organism.

  b. Findings include:

    i. Localized area of dead bone (sequestrum) with a surrounding area of new bone formation (involucrum).

    ii. Draining sinus tract to the skin surface (associated with increased risk of squamous cell carcinoma at cutaneous drainage site).

4. Laboratory and radiologic findings

  a. Elevated white blood cell count.

  b. Elevated systemic markers of inflammation (e.g., erythrocyte sedimentation rate [ESR] and C-reactive protein [CRP]).

  c. Blood and bone cultures often positive.

  d. Imaging shows a lytic area of necrotic bone (sequestrum) surrounded by the sclerotic rim of new bone (involucrum).

E. Osteopenia/osteoporosis

1. Overview

  a. Osteopenia is defined as a reduction in bone mass to between 1 and 2.5 standard deviations below average peak bone mass of young adulthood.

    i. Bone mass peaks by 30 years of age and is somewhat greater in men than women.

  b. Osteoporosis is a more severe form of osteopenia (Fig. 24.1).

    i. Bone mass $\geq$2.5 standard deviations below average peak bone mass of young adulthood.

2. Risk factors

  a. Increasing age (reduced osteoblastic activity with aging).

  b. Sedentary lifestyle (weight-bearing exercises stimulate bone remodeling).

  c. Estrogen deficiency (enhanced bone resorption).

  d. Calcium and/or vitamin D deficiency.

  e. Ethnicity (Whites and Asians).

  f. Use of corticosteroids, hyperparathyroidism, and heavy alcohol intake.

3. Clinical manifestations

  a. Increased fracture risk (e.g., vertebral bodies and hip)

    i. Vertebral compression fractures can lead to a loss of height and/or radiculopathy secondary to nerve compression (Fig. 24.2).

  b. Kyphosis caused by advanced osteoporosis, may interfere with chest wall movement/respiration (Fig. 24.2B and C).

4. Diagnosis

  a. Dual-energy X-ray absorptiometry scan

    i. Evaluates bone mineral density.

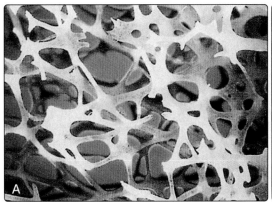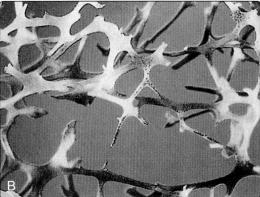

24.1: Osteoporosis. Bone showing normal trabeculae (A) and bone showing loss of trabeculae in osteoporosis (B). *(From Gaw A, Murphy MJ, Srivastava R, Cowan RA, O'Reilly Denis St J: Clinical biochemistry: an illustrated colour text, ed 5, 2013, Churchill Livingstone Elsevier, p 78, Fig. 39.1.)*

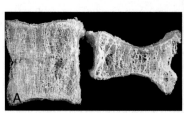
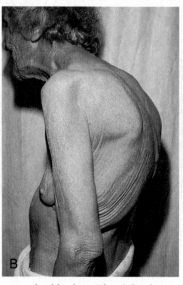
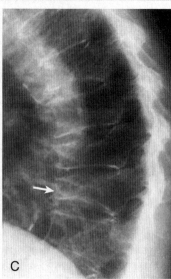

24.2: (A) Osteoporosis of the vertebral column. The vertebral body on the right shows decreased bone mass caused by compression fractures compared with a normal vertebral body on the left. (B) Older woman with osteoporosis. (C) Radiograph of the spine showing radiolucency (loss of bone mass), compression fractures (*white arrow*), and kyphosis of the spine in a patient with osteoporosis. (A, From Kumar V, Fausto N, Abbas A: Robbins and Cotran pathologic basis of disease, ed 7, Philadelphia, 2004, Saunders, p 1284, Fig. 26.12; B, from Seidel HM, Ball JW, Danis JE, Benedict GW: Mosby's guide to physical examination, ed 6, St. Louis, 2006, Mosby Elsevier, p 756, Fig. 21.78; C, from Ashar BH, Miller RG, Sisso SD: The Johns Hopkins internal medicine board review, ed 4, 2012, Elsevier, p 316, Fig. 39.6; taken from Goldman L, Bennett JC, Ausiello D: Cecil medicine, ed 22, Philadelphia, 2004, Elsevier Saunders, Fig. 258.4.)

F. Osteonecrosis (avascular necrosis)
 1. Definition
    a. Ischemic necrosis of bone and bone marrow.
 2. Risk factors
    a. Use of corticosteroids, heavy alcohol intake, fracture, sickle cell anemia, and decompression sickness.
 3. Sites of involvement
    a. Femoral head (the most common site)
       i. Trochanteric fractures are less likely to impair the blood supply (Fig. 24.3).
       ii. Femoral neck fractures interrupt the blood supply (retinacular arteries from medial circumflex femoral artery) and are therefore more likely to cause avascular necrosis.
    b. Scaphoid bone
       i. The scaphoid, located on the radial aspect (thumb side) of the wrist, is perfused from distal to proximal. For this reason, a fracture (e.g., falling on outstretched hand) may disrupt the flow of blood to proximal aspects of the bone resulting in osteonecrosis.
    c. Metacarpal bones
       i. Sickled red blood cells (sickle cell anemia) can occlude the small vasculature of the metacarpal bones causing infarction with pain and swelling.
 4. Diagnosis
    a. Plain X-rays are insensitive in early phases. In later phases, as dead bone is resorbed, a radiolucency is noted with surrounding sclerotic (increased density) border secondary to the formation of reactive bone.
    b. To detect early osteonecrosis, magnetic resonance imaging (MRI) is best.
 5. Legg–Calvé–Perthes disease
    a. Idiopathic avascular necrosis of the femoral head arising in children (peak incidence 5–7 years).
    b. More common in males; typically presents with a limp.
G. Osgood–Schlatter disease
 1. Definition
    a. Overuse injury secondary to repetitive traction on the tibial tubercle (the site of insertion of patellar tendon onto tibia).
 2. Epidemiology
    a. Usually seen in children between the age of 10 and 15 years who are athletically active (e.g., running and jumping).
    b. More common in males (3:1).
 3. Clinical manifestations
    a. Pain and swelling at tibial tubercle; exacerbated by squatting, climbing stairs, or knee extension against resistance.
    b. Relieved by rest.
    c. Thickening and tenderness of the tibial tuberosity.
    d. Manifestations resolve following closure of the tibial growth plate (by 18 years in most cases).

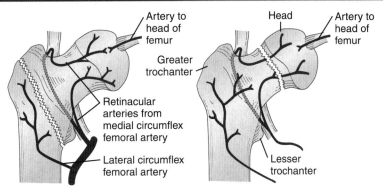

24.3: Schematic showing a trochanteric fracture (*left*) and a femoral neck fracture (*right*). See text for discussion. (*From Moore NA, Roy WA: Rapid review gross and developmental anatomy, ed 2, Philadelphia, 2007, Mosby Elsevier, p 147, Fig. 5.4.*)

H. Paget disease of bone (osteitis deformans)
  1. Definition
     a. Localized disorder of bone metabolism associated with accelerated bone remodeling and overgrowth (abnormal osteoclast function).
     b. May occur at one (monostotic) or multiple (polyostotic) sites.
     c. Commonly involves axial skeleton (skull, pelvis, and spine) as well as long bones of the lower extremity (e.g., femur).
  2. Epidemiology
     a. Relative common in older individuals; typically arising after the age of 55 years.
  3. Clinical manifestations
     a. Most are asymptomatic; some develop bone pain, deformity, and/or fracture (lesions are weak).
     b. Elevated alkaline phosphatase (due to the increased osteoblastic activity).
  4. Complications
     a. Nerve compression (causing radiculopathy and hearing loss).
     b. Headaches, increased hat size (with involvement of the skull).
     c. Increased risk bone tumors (particularly osteosarcoma).
  5. Pathology
     a. Involved bones show haphazard osteoid deposition in a "mosaic" pattern (Fig. 24.4).
  6. Diagnosis
     a. Elevated serum alkaline phosphatase.
     b. Bone thickening on imaging studies.
 I. Fibrous dysplasia
  1. Definition
     a. Developmental anomaly characterized by replacement of the marrow by fibrous connective tissue and poorly formed trabecular bone.
     b. May involve one (monostotic) or multiple (polyostotic) bones.
     c. Due to somatic gain-of-function mutation in the guanine nucleotide stimulatory protein (*GNAS1*) gene.
        i. G stimulatory protein becomes constitutively active. Sustained activation of adenylate cyclase results in overproduction of cyclic adenosine monophosphate (impairs osteoblast maturation).
  2. Epidemiology
     a. Usually presents during early to mid-teens (i.e., during the period of active bone growth).
  3. Pathology
     a. Medullary bone replaced by fibrous tissue with cyst formation.
     b. Lesions characterized by irregular, curvilinear, or serpiginous trabecular bone ("C" or "S"-shaped bone).
  4. Clinical manifestations
     a. Often asymptomatic; may cause physical deformities (e.g., leg-length discrepancy; facial asymmetry with involvement of facial bones).
     b. Pathologic fracture is the most common complication.
     c. Small risk of malignant transformation (into various sarcomas).
     d. McCune–Albright syndrome refers to the presence of fibrous dysplasia in conjunction with pigmented skin lesions and endocrine dysfunction (e.g., precocious puberty).
 J. Neoplastic disorders of bone
  1. Osteoid osteoma
     a. Benign bone neoplasm, most common in patients between 10 and 30 years of age; 2:1 male-to-female ratio.
     b. Characterized by intense pain, often more severe at night, relieved by nonsteroidal antiinflammatory drugs (NSAIDs).
  2. Enchondroma
     a. Benign, relatively common; asymptomatic cartilage-forming tumors within the marrow cavity of long bones.

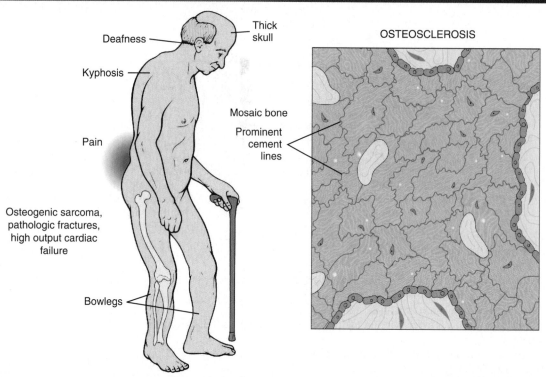

OSTEOSCLEROSIS

Deafness

Thick skull

Kyphosis

Mosaic bone
Prominent cement lines

Pain

Osteogenic sarcoma, pathologic fractures, high output cardiac failure

Bowlegs

24.4: Paget disease. Clinical features are caused by bone deformities. The mosaic pattern of dense but structurally weak mosaic bone is seen on the histologic examination. *(From Ivan Damjanov, MD, PhD: Pathology for the health professions, ed 4, Philadelphia, 2012, Saunders Elsevier, p 421, Fig. 19.8.)*

      b. Comprised of lobules of mature hyaline cartilage with partial to complete encasement by bone.
   3. Primary malignant tumors of bone, in descending order of frequency, include multiple myeloma (see Chapter 14), osteosarcoma, and chondrosarcoma.
   4. Osteosarcoma
      a. Primary malignant bone tumor with a bimodal age distribution (early adolescence, adults over 65 years).
      b. Most common bone cancer under the age of 20 years.
      c. Usual arises within the metaphysis of long bones (distal femur, proximal tibia, and proximal humerus).
         i. In adults, they often arise from preexisting bone lesions (e.g., chronic osteomyelitis, Paget disease of bone, and fibrous dysplasia).
      d. Risk factors include:
         i. Inherited mutations in tumor suppressor genes (e.g., *TP53* and *RB1*).
      e. Clinical manifestations
         i. Pain, mass lesion, and pathologic fracture.
         ii. Elevated lactate dehydrogenase and elevated alkaline phosphatase.
         iii. Propensity for hematogenous metastasis, particularly to the lungs.
      f. Imaging
         i. Sunburst pattern with the elevation of periosteum (Fig. 24.5).
      g. Pathology
         i. Malignant appearing osteoblasts forming bone.
   5. Chondrosarcoma
      a. Malignant bone tumor characterized by the production of cartilage; may arise from underlying precursor lesion (e.g., enchondroma or osteochondroma).
      b. Usually arise within the metaphysis of the proximal femur, proximal humerus, or pelvic bones (particularly the ilium).
      c. Most common in older adults.
  K. Overall most common malignancy of bone is metastasis from elsewhere (e.g., breast, lung, thyroid, kidney, and prostate).
II. Joint Disorders
  A. Signs and symptoms of joint disease
   1. Arthralgia (joint pain).
   2. Arthritis (inflammation of joint); presents with redness, swelling, pain, and warmth.
   3. Morning stiffness (prolonged stiffness to the joint).

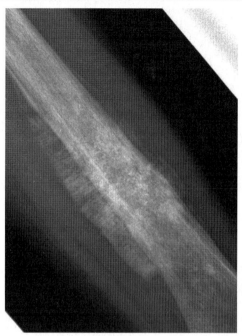

24.5: Radiograph showing a "sunburst" appearance representing a periosteal reaction to osteosarcoma. *(From West SG: Rheumatology secrets, ed 3, St. Louis, 2015, Elsevier Mosby, p 499, Fig. 67.8.)*

4. Abnormal joint mobility (e.g., ligament injury).
5. Swelling of the joint (effusion; due to increased joint fluid).

B. **Synovial fluid analysis**
   1. Used to evaluate for joint infection (septic joint) or crystal-induced arthritis (e.g., gout); includes a white blood cell count with differential, a Gram stain with culture, and crystal analysis.
   2. Normal synovial fluid is clear and essentially acellular.
   3. Inflammatory or septic joint fluid appears yellow or yellow-green (due to the abundance of white blood cells, particularly neutrophils).
   4. Bright red or chocolate-brown color (indicative of fresh or old blood, respectively).
   5. Crystal analysis
      a. Monosodium urate (MSU) crystals are needle-shaped with negative birefringence on polarization microscopy.
         i. Yellow when parallel to the slow ray of the compensator (Fig. 24.6A).
      b. Calcium pyrophosphate crystals are rectangular to rhomboid in shape, positive birefringence on polarization microscopy.
         i. Blue when parallel to the slow ray of the compensator (Fig. 24.6B).

C. **Osteoarthritis (OA)**
   1. Definition
      a. Degenerative process of articular cartilage and subchondral bone.
      b. Historically believed primarily degenerative in nature in relation to mechanical forces (obesity and trauma); recent studies however, reveal an inflammatory component as well, characterized by the release of pro-inflammatory cytokines and proteases into the joint.
   2. Epidemiology
      a. Increased incidence with aging.
      b. Primarily affects weight-bearing joints (e.g., knees, hips, cervical and lumbosacral spine, and feet) and those used frequently (e.g., hands).
   3. Risk factors
      a. Advanced age, obesity, joint trauma/injury, and neuropathic joint.
      b. Endocrine or metabolic conditions (e.g., acromegaly, chondrocalcinosis, hemochromatosis, and alkaptonuria).
         i. Alkaptonuria is an autosomal recessive disorder due to a deficiency of homogentisic acid oxidase and characterized by the accumulation of homogentisic acid within cartilage. Associated with blue-black discoloration of affected tissues, increased risk of OA.
   4. Joint findings
      a. Erosion and clefts in articular cartilage (Fig. 24.7). Bone eventually rubs on bone.
      b. Reactive bone formation at the joint margins (osteophytes) and subchondral bone cysts.
      c. No ankylosis (fusion) of the joint.

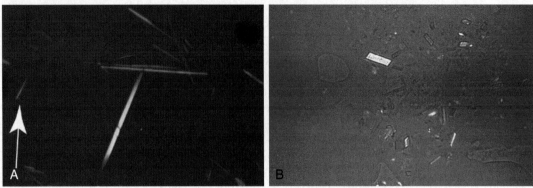

24.6: Radiographic image of osteoarthritis with joint space narrowing (*arrows*), sclerotic bone, osteophytes, and subchondral cysts. *(From Kelly IC, Bickle BE: Crash course imaging, Philadelphia, 2007, Elsevier.)*

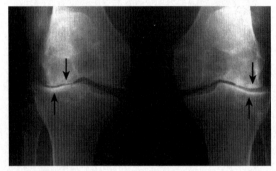

24.7: Osteoarthritis (OA). Comparison of Heberden nodes with Bouchard nodes (seen in patients with OA). *(From Copstead LE, Banasik JL: Pathophysiology, ed 5, Philadelphia, 2013, Elsevier Saunders, p 1041, Fig. 52.3.)*

     5. Clinical manifestations
       a. Deep achy joint pain; exacerbated with the movement of joint (most common manifestation).
       b. Joint stiffness following the period of inactivity (e.g., upon awaking).
       c. Reduced range of motion.
       d. Crepitus of the joint with movement.
       e. OA of the hand (Fig. 24.8)
         i. Osteophytes of the distal interphalangeal (DIP) joint (Heberden nodes).
         ii. Osteophytes of the proximal interphalangeal (PIP) joint (Bouchard nodes).
       f. Degeneration of intervertebral disks may be complicated by compression of nerve roots, causing pain, paresthesia, and weakness.
     6. Diagnosis
       a. Plain radiographs show loss of joint space, subchondral bone cysts, and sclerosis.
       b. Synovial fluid is noninflammatory with a lack of crystals.
       c. Gram stain and culture are negative.
D. Neuropathic arthropathy (Charcot joint)
     1. Joint damage (arthropathy) occurring as a result of repeated joint trauma; usually seen in association with a loss of pain sensation (e.g., diabetic neuropathy).
     2. Cause of foot/ankle pain and deformity.
E. Rheumatoid arthritis (RA)
     1. Definition
       a. Chronic, systemic inflammatory disease of joints (e.g., hands, feet, and cervical spine) and other tissues (e.g., heart and lungs).
     2. Epidemiology
       a. Prevalence of ~1%; more common in females (3:1).
       b. Usual presentation between 30 and 50 years of age.
     3. Pathogenesis
       a. Not completely understood, likely involves a combination of environmental exposure (e.g., tobacco and infectious agents) and genetic susceptibility.

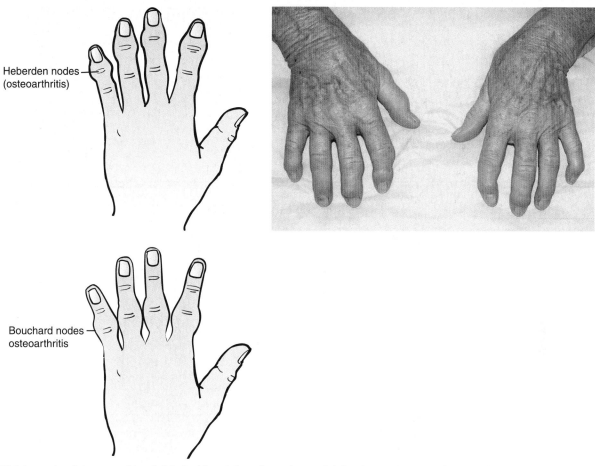

Heberden nodes
(osteoarthritis)

Bouchard nodes
osteoarthritis

24.8: (A) Schematic of rheumatoid arthritis (RA) in a joint. The red material that is growing over the articular cartilage and destroying it is called the "pannus." Note that fibrous ankylosis is beginning at the margin of the joint. (B) A patient with RA showing bilateral ulnar deviation of the hands and prominent swelling of the metacarpophalangeal joints. (C) Swan neck deformity of the fingers (flexion of distal interphalangeal [DIP] joint and extension of proximal interphalangeal [PIP] joint). (D) Boutonnière deformity of the index finger (extension of DIP joint, flexion of PIP joint; index finger), with swan neck deformity of the other fingers (*the third through the fifth finger*). (E) Baker cyst. *(A, From Kumar V, Abbas AK, Fausto N, Mitchell RN: Robbins basic pathology, ed 8, Philadelphia, 2007, Saunders Elsevier, p 820, vFig. 7.18 on the left; B, from Forbes C, Jackson W: Color atlas and text of clinical medicine, ed 2, London, 2002, Mosby, p 121, Fig. 3.3; C–E, from Marx J: Rosen's emergency medicine concepts and clinical practice, ed 7, Philadelphia, 2010, Mosby Elsevier, pp 514, 664, respectively, Figs. 47.51, 47.52, 54.12, respectively.)*

  b. Complex interplay between innate and adaptive immunity.
   i. Innate immunity
       (1) Cytokines (e.g., interleukin-1 [IL-1], IL-6, and tumor necrosis factor-α [TNF]) released from tissue-resident macrophages appear to play a central role.
   ii. Adaptive immunity
       (1) Autoantibodies against anticitrullinated proteins are relatively specific to RA. Represent antibodies against extracellular proteins that have been altered by the enzyme peptidyl-arginine-deiminase (to form "citrullinated" proteins).
       (2) Antibodies against the Fc portion of IgG (rheumatoid factor—RF).
       (3) Deposition of immune complexes within joints (Type III hypersensitivity reaction [HSR]) activates complement, causes joint inflammation (synovitis) with pannus formation (Fig. 24.9A).
           (a) Pannus refers to fibroblast-like cells, derived from the synovial membrane; causes joint damage.
  4. Clinical manifestations
   a. Malaise, fatigue, and prolonged morning stiffness (>1 hour).
   b. Joint manifestations
    i.   Warm, painful, and swollen joints.
    ii. Symmetrical involvement of metacarpophalangeal and PIP joints.
    iii. Bilateral ulnar deviation of hands (Fig. 24.9B).
    iv. Swan neck deformity (flexion of the DIP joint and extension of the PIP joint, see Fig. 24.9C).
    v.   Boutonnière deformity (extension of the DIP joint and flexion of the PIP joint, see Fig. 24.9D).

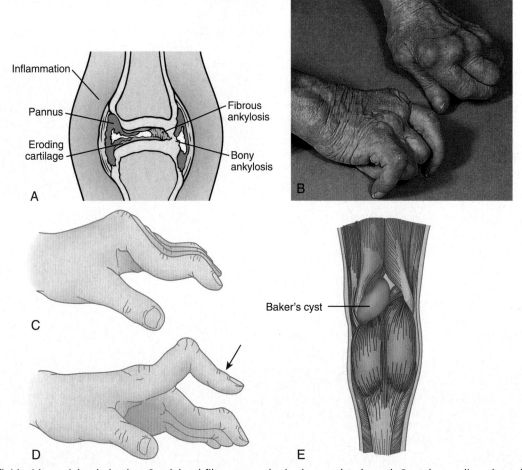

24.9: (A) Synovial fluid with special polarization. Special red filter causes the background to be red. Crystals are aligned parallel to the slow ray (axis) of the compensator (*arrow*). If the crystal is yellow when parallel to the slow ray, as in this figure, the crystal demonstrates negative birefringence indicating gout. If the crystal is blue when parallel to the slow ray, the crystal demonstrates positive birefringence. (B) Calcium pyrophosphate crystal from a patient with pseudogout. Compensated polarized light normally shows positive birefringence in polarized light when it is parallel to the slow ray of analyzer. It is not evident in this photograph. (*A, From Henry JB: Clinical diagnosis and management by laboratory methods, ed 20, Philadelphia, 2001, Saunders, Plate 19-7; B, from McPherson RA, Pincus MR: Henry's clinical diagnosis and management by laboratory methods, ed 23, 2017, p 496, Fig. 29.14; taken from Kjeldsberg CR, Knight JA: Body fluids: laboratory examination of amniotic, cerebrospinal, seminal, serous, and synovial fluids, ed 3, Chicago, 1993, © American Society for Clinical Pathology.*)

     vi. Involvement of cervical spine is associated with the risk of subluxation of atlantoaxial joint, causing cord compression or stroke.

     vii. Involved joints may become fused (ankylosis). Risk of popliteal synovial cyst (Baker cyst, see Fig. 24.9E).

  c. Pulmonary manifestations

     i. Pleuritis with effusions (low pleural fluid glucose is characteristic) and interstitial fibrosis.

     ii. Caplan syndrome refers to the presence of RA and a pneumoconiosis (e.g., silica).

  d. Hematologic manifestations

     i. Anemia of chronic disease.

     ii. Felty syndrome (triad of neutropenia, RA, and splenomegaly).

     iii. Autoimmune hemolytic anemia.

  e. Rheumatoid nodules

     i. Nodules on the extensor surface of the fingers, forearms, and pressure points (Achilles tendon and olecranon process) and other locations.

     ii. Seen in 20% of patients; presence correlates with high titers of RF.

 5. Laboratory findings

  a. Autoantibodies

     i. RF (antibodies against the Fc component of IgG).

     ii. Anticyclic citrullinated peptide

  b. Elevated white blood cells (largely neutrophils) within synovial fluid of involved joints.

  c. Systemic markers of inflammation (ESR; CRP) often elevated.

F. Sjögren syndrome

 1. Definition

a. Autoimmune disease characterized by the destruction of exocrine (e.g., salivary and lacrimal) glands.
   2. Epidemiology
      a. Marked female dominance (~10 to 15:1), often presenting during the fourth to fifth decades of life.
   3. Pathogenesis
      a. Environmental trigger (e.g., viral infection) in a genetically susceptible individual is believed to trigger the auto-immune reaction.
   4. Clinical manifestations
      a. Keratoconjunctivitis sicca (dry eyes) is often characterized as a gritty sensation ("sand") in the eyes.
      b. Xerostomia (dry mouth) manifests with difficulty swallowing dry foods (e.g., crackers), increased incidence of dental caries.
   5. Laboratory findings
      a. Anti-SS-A antibodies (anti-Ro) and anti-SS-B antibodies (anti-La).
      b. Lip biopsy shows lymphoid destruction of the minor salivary glands (confirmatory test).
G. Gout
   1. Definition
      a. Inflammatory disease of joints occurring in response to the intra-articular formation of MSU crystals.
   2. Epidemiology
      a. Usually presents by the fourth to the fifth decade in males, somewhat later in females (postmenopausal) due to the effect of estrogen to increase the excretion of uric acid (uricosuric effect).
   3. Pathogenesis
      a. Hyperuricemia, over years, results in supersaturation of the joint fluid and the formation of MSU crystals within the joint space. MSU triggers the release of cytokines (e.g., IL-1, IL-6, IL-8, and TNF), leading to an influx of neutrophils which then engulf the crystals and rupture, releasing various inflammatory mediators into the joint (Fig. 24.10).
   4. Causes of hyperuricemia
      a. Underexcretion (80%–90% of cases)
         i. Renal insufficiency, volume depletion, lead nephropathy, metabolic acidosis, alcohol, low-dose salicylates, and diuretics.
      b. Overproduction (increased cell turnover).
         i. Tumor lysis syndrome, hemolysis, myeloproliferative neoplasms, and diffuse psoriasis.
      c. Inherited conditions
         i. Lesch–Nyhan syndrome (inherited deficiency of hypoxanthine-guanine phosphoribosyl transferase), charac-terized by gout, intellectual disability, and self-mutilating behavior.
   5. Clinical manifestations
      a. Sudden onset of joint inflammation (e.g., pain, erythema, edema, and warmth), most commonly involving the first metatarsophalangeal joint (Fig. 24.11).
         i. Other sites include the foot, ankle, wrist, fingers, and knees.
   6. Laboratory findings (acute gout)
      a. Hyperuricemia (urate concentration may have returned to normal at the time of gout flare).

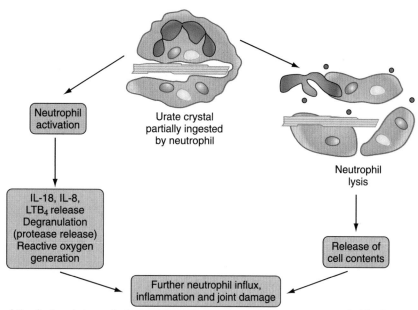

24.10: Podagra, painful swelling of the first metatarsophalangeal joint, in a patient with acute gouty arthritis. *(From Luqmani R, Robb J, Porter D: Textbook of orthopaedics, trauma, and rheumatology, Philadelphia, 2008, Elsevier.)*

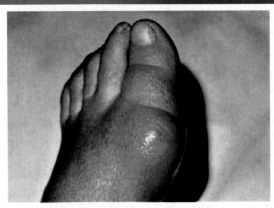

24.11: Propagation of the acute gouty arthritis response by activated neutrophils. Neutrophils entering the joint space migrate toward and phagocytose the crystals. In the case of crystals coated with immunoglobulins, the resultant activation results in synthesis and release of inflammatory mediators such as interleukins (ILs) as well as proteases and reactive oxygen species. In the case of uncoated crystals, the crystal frequently interacts with, and lyses, the phagolysosome, spilling toxic contents, leading to cell lysis. In both cases, the result is local tissue damage and recruitment of additional neutrophils from the bloodstream, leading to acute inflammation. *LTB4*, Leukotriene B4. *(From Firestone GS, et al: Kelley's textbook of rheumatology, ed 9, Philadelphia, 2013, Elsevier Saunders, p 1549, Fig. 94.12.)*

    b. Neutrophilic leukocytosis.
    c. Elevated systemic markers of inflammation (e.g., ESR and CRP).
    d. Joint fluid shows MSU crystals (needle-shaped, negatively birefringent) and increased neutrophils (Fig. 24.6A).
  7. Chronic tophaceous gout
    a. Deposits of MSU crystals within various tissues of the body (e.g., skin, cartilage, tendon, ligament, and kidney); forms a "tophus" comprised of urate deposits and associated granulomatous host response.
    b. Microscopic sections reveal numerous multinucleated giant cells containing polarizable MSU crystals.
    c. Subjacent bone damage results in "overhanging" edges on imaging studies.
H. Calcium pyrophosphate dihydrate crystal deposition (CPPD) disease
  1. Definition
    a. Clinical manifestations associated with the precipitation of calcium pyrophosphate dihydrate crystals.
  2. Manifestations
    a. Pseudogout (acute CPPD synovitis) refers to a gout-like inflammatory process of the joint due to the presence of calcium pyrophosphate dihydrate crystals within the joint space.
      i. CPPD crystals are positively birefringent (blue), rectangular or rhomboid-shaped crystals; Fig. 24.6B.
    b. Chondrocalcinosis refers to the radiologic finding of linear calcifications of the articular cartilage (commonly the knee).
I. Spondyloarthritis
  1. Family of disorders that share several characteristic clinical findings, including:
    a. Positivity for HLA-B27.
    b. Inflammation of the sacroiliac (SI) joint
    c. Inflammation at sites of attachment of ligaments and tendons to bone (enthesitis).
    d. Sausage-shaped digits (dactylitis).
  2. Specific entities include:
    a. Ankylosing spondylitis.
    b. Psoriatic arthritis.
    c. Reactive arthritis.
  3. Ankylosing spondylitis
    a. Definition
      i. Spondyloarthropathy primarily involving the SI joint and spine.
    b. Epidemiology
      i. More common in males, as well as populations in which HLA-B27 is common (e.g., Northern European descent).
      ii. Typical age of onset between 15 and 35 years.
    c. Clinical manifestations
      i. Low back and buttock pain due to sacroiliitis; improves with exercise.
      ii. Eventually involves vertebral column; ultimately resulting in fusion of vertebrae (radiologic appearance of "bamboo spine"); forward curvature of the spine (kyphosis).
      iii. Enthesitis (inflammation of enthesis, site of tendon, and ligament insertion onto bone).
      iv. Dactylitis (diffuse swelling of toes/fingers causing "sausage-shaped" digits).
      v. Extraarticular manifestations include:
        (1) Acute anterior uveitis (characterized by pain, photophobia, and blurred vision).

       (2) Restrictive lung disease (mechanisms include impaired movement of chest wall secondary to kyphosis, spinal immobility; pulmonary fibrosis).

       (3) Cardiovascular manifestations (aortitis, aortic regurgitation, and increased risk ischemic heart disease).

  4. Reactive arthritis

    a. Definition

      i. Arthritis that follows an infection elsewhere in the body but in which there are no microorganisms within the joint.

      ii. Usually follows a genitourinary (e.g., *Chlamydia trachomatis* urethritis) or gastrointestinal (e.g., *Salmonella*, *Shigella*, *Campylobacter*) infection.

    b. Epidemiology

      i. Relative rare, usually young adults (20–40 years).

      ii. HLA-B27 positive (up to 50% of cases).

    c. Clinical manifestations

      i. Triad of arthritis, conjunctivitis, and history of infection (classically *C. trachomatis* urethritis).

        (1) Arthritis is characteristically asymmetric and involves peripheral joints (especially the knees).

        (2) Dactylitis and enthesitis (commonly involving the Achilles tendon).

      ii. Extraarticular manifestations include conjunctivitis and circinate balanitis (painless erythematous ulceration of glans penis).

  5. Psoriatic arthritis

    a. Definition

      i. Arthritis associated with psoriasis (present in ~20% of patients with psoriasis).

    b. Epidemiology

      i. Men and women are affected equally.

    c. Clinical manifestations

      i. Skin lesions of psoriasis usually precede the arthritic manifestations (70% of cases).

      ii. Arthritis may involve peripheral joints (e.g., DIP joints), axial joints (e.g., sacroiliitis), or both.

      iii. Classic "pencil-in-cup" radiologic finding.

      iv. Sausage-shaped digits (dactylitis).

      v. Nail findings include "pitting" and onycholysis (separation of the nail from the nail bed).

  6. Enteropathic arthritis

    a. Definition

      i. Arthritis associated with inflammatory bowel disease (i.e., ulcerative colitis and Crohn disease) and other gastrointestinal disease/infection.

    b. Epidemiology

      i. Men and women are affected equally, often in association with HLA-B27.

    c. Clinical manifestations

      i. Arthritis may manifest with axial involvement (e.g., spondylitis and sacroiliitis), peripheral involvement, or both.

      ii. Enthesitis and dactylitis, as described above, are also common accompaniments.

J. Septic (infectious) arthritis

  1. Definition

    a. Infection of a joint, usually bacterial.

    b. Overall, the most common etiologic agent is *S. aureus*.

  2. Routes of infection

    a. Hematogenous seeding

      i. Risk factors include any cause of bacteremia (e.g., infection elsewhere in the body, IV drug abuse, and indwelling catheters).

    b. Direct inoculation into joint

      i. Penetrating injury (e.g., dog or cat bites often cause an infection by *Pasteurella multocida*).

  3. Risk factors

    a. Older age.

    b. Immunosuppression.

    c. Preexisting joint disease.

  4. Diagnosis

    a. Arthrocentesis (joint fluid has markedly elevated white cells, mostly neutrophils), culture of joint fluid.

K. Lyme disease

  1. Definition

    a. Systemic inflammatory illness caused by *Borreliella burgdorferi*, a spirochete transmitted to humans via tick bite.

  2. Clinical manifestations

    a. Erythema migrans (Fig. 24.12)

      i. Characteristic skin lesion; develops within the first month following infection.

      ii. Manifests as a slowly expanding area of erythema with central clearing ("bull's eye" lesion).

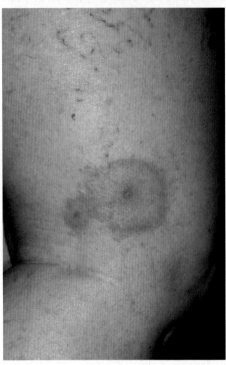

24.12: Erythema migrans. Characteristic lesion of Lyme disease. *(From Habif's clinical dermatology, ed 7, © 2021 Elsevier, Fig. 15.37.)*

    iii. Dissemination of disease, occurring over weeks to months, may result in additional manifestations:
        (1) Arthritis (primarily affects large joints—especially the knee).
        (2) Cardiac manifestations (e.g., atrioventricular block, myocarditis, and pericarditis).
        (3) Neurologic manifestations (e.g., cranial nerve palsy, meningeal irritation, peripheral neuropathy, and encephalomyelitis).

III. Muscle Disorders
A. Muscular dystrophy
  1. Definition
    a. X-linked recessive disorder characterized by the progressive degeneration of muscle fibers.
    b. Due to a mutation in the dystrophin (DMD) gene.
    c. Presents with progressive muscle weakness.
  2. Types
    a. Duchenne muscular dystrophy (more severe) presents by 2–3 years of age, causing loss of ambulation by about 12 years and death by early 20s (from respiratory insufficiency or cardiomyopathy).
    b. Becker muscular dystrophy is characterized by a less severe reduction in dystrophin, a later onset (between 5 and 15 years), a more benign course, and a longer life expectancy.
  3. Clinical manifestations
    a. Muscle weakness of limbs (proximal > distal); lower extremities affected before upper extremities.
    b. Difficulty running, jumping, and climbing steps.
    c. Gower's sign (child pushes themselves up off the floor with their hands due to the lower limb weakness).
    d. Waddling (duck-like) gait and calf enlargement on examination.
  4. Pathogenesis
    a. An absence (Duchenne muscular dystrophy) or deficiency (Becker muscular dystrophy) of dystrophin impairs the integrity of the sarcolemmal membrane ultimately, resulting in the necrosis of muscle fibers and replacement by fibrous tissue.
  5. Diagnosis
    a. Serum creatine kinase rises as muscle cells die (progressively declines as muscle tissue is lost).
    b. Muscle biopsy, electromyography (EMG), and DNA testing.
B. Myasthenia gravis
  1. Definition
    a. Acquired autoimmune disorder of postsynaptic neuromuscular transmission resulting in fatigable muscle weakness.

   2. Epidemiology
      a. Relatively uncommon, may present at any age (commonly the second to third decades in females; the sixth to eighth decades in males).
   3. Pathogenesis
      a. Autoantibody-mediated destruction (Type II HSR) of the acetylcholine (ACh) receptor at the neuromuscular junction.
      b. Reduces the number of functioning ACh receptors.
         i. Antibodies are synthesized within the thymus.
         ii. A thymic disorder (thymic hyperplasia or thymoma) is present in most cases.
      c. A minority of cases are associated with antibodies against muscle-specific receptor tyrosine kinase (MuSK), a component of the postsynaptic neuromuscular junction.
   4. Clinical manifestations
      a. Fluctuating muscle weakness; worsened with exercise and improved with rest (i.e., fatigable).
      b. Often initially involves the ocular musculature, causing ptosis and diplopia.
      c. Additional muscle groups usually become involved as well, resulting in a variety of manifestations, including:
         i. Dysphagia and dysarthria (due to weakness involving the musculature of the oropharynx).
         ii. Lack of facial expression (facial muscle weakness).
         iii. Respiratory failure (respiratory muscle weakness).
   5. Diagnosis
      a. Ice pack test
         i. Placement of an ice pack over eyelids for a couple of minutes leads to the improvement of ptosis (neuromuscular transmission improved at lower muscle temperature).
      b. Edrophonium ("Tensilon") test
         i. Historical, no longer available in the United States.
         ii. Edrophonium, a short-acting inhibitor of acetylcholinesterase, prolongs the presence of ACh within the synapse (causing an immediate increase in muscle strength).
      c. Serology
         i. Anti-ACh receptor antibodies.
         ii. Anti-MuSK antibodies.
      d. Electrophysiologic studies (e.g., repetitive nerve stimulation, EMG) can be confirmatory in those with negative serology.
   6. Once the diagnosis is confirmed, chest imaging (e.g., computed tomography and MRI) should be performed to evaluate for thymoma (which is present in 15% of cases).

IV. **Soft Tissue Disorders**
   A. **Fibromyalgia**
      1. Definition
         a. Chronic pain syndrome of unknown etiology.
      2. Epidemiology
         a. More common in females; typically, young to middle-aged.
      3. Pathogenesis
         a. Etiology unknown, thought likely secondary to disordered pain sensation.
      4. Clinical manifestations
         a. Widespread musculoskeletal pain, fatigue, and sleep disturbances.
         b. Psychiatric symptoms (e.g., anxiety and depression).
         c. Impaired cognition (impaired attention and problem solving).
         d. No evidence of muscle inflammation (i.e., inflammatory markers and levels of muscle enzymes are normal).
   B. **Fibromatosis**
      1. Definition
         a. Disorder characterized by a nonneoplastic proliferation of fibrous tissue.
      2. Dupuytren contracture
         a. Benign, slowly progressive (years to decades) fibrosing process of the palmar fascia.
         b. Causes nodular thickening in the palm, eventual development of fibrous bands that impair finger extension.
         c. Most common in White males over the age of 50 years.
         d. Etiology unknown; increased in those with diabetes mellitus and those who experience repetitive hand vibration (e.g., use of jackhammer).
         e. Similar process involving the tunica albuginea of penis (Peyronie's disease) causes curvature of the penis.
      3. Desmoid tumor (musculoaponeurotic fibromatosis)
         a. Definition
            i. Aggressive form of fibromatosis thought secondary to dysregulated wound healing.
         b. Epidemiology

   i. Most arise in sporadic fashion; however, up to 15% are seen in those with familial adenomatous polyposis (FAP).
   ii. Usually arises between the ages of 30 and 40 years.
   iii. More common in females (especially during and following pregnancy).
c. Clinical manifestations
   i. Painless (or minimally painful) slow growing mass; commonly involving the trunk (e.g., chest or abdominal wall, hip/buttocks).
   ii. Intraabdominal lesions may involve bowel and mesentery (more likely in those with FAP).
d. Prognosis is poor.
   i. Aggressive with propensity for recurrence.
   ii. Although there is no risk of metastasis, lesions may be fatal secondary to involvement/destruction of tissues/organs.

CHAPTER
25 Skin Disorders

I. **Skin Histology and Terminology**
   A. **Layers of the epidermis (Fig. 25.1)**
      1. Stratum basalis is comprised of mitotically active stem cells.
      2. Stratum spinosum exhibits prominent intercellular processes known as desmosomes.
      3. Stratum granulosum exhibits prominent keratohyalin granules.
      4. Stratum lucidum is a subdivision of the stratum corneum only present in thick skin.
      5. Stratum corneum is the most superficial layer and is comprised of anucleate cells filled with keratin filaments.
   B. **Layers of the dermis**
      1. The superficial (papillary) dermis contains loose connective tissue, blood vessels, and nerve fibers.
      2. The deeper and thicker dermal layer (reticular dermis) is comprised of dense Type I collagen.
   C. **Melanocytes**
      1. Derived from the neural crest, located in the basal layer of the epidermis.
      2. Stimulated by melanocyte-stimulating hormone, produce melanin.
         a. Melanin is synthesized within organelles (melanosomes) via the oxidation of tyrosine by tyrosinase.
            i. Tyrosine → DOPA → melanin.
      3. Melanin functions to protect against ultraviolet (UV) radiation.
      4. Melanocytes of darkly skinned individuals contain more melanin; however, the number of melanocytes is equal among individuals.
   D. **Langerhans cells**
      1. Antigen-presenting cells of the epidermis.
      2. Not recognizable on routine histologic sections.
      3. Contain tennis racquet-shaped Birbeck granules (electron microscopy).
II. **Morphologic Description of Skin Lesions**
   A. **Macule:** Flat, circumscribed lesion differing in color from surrounding skin (<1 cm in diameter).
   B. **Patch:** Flat, circumscribed lesion differing in color from surrounding skin (>1 cm in diameter).
   C. **Papule:** Palpable (elevated) circumscribed lesion <1 cm diameter.
   D. **Nodule:** Palpable (elevated) circumscribed lesion >1 cm in diameter.
   E. **Vesicle:** Elevated, circumscribed lesion of <1 cm in diameter filled with fluid (may be clear, serous, or bloody).
   F. **Bulla:** Elevated, circumscribed lesion of >1 cm in diameter filled with fluid (may be clear, serous, or bloody).
   G. **Pustule:** Elevated, circumscribed lesion, usually <1 cm in diameter, filled with pus.
   H. **Erosion:** Partial loss of the epidermis (epithelium).
   I. **Ulcer:** Full-thickness loss of the epidermis (epithelium).
   J. **Crust:** Dried secretions (serum, blood, and pus) on the skin surface.
III. **Selected Viral Disorders of the Skin**
   A. **Verrucae vulgaris (common wart)**
      1. Benign proliferative lesion of squamous cells; caused by human papillomavirus.
      2. Most common in children and adolescence, especially on the hands (transmission by direct skin contact).
      3. Gray-white, convex papules with the rough surface.
      4. Spontaneous regression typical in immunocompetent individuals; may take a few years.

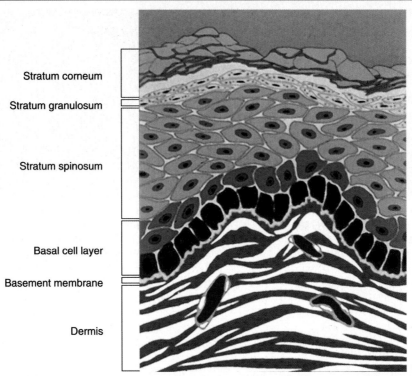

Stratum corneum

Stratum granulosum

Stratum spinosum

Basal cell layer

Basement membrane

Dermis

25.1: Epidermal layers and papillary dermis. *(From Fitzpatrick JE, Morelli JG: Dermatology secrets plus, ed 4, Philadelphia, 2011, Elsevier Mosby, p 7, Fig. 1.2.)*

B. **Molluscum contagiosum**
   1. Pink to skin-colored umbilicated papules (central depression filled with keratin); caused by a poxvirus.
   2. Most common in children, spontaneous regression is typical.
   3. Cytoplasmic inclusions containing viral particles are known as "molluscum bodies."
C. **Erythema infectiosum (fifth disease, slapped cheek disease)**
   1. Illness due to infection by parvovirus B19.
   2. Presents with mild fever, myalgia, and headache, followed by bright red macular rash on cheeks ("slapped cheek").
   3. Tropism of virus for erythroid progenitor cells via binding to the "P" antigen; causes transient suppression of erythropoiesis.
      a. Though not severe in healthy individuals, parovovirus may cause severe anemia in those with chronic hemolysis (e.g., sickle cell anemia) who may develop an acute worsening of anemia ("aplastic crisis").
   4. Parvovirus infection during pregnancy may cause fetal anemiap that can be lethal.
D. **Roseola infantum**
   1. Common febrile illness of infants and young children due to human herpesvirus 6.
   2. High fever for 3–5 days followed by a maculopapular rash involving the trunk before spreading to the extremities and face.
E. **Varicella (chickenpox)**
   1. Mild fever and malaise followed by the development of pruritic, erythematous papules due to an infection with Varicella–Zoster virus (VZV).
   2. Skin lesions begin on the scalp and face, then spread to the trunk and extremities.
   3. Lesions progress from papules to vesicles/pustules; lesions at all stages of development are present simultaneously.
      a. Infection remains latent in the sensory ganglia.
   4. Predominantly a disease of childhood (becoming less common since the introduction of varicella vaccine).
   5. Risk of severe disease in adults and immunosuppressed patients (e.g., hepatitis, pneumonia, and encephalitis).
F. **Herpes zoster (shingles)**
   1. Reactivation of latent VZV infection.
   2. Presents with prodrome of pruritus and tingling followed by painful eruption of grouped vesicles on an erythematous base in a dermatomal distribution (Fig. 25.2).
   3. May occur at any time after the initial infection; particularly common in those over 50 years, as well as immuno-suppressed (e.g., HIV and transplant recipients).
G. **Herpes gingivostomatitis**
   1. Acute, self-limiting, painful vesicular eruption of the gingiva and oropharyngeal mucosa due to herpes simplex virus (HSV)-1 infection.
   2. Transmission is by direct contact with infected secretions (saliva and/or vesicles).

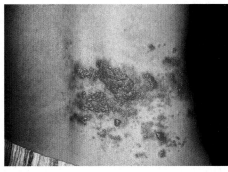

25.2: Herpes zoster eruption. Note the dermatomal distribution. *(From Mandell, Douglas, and Bennett's principles and practice of infectious diseases, ed 9, Copyright © 2020 by Elsevier, Fig. 136.2.)*

3. Infection is followed by retrograde movement of the virus to the sensory ganglia where it remains latent indefinitely.
4. May have intermittent episodes of reactivation (typically less severe and of shorter duration than the initial infection).

H. **Herpes labialis**
1. Refers to recurrent HSV-1 infection localized to the lips and perioral region (fever blisters, cold sores).
2. Reactivation triggers include stress, sunlight, and menses.

I. **Hand-foot-and-mouth disease**
1. Vesicular eruption of the hands and feet, mouth erosions.
2. Due to coxsackievirus A16 and primarily seen in children.

IV. **Selected Bacterial Disorders of the Skin**
A. **Impetigo**
1. Highly contagious, superficial bacterial infection of skin; usually caused by *Staphylococcus aureus*.
   a. Group A streptococcus is less common.
2. More common in children, particularly in hot humid conditions.
3. Initially presents as vesicles and papules. Evolves to form pustules that then break down leaving golden-crusted lesions (nonbullous impetigo).
   a. Lesions do not involve dermis and therefore heal without scarring.

B. **Staphylococcal scalded skin syndrome**
1. Febrile, superficial blistering disease caused by bacterial toxins (exfoliative toxins A and B) released by certain strains of *S. aureus*.
2. Primarily seen in children <5 years; less common in adults.
3. Exfoliative toxins A and B cleave desmoglein 1, causing loss of cell-to-cell adhesion within the stratum granulosum; results in superficial blistering and peeling of the skin (Fig. 25.3).
4. Complications include secondary infection, sepsis, hypovolemia, electrolyte imbalances, and death.

C. **Pseudomonal (hot tub) folliculitis**
1. Follows exposure to hot tubs and swimming pools contaminated with *Pseudomonas aeruginosa*.
2. Presents 1–2 days after exposure; self-limited erythematous perifollicular papules and pustules.

D. **Scarlet fever**
1. Diffuse erythematous rash usually occurring in association with infection by group A β-hemolytic streptococci.
2. Due to bacterial toxins, presents as a diffuse erythematous blanching rash with "sandpaper" quality.
3. Rash usually begins on the chest before spreading to trunk and extremities. After several days, the rash fades and then there is desquamation (peeling) of the skin.
   a. Tongue is beefy red in appearance (strawberry tongue).

E. **Erysipelas**
1. Syndrome of a rapidly spreading well-demarcated erythematous rash, usually on the face; often with accompanying systemic manifestations (e.g., fever, chills, headache, and malaise).
2. Most commonly due to group A streptococci (*Streptococcus pyogenes*).
3. Lesions are painful with elevated border; peeling (desquamation) in some cases. May be accompanied by lymphangitis and regional lymphadenopathy.

F. **Acne vulgaris**
1. Chronic or recurrent inflammatory disorder of the hair follicle and sebaceous gland; usually on the face and neck of adolescents and young adults.
2. Complex pathogenesis involves keratin plugging of follicles, increased sebum production, and bacterial infection.
   a. Androgens stimulate sebaceous glands to increase sebum production (acne more common in adolescent males).
3. Sebum is a good growth medium for *Cutibacterium acnes* (previously *Propionibacterium acnes*) which uses the triglycerides in sebum as a nutrient source.

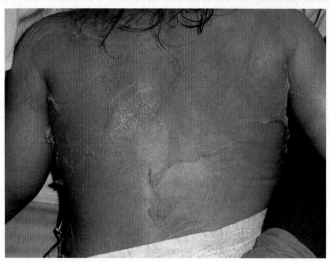

25.3: Staphylococcal scalded skin syndrome. *(From Andrews' diseases of the skin, ed 13, © 2020, Elsevier, Fig. 14.12.)*

4. Clinical manifestations
   a. Inflammatory papules, pustules, nodules, and cysts.
   b. Skin lesions (comedones): open (blackhead) and closed (whitehead).

V. **Selected Fungal Disorders of the Skin**
   A. **Superficial mycoses (dermatophytoses)**
      1. Overview
         a. Fungal diseases confined to the stratum corneum and adnexal structures.
         b. Excessive heat and humidity are predisposing factors.
         c. Tinea refers to superficial fungal infections; further characterized by location (e.g., capitis [head], pedis [foot], corporis [body], and cruris [groin]).
         d. Dermatophytes include fungi in the genera *Trichophyton*, *Microsporum*, and *Epidermophyton*.
      2. Diagnostic testing
         a. Wood lamp
            i. Handheld UV light-emitting device used to highlight various skin diseases based on characteristic fluorescent patterns.
            ii. Normal skin has a blue, fluorescent appearance.
         b. Potassium hydroxide (KOH) preparation
            i. KOH added to skin scrapings is used to identify fungal yeast and hyphae (Fig. 25.4).
      3. Tinea capitis
         a. Superficial fungal infection of the scalp.
         b. Due to infection by dermatophyte fungi (*Trichophyton* and *Microsporum* are major etiologies).
         c. More common in children and those of African descent.
         d. Acquired through direct contact; causes areas of pruritus (itching), scaling, and hair loss (alopecia).
         e. *Trichophyton tonsurans*, the most common cause, invades the hair shaft (endothrix) and is nonfluorescent under UV light.
         f. *Microsporum canis* is present on the outside of the hair shaft (ectothrix) and can be highlighted by UV light (green-yellow fluorescence).
      4. Tinea corporis
         a. Superficial dermatophyte infection of the skin; usually due to *Trichophyton* or *Microsporum* species.
            i. *Trichophyton rubrum* is the most common cause.
         b. Acquired through direct contact (e.g., contact with infected pets).
         c. Presents as a raised circular or oval, erythematous scaling plaque.
            i. "Ring-shaped" appearance explains the common name of "ringworm."
      5. Tinea pedis (athlete's foot)
         a. Dermatophyte infection involving the skin of the foot, mostly in adolescents and adults.
         b. Often caused by *Trichophyton* species (e.g., *T. rubrum*); may be acquired from walking barefoot in locker rooms and gyms.
         c. Presents as scaling rash between one or more toes.
      6. Tinea cruris (jock itch)
         a. Far more common in males; most common cause is *T. rubrum*.
         b. Risk factors include excessive sweating, obesity, and diabetes mellitus.

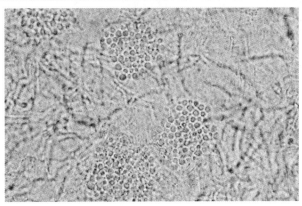

25.4: Tinea versicolor. Potassium hydroxide (KOH) prep showing the classic "spaghetti and meatballs" appearance. *(From Zitelli and Davis' atlas of pediatric physical diagnosis, ed 7, Copyright © 2018 by Elsevier, Fig. 8.40.)*

    c. Presents as erythematous rash involving the upper inner thigh that spreads outward. Border is slightly elevated and well demarcated with central area of clearing.

    d. May spread to perineum and buttocks, usually spares scrotum.

7. Onychomycosis
    a. Chronic fungal infection of nails; usually in adults.
    b. Causes discoloration and/or separation of the nail from nailbed (onycholysis).
    c. *T. rubrum* is the most frequent dermatophyte; nondermatophytes include *Candida, Aspergillus* spp.

8. Tinea versicolor (pityriasis versicolor)
    a. Common superficial fungal infection secondary to the lipid-dependent yeast *Malassezia* (most commonly *Malassezia globosa*).
      i. Growth dependent on lipids from sebum.
    b. More common in adolescence and young adulthood; especially in tropical regions (exacerbated by hot and humid weather).
    c. Manifests as hyperpigmented or hypopigmented macules on the trunk and proximal upper extremities.
      i. The greater density of sebaceous glands, and thus sebum production, on the upper body explains the predilection for this region.
      ii. Azelaic acid from the organism is damaging to melanocytes, hence the hypopigmentation. Inflammatory response to the yeast explains the hyperpigmentation.
    d. Yellow-green fluorescence under Wood lamp.
    e. KOH prep of skin scrapings shows hyphae and yeasts ("spaghetti and meatballs") appearance (Fig. 25.4).

9. Intertrigo (intertriginous dermatitis)
    a. Inflammatory condition of skin folds (areas of excessive moisture and friction), such as below the breasts (inframammary) and groin.
    b. Often secondary to *Candida*.
    c. Additional risk factors include obesity, incontinence, poor hygiene, and immune deficiencies (e.g., diabetes mellitus and human immunodeficiency virus).

10. Seborrheic dermatitis
    a. Chronic relapsing mild dermatitis, usually in areas rich in sebaceous glands (e.g., scalp, eyebrows, and nasal creases).
      i. Ranges from fine, white, scaliness (dandruff) to erythematous plaques with yellow scales.
    b. Etiology is unknown; however, the predilection for areas rich in sebaceous glands suggests an association with *Malassezia*.
    c. Called "cradle cap" in newborns.

11. Sporotrichosis
    a. Chronic infection of the skin and subcutaneous tissue by *Sporothrix schenckii*, a dimorphic fungus.
    b. Transmitted via traumatic implantation from the soil into the skin
      i. Explains the increased risk in landscapers, rose gardeners.
    c. Causes "lymphocutaneous disease"
      i. Papule at inoculation site is followed by the development of nodules along draining lymphatics.

VI. **Melanocytic Disorders**
  A. **Overview**
    1. Solar lentigo
      a. Oval, evenly pigmented, brown macules caused by the proliferation of melanocytes and the accumulation of melanin in sun-exposed sites (e.g., dorsal aspects of the hands, forearms, and face) of older adults.

2. Vitiligo
   a. Disorder of depigmentation believed secondary to autoimmune destruction of melanocytes.
      i. Coexisting autoimmune disorders (e.g., autoimmune thyroiditis, Type I diabetes mellitus) are common.
   b. Arises at any age, peaks in the second and third decades of life.
   c. No racial predilection; affects females and males equally.
   d. Depigmentation may be either localized or extensive (Fig. 25.5).
   e. Highlighted with Wood lamp.
3. Melasma
   a. Irregular light brown hyperpigmented macules, particularly in sun-exposed areas (e.g., face) of women (often associated with pregnancy or the use of oral contraceptives).
      i. "Mask of pregnancy"
   b. Due to the excessive deposition of melanin by hyperfunctioning melanocytes.
4. Melanocytic nevi (mole)
   a. Benign proliferations of neoplastic melanocytes ("nevus cells").
   b. Normal melanocytes reside in the basal layer of the epidermis. Nevus cells, however, form small clusters (nests) within the lower epidermis and/or dermis.
   c. Nevi may begin to develop as early as 6 months of age as a "junctional" nevus ("junctional" indicating the junction of epidermis and dermis).
   d. Over time, the nevus cells migrate downward into the dermis forming a "compound nevus" and then ultimately an "intradermal nevus."
      i. Junctional nevi exhibit nests of melanocytes at the dermal–epidermal junction.
      ii. Compound nevi exhibit nests of melanocytes at the dermal–epidermal junction as well as the dermis.
      iii. Intradermal nevi exhibit nests of melanocytes only within the dermis.
   e. Intradermal nevi, the most common type in adults, develop when a compound nevus loses its junctional component.
5. Atypical (dysplastic) nevus
   a. Benign acquired neoplasm of melanocytes with atypical ("dysplastic") gross and histologic features.
   b. Lesions begin during puberty and develop throughout life.
   c. Although benign, they exhibit some clinical features of melanoma (e.g., asymmetry, irregular borders, color variegation, and diameter >5 mm) and are a potential precursor to melanoma.
   d. "Familial atypical multiple mole and melanoma (FAMMM) syndrome."
      i. Autosomal dominant disorder characterized by many (>50) nevi (both common and dysplastic) and family history of melanoma.

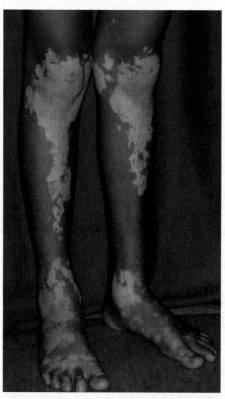

25.5: Vitiligo. Symmetrical depigmentation of the knees and lower extremities. *(From Paller AS, Mancini AJ: Hurwitz clinical pediatric dermatology, a textbook of skin disorders of childhood and adolescence, ed 5, Philadelphia, 2016, Elsevier.)*

     ii. Due to mutations in the *CDKN2A* gene (important in the regulation of the cell cycle).

     iii. Increased risk of melanoma and pancreatic cancer.

6. Melanoma

  a. Malignancy of melanocytes.

  b. Usually arising on the skin (cutaneous) but may rarely be seen in other locations (e.g., conjunctiva, vagina, eye, or meninges).

  c. Most rapidly increasing malignancy in Whites.

  d. Risk factors

     i. Excessive exposure to UV light (sunlight and tanning booths); especially at an early age.

     ii. Family history of melanoma.

     iii. FAMMM syndrome.

  e. Some melanomas, particularly those arising in locations without chronic sun exposure, exhibit mutations in genes of the mitogen-activated protein kinase (MAPK) and phosphoinositide 3-kinase (PI3K) signaling pathways (e.g., *BRAF*).

  f. Tumor growth

     i. Most have initial "radial" growth phase in which the tumor grows laterally along the epidermal–dermal border.

     ii. Over time, if not excised, tumor cells acquire the ability, through additional genetic mutations, to grow downward into the dermis (called "vertical" growth phase).

  g. Histologic subtypes

     i. Superficial spreading melanoma (Fig. 25.6)

       (1) Most common type (~75%); usually located on the legs, arms, or upper back.

     ii. Nodular melanoma

       (1) Second most common type of melanoma.

       (2) Characterized by the lack of radial growth phase (i.e., only has a vertical growth phase).

       (3) Located in any sun-exposed area (commonly the trunk), nodular melanomas have an overall less favorable prognosis (tend to present at higher stage).

     iii. Lentigo maligna melanoma

       (1) Arises in sun-damaged skin (e.g., face) of older individuals.

       (2) Appears as a tan-brown macule; indolent (long radial growth phase, favorable prognosis).

     iv. Acral lentiginous melanoma

       (1) Least common variant: typically located on the palms, soles, or under the nailbed (may be mistaken for a subungual hematoma) of dark-skinned individuals. Less favorable prognosis.

  h. Biological behavior of a melanoma is most dependent upon the depth of invasion (invasion of ≥1 mm worse prognosis).

  i. ABCDE criteria for malignancy include:

     i. Asymmetry of shape

     ii. Border irregularity

     iii. Color variation

     iv. Diameter >5 mm

     v. Evolving (increase in size and change in color)

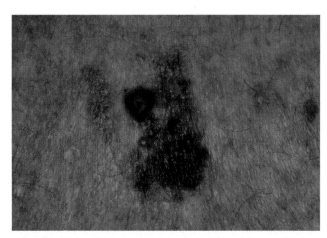

25.6: Melanoma, superficial spreading subtype. Note the asymmetric, irregular border with variegated coloring. *(From Habif's clinical dermatology, ed 7, © 2021 Elsevier, Fig. 22.34B.)*

VII. **Benign Epithelial Tumors**
  A. **Seborrheic keratosis**
    1. Benign proliferation of epidermal keratinocytes.
    2. Pigmented round to oval, raised lesions with a "stuck-on" appearance.
    3. Common, especially after the age of 50 years; often on face and shoulders.
    4. Sign of Leser–Trélat refers to the abrupt development of multiple seborrheic keratoses; may be a sign of malignancy (e.g., gastric adenocarcinoma).
  B. **Acanthosis nigricans**
    1. Velvety, hyperpigmented, papillomatous, "dirty-appearing" lesion; typically involves axilla and/or posterior neck.
    2. Associated with insulin resistance (i.e., obesity and diabetes) or sometimes with an internal malignancy (e.g., gastric adenocarcinoma).
  C. **Fibroepithelial polyp (skin tag)**
    1. Flesh-colored tag of the skin attached to the body by a narrow stalk.
    2. Common with increasing age; particularly on neck, axilla, and upper back.
VIII. **Premalignant and Malignant Epithelial Tumors**
  A. **Actinic keratosis**
    1. Dysplastic lesion of epidermal keratinocytes; either partial- or full-thickness.
    2. Due to excessive sunlight exposure; may transform into an invasive squamous cell carcinoma.
    3. Hyperkeratotic, gray, white; located on sun-exposed areas of the skin (e.g., face, neck, and back of hands or forearms).
  B. **Basal cell carcinoma**
    1. Malignant neoplasm of epidermal basal cells; most common primary skin cancer.
    2. Commonly seen on face and/or ears due to strong correlation with chronic excessive sun exposure.
    3. Appears as a raised nodule with a central crater (Fig. 25.7)
       a. Periphery of crater often exhibits dilated (telangiectatic) vessels.
    4. Locally aggressive and invasive but rarely metastasizes.
    5. Histology reveals cords of basophilic-staining (dark blue) basal cells infiltrating the underlying dermis.
  C. **Squamous cell carcinoma**
    1. Malignancy of epidermal keratinocytes; second most common primary skin cancer.
    2. Risk factors
       a. Chronic excessive exposure to sunlight (major factor), often arising from an actinic keratosis.
       b. Additional factors include:
          i.   History of arsenic exposure
          ii. Third-degree burn wounds
          iii. Chronically draining sinus tracts (e.g., osteomyelitis)
          iv. Immunosuppression
       c. Presents as scaly to nodular lesions of sun-exposed skin (e.g., ears, lip, and dorsum of hands).
       d. Usually well differentiated with squamous pearls.
       e. Minimal risk of metastatic spread.
IX. **Selected Miscellaneous Skin Disorders**
  A. **Atopic dermatitis (eczema)**
    1. Chronic, pruritic, inflammatory skin disease; usually of children.
    2. May be associated with an elevated serum immunoglobulin E (IgE), personal or family history of atopy.
    3. Sites of involvement include cheeks and flexural surfaces.

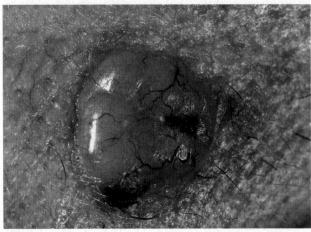

25.7: Basal cell carcinoma. *(From Habif's clinical dermatology, ed 7, © 2021 Elsevier, Fig. 21.2.)*

B. Contact dermatitis
1. Inflammatory condition arising after direct contact of a substance with the skin.
2. Two broad categories
   a. Irritant contact dermatitis
      i. A substance (e.g., laundry detergent) causes immediate inflammation of the skin.
   b. Allergic contact dermatitis (e.g., poison ivy).
      i. Delayed-type (Type IV) hypersensitivity reaction (HSR).
      ii. Vesicular pruritic rash triggered by contact with chemical to which the individual has been previously sensitized.
      iii. An example is urushiol (present within the sap of poison ivy, poison oak, and poison sumac).

X. Autoimmune Skin Disorders
A. Pemphigus vulgaris
1. Definition
   a. Autoimmune disorder characterized by the development of vesicles and bullae affecting skin and mucous membranes.
2. Pathogenesis
   a. IgG autoantibodies against "desmoglein" with disruption of intercellular adhesion.
   b. Causes loss of cell-to-cell adhesion between keratinocytes (called acantholysis) and hence the formation of vesicles and bullae.
3. Pathology
   a. Intraepithelial vesicles located above the basal layer (suprabasal).
   b. Linear row of intact basal cells resembles tombstones, acantholysis of keratinocytes (Fig. 25.8).
   c. Direct immunofluorescence shows "net-like" pattern of IgG deposits between keratinocytes (i.e., intercellular).
4. Clinical manifestation
   a. Vesicles and bullae on the skin and oral mucosa.
   b. Positive Nikolsky sign: Outer epidermis separates from the basal layer with minimal pressure.

B. Bullous pemphigoid
1. Definition
   a. Autoimmune subepidermal blistering disease; usually in older adults.
2. Pathogenesis
   a. Autoantibodies against "bullous pemphigoid antigen" of hemidesmosomes; causes loss of adhesion between the epidermis and the dermis (or the mucosa from the submucosa, Fig. 25.9).
3. Clinical manifestations
   a. Multiple, tense bullae of varying size.

C. Dermatitis herpetiformis
1. Definition
   a. Rare, chronic, subepidermal blistering disorder often associated with celiac disease.
   b. Strong genetic component (HLA DQ2 and/or HLA DQ8).
2. Pathology
   a. Granular deposits of IgA in the dermal papillae
      i. IgA antibodies against epithelial transglutaminase form complexes in the papillary dermis; results in the recruitment of neutrophils and complement activation.
3. Clinical manifestations
   a. Pruritic inflammatory papules and vesicles on the forearms, knees, scalp, or buttocks.
4. Treatment
   a. Gluten-free diet, dapsone.

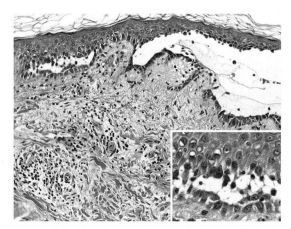

25.8: Pemphigus vulgaris. Note the suprabasal blister that forms as the basal cells lose their intercellular bridges but remain attached to the dermis, giving a "tombstone appearance." *(Courtesy, Lorenzo Cerroni, MD.)*

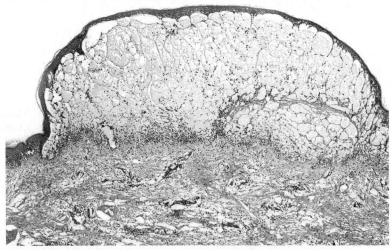

25.9: Bullous pemphigoid. *(From McKee's pathology of the skin, ed 5, © 2020, Elsevier, Fig. 4.59.)*

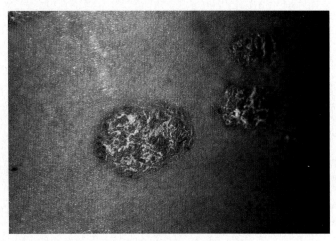

25.10: Psoriasis. *(From Andrews' diseases of the skin, ed 13, © 2020, Elsevier, Fig. 10.3.)*

D. Psoriasis
1. Definition
   a. Chronic immune-mediated skin disorder characterized by excessive proliferation of keratinocytes with cutaneous plaques and silvery scales.
2. Epidemiology
   a. Common worldwide; particularly in adults. No sex predilection.
3. Pathogenesis
   a. Complex interplay of T-lymphocytes and cytokines leading to excessive proliferation of keratinocytes.
4. Clinical manifestation
   a. Well-demarcated erythematous plaques with adherent white to silver-colored scales (Fig. 25.10); commonly involves the scalp, elbows, knees, and gluteal cleft.
   b. Auspitz sign (bleeding after the removal of psoriatic scale).
   c. Pitting of nails.
   d. Associated with arthritis in some cases ("psoriatic arthritis").

E. Pityriasis rosea
1. Definition
   a. Acute, self-limited skin disorder of older children and young adults.
2. Clinical manifestation
   a. Initially, a single round or oval, sharply delimited, pink or salmon-colored lesion on the chest, neck, or back ("herald" patch).
   b. Days or weeks later, smaller lesions appear on the trunk; long axis of lesions are perpendicular to lines of cleavage ("Christmas tree" distribution).

F. **Erythema nodosum**
  1. Definition
     a. Acute inflammatory disorder of subcutaneous fat (panniculitis).
  2. Epidemiology
     a. More common in women, especially the second to the fourth decade.
     b. Often idiopathic, sometimes seen in association with another condition (e.g., infection, sarcoidosis, and drugs).
  3. Clinical manifestation
     a. Tender, erythematous nodules on the anterior lower legs.
G. **Urticaria (hives)**
  1. Definition
     a. Localized areas of skin edema; typically, transient and self-limited.
  2. Pathogenesis
     a. Release of histamine and other mediators from mast cells in the superficial dermis (Type I HSR) causing leakage of plasma into the dermis from capillaries and small postcapillary venules.
     b. Associated with a variety of exposures (e.g., tomatoes, strawberries, insect bites, penicillin, morphine, and aspirin).
H. **Rosacea**
  1. Definition
     a. Inflammatory papules and pustules involving the central face with flushing (increased blood flow to the skin occurring spontaneously) and telangiectasia (dilated cutaneous blood vessels).
  2. Pathogenesis
     a. Unclear; proposed relationship with *Demodex* mites, immune dysfunction, and vascular hyperreactivity.
  3. Clinical manifestation
     a. Facial papules and pustules and excessive redness.
I. **Necrotizing fasciitis**
  1. Rapidly progressive (hours to a few days) necrotizing infection of the deep soft tissues with spread of infection along fascial planes.
  2. Variety of etiologic agents (often group A β-hemolytic streptococcus); may be polymicrobial.
  3. Risk factors include a breach in the skin surface (e.g., penetrating trauma and parenteral drug use), diabetes mellitus, and alcoholism.
  4. Initially erythematous, swollen, hot, and exquisitely tender (may become painless after a few days due to the destruction of superficial nerves).
  5. Nearly always fatal without prompt therapy (debridement and systemic antibiotics).

XI. **Dermal and Subcutaneous Growths**
  A. **Dermatofibroma (benign fibrous histiocytoma)**
    1. Benign proliferation of fibroblasts in dermis of unknown etiology; sometimes follows trauma or insect bites.
    2. Presents as a solitary, firm nodule, usually on the lower extremities of adults.
    3. Often asymptomatic; characteristically dimple when pinched (a key finding).
  B. **Epidermal inclusion cyst**
    1. Benign keratin-containing dermal cyst lined by stratified squamous epithelium.
    2. May arise anywhere on the body, presents as a fluctuant skin-colored dermal nodule.
    3. Usually asymptomatic, may communicate with the skin surface through a narrow opening.
    4. Potential for rupture and/or secondary infection.
    5. May be associated with Gardner syndrome.

I. **Cerebrospinal Fluid**
   A. **Produced by the choroid plexus within the ventricles of the brain (~500 mL daily).**
   B. **Total cerebrospinal fluid (CSF) volume averages 125–150 mL.**
   C. **Functions include:**
      1. Physical support and protection of the brain and spinal cord.
      2. Removal of waste products (brain lacks lymphatics).
      3. Chemical communication within the central nervous system (CNS).
   D. **Flow of CSF**
      1. Lateral ventricles → interventricular foramen of Monro → third ventricle → cerebral aqueduct → fourth ventricle (Fig. 26.1).
      2. From the fourth ventricle, CSF flows through the two lateral foramina of Luschka or the single medial foramen of Magendie into the subarachnoid space.
         a. Subarachnoid space contains CSF and blood vessels (Fig. 26.2).
      3. Resorption of CSF is by arachnoid granulations, mostly into the superior sagittal sinus.
   E. **CSF analysis**
      1. CSF is obtained by a lumbar puncture (LP); usually in the L3–L4 or the L4–L5 interspace (below the conus medullaris at L1).
         a. Primary indication for performing an LP is suspected cases of CNS infection (e.g., meningitis).
         b. May also be used, following a normal computed tomography (CT) scan, in suspected cases of subarachnoid hemorrhage (SAH).
      2. Normal CSF opening pressure is <150 mm H_2O.
         a. Elevated opening pressure signifies increased intracranial pressure (ICP) ("intracranial hypertension").
      3. CSF is normally clear but will appear cloudy (turbid) in the presence of increased cells and/or protein (e.g., inflammation and hemorrhage).
         a. Blood within the CSF may be seen with either:
            i. Traumatic tap (the most common cause); CSF clears between the first and third collection tubes.
            ii. SAH (e.g., following ruptured berry aneurysm); CSF remains bloody in all collection tubes.
         b. Inflammation of the meninges/subarachnoid space (meningitis) is characterized by an increased number of white blood cells (WBCs) within the CSF.
      4. CSF protein (normal 15–60 mg/dL)
         a. Elevated protein levels in the CSF may be seen with infectious (e.g., meningitis) as well as noninfectious (e.g., SAH) processes.
      5. CSF immunoglobulins
         a. In health, immunoglobulins are almost entirely excluded from the CSF.
         b. Specific immunoglobulin clones present within the CSF, but not in circulation, represent intrathecal production of antibodies.

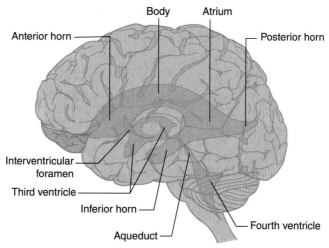

26.1: Ventricular system. *(From Nolte J: Elsevier's integrated neuroscience, St. Louis, 2007, Mosby Elsevier, p 78, Fig. 7.9.).*

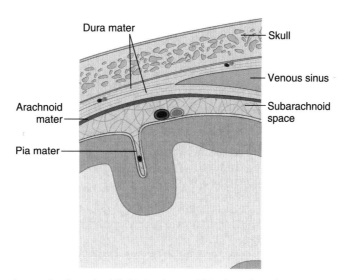

26.2: Basic arrangement of the meninges. Cerebrospinal fluid circulates within the subarachnoid space. *(From Nolte J: Elsevier's integrated neuroscience, St. Louis, 2007, Mosby Elsevier, p 73, Fig. 7.1.).*

       i. Called "oligoclonal bands."

      ii. Although nonspecific, oligoclonal bands are a characteristic finding in demyelinating disorders (e.g., multiple sclerosis [MS]).

  6. CSF glucose (normal 40–80 mg/dL)

    a. Normal CSF glucose is 60% of serum glucose concentration.

    b. Low CSF glucose (<40 mg/dL) may be caused by increased cellular uptake (e.g., neutrophils in those with bacterial meningitis).

    c. CSF glucose concentrations are usually normal in viral meningitis.

  7. CSF WBC count

    a. Normally no more than five WBC per μL (lymphocytes and monocytes).

    b. Increased WBCs in the CSF are seen with meningitis.

II. Intracranial Pressure

  A. Definition

    1. Pressure within the cranial cavity (normally <20 mm Hg).

    2. Intracranial contents include the brain, CSF, and blood.

    3. Intracranial volume is fixed; therefore, an increase in the volume of one component must be accompanied by a decrease in the volume of another component, otherwise, ICP will rise ("intracranial hypertension").

  B. Etiologies of intracranial hypertension (↑ ICP)

    1. Cerebral edema

a. Increased fluid in the brain; may be secondary to a variety of brain disorders (e.g., infection, tumor, stroke, and trauma).
b. Vasogenic edema (increased extracellular fluid)
i. Due to increased vascular permeability (i.e., "leaky vessels").
ii. May be localized (e.g., trauma and tumor) or generalized (e.g., encephalitis).
c. Cytotoxic edema (increased intracellular fluid)
i. Occurs when there is an osmotic shift of fluid into cells (e.g., severe hyponatremia) or when energy-requiring membrane pumps (Na^+/K^+-ATPase) fail (e.g., cerebral ischemia).
2. Increased CSF volume (hydrocephalus, see later discussion).
3. Increased cerebral blood volume
a. Due to either an increase in cerebral blood flow (e.g., hypercarbia-induced cerebral vasculature dilatation) and/or impaired venous outflow (e.g., venous sinus thrombosis or heart failure).
4. Intracranial mass lesions
a. Tumor, hematoma, and abscess.
5. Idiopathic intracranial hypertension (pseudotumor cerebri)
a. Syndrome of increased ICP (headache, papilledema, and visual changes) in the absence of an identifiable lesion.
b. Primarily seen in overweight females of childbearing age.
c. Pathogenesis is unknown, risk factors include obesity, growth hormone therapy, and excessive vitamin A.
C. **Manifestations of intracranial hypertension**
1. Flattening of gyri, narrowing of sulci, and ventricular compression (Fig. 26.3A).
2. Papilledema (swelling of the optic disk, see Fig. 26.3B).
3. Headache, vomiting, and depressed consciousness.
4. Bradycardia, respiratory depression, and hypertension (Cushing triad).
5. Herniation.
III. **Herniation**
A. **Definition**
1. Displacement of brain tissue across dural partitions (e.g., under the falx cerebri and across tentorium cerebelli) or openings in the skull (foramen magnum) due to elevated ICP (Fig. 26.4).
B. **Types**
1. Subfalcine herniation
a. Herniation of the cingulate gyrus under the falx cerebri.
b. May compress the anterior cerebral artery causing ischemic injury and associated clinical manifestations (e.g., contralateral lower leg weakness and urinary incontinence).
2. Transtentorial (uncal) herniation
a. Herniation of the medial temporal lobe (including the uncus) medially over the edge of the tentorium cerebelli.
b. Compression of ipsilateral third cranial (oculomotor) nerve causes pupillary dilation and impaired ocular movement (ipsilateral "down and out" eye).
c. Potential for compression of the posterior cerebral artery with associated tissue ischemia (e.g., visual field deficits).
3. Tonsillar herniation
a. Herniation of cerebellar tonsils through the foramen magnum.
b. Compression of medullary cardiac and respiratory centers results in death.
c. Downward displacement of brainstem tears penetrating arteries, causing hemorrhage within the midbrain and pons ("Duret hemorrhages").

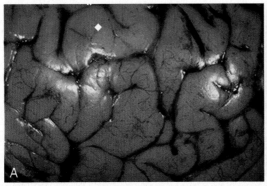
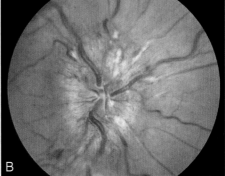

26.3: (A Cerebral edema. Note the widening and flattening of the gyri and the narrowing of the sulci. B. Optic disk with papilledema showing loss of the disk margin and hard exudates (*white streaks*). (A, *From Klatt E:* Robbins and Cotran atlas of pathology, *Philadelphia, 2006, Saunders, p 449, Fig. 19-11; B, from Perkin GD:* Mosby's color atlas and text of neurology, *St. Louis, 2002, Mosby, p 160, Fig. 9.4.)*

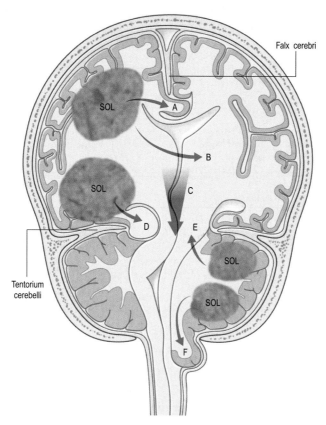

A Cingulate herniation under falx, potential anterior cerebral artery damage
B Herniation into opposite hemisphere, potential decorticate posturing
C Transtentorial or central herniation, potential decerebrate posturing, somnolence
D Uncal/parahippocampal gyrus herniation, pupillary signs, hemiparesis, somnolence, stupor
E Upward cerebellar herniation, increased intracranial pressure, hydrocephalus, impaired upward gaze
F Tonsillar herniation, potential cardiac and respiratory arrest

26.4: Herniation patterns. See text for further explanation. *SOL*, Space-occupying lesion. *(From Gray's anatomy, ed 42, © 2021, Elsevier, Fig. 28.23.)*

IV. Hydrocephalus
A. Definition
1. Excessive CSF accumulation causing ventricular dilation.
B. Types
1. Communicating hydrocephalus
   a. Pathogenesis
      i. Impaired CSF resorption, usually secondary to scarring of arachnoid granulations (e.g., SAH or meningitis).
      ii. Overproduction of CSF (by choroid plexus tumor, rare).
   b. Ventricles and subarachnoid space remain in open communication with one another (i.e., no intraventricular obstruction); all ventricles are enlarged.
2. Noncommunicating hydrocephalus
   a. Pathogenesis
      i. Obstruction to CSF flow, causes accumulation of CSF, and ventricular dilatation behind the obstruction (Fig. 26.5).
   b. Etiologies
      i. Disruption of ventricular anatomy by mass
         (1) As an example, tumors near the cerebral aqueduct may cause enlargement of the lateral and third ventricles (upstream to the obstruction) while the fourth ventricle (downstream) remains normal.
      ii. Impaired CSF flow secondary to scarring at the base of the brain (characteristic of tuberculous meningitis).
3. Hydrocephalus ex vacuo
   a. Dilated ventricles secondary to cerebral atrophy (e.g., advanced Alzheimer disease [AD]).
C. In infancy, prior to the closure of the cranial sutures, hydrocephalus is associated with an increased head circumference.

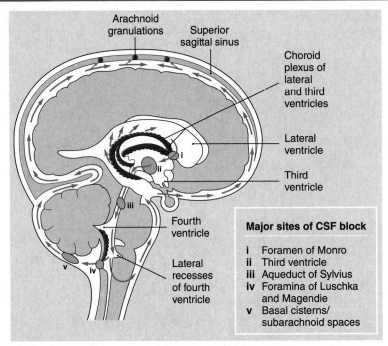

Major sites of CSF block

i   Foramen of Monro
ii Third ventricle
iii Aqueduct of Sylvius
iv Foramina of Luschka
    and Magendie
v   Basal cisterns/
    subarachnoid spaces

26.5: Diagram showing the normal cerebrospinal fluid (CSF) pathways and indicating the principal sites of obstruction (*blue circles*) in hydrocephalus. *(From Ellison D, Love S, Cardao Chimelli LM, et al: Neuropathology: a reference text of CNS pathology, ed 3, St. Louis, 2013, Mosby Elsevier, p 120, Fig. 4.3.)*

D.   Conversely, once the cranial sutures have fused, the ventricles dilate and ICPs rise (head circumference does not change).

V.   **Malformations and Developmental Disorders**

A.   **Neural tube defects (NTDs)**

1.   Midline malformation involving a combination of neural tissue, meninges, and overlying bone or soft tissue.
2.   Major risk factor is maternal folate deficiency.
3.   Prenatal screening for NTD
     a.   Ultrasound (best).
     b.   Elevated maternal serum alpha-fetoprotein (MSAFP).
4.   Types of open NTDs (Fig. 26.6)
     a.   Anencephaly
          i.   Malformation of the anterior neural tube with an opening in the calvaria and skin.
          ii. Brain is absent/maldeveloped (incompatible with survival).
          iii. Polyhydramnios (excess amniotic fluid) is seen due to the inability to swallow.
     b.   Spina bifida occulta
          i.   Defect in the closure of the posterior vertebral arch (bony defect).
          ii. May be accompanied by a dimple or tuft of hair in the skin overlying the lumbosacral spine. No increase in MSAFP.
     c.   Meningocele
          i.   Open NTD with protrusion of meninges through the bony defect, usually within the lumbosacral region. Increased MSAFP.
     d.   Myelomeningocele
          i.   Open NTD in which both meninges and neural tissue of the spinal cord herniate through the bony defect.
          ii. Typically, seen in the lumbosacral region; associated with motor and sensory deficits of lower extremities, impaired bowel, and bladder control. Increased MSAFP.
     e.   Encephalocele

Normal pressure hydrocephalus (NPH)

- Pathologically enlarged ventricles in the presence of normal CSF pressure.
- Clinical manifestations include urinary incontinence, dementia, and gait ataxia ("wet, wacky, and wobbly").
- Potentially reversible cause of dementia, most commonly idiopathic (50%).
- Imaging (MRI) shows ventricular enlargement in the absence of, or out of proportion to, sulcal enlargement with no evidence of obstruction.
- Treatment with ventricular shunting, usually into the peritoneum (called ventriculoperitoneal shunt).

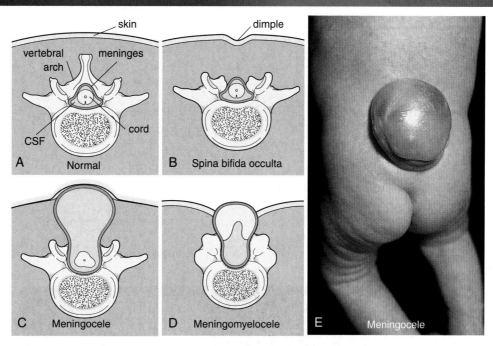

26.6: Spinal neural tube defects. (A) Normal. (B) Spina bifida occulta. (C) Meningocele. (D) Meningomyelocele. (E) Meningocele in a newborn child. *CSF,* Cerebrospinal fluid. *(From Stevens A, Lowe J, Scott I: Core pathology, ed 3, St. Louis, 2009, Mosby Elsevier, p 477, Fig. 21.38.)*

     i. Protrusion of the brain and/or meninges through a defect in the skull (usually in the occiput region); covered with skin.
- **B. Chiari malformations**
  1. Chiari I malformation
     a. Characterized by abnormally shaped cerebellar tonsils that extend down below the level of the foramen magnum.
     b. May be asymptomatic; however, symptoms arise if/when CSF flow is impaired. Increased risk of syringomyelia (see later).
  2. Chiari II malformation (Arnold–Chiari malformation)
     a. Severe condition characterized by a small posterior fossa with downward displacement of the cerebellar vermis and brainstem with associated hydrocephalus.
     b. Most patients have coexisting myelomeningocele.
     c. Risk of brainstem compression and associated respiratory failure.
- **C. Dandy–Walker malformation**
  1. Developmental anomaly of the cerebellar vermis (agenesis or hypoplasia) accompanied by cystic dilatation of the fourth ventricle and enlargement of the posterior fossa.
- **D. Syringomyelia**
  1. Fluid-filled cavity (syrinx) within the spinal cord, usually within the cervical/thoracic region (C2–T9).
  2. Most commonly found in association with the Chiari malformation; other etiologies include spinal trauma or neoplasms.
  3. Manifestations include loss of pain and temperature sensation in a "cape-like" distribution across the shoulders, upper torso, and arms.
  4. Imaging (magnetic resonance imaging [MRI]) reveals enlarged cervical cord with central cystic cavity.
- **VI. Traumatic Injuries (Fig. 26.7)**
  - **A. Cerebral contusion**
    1. Analogous to a bruise, due to blunt force trauma.
    2. *Coup* injuries occur at the site of the impact.
    3. *Contrecoup* injury occurs on the side of the brain opposite the site of impact.
  - **B. Epidural hematoma**
    1. Definition
       a. Arterial bleed into the potential space between the dura and skull.
    2. Mechanism
       a. Fracture of the temporal bone with tearing of the middle meningeal artery; often follows a blow to the side of the head (e.g., baseball bat, hammer, etc.).
    3. Clinical findings
       a. Classic presentation is a transient loss of consciousness, followed by a "lucid interval" of minutes to hours, before lapsing into a coma as hematoma volume and ICP rise.

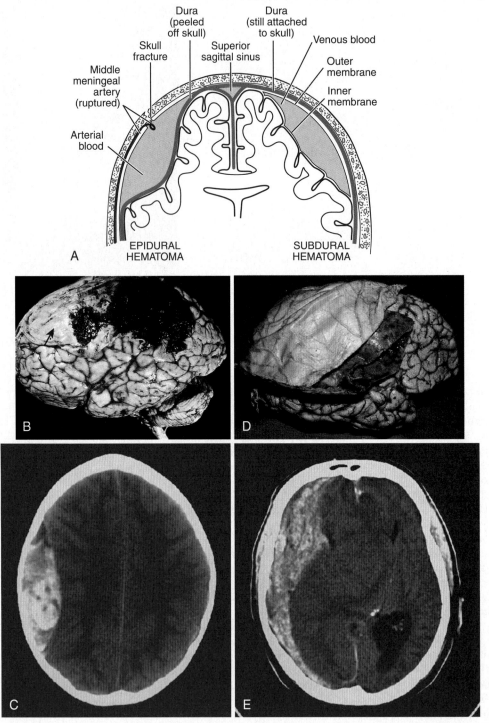

26.7: (A) Schematic of epidural hematoma (*left side*) and subdural hematoma (*right side*). (B) Epidural hematoma. Note the blood is located on top of the dura (*arrow*). (C) Noncontrast computed tomography (CT) scan of an acute epidural hematoma with mass effect and midline shift. (D) Subdural hematoma. The reflected dura shows the outer membrane of an organized venous clot covering the convexity of the brain. (E) Noncontrast CT scan of a right temporal subdural hematoma with a massive midline shift right to left. The right lateral ventricle has been obliterated. (A, *From Kumar V, Abbas AK, Fausto N, Mitchell RN:* Robbins basic pathology, *ed 8, Philadelphia, 2007, Saunders Elsevier, p 871, Fig. 23-13A; B, courtesy of Dr. Raymond D. Adams, Massachusetts General Hospital, Boston; C, and E from Marx J:* Rosen's emergency medicine concepts and clinical practice, *ed 7, Philadelphia, 2010, Mosby Elsevier, pp 306, 320, respectively, Figs. 38.7 and 38.9, respectively; D, from Ivan Damjanov, MD, PhD, Linder J:* Pathology: a color atlas, *St. Louis, 2000, Mosby, p 405, Fig. 19.20.)*

    4. Diagnosis
       a. Noncontrast CT of the head
          i. Lens-shaped bleed at the periphery of the brain (Fig. 26.7C); blood does not cross suture lines.
    5. Treatment is a surgical evacuation of the hematoma.

C. **Subdural hematoma**
1. Definition
   a. Collection of blood within the potential space between the dura and arachnoid.
2. Mechanism
   a. Tearing of bridging veins between the brain and dural sinuses.
   b. Since the bleed is of venous origin, blood accumulates slowly over the convexity of the brain.
   c. Most commonly follows head trauma (e.g., motor vehicle accidents or falls).
3. Risk factors
   a. Cerebral atrophy
      i. Atrophy of the brain, characteristically seen in older adults or alcoholics, causes excessive traction on bridging veins (making them prone to rupture).
   b. Infants
      i. "Shaken baby syndrome" where the back-and-forth movement of the child's head causes tearing of bridging veins.
4. Clinical manifestations
   a. Onset varies; depends on the severity of the bleed.
   b. In severe cases, patients may develop an acute loss of consciousness.
   c. With less severe bleeding, patients may have delayed onset of ataxia, headache, cognitive changes (days to weeks after traumatic event).
5. Diagnosis:
   a. Noncontrast CT of the head shows a crescent-shaped collection of blood over cerebral convexity.

Imaging of brain bleeds

- Noncontrast CT is a useful and rapid method of identifying brain bleeds.
- Over time, as the hemoglobin degrades, the radiologic appearance changes.
- Acute bleeds are hyperdense (bright white), becoming less dense over time.
- Hyperdense → isodense → hypodense.

VII. **Cerebrovascular Disease**
A. **Overview**
1. Brain injury secondary to cerebral hypoxia occurring in a setting of altered blood flow (may be localized or generalized).
B. **Pathophysiology**
1. Lack of adequate blood flow (ischemia) reduces the amount of oxygen delivered to the brain and thus the amount of energy (adenosine triphosphate [ATP]) generated.
   a. As energy-dependent ion pumps (Na^+, K^+-ATPase) fail, intracellular sodium levels rise. Causes an osmotic shift of fluid into cells (cell swelling).
   b. Reduced protein synthesis.
   c. Excessive release of excitatory neurotransmitters (e.g., glutamate), causing "excitotoxicity."
      i. Unregulated opening of calcium channels allows the influx of calcium, activating various destructive enzymes (proteases, lipases, and endonucleases), and increasing the generation of free radicals.
2. The net result is cell injury/death.
   a. Hypoglycemia has similar effects (neurons are highly dependent upon glucose as an energy source).
C. **Complications**
1. Cerebral atrophy
   a. Neurons are more susceptible to ischemia/hypoxia than other cells within the CNS.
   b. Ischemic neurons appear red within about 12–24 hours after the event ("dead reds"); see Fig. 26.8.
   c. Regions of the brain most prone to ischemia:
      i. CA1 sector of the hippocampus.
      ii. Purkinje cells of the cerebellum.
      iii. Third and fifth layers of the cortex (laminar necrosis).
      iv. Watershed zones (regions near the junctions of arterial territories).
         (1) For example, just lateral to the interhemispheric fissure is a watershed zone between the vascular territories of the anterior cerebral and middle cerebral arteries (Fig. 26.9).
2. Stroke
   a. Definition
      i. Focal disturbance of blood flow into or out of the brain resulting in either tissue ischemia or hemorrhage.
   b. Epidemiology
      i. Incidence increases with age, more common in men.
      ii. Ischemic strokes are far more common (~87%) than hemorrhagic strokes (~13%).

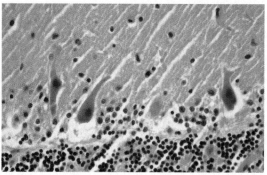

26.8: Hypoxic change in cerebral Purkinje cells. High-power view of showing eosinophilic Purkinje cells in the cerebellum. *(From Ellison D, Love S, Cardao Chimelli LM, et al: Neuropathology: a reference text of CNS pathology, ed 3, St. Louis, 2013, Mosby Elsevier, p 177, Fig. 8.8d.)*

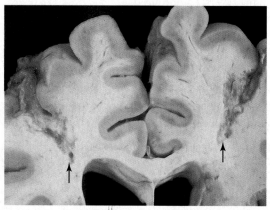

26.9: Watershed infarct. Asymmetric anterior cerebral artery–middle cerebral artery watershed zone infarcts *(arrows)*, with wedge-shaped areas of old necrosis extending from cortex into deep white matter. *(From Ellison D, Love S, Cardao Chimelli LM, et al: Neuropathology: a reference text of CNS pathology, ed 3, St. Louis, 2013, Mosby Elsevier, p 228, Fig. 9.64a.)*

   c. Risk factors
     i.   Increasing age (half of all strokes arise after the age of 75 years).
     ii. Systemic hypertension.
     iii. History of a previous stroke.
     iv. Smoking.
     v.   Atherosclerotic vascular disease.
     vi. Atrial fibrillation (embolic stroke).
     vii. Use of illicit drugs (e.g., cocaine).
     viii. Hypercoagulable states (e.g., antiphospholipid syndrome).
   d. Ischemic stroke
     i.   Cell death within the brain or spinal cord due to a reduction in blood flow (↓ delivery of oxygen and other nutrients).
     ii. Causes of ischemia include:
       (1) Thrombosis
          (a) Blood clots commonly develop in relation to atherosclerotic plaque rupture; cause pale infarction (no reperfusion).
       (2) Emboli
          (a) Most emboli originate from the left side of the heart, usually in association with a predisposing condition (e.g., atrial fibrillation or reduced myocardial contractility).
          (b) Other sources of emboli include fragments of atherosclerotic plaque ("atheroemboli"), fat (following traumatic bone fracture), and air (e.g., decompression sickness).
          (c) "Paradoxical" emboli refer to venous thrombi that have crossed into the arterial system via a right-to-left shunt (e.g., patent foramen ovale, atrial septal defect).
          (d) Emboli most commonly lodge within the distribution of the middle cerebral artery (MCA).
          (e) Embolic infarcts are initially pale; however, lysis of the clot may be followed by secondary hemorrhage into the ischemic region.
          (f) Clinical manifestations of embolic strokes are maximal from the onset (i.e., not progressive).

(3) Small vessel strokes
    (a) Small (<1 cm) infarcts with secondary cyst formation ("lacunar infarcts").
    (b) Often deep within the brain parenchyma (e.g., basal ganglia).
    (c) Caused by narrowing of small blood vessels by hyaline arteriolosclerosis, usually in association with chronic hypertension or diabetes mellitus.
iii. Pathology
    (1) Ischemic neurons become eosinophilic (red) by about 12–24 hours after the infarct.
    (2) Neutrophils are the predominant inflammatory cell initially, becoming very prominent by about 2–3 days after the infarct.
    (3) By days 5–7, macrophages become the most prominent cell type. As the necrotic cellular debris is slowly phagocytosed over a period of weeks, a cystic cavity forms at the site due to liquefactive necrosis.
    (4) Fibrosis, as seen elsewhere following tissue injury, does not occur due to the lack of fibroblasts within the brain.
e. Hemorrhagic stroke
  i. Intracerebral hemorrhage
    (1) Definition
      (a) Bleed into the brain parenchyma.
    (2) Manifestations
      (a) Altered consciousness, nausea, vomiting, headache, seizures, and focal neurological deficits.
      (b) Potential for herniation secondary to elevated ICP.
    (3) Etiologies
      (a) Hypertension (the most common cause).
        • High pressures weaken small blood vessels, forming so-called "Charcot–Bouchard" microaneurysms.
        • Most susceptible are those vessels that branch at 90 degrees off the feeding vessel.
        • Commonly affects lenticulostriate vessels that branch off the MCA, with bleeding into the basal ganglia.
      (b) Cerebral amyloid angiopathy (CAA)
        • Less common, older individuals.
        • Due to the deposition of β-amyloid within walls of small- to medium-sized arteries within the cortex and leptomeninges (causes vessels to become fragile and prone to rupture).
        • Results in "lobar hemorrhage" (i.e., cortical, subcortical).
  ii. SAH
    (1) Definition
      (a) Hemorrhage into the subarachnoid space.
    (2) Mechanism
      (a) Usually secondary to a ruptured saccular (berry) aneurysm.
      (b) Although not present at birth, these aneurysms are believed to be a developmental anomaly (i.e., lack of internal elastic lamina and smooth muscle), usually at branch points around the Circle of Willis (Fig. 26.10).
      (c) Rupture of the aneurysm causes hemorrhage into the subarachnoid space.
      (d) Increased incidence with hypertension, autosomal dominant polycystic kidney disease.
    (3) Pathology
      (a) Blood on the surface of the brain.

• SAHs classically present with the abrupt onset of a severe headache ("worst ever") and other manifestations (e.g., neck stiffness, cranial nerve palsies, confusion, syncope, and coma).

    (4) Complications
      (a) Rebleeding (often within the first 24 hours).
      (b) Hydrocephalus (blood impedes the resorption of CSF and/or obstructs the flow of CSF).
      (c) Vasospasm (blood within CSF is irritating to blood vessels, may cause secondary ischemic injury).
  iii. Arteriovenous malformation (AVM)
    (1) AVMs are comprised of enlarged aberrant vascular channels with intervening gliotic brain tissue.
    (2) Rupture leads to intracerebral and/or SAH.
f. Stroke diagnosis
  i. CT scan without contrast
    (1) Best first test because it can be performed in a timely fashion; distinguishes between ischemic and hemorrhagic strokes.

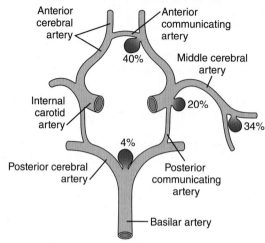

26.10: Schematic of locations of saccular (*berry*) aneurysms in the circle of Willis. *(From Kumar V, Abbas AK, Fausto N, Mitchell RN: Robbins basic pathology, ed 8, Philadelphia, 2007, Saunders Elsevier, p 867, Fig. 23-9.)*

VIII. Central Nervous System Infections
A. Overview
1. Infection of the CNS (brain and spinal cord) can cause cellular injury either directly or indirectly via the host immune response.
2. Routes of transmission
   a. Hematogenous dissemination (most common).
   b. Direct implantation (e.g., penetrating trauma).
   c. Extension from the adjacent infection (e.g., sinusitis or otitis media).
   d. Ascending via peripheral nerves (e.g., rabies and herpes).
B. Meningitis
1. Definition
   a. Inflammation of the meninges (pia-arachnoid) and CSF.
2. Risk factors
   a. Extremes of age (children <1 year; adults >60 years).
   b. Immunosuppression (e.g., congenital immunodeficiency states, human immunodeficiency virus, and organ transplantation).
   c. Crowded living conditions (e.g., prisons, college dormitories, and military barracks).
   d. Underlying illness (e.g., diabetes mellitus, chronic kidney disease, chronic liver disease, and alcoholism).
   e. Splenic dysfunction (e.g., sickle cell anemia, postsplenectomy).
3. Clinical manifestations
   a. Fever, headache, nuchal rigidity, and reduced level of consciousness (e.g., drowsiness).
   b. Kernig sign: resistance to passive knee extension following hip flexion to 90 degrees.
   c. Brudzinski sign: hip or knee flexion following passive neck flexion.
4. Pathogens by age
   a. Newborns
      i. Group B *Streptococcus* and *Escherichia coli*.
   b. Older infants and children:
      i. *Streptococcus pneumoniae* and *Neisseria meningitides*.
   c. Teens and young adults
      i. *N. meningitidis* and *S. pneumoniae*.
   d. Older adults
      i. *S. pneumoniae*, *N. meningitidis*, and *Listeria monocytogenes*.
5. Complications
   a. Seizures (focal or generalized).
   b. Cerebral edema and increased ICP.
   c. Focal neurologic deficits (e.g., cranial nerve palsies).
   d. Sensorineural hearing loss.
   e. Hydrocephalus.
6. CSF findings
   a. Viral meningitis
      i. Increased protein, increased WBC count (neutrophils early, predominantly lymphocytes by 24 hours), and normal glucose.
   b. Bacterial meningitis

   i. Increased protein, increased WBC count (neutrophil predominant), and decreased glucose.

  c. Fungal meningitis

   i. Increased protein, increased WBC count (lymphocyte predominant), and decreased glucose.

  d. *Mycobacterium tuberculosis* meningitis

   i. Increased protein, increased WBC count (lymphocyte predominant), and decreased glucose.

C. Encephalitis

 1. Definition

  a. Inflammation of the brain parenchyma; commonly secondary to viral infection.

   i. Arboviruses (e.g., West Nile virus, Eastern equine, Western equine, and St. Louis encephalitis).

    (1) Summer months (when mosquitoes are active).

    (2) West Nile most common in the United States, can also cause an acute flaccid paralysis syndrome similar to that seen with poliovirus.

  b. Clinical manifestations

   i. Fever, headache, focal or diffuse neurologic deficits, impaired cognition/arousal, disorientation, and behavioral changes.

  c. Complications

   i. Seizures, coma, and increased ICP.

D. Cerebral abscess

 1. Definition

  a. Focal space-occupying infection by bacterial (most common), fungal, or parasitic organisms.

 2. Pathogenesis

  a. Hematogenous dissemination from a distant site (e.g., pneumonia or endocarditis).

  b. Direct extension from an adjacent infection (e.g., sinusitis, otitis media, mastoiditis).

 3. Clinical manifestations

  a. Headache, fever, focal neurologic deficits (depending upon the site of abscess), and seizures.

  b. Signs and symptoms associated with the elevated ICP (e.g., nausea, vomiting, and papilledema).

IX. Demyelinating Disorders

 A. Multiple sclerosis (MS)

  1. Definition

   a. Immune-mediated inflammatory disease of the CNS causing a loss of myelin (and axons to a variable degree).

  2. Epidemiology

   a. Female > male (2:1).

   b. Onset usually between 15 and 45 years of age (mean 30 years).

  3. Pathology

   a. Demyelinating plaques in the white matter of the brain and/or spinal cord (Fig. 26.11).

   b. Active plaques contain mostly CD4 helper T cells.

   c. Damage thought secondary to cytokines released from Th1 (interferon-γ) and Th17 (IL-17 and TNFα) cells.

  4. Clinical variants

   a. "Relapsing, remitting" MS: each episode followed by partial to complete recovery.

   b. "Secondary progressive" MS: describes accumulating neurologic deficits following an initial period of relapsing and remitting disease.

   c. "Primary progressive" MS: uncommon type, characterized by progressive deficits from the outset without periods of remission.

  5. Clinical manifestations

   a. Vary according to the site of demyelination.

    i. Fatigue, weakness, visual changes, sensory loss, and ataxia.

    ii. Lhermitte sign—electric shock-like sensation running down the back and/or limbs following neck flexion.

    iii. Upper motor neuron dysfunction

     (1) Exaggerated deep tendon reflexes (DTRs).

     (2) Extensor plantar response (positive Babinski).

    iv. Autonomic dysfunction

Herpes simplex virus (HSV) encephalitis

- Most cases are associated with HSV-1, often secondary to reactivation of latent infection.
- Most common identified cause of sporadic fatal encephalitis.
- Characteristically causes hemorrhage and necrosis, primarily of the medial temporal and inferior frontal lobes.
- Presents with fever, headache, altered consciousness, personality changes, seizures, memory disturbances, aphasia, and motor deficits.
- Diagnosis depends on CSF examination (polymerase chain reaction assay).
- High morbidity and mortality, even with treatment (acyclovir).
- Histology reveals "Cowdry A" intranuclear inclusions.

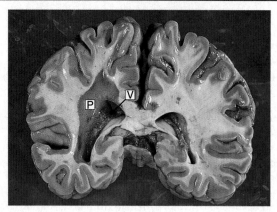

26.11: Multiple sclerosis. A large plaque (P) is seen adjacent to the lateral ventricle (V). Histologically, areas of myelin loss would be apparent on myelin stains. *(From Stevens A, Lowe J, Scott I: Core pathology, ed 3, St. Louis, 2009, Mosby Elsevier, p 470, Fig. 21.28.)*

            (1) Bladder and/or bowel problems, sexual dysfunction.
      v. Optic neuritis
            (1) Inflammation of the optic nerve.
            (2) Common initial manifestation of MS; causes blurry vision and pain with movement or palpation of globe.
      vi. Bilateral internuclear ophthalmoplegia
            (1) Impaired horizontal eye movements; due to demyelination of the medial longitudinal fasciculus.
   6. Laboratory and radiologic findings
     a. CSF WBC count often increased (primarily T lymphocytes).
     b. CSF protein may be increased (increased immunoglobulins).
     c. Presence of oligoclonal bands.
     d. Evidence of demyelination on MRI.
   7. Diagnosis
     a. MRI with gadolinium (the most sensitive test).
     b. LP in equivocal cases to exclude infectious and/or neoplastic processes.
   8. Prognosis varies greatly.
  B. Osmotic demyelination syndrome
   1. Definition
     a. Disorder of central demyelination occurring as a complication of too rapid correction of severe and prolonged hyponatremia. Often affects the pons, thus the alternative moniker of "central pontine myelinolysis."
   2. Pathogenesis
     a. Hyponatremia-induced decrease in serum tonicity causes the movement of water into cells (cytotoxic edema).
     b. Over a period of 2–3 days, the brain adapts to the change in tonicity. Afterward, sudden changes in osmolality (e.g., rapid correction of hyponatremia) cause an efflux of water out of the cells and demyelination.
   3. Clinical manifestations
     a. Generalized encephalopathy with behavioral changes, cranial nerve palsies, and progressive weakness.
     b. Potential for the development of quadriplegia and the "locked-in" syndrome.
  C. Leukodystrophies
   1. Adrenoleukodystrophy
     a. X-linked disorder due to loss-of-function mutation in the *ABCD1* gene (encodes for a transport protein necessary for the transport of fatty acids into peroxisomes).
     b. Results in an inability to catabolize very long-chain fatty acids and a generalized loss of myelin in the brain as well as adrenocortical insufficiency.
   2. Metachromatic leukodystrophy
     a. Autosomal recessive; due to a deficiency of the lysosomal enzyme, arylsulfatase A.
     b. Causes demyelination due to the accumulation of toxic sulfatides.
     c. Manifestations, which begin in childhood, include gait abnormalities, seizures, ataxia, hypotonia, and ultimately death.
   3. Krabbe disease (globoid cell leukodystrophy)
     a. Autosomal recessive; due to a deficiency of galactocerebroside β-galactocerebrosidase.
     b. Results in the accumulation of galactocerebroside which is then catabolized to galactosylsphingosine, a toxic compound causing demyelination of the central and peripheral nervous system.
     c. Muscle stiffness and weakness by 3–6 months; death during early childhood.
X. Neurodegenerative Disorders
  A. Alzheimer disease (AD)
   1. Definition

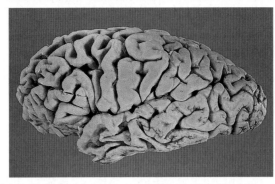

26.12: Alzheimer's disease. Lateral view shows severe atrophy of the temporal lobe with less severe atrophy of the parietal and frontal lobes. Note enlargement of the sulci between the atrophied gyri. The occipital lobe is spared. *(From Ellison D, Love S, Cardao Chimelli LM, et al: Neuropathology: a reference text of CNS pathology, ed 3, St. Louis, 2013, Mosby Elsevier, p 611, Fig. 31.2a.)*

      a. Neurodegenerative disease characterized by a progressive loss of memory, judgement, language, problem solving, and other cognitive skills.
2. Epidemiology
      a. Most common cause of dementia; primarily affecting older adults (>65 years).
      b. Uncommon before the age of 60 years except in rare inherited cases.
      c. Familial cases may begin in the fifth decade; mutations include:
         i. Amyloid precursor protein (*APP*)
         ii. Presenilin 1 (*PSEN1*)
         iii. Presenilin 2 (*PSEN2*)
      d. Down syndrome (trisomy 21) strongly associated with AD.
         i. *APP* gene located on chromosome 21.
         ii. Essentially all patients develop early onset AD.
3. Pathogenesis
      a. Neuronal degeneration begins within medial temporal lobes (especially the entorhinal cortex and hippocampus), later involving other regions of the cerebral cortex.
      b. Characteristic abnormal protein aggregates
         i. Amyloid plaques (beta-amyloid [Aβ] peptides)
           (1) Aβ formed from the proteolytic cleavage of APP.
           (2) ApoE ε4 allele promotes the generation and deposition of Aβ (increasing one's risk of AD).
         ii. Neurofibrillary tangles (hyperphosphorylated tau protein).
4. Pathology
      a. Cerebral atrophy (Fig. 26.12), eventually causing ventricular dilatation (*hydrocephalus ex vacuo*) due to the loss of neurons in the temporal, frontal, and parietal lobes.
      b. Histologic findings
         i. Neurofibrillary tangles (Fig. 26.13A) comprised of hyperphosphorylated tau.
         ii. Neuritic (senile) plaques (Fig. 26.13B) comprised of Aβ.
         iii. Note that neither are specific for AD as each may be found, albeit to a lesser degree, in otherwise normal older adults.
5. Clinical manifestations
      a. Patients initially have a loss of memory for recent events.
      b. Over time, deficits involve other cognitive domains; causing changes in behavior, judgment, language, and abstract thought.
      c. Eventually, patients lose the ability for self-care, become bedridden, and die (usually ~10 years after diagnosis).
      d. High incidence of associated CAA
         i. β-Amyloid deposits within the walls of small- and medium-sized arteries of the cortex and leptomeninges; risk of lobar hemorrhages (see previous discussion).
6. Diagnosis
      a. Presumptive diagnosis with mental status testing and exclusion of other causes of dementia.
      b. Neuroimaging with amyloid and tau positron emission tomography are newer techniques used in research settings.
      c. Historically, the examination of brain at autopsy was required for the confirmation of diagnosis.
B. Parkinson disease
1. Definition
      a. Progressive neurodegenerative movement disorder.
2. Epidemiology
      a. Affects ~1% of older adults, beginning at an average age of ~60 years, slight male predominance.

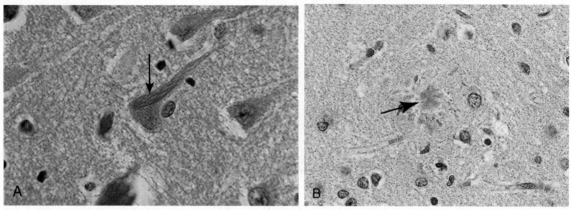

26.13: (A) Neurofibrillary tangle (NFT). The stain shows a neuron with neurofilaments (*arrow*) composed of hyperphosphorylated tau protein. These are present in Alzheimer disease (AD). (B) Senile plaque (*arrow*) shows an eosinophilic center with peripherally located distended neuronal processes (neurites). Similar to NFTs, these are present in AD. (*A, From Klatt E:* Robbins and Cotran atlas of pathology, *Philadelphia, 2006, Saunders, p 481, Fig. 19-110; B, from Burger PC, Scheithauer BW, Vogel KS:* Surgical pathology of the nervous system, *ed 4, London, 2002, Churchill Livingstone, p 428, Fig. 8.9.)*

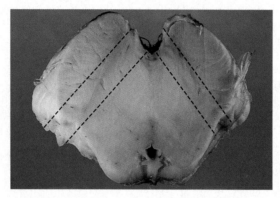

26.14: Parkinson disease. In this section through the midbrain, pigmented neurons have been lost from the substantia nigra (*between the lines*), which is abnormally pale. *(From Stevens A, Lowe J, Scott I:* Core pathology, *ed 3, St. Louis, 2009, Mosby Elsevier, p 472, Fig. 21.30.)*

    3. Pathogenesis
       a. Degeneration of dopaminergic neurons in the substantia nigra pars compacta (Fig. 26.14) due to unclear mechanisms (theorized to involve mitochondrial dysfunction, oxidative stress, and abnormal protein processing).
       b. Neuronal aggregates of α-synuclein (called "Lewy bodies").
    4. Clinical manifestations
       a. Cardinal manifestations (unilateral initially, becoming bilateral and worse with time)
         i. Resting tremor ("pill rolling").
         ii. Muscle rigidity/stiffness.
         iii. Bradykinesia (slowed voluntary muscle movement).
       b. Other
         i. Visual hallucinations.
         ii. Rapid eye movement (REM) sleep behavior disorder ("acting out one's dreams").
         iii. Lack of facial expression ("masked facies").
         iv. Stooped posture, difficulty initiating movement.
         v. Autonomic dysfunction (e.g., erectile dysfunction, constipation, urinary frequency, and orthostatic hypotension).
         vi. Dementia in some cases.
    5. Diagnosis
       a. Characteristic history and physical examination findings in conjunction with clinical improvement following dopaminergic therapy.
  C. Dementia with Lewy bodies
    1. Neurodegenerative disorder characterized by dementia along with parkinsonism.
    2. Key distinguishing features include the presence of recurrent vivid visual hallucinations and REM sleep behavior disorder (along with presence of Lewy bodies on pathologic exam).
    3. Male predominant, average age onset 75 years.

D. Huntington disease (HD)
   1. Definition
      a. Autosomal dominant neurodegenerative disorder characterized by the triad of chorea (dance-like involuntary movements), cognitive changes, and psychiatric disturbances.
   2. Pathogenesis
      a. CAG (trinucleotide) repeat expansion in exon 1 of the huntingtin gene (*HTT*).
         i. Greater than or equal to 36 CAG repeats are diagnostic.
         ii. Age of onset inversely related to the number of CAG repeats (increased repeats = earlier onset).
      b. Mutant huntingtin protein causes neuronal cell loss and atrophy of the caudate and putamen (mechanism unclear).
   3. Clinical manifestations
      a. Usually presents by the middle age with chorea (irregular, rapid, and nonstereotyped involuntary movements).
      b. Cognitive changes (e.g., diminished ability to make decisions and decreased ability to multitask).
      c. Psychiatric manifestations (e.g., depression and irritability).
      d. Death within ~15 years of symptom onset.
   4. Diagnosis
      a. Genetic testing.
      b. Imaging studies show atrophy of the caudate and putamen.

E. Friedreich ataxia
   1. Definition
      a. Autosomal recessive disorder characterized by ataxia, cardiomyopathy, and, in some cases, diabetes mellitus.
   2. Pathogenesis
      a. GAA trinucleotide repeat in *FXN* gene (encodes for frataxin, a mitochondrial protein involved in iron transport).
      b. Reduced levels of frataxin → degenerative changes of the spinal cord, peripheral nerves, cerebellum, and other sites.
   3. Clinical manifestations
      a. Gait ataxia (clumsy walking/running) usually beginning in childhood (peak onset between 8 and 15 years).
         i. Loss of ability to ambulate, becoming wheelchair bound within a few years.
      b. Hypertrophic cardiomyopathy
         i. Conduction defects, arrhythmias, and heart failure.
         ii. Common cause of death, usually between 40 and 50 years of age.
      c. Diabetes mellitus or glucose intolerance (some cases).
   4. Diagnosis
      a. Genetic testing

F. Amyotrophic lateral sclerosis (ALS)
   1. Definition
      a. Relentlessly progressive degenerative disease of motor neurons.
   2. Epidemiology
      a. Usually, a disease of middle-aged to older adults (mean ~60 years); slightly more common in males.
      b. Risk factors include aging and family history.
      c. Sporadic in most cases (>80%).
   3. Pathogenesis
      a. Degeneration of upper and lower motor neurons by an unclear mechanism (causing loss of muscle innervation).
      b. Various genetic mutations (e.g., *SOD1*) in familial cases.
   4. Clinical manifestations
      a. Upper motor neuron signs include hyperreflexia and spasticity.
      b. Lower motor neuron signs include cramps, fasciculations, and muscle atrophy.
      c. Slowly progressive muscle weakness involving one or more regions of the body.
         i. Dropping objects, inability to button clothing.
         ii. Difficulty walking/running, speaking (dysarthria), and swallowing (dysphagia).
      d. Pseudobulbar affect (sudden bursts of uncontrollable laughing and/or crying).
      e. Extraocular eye movements and sensation remain intact.
   5. Diagnosis
      a. Electromyography (EMG) and nerve conduction studies (NCS).
   6. Prognosis
      a. Progressive disorder with average survival of 3–5 years.
      b. Death often secondary to respiratory complications (e.g., aspiration or respiratory failure).

G. Frontotemporal dementia
   1. Neurodegenerative disorder characterized by changes in behavior and personality (inappropriate sexual remarks, invasion of other's personal space, and impulsive behavior), apathy, and loss of empathy.
   2. Early onset dementia (an average age of 58 years).
   3. May have manifestations of ALS, pseudobulbar affect.
   4. Pathologic protein inclusions include TAR DNA-binding protein with molecular weight 43 kDa (TDP-43), microtubule-associated protein tau (MAPT), or fused-in-sarcoma protein (FUS).

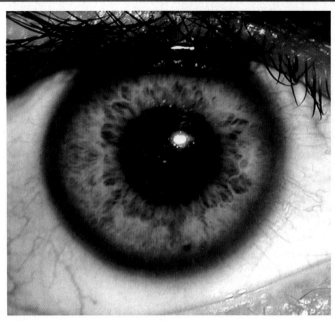

26.15: Kayser–Fleischer ring. *(From Bowling B:* Kanski's clinical ophthalmology, a systemic approach, *ed 8, Philadelphia, 2016, Elsevier.)*

H. **Creutzfeldt–Jakob disease CJD**
1. Rare, incurable, and progressive neurodegenerative disease due to the accumulation of misfolded prion proteins.
2. Most cases (~85%) are sporadic, an average age of presentation is 60 years.
3. Manifestations include rapidly progressive dementia, ataxia, involuntary movements (myoclonus), exaggerated startle reflex, disability, and death within several (6–7) months.
   a. New-variant CJD, due to the ingestion of beef contaminated with bovine spongiform encephalopathy, presents at a younger age (an average of 29 years) but with a slower progression to death (~13 months).
4. Histology reveals "spongiform" change (vacuolization).
5. Electroencephalogram (EEG) shows periodic sharp wave complexes.

XI. **Toxic and Metabolic Disorders**
A. **Wilson disease (see Chapter 19), summary**
1. Autosomal recessive disorder of copper metabolism.
2. Due to mutation in copper-transporting ATPase (*ATP7B*); impairs biliary copper excretion.
3. Copper progressively accumulates within tissues (e.g., liver, brain, and cornea).
4. Clinical manifestations
   a. Kayser–Fleischer ring (gold-yellow ring at periphery of the iris, see Fig. 26.15).
   b. Chronic liver disease/cirrhosis.
   c. Movement disorder (e.g., tremors and ataxia).
B. **Acute intermittent porphyria (AIP)**
1. Definition
   a. Autosomal dominant disorder of heme biosynthesis resulting in various neuropsychiatric manifestations.
2. Pathogenesis
   a. Decreased porphobilinogen deaminase activity leading to the accumulation of various neurotoxic heme biosynthetic intermediates.
3. Laboratory findings
   a. Increased urinary porphobilinogen.
4. Clinical presentation
   a. Periodic attacks of abdominal pain, psychiatric symptoms (e.g., depression), and neurologic manifestations (e.g., peripheral neuropathies, seizures, and delirium).
   b. Attacks may be triggered by certain medications (e.g., progesterone), infections, surgery, and dieting.
C. **Subacute combined degeneration of the spinal cord**
1. Definition
   a. Demyelinating disorder of the lateral corticospinal and posterior columns of the spinal cord secondary to vitamin B12 deficiency (the cause of myelin abnormality is unclear).
2. Clinical manifestations
   a. Bilateral, symmetric loss of vibratory and position sense, numbness, tingling, and ataxia of lower extremities developing over weeks.
      i. Neurologic changes may occur in the absence of characteristic hematologic changes (i.e., macrocytosis and megaloblastic anemia).

b. Vitamin B12 supplementation stops progression and improves symptoms.

D. Wernicke–Korsakoff syndrome

1. Definition
   a. Neurologic complications associated with a deficiency of thiamine.
2. Stages of disease
   a. Wernicke encephalopathy refers to the triad of acute changes:
      i. Encephalopathy (e.g., disorientation and inattentiveness).
      ii. Oculomotor dysfunction (e.g., nystagmus and conjugate gaze palsies).
      iii. Ataxia (e.g., wide-based gait and slow short steps).
   b. Korsakoff syndrome refers to the long-term effects of chronic thiamine deficiency.
      i. Amnesia, both retrograde and anterograde (loss of memory for events both before and after the causative event, respectively).
      ii. Confabulation (fabrication of stories to fill gaps in memory).
3. Pathology
   a. Vascular congestion and petechial hemorrhages involving structures around the third ventricle, aqueduct, and fourth ventricle.
   b. Atrophy of the mamillary bodies (highly specific finding).

XII. Central Nervous System Tumors

A. Overview

1. Primary brain tumors in adults most commonly arise above the tentorium cerebelli (i.e., supratentorial).
2. Primary brain tumors in children most commonly arise below the tentorium cerebelli (i.e., infratentorial).
3. Most primary CNS tumors are sporadic; small percentage associated with hereditary syndromes.
4. Metastatic tumors are far more common than primary tumors.
5. Clinical manifestations may be secondary to neural invasion, compression of adjacent structures, and/or elevation of ICP.
6. Tumor categorization
   a. World Health Organization (WHO) grading system: Grades I through IV (low to high grade).

B. Risk factors

1. Exposure to ionizing radiation (major environmental risk factor).
2. Inherited disorders (e.g., neurofibromatosis, von Hippel–Lindau syndrome, Li–Fraumeni syndrome, and tuberous sclerosis).

C. Clinical manifestations

1. Headache (classically at night and early morning).
2. Nausea and vomiting (particularly with the posterior fossa tumors due to associated obstructive hydrocephalus).
3. Seizures (especially with low-grade supratentorial tumors).
4. Cranial nerve palsies (with brainstem involvement).
5. Papilledema (swelling of optic disk, due to elevated ICP).
6. Herniation syndromes (due to elevated ICP).

D. Diagnosis

1. Imaging studies (primarily MRI) and tissue biopsy.

E. Tumor types

1. Astrocytoma
   a. Definition
      i. Primary CNS tumor characterized by a proliferation of cells that differentiate down the astrocytic cell lineage.
   b. Grade I (pilocytic astrocytoma)
      i. Slow-growing, well-circumscribed tumor of children.
      ii. Solid and cystic, usually within the cerebellum.
      iii. Histology reveals "hair-like" processes; positive staining for glial fibrillary acidic protein, an intermediate filament protein of astrocytes.
      iv. Often curable with surgical resection.
   c. Grades II through IV astrocytomas are infiltrative (and therefore unresectable).
   d. Glioblastoma (WHO grade IV astrocytoma)
      i. Most common primary malignant brain tumor of adults, usually arising in older adulthood.
      ii. Most arise de novo; however, some arise through dedifferentiation of a lower grade astrocytoma (more likely in younger individuals).
      iii. Characterized by areas of necrosis and microvascular proliferation (key histologic findings for the diagnosis).
      iv. May cross the corpus callosum into adjacent hemisphere (Fig. 26.16—"butterfly lesion").
      v. Despite their highly infiltrative and aggressive nature, they rarely metastasize outside the CNS.
      vi. Manifestations depend on location of tumor, include:
         (1) Headache, seizures, symptoms of increased ICP, weakness, sensory deficits, and cognitive disturbances.
      vii. Poor prognosis (1-to-2-year survival), even with treatment.
         (1) Due to inability to completely resect as tumor cells diffusely infiltrate into surrounding normal-appearing brain tissue.

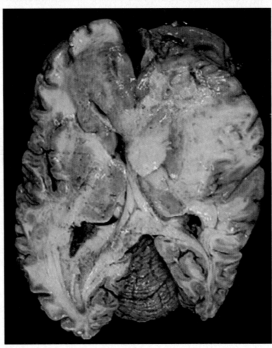

26.16: "Butterfly" glioblastoma. Glioblastoma has extended across the corpus callosum into the opposite hemisphere. Appearance resembles two wings of a butterfly (*circle*). *(From Ellison D, Love S, Cardao Chimelli LM, et al: Neuropathology: a reference text of CNS pathology, ed 3, St. Louis, 2013, Mosby Elsevier, p 715, Fig. 35.14.)*

2. Meningioma
   a. Definition
      i. Tumor arising from meningothelial cells within the arachnoid; attached to the dura.
   b. Epidemiology
      i. Most common primary benign tumor of the CNS.
      ii. Most arise in adulthood, more common in females.
      iii. Risk factors
         (1) History of radiation.
         (2) Neurofibromatosis type 2 (NF2).
   c. Pathology
      i. Slow-growing dural-based mass of the brain or spinal cord.
      ii. Variable histologic appearance; often with swirling masses of meningothelial cells with psammoma bodies.
      iii. Genetic mutation in *NF2* common (in both sporadic as well as those associated with NF2).
      iv. MRI shows increased density and a "dural tail" due to thickening of the dura related to the tumor.
3. Ependymoma
   a. Low-grade tumors of ependymal cell differentiation.
   b. Typically, originate near the ventricular system (e.g., floor of the fourth ventricle in children; spinal cord in adults).
   c. Those near the fourth ventricle may obstruct the flow of CSF, causing hydrocephalus, headache, nausea, vomiting, ataxia, and papilledema.
   d. Tumor cells form round "gland-like" structures around a central vessel ("perivascular pseudorosettes").
4. Medulloblastoma
   a. Primitive undifferentiated embryonal tumor of the cerebellum.
   b. Most cases occur in children; the most common malignant brain tumor of childhood.
   c. Highly aggressive (WHO grade IV) with propensity for spread throughout the subarachnoid space onto the surface of the cord and cauda equina ("drop metastases").
   d. Tumor growth within the cerebellum in proximity to the fourth ventricle can obstruct the flow of CSF.
   e. Manifestations include nausea, vomiting, headache, ataxia, loss of balance, and incoordination.
   f. Variable prognosis based on molecular and histologic subtypes.
   g. Treatment involves combination of surgery, radiation therapy, and chemotherapy.
5. Oligodendroglioma
   a. Rare, low-grade (WHO grade II) tumor with differentiation down the oligodendrocyte lineage.
   b. Usually arise within middle-aged adults (25–45 years).
   c. Commonly arise within frontal lobes; often presents with seizures.
   d. Frequently calcify, with a "fried egg" appearance histologically.

e. Combined deletions of the short arm of chromosome 1 (1p) and the long arm of chromosome 19 (19q) are hallmark findings.
6. Primary CNS lymphoma (PCNSL)
a. Rare form of non-Hodgkin lymphoma arising within the CNS.
b. Associated with Epstein–Barr virus in some cases.
c. Risk factors
i. Immunosuppression (e.g., acquired immunodeficiency syndrome [AIDS])
ii. Older age (>65 years)
d. PCNSL is an AIDS-defining criterion.
e. Characteristically of B-cell lineage; will therefore exhibit B-cell markers (e.g., CD19).
F. **Familial tumor syndromes**
1. Neurofibromatosis type 1 (NF1)
a. Autosomal dominant disorder due to mutations in the *NF1* gene.
b. *NF1* encodes for neurofibromin, a tumor suppressor protein.
c. Common (~1 in 3000 individuals).
d. Clinical manifestations
i. Café au lait spots.
ii. Axillary and inguinal freckling.
iii. Cutaneous neurofibromas, may be painful/disfiguring.
iv. Pigmented hamartomas of iris (Lisch nodules).
v. Increased risk of neoplasms (e.g., optic nerve glioma, malignant peripheral nerve sheath tumors, and others).
vi. Genetic testing available.
2. Neurofibromatosis type 2 (NF2)
a. Autosomal dominant disorder due to a mutation in the *NF2* gene.
b. *NF2* encodes for merlin, a tumor suppressor protein.
c. Uncommon, frequency of roughly 1 in 50,000 individuals.
d. Characterized by vestibular schwannomas (often bilateral); usual presentation in young adulthood.
i. Associated symptoms include tinnitus, hearing loss, and imbalance.
e. Patients also at increased risk of meningiomas, ependymomas, and juvenile onset cataracts.
f. Genetic testing available.
3. Tuberous sclerosis complex (TSC)
a. Autosomal dominant syndrome affecting multiple organ systems.
b. Due to mutations involving *TSC1* (protein hamartin) or *TSC2* (protein tuberin).
c. Clinical manifestations
i. Skin lesions
(1) Angiofibroma.
(2) Hypopigmented skin lesions ("ash leaf spots").
(3) Subungual and periungual fibromas.
ii. CNS lesions
(1) Seizures, intellectual disability, developmental delay, and subependymal astrocytoma.
iii. Renal angiomyolipoma
(1) Benign tumor comprised of blood vessels, smooth muscle, and adipose tissue.
iv. Cardiac rhabdomyomas
(1) Usually present at birth, typically regress over time.
XIII. Headaches
A. **Primary**
1. Tension headache
a. Most common type of headache; female > males.
b. Bilateral, pressure or tightening quality, of mild-to-moderate intensity.
2. Migraine headache
a. Recurrent episodic, moderate to severe, and pulsating quality.
b. Accompanied by nausea, vomiting, photophobia, phonophobia, and exacerbated by movement.
i. Patients prefer to lie in bed motionless in dark quiet room.
c. May or may not have aura (e.g., flickering lights and loss of vision).

Metastatic disease

- Most common CNS malignancy.
- Often characterized by the presence of multiple lesions.
- Within the cerebral hemispheres, the tumors often appear at the gray-white junction (decreased diameter of blood vessels with trapping of tumor emboli).
- Most common primary tumors, in decreasing frequency:
  - Lung > breast > skin (melanoma) > renal > colon.

       d. More common in females; usually, beginning in young adulthood.
   3. Cluster headache
       a. Severe, unilateral orbital or supraorbital pain, lasting minutes to a few hours.
       b. May occur several times per day over a span of weeks to months.
       c. Associated manifestations include ipsilateral conjunctival injection, lacrimation, nasal congestion, and rhinorrhea.
       d. Restless during an attack (patient paces around).
       e. More common in males, usually young adulthood.
       f. 100% oxygen often aborts attacks.
 B. Secondary
   1. Headache arising as a manifestation of another disease process (e.g., temporal arteritis, meningitis, brain tumor, SAH, etc.).

XIV. Peripheral Nervous System Disorders
 A. Peripheral neuropathy
   1. Broadly defined as a disease of peripheral nerves; may be localized or generalized.
       a. Localized (mononeuropathy) is commonly secondary to trauma or compression.
          i. For example, compression of the median nerve within the wrist causes "carpal tunnel syndrome."
       b. Generalized (i.e., polyneuropathy) is more likely with systemic disorders (e.g., alcohol, diabetes mellitus, and nutritional deficiencies).
   2. May affect primarily motor pathways, sensory pathways, or both.
       a. Sensory manifestations may be "negative" (e.g., numbness) or "positive" (e.g., burning, pain, and tingling).
       b. Motor involvement can lead to muscle atrophy and weakness.
   3. Pathology reveals segmental demyelination and axonal degeneration.
   4. Etiologies
       a. Diabetes mellitus
          i. Most common cause of peripheral neuropathy; affects ~50% of diabetics.
          ii. Affects both sensory (primarily) and motor fibers in a symmetrical fashion beginning in the distal extremities (i.e., "distal sensorimotor symmetrical polyneuropathy").
             (1) Sensory manifestations include numbness and tingling (paresthesia) in a "stocking and glove" distribution.
          iii. Involvement of autonomic nerves (autonomic neuropathy)
             (1) Impaired gastric emptying (gastroparesis).
             (2) Impaired bladder emptying; causing urinary stasis (and increasing one's risk of developing cystitis).
             (3) Postural hypotension.
             (4) Silent myocardial ischemia/infarction.
          iv. Multiple mechanisms
             (1) Nonenzymatic glycosylation of various cellular components (e.g., proteins and lipids) to form "Advanced glycosylation end products" (AGEs) that bind with receptors (RAGEs) to initiate inflammatory pathways.
             (2) Polyol pathway (glucose reduced to sorbitol by the enzyme aldose reductase) causes swelling due to osmotic effect and impairs the production of glutathione (thereby contributing to oxidative stress).
          v. Onset and progression of disease is highly correlated with blood glucose levels (i.e., poor glucose control is associated with an earlier onset and worse manifestations).
       b. Various toxins/medications
          i. Vinca alkaloids (e.g., vincristine, an antineoplastic agent).
          ii. Heavy metals (e.g., lead; causes foot and wrist drop).
          iii. Alcohol (causes both direct and indirect nerve injury, the latter related to nutritional deficiencies).
       c. Charcot–Marie–Tooth (CMT) disease
          i. Inherited (usually autosomal dominant) form of motor and sensory neuropathy.
          ii. Presents during childhood with weakness and atrophy of distal lower extremities (e.g., foot drop, pes cavus, and hammertoe deformity).
          iii. Eventually, the upper extremities may be involved as well.
          iv. Sensory symptoms less prominent.
          v. Pathogenesis related to inherited mutations in various genes necessary for peripheral myelination.
          vi. Most common type (CMT1A) is associated with mutations in the peripheral myelin protein 22 (*PMP22*) gene.
       d. Guillain–Barré syndrome (GBS)
          i. Acquired immune-mediated disease characterized by rapidly progressive ascending motor weakness.
          ii. Often follows an infection of the gastrointestinal or respiratory tract (the most common causative pathogen is *Campylobacter jejuni*).
             (1) Pathogenesis believed related to a cross-reaction of the host immune response against the infectious agent and components of the peripheral nerve (molecular mimicry).
          iii. The net result is demyelination and/or axonal degeneration.
          iv. Clinical manifestations

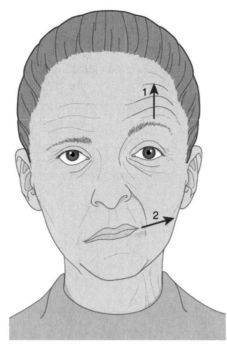

26.17: Right facial nerve paralysis. Numbers 1 and 2 on the left side show the normal facial muscle response when the patient is asked to smile and when asked to wrinkle the forehead muscles. In a right facial nerve paralysis, note that the patient is unable to smile (note sagging of the mouth) or furrow his brow (note the absence of wrinkling of the forehead muscles). *(Taken from FitzGerald MJT, Gruener G, Mtui E: Clinical neuroanatomy and neuroscience, ed 6, Philadelphia, 2011, Saunders.)*

    (1) Progressive ascending weakness beginning in the lower extremities over 2–4 weeks.
    (2) Diminished to absent DTRs.
    (3) Sensory changes (e.g., paresthesia and pain) present but often less prominent.
    (4) Involvement of respiratory musculature may necessitate mechanical ventilation (up to 30% of patients).
  v. Diagnosis
    (1) LP shows normal glucose, elevated CSF protein but normal WBC count ("albuminocytologic dissociation").
    (2) NCS and EMG.
  vi. Prognosis
    (1) Partial or complete resolution over months in most patients.
    (2) Fatal in small percent of cases, usually secondary to respiratory complications (e.g., acute respiratory distress syndrome or pulmonary emboli).
 e. Bell palsy
  i. Acute facial nerve palsy causing ipsilateral weakness of the upper and lower facial musculature (Fig. 26.17).
  ii. Drooping of the corner of the mouth, difficulty speaking.
  iii. Inability to close the eye and inability to wrinkle the forehead muscles.
  iv. Pathogenesis believed secondary to inflammation of facial nerve in association with reactivated herpes simplex virus (HSV) infection.
  v. No racial or gender predilection; however, there is an increased risk during pregnancy.
  vi. Glucocorticoids reduce inflammation and hasten recovery.

B. Myasthenia gravis (review, see discussion Chapter 24)
1. Autoimmune disorder of neuromuscular transmission due to immune-mediated destruction of the nicotinic acetylcholine receptor (AChR) at the neuromuscular junction by anti-AChR antibodies.
  a. Less common are anti-muscle-specific tyrosine kinase (MuSK) antibodies.
2. Causes "fatigable weakness" (worse with repeated stimulation), often presenting with ptosis or diplopia.
3. Other manifestations include difficulty chewing, swallowing, or talking.
4. Associated with thymic hyperplasia or thymoma.

C. Lambert–Eaton myasthenic syndrome (LEMS)
1. Autoimmune disorder of neuromuscular transmission.
2. Secondary to antibodies against presynaptic voltage-gated P/Q calcium channels on motor and autonomic nerve terminals.
3. Presents with weakness of proximal lower-extremity muscles (transiently improves with repeated stimulation).
4. Often a paraneoplastic phenomenon, usually in association with small cell lung carcinoma.

D. Schwannoma
1. Benign tumor of Schwann cells.
2. Histology reveals biphasic architecture of dense (Antoni A) and loose (Antoni B) cell growth with areas of nuclear palisading (Verocay bodies).
3. Most are sporadic and single in number; however, individuals with NF2 are predisposed to bilateral tumors.
   a. Arise most commonly at the cerebellopontine angle involving the eighth cranial nerve with manifestations of tinnitus, sensorineural hearing loss, and unsteady gait.

Appendix: Acid–Base Disorders

I. Formulas for Calculations of Acid–Base Disorders
   A. Calculation of expected compensation can help to determine whether there is more than one primary acid–base disorder in a patient (called a mixed disorder; see later).
   B. If the calculated expected compensation closely approximates the measured compensation, then a single primary disorder is present.
   C. Conversely, if there is an obvious disparity between the calculated expected compensation and the measured compensation, then a second primary disorder is present.
   D. Recall that respiratory compensation for metabolic disorders is rapid (within minutes) and that metabolic compensation of respiratory disorders takes time, with complete compensation requiring a few (~2–3) days.

II. Expected Compensation in Acute Respiratory Acidosis
   A. In acute respiratory acidosis, expected HCO_3^- compensation $= 0.10 \times \Delta P_{CO_2}$ (difference from normal of 40 mm Hg).
   B. Recall (refer to Chapter 5) that the expected compensation in respiratory acidosis is metabolic alkalosis ($\uparrow HCO_3^-$).
   C. Example: pH 7.20, P_{CO_2} 74 mm Hg, HCO_3^- 27 mEq/L
      1. Expected HCO_3^- compensation $= 0.10 \times (74 - 40) = 3.4$ mEq/L increase above normal.
      2. Expected HCO_3^- compensation $= 24$ mEq/L (mean HCO_3^-) $+ 3.4 = 27.4$ mEq/L.
      3. Note that measured and expected calculated HCO_3^- are similar; therefore a single disorder is present.

III. Expected Compensation in Chronic Respiratory Acidosis
   A. Expected HCO_3^- compensation $= 0.40 \times \Delta P_{CO_2}$.
   B. Example: pH 7.34, P_{CO_2} 60 mm Hg, HCO_3^- 32 mEq/L.
   C. Expected HCO_3^- compensation $= 0.40 \times (60 - 40) = 8$ mEq/L increase above normal.
   D. Expected HCO_3^- compensation $= 24 + 8 = 32$ mEq/L.
      1. Note that measured and expected calculated HCO_3^- are similar; therefore a single disorder is present.

IV. Expected Compensation in Acute Respiratory Alkalosis
   A. Expected HCO_3^- compensation $= 0.20 \times \Delta Pa_{CO_2}$ (difference from normal of 40 mm Hg).
   B. Recall that the expected compensation in respiratory alkalosis is metabolic acidosis ($\downarrow HCO_3^-$).
   C. Example: pH 7.56, Pa_{CO_2} 24 mm Hg, HCO_3^- 21 mEq/L.
   D. Expected HCO_3^- compensation $= 0.20 \times (40 - 24) = 3.2$ mEq/L less than the normal.
   E. Expected HCO_3^- compensation $= 24$ mEq/L (mean HCO_3^-) $- 3.2 = 20.8$ mEq/L.
      1. Note that measured and expected calculated HCO_3^- are similar; therefore a single disorder is present.

V. Expected Compensation in Chronic Respiratory Alkalosis
   A. Expected $HCO_3^- = 0.50 \times \Delta Pa_{CO_2}$.
   B. Example: pH 7.47, Pa_{CO_2} 18 mm Hg, HCO_3^- 13 mEq/L.
   C. Expected HCO_3^- compensation $= 0.50 \times (40 - 18) = 11$ mEq/L less than the normal.
   D. Expected HCO_3^- compensation $= 24 - 11 = 13$ mEq/L.
      1. Note that measured and expected calculated HCO_3^- are similar; therefore a single disorder is present.

VI. Expected Compensation in Metabolic Acidosis (Either High or Normal Anion Gap Type)
   A. Expected $Pa_{CO_2} = 1.2 \times \Delta HCO_3^- \pm 2$.
   B. ΔHCO_3^- is measured HCO_3^- subtracted from the mean HCO_3^- of 24 mEq/L.
   C. Recall that the expected compensation in metabolic acidosis is respiratory alkalosis ($\downarrow Pa_{CO_2}$).
   D. Example: pH 7.27, Pa_{CO_2} 27 mm Hg, HCO_3^- 12 mEq/L.
   E. Expected Pa_{CO_2} compensation $= 1.2 \times (24 - 12) = 14.4$ mm Hg less than the normal.

F. Expected $Paco_2 = 40$ (mean $Paco_2$) $- 14.4 = 25.6$ mm Hg (23.6–27.6).
   1. Note that measured $Paco_2$ is within the calculated range; therefore only a single disorder is present.

VII. **Expected Compensation in Metabolic Alkalosis**
   A. Expected $Paco_2 = 0.7 \times \Delta HCO_3^- \pm 2$.
   B. Recall that the expected compensation in metabolic alkalosis is respiratory acidosis ($\uparrow Paco_2$).
   C. Example: pH 7.58, $Paco_2$ 49 mm Hg, HCO_3^- 39 mEq/L.
   D. Expected $Paco_2$ compensation $= 0.7 \times (39 - 24) = 10.5$ greater than the normal.
   E. Expected $Paco_2$ compensation $= 40 + 10.5 = 50.5$ mm Hg (48.5–52.5).
      1. Note that measured $Paco_2$ is within the calculated range; therefore only a single disorder is present.

VIII. **Examples of How Formulas Help Identify a Mixed Disorder**
   A. pH 7.26, $Paco_2$ 38 mm Hg, HCO_3^- 17 mEq/L
      1. Presumptive diagnosis: metabolic acidosis (HCO_3^- <22 mEq/L) without compensation ($Paco_2$ in normal range).
      2. Formula for calculating expected compensation in metabolic acidosis:
         a. Expected $Paco_2 = 1.2 \times \Delta HCO_3^- \pm 2$.
         b. Expected $Paco_2 = 1.2 \times (24 - 17) = 8.4$ mm Hg less than the normal value.
         c. Expected $Paco_2 = 40$ (mean $Paco_2$) $- 8.4 = 31.6$ (29.6–33.6).
         d. The measured $Paco_2$ is 38 mm Hg, which is higher than it should be, indicating that a primary respiratory acidosis (retention of CO_2) must also be present.
   B. pH 7.38, $Paco_2$ 70 mm Hg, HCO_3^- 41 mEq/L.
      1. Presumptive diagnosis: mixed disorder (because the pH is normal) with chronic respiratory acidosis ($Paco_2$ >45 mm Hg, HCO_3^- >30 mEq/L) and primary metabolic alkalosis (HCO_3^- >28 mEq/L).
      2. Using either the formula for metabolic alkalosis or chronic respiratory acidosis will prove the presence of a mixed disorder.
      3. Using the chronic respiratory acidosis formula (expected $HCO_3^- = 0.40 \times \Delta Paco_2$).
         a. Expected HCO_3^- compensation $= 0.40 \times (70 - 40) = 12$ mEq/L increase above normal.
         b. Expected HCO_3^- compensation $= 24 + 12 = 36$ mEq/L.
         c. Measured HCO_3^- is 41 mEq/L, which is higher than the expected compensation indicating the presence of an additional primary metabolic alkalosis (more HCO_3^- than there should be for compensation).
      4. Using the metabolic alkalosis formula (expected $Paco_2 = 0.7 \times \Delta HCO_3^- \pm 2$)
         a. Expected $Paco_2 = 0.7 \times (41 - 24) = 11.9$ mm Hg increase from the normal.
         b. Expected $Paco_2 = 40 + 11.9 = 51.9$ mm Hg (49.9–53.9).
         c. The measured $Paco_2$ is 70 mm Hg, which is much higher than it should be indicating the presence of an additional primary respiratory acidosis.

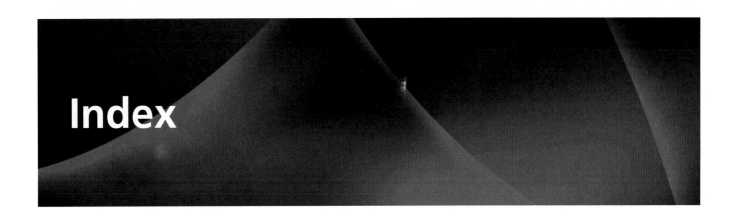

Index

Note: Page numbers followed by "*f*" indicate figures, "*t*" indicate tables, and "*b*" indicate boxes.

A

Abdominal aortic aneurysm (AAA), 96
Abnormal uterine bleeding (AUB),
    296–297
ABO blood group
    antigens, 182–184, 183*f*
        definition of, 182
    back type, 183–184
        identification of, 183*f*
    determination of, 183–184
    forward type, 183
        identification of, 183*f*
    genotypes and serum reactivity, 184,
        184*t*
    summary of, 182*b*
ABO HDN, 186–187
    clinical and laboratory findings of, 187
    complications, 187
    definition, 186
    epidemiology of, 186
    pathogenesis of, 186–187
    treatment, 187
ABO hemolytic disease, Rh hemolytic disease
    (comparison), 189*t*
Abruptio placenta, 305–306
    clinical findings of, 305
    definition, 305
    diagnosis of, 305–306
    pathogenesis, 305
    risk factors, 305
Absolute leukocytosis, with left shift, 26*f*
ACA. *See* Anterior cerebral artery
Academia, 49
Acanthosis nigricans (AN), 358
Accuracy, of test results, 2–3, 2*f*
ACD. *See* Anemia of chronic disease
Acetaminophen metabolism, 242*f*
Acetaminophen toxicity, 242
Acetylcholine (ACh) receptors, autoantibodies
    (impact), 349
Achalasia, 218
    barium study for, 217*f*
    Chagas' disease, 218
    clinical manifestations, 218
    diagnosis of, 218
    epidemiology of, 218
Achilles tendon xanthoma, 94*f*
Achondroplasia, 336

Acid-base disorders, 49–52
    interpretation, 49–50
    metabolic acidosis, 51
    metabolic alkalosis, 52
    mixed, 52
    overview, 49
    respiratory acidosis, 50–51
    respiratory alkalosis, 51
Acid-base homeostasis, maintenance of, 256
Acne vulgaris, 353–354
Acquired (adaptive) immunity, 28
Acquired immunodeficiency syndrome (AIDS),
    42, 44*b*
Acquired valvular heart disease, 117–123
Acral lentiginous melanoma (ALM), 357
Acromegaly
    in adults, 316
    facial characteristics, 316*f*
Actinic (solar) keratosis, 358
    hyperkeratotic lesion in, 358
Activated partial thromboplastin time (aPTT), 174
Acute anterior myocardial infarction,
    electrocardiogram for, 113*f*
Acute appendicitis, 232
Acute bacterial endocarditis, vegetation (presence)
    of, 122*f*
Acute bacterial prostatitis, 281
Acute blood loss, 143
Acute chest syndrome (ACS), 148
Acute cholecystitis, 252
Acute coronary syndromes, 111*f*
Acute cystitis, 274–275
Acute endocarditis, 122–123
Acute endometritis, 298
Acute epidural hematoma, non-contrast-enhanced
    computed tomography (CT) scan for, 368*f*
Acute gastritis, 220
Acute gout, 345–346
Acute gouty arthritis, 345*f*, 346*f*
Acute hemolytic transfusion reaction (HTR), 186
Acute hemorrhagic erosive gastropathy, 222
Acute immune thrombocytopenia, 177*t*
Acute inflammation (AI), 17–27
    cardinal sign of, 17*t*
    circulatory changes, 18*f*
    components of, 17–19
    definition of, 17
    edema, 17, 18*f*

Acute inflammation (AI) *(Continued)*
    fever, 20
    fibrinous, 19–20, 21*f*
    granulomatous, 21, 22*f*
    innate immune response, 17
    laboratory findings, 24–26
        Döhle bodies, 26, 26*f*
        neutrophilic leukocytosis, 24–26, 26*f*
        serum IgM, 26
        toxic granulation, 26
    neutrophil events, 19*f*
    purulent (suppurative), 19, 21*f*
    serous, 20
    serum protein electrophoresis for, 27, 27*f*
    stimuli for, 17
Acute intermittent porphyria (AIP), 378
Acute kidney injury (AKI), 266
Acute lung injury, 192–194
Acute lymphoblastic leukemia (ALL), 160
    clinical manifestations, 160
    definition, 160
    diagnosis, 160
    epidemiology, 160
    lymphoid blasts, 160*f*
    pathogenesis, 160
Acute mountain sickness, 72
Acute myelogenous leukemia (AML), 162
Acute myocardial infarction (AMI), 110–112, 113*b*
    causes of, 110
    classification, 110–112
    complications, 112
    diagnosis of, cardiac enzymes (usage), 111*f*
    ECG findings, 112, 113*f*
    gross changes, 112
    ischemia/reperfusion injury, 112
    laboratory diagnosis, 112
    microscopic findings, 112
Acute osteomyelitis, 336–337
Acute pancreatitis, 253–254
    clinical manifestations, 253–254
    complications of, 254
    definition, 253
    diagnosis, 254
    etiologies, 253
    imaging studies for, 254
    pathogenesis, 253
Acute phase reactants (APRs), synthesis/release
    of, 20–21